Nutrition and Physical Fitness

ninth edition

The Late L. JEAN BOGERT, Ph.D.

Formerly, Instructor in Experimental Medicine, Yale
Medical School, New Haven; Professor of Food
Economics and Nutrition, Kansas State University,
Manhattan; Research Chemist, Obstetrical
Department, Henry Ford Hospital, Detroit;
Instructor in the Department of Medicine,
University of Chicago

GEORGE M. BRIGGS, Ph.D.

Professor of Nutrition, Department of
Nutritional Sciences, University of California
at Berkeley

DORIS HOWES CALLOWAY, Ph.D.

Professor of Nutrition, Department of
Nutritional Sciences, University of California
at Berkeley

1973 — W. B. Saunders Company — PHILADELPHIA – LONDON – TORONTO

W. B. Saunders Company: West Washington Square
Philadelphia, Pa. 19105

12 Dyott Street
London, WC1A 1DB

833 Oxford Street
Toronto 18, Ontario

Nutrition and Physical Fitness

ISBN 0-7216-1817-0

Print No.: 9   8   7   6   5   4   3   2   1

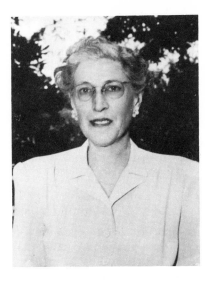

Publisher's Foreword

Lydia Jean Bogert, Ph.D., died on August 22, 1970, just after she participated actively in the construction of the outline for this ninth edition of *Nutrition and Physical Fitness*. There are two stories embodied in that statement: one, the tale of a woman who retained her vigor and will into her eighty-third year; the other, the progress of an intellectual concept that is still strong and valid more than 40 years after it was first introduced.

Lydia Jean Bogert was born on June 17, 1888, in a town called Scotland, South Dakota. It must have been virtually frontier then; even the 1970 census found only 1095 inhabitants. Miss Bogert persevered, and in 1910 she obtained her A.B. from Cornell University. Six years later, she received her Ph.D. in physiological chemistry from Yale, and the sociological feat is perhaps more significant than the intellectual; women would not have the right to vote until four years later.

For the next 13 years, Dr. Bogert pursued a varied and thoroughly remarkable career: Instructor at the Yale University School of Medicine, Professor of Food Economics and Nutrition at Kansas State University, Research Chemist in the Department of Obstetrics and Gynecology at the Henry Ford Hospital in Detroit, and Instructor in Medicine at the University of Chicago.

In addition, she began to write texts. In 1924, while she worked at the Ford Hospital, she wrote a book called *Fundamentals of Chemistry*, a text intended for nurses and other people interested in the application of chemistry to health-oriented areas. The first edition of a laboratory manual followed in 1927, while she taught at the University of Chicago. The ninth and last edition of the chemistry text was published successfully in 1963, having survived the discoveries of the wave equation, atomic fission, free radicals, spectroscopy, and the hundreds of other revolutions that occurred in chemistry in the twentieth century.

But this is running ahead of the story. In 1929, Dr. Bogert decided to leave the academic world and concentrate on writing, a career she was to follow for the next 41 years. She produced the first edition of *Nutrition and*

Physical Fitness in 1931, and we can comprehend part of the reason for the book's durability by realizing that its basic *raison d'être* has never changed: Dr. Bogert started her preface as follows:

The purpose of the author in writing this book has been three-fold.

(1) To gather into a single volume facts useful in meeting every day nutritional problems, which have been gleaned from the fields of food composition and economics, the chemistry and physiology of body processes, dietetics, and medicine.

(2) To make this information available to a comparatively large group by presenting it in such simple language as to be understandable to those with no previous knowledge of chemistry.

(3) To point out, in every instance possible, how such knowledge may be utilized for preventing ill health and promoting a high degree of physical fitness.

The fact that the aims of this ninth edition are virtually identical to those of the first should not conceal the fact that the science of nutrition is now far different from what it used to be. The first edition contained a single 30 page chapter on vitamins among its more than 550 pages. In this edition, vitamins are discussed in over 150 pages in four chapters. Nowhere in the first edition do we learn any quantitative facts about vitamins, either in terms of dietary needs or in terms of their occurrence in foods; it was not until after the publication of the first edition that such studies commenced. The fantastic proliferation of acknowledged trace minerals had barely begun in 1931, and the increasing concern for nutrition problems abroad and distribution problems at home is a phenomenon of the last decade.

Even as the scientific facts grew in number and complexity, however, Dr. Bogert kept this book on a steady course. Through all nine editions, this book has simply endeavored to teach people how to eat wisely. That aim reveals itself as strongly today as it did in the 1930's, and it has taken a strong will and intellect to keep the book focused that clearly.

Now the technical problems of authorship have passed to Professors George M. Briggs and Doris H. Calloway, who collaborated with Dr. Bogert on the eighth edition. The writing of this edition became solely their responsibility, and they will carry that responsibility into future editions. But the distinctive stamp of Lydia Jean Bogert's ideas is still on this book and will be for a long time to come.

She was an indomitable lady, and she will be missed.

W. B. SAUNDERS COMPANY

Preface

The aim of this book has always been to present the basic facts and principles of nutrition in as simple and interesting a manner as possible, and to point out how such knowledge may be utilized to build strong bodies and maintain a high degree of health and vigor. With each revision, we have endeavored to include and interpret for students the progressive findings of nutritional research. However, research has concentrated more and more on the study of the basic life processes—the chemistry of the cell, the chemical changes that take place in the various tissues, and the role of enzymes, vitamins, and mineral elements in catalyzing these processes. This deeper inquiry into the need for and functions of the various nutrients is often a team effort, involving the collaboration of biochemists with physiologists and microbiologists. Looking at the vast amount of data and numerous fundamental discoveries which have been accumulated by this type of research, it becomes apparent that even though this material may be difficult to translate into terms which are understandable to less advanced college students, it cannot be ignored; to be as meaningful as it should be, nutrition must be treated in greater depth than was formerly the case.

Fortunately, because of increased emphasis on science in secondary schools, most present-day college students have already acquired some knowledge of fundamental scientific terms and concepts through courses (general science, biology, chemistry, physics) in high school or even at grade school levels. Hence, college students may be expected to comprehend a presentation of nutrition which relies on an elementary understanding of science.

The dependence upon the scientific method for providing proven facts about foods and nutrition is often a difficult concept for today's student to accept. The student today has seen evidence of certain segments of the food industry putting the consumer at the low end of the priority list. The student has learned, rightly or wrongly, to mistrust intentional food additives, highly processed foods, foods treated with synthetic "chemicals," certain food advertising, high food prices, and even college teachers of a different generation. We recommend that teachers using this book in classes comprised mainly of nonscience-trained students spend the first few days or so of class discussing the meaning of science, the scientific method, a controlled experiment, the placebo, and the difference between a true scientific publication (with its system of peer review) and a scare magazine or newspaper article. (Chapter 1 will assist you somewhat in this.)

This book gives considerable weight to the 1968 recommended dietary allowances of the Food and Nutrition Board. The authors suggest that when the proposed revised values of 1973 are available they be used to supplement the information in this book.

We believe the book to be considerably improved by the new arrangement of the chapters, the new chapters on physical activity, dental health, infant nutrition, and food habits and beliefs, a section on appetite regulation, and consolidation of much material in the later sections of the previous edition. We have attempted to focus directly on nutrition problems existing today that are of concern to students in their own lives and future careers.

The information in the book is accurate and as up-to-date as possible within publication time lags. More than two thirds of the book has been completely rewritten. We have attempted, as did Dr. Bogert, not to straddle the fence on controversial issues but to give our informed opinion on such issues when valid information exists. We hope you will find the book better able to meet your needs than ever before. Your comments are always most welcome.

Berkeley, California   GEORGE M. BRIGGS
                                                             DORIS HOWES CALLOWAY

Acknowledgments

First we wish to acknowledge our deep gratitude to the late Dr. L. Jean Bogert, whose writing ability and dedication to this book was, and still is, an inspiration to us. Several weeks before her death, on August 22, 1970, she had evaluated the proposed changes in the Table of Contents of this edition and given her approval, as well as making several valuable suggestions. She had stated that she could not take an active part in the revision of any of the chapters for this edition but was prepared to read the new chapters and offer advice. We feel fortunate to have worked with her and are happy to dedicate this edition to her.

We are greatly indebted to Miss Morissa White, nutrition student, dietetic intern, and anthropologist, whose help was invaluable in preparation of this edition. She not only typed the entire manuscript, but also edited galleys and page proofs, and helped considerably in collecting references from our files. She is mainly responsible for Chapter 17 (Food: From the Producer to the Consumer), and contributed to other sections of the book (including the new Table 3 of the Appendix).

We are indebted, too, to Dr. Christine Wilson, nutritional anthropologist, for writing Chapter 16 (Food Habits and Beliefs) and to Dr. Marilyn Crim for a major role in Chapter 14 (Metabolism and Excretion). Writing the two new chapters on Nutrition in Infancy and Preschool Years (Chapter 20) and Dental Health, Nutrition, and Diet (Chapter 22) were the primary responsibility of Catherine Briggs, M.D., M.P.H., to whom we are also greatly indebted.

Many others have helped in various phases in the writing of this edition, including Dr. Mary Ann Williams, Mrs. Marilyn Nebeker, R. D., and Mrs. Eleanor Briggs, who have read many of the drafts of the chapter.

Special thanks, too, go to the W. B. Saunders Company, the publishers, who have done an exceptional job, we feel, in preparing and editing the proofs and in assisting the authors in many ways. The Biology Editor, Richard Lampert, has been unusually cooperative and able.

We acknowledge, too, the help of many who have supplied photographs and other material for the book. Many readers have offered constructive criticism about the last edition which was of great help to us in revision.

GEORGE M. BRIGGS

DORIS HOWES CALLOWAY

Contents

Part Two
*Food
Intake
and
Utilization*

Part Three
*Applied
Nutrition*

Part One

Nutrients and Their Functions

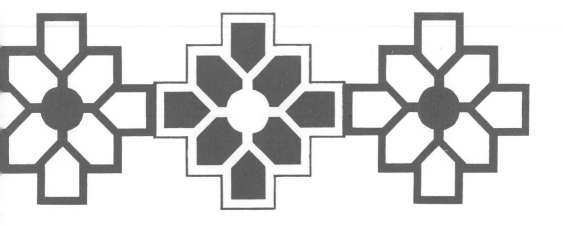

one

Functions of Food and Its Relation to Health

Why do we need to eat? What should we eat? The answers to these questions are what nutrition—and this book—is all about.

The foods we eat contain about 40 to 45 highly important substances (the "nutrients") *which each of us must consume in adequate amounts in order to grow, reproduce, and lead a full healthy life.* Water, another form of food, and the oxygen of the air we breathe, are equally essential.

Starting only with these 40 or so essential nutrients that we must get from our food, the body then makes literally thousands of substances necessary for life and physical fitness. Most all of these substances are far more complicated in structure than the original starting nutrients. If our bodies could manufacture, in some manner, these 40 nutrients that we now get from our food, we would not have to eat at all.

But, of course, this is impossible. In common with green plants and all other forms of life, we must be provided first with 12 to 15 minerals from some outside source (see Chapters 11 to 14). However, our bodies are far more complicated and delicately balanced than green plants. We must have still additional nutrients from our food which make possible normal human life as we know it. With these, we can move about, see, hear, taste, speak, smell, feel, think, learn and remember, sing, walk, run, play, enjoy pleasures, and be innovative and creative. All of these things, and more, are possible only if we first consume in our food *all* the essential nutrients in some form or another on a regular basis. Without all the 40 to 45 nutrients none of these things so characteristic of human life is possible.

Nutrition, then, may be defined as *the science of food as it relates to optimal health and performance.*

We all are, or should be, vitally interested in promoting or protecting our own health, since upon it depends our happiness, capacity for rewarding work, and even our length of life. The rapidly developing science of nutrition has accumulated a mass of facts about

3

what constitutes the best type of diet and how foods are used for building strong bodies.

Some knowledge of the basic facts of nutrition is helpful to anyone, while a more detailed and scientific background of knowledge is essential for those who have the responsibility of feeding others and participating in health education—such as homemakers, dietitians, nurses, doctors, dentists, home economists, social workers, health and physical education teachers, teachers and extension workers in the field of nutrition, public health workers, food scientists, food industry and advertising personnel, and managers of public eating places and school lunchrooms.

People in the United Nations food and health agencies are concerned with attempting to bring more of the right kinds of food to countries all over the world, many of whose people now exist at a semistarvation level. It should be clear to all, including our national leaders, that no country can achieve the vigor essential for economic, social, and political stability without adequate nutrition for all its people. This is equally true for developed nations as well as the developing nations.

People in countries, such as our own, with a plentiful supply of a wide variety of foods do not necessarily have a high general level of health.

While it is true that children of the present generation grow faster and taller and weigh more (on the average) than did those of comparable ages several generations ago, signs of malnutrition, hunger, and poor eating practices exist all around us. Many of our health problems stem from overeating or from eating too freely of certain types of food (sugar, fats, and alcohol), with the inevitable overweight and the diseases that are often associated with it (diabetes, high blood pressure, heart disease, etc.).

Moreover, although proper nutrition provides an essential basis for health, good health also depends on many other factors. Factors of heredity, disease, environment, stress, and emotional instability may counterbalance the effects of a good diet. Persons who do not eat luxuriously but whose mode of life often involves more exercise (much like our farmer forebears) may often be more healthy. Less physical work in factory and home, together with the almost universal use of the automobile for getting about, results in the average American getting much less exercise than formerly. A survey of pupils in New York City public schools has served to point up the need for regular programs to improve physical fitness. Nearly a third of the pupils failed to qualify at initial testing, but

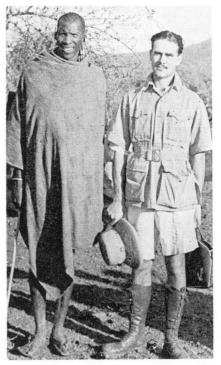

Figure 1–1. Members of the African Masai tribe illustrate the fine nutrition provided by their herds of cattle and goats—using milk, meat, and blood, reinforced by some vegetables and fruit. The chief, seen here, towers above the European man beside him, although the latter is nearly six feet tall. (From Price, W. A.: *Nutrition and Physical Degeneration,* Paul B. Hoeber, Inc.)

after about six weeks of the physical activity program, nearly two-thirds of those who had previously failed were now able to qualify.[1] The young respond quickly to the right conditions; unfortunately, the reconditioning of a sedentary (and perhaps overweight) adult is of necessity a slower and more gradual process.

Instinctive Selection of Foods Does Not Always Lead to Good Nutrition

It is true that in many parts of the world peoples who know little or nothing of the science of nutrition have subsisted for generations on diets that maintained strong bodies. Sometimes, with even a limited variety of foods, those available were such that all the requirements for good nutrition were provided. Other primitive peoples were not so fortunate; either the food supply was inadequate or the cultural habits prompted selection of foods that made an improperly balanced diet which lacked some factors necessary for growth and health.

McCarrison made some early studies on diets used in different sections of India and their relation to the health of the respective tribes.[2] In the southern sections of the country, the diet consisted chiefly of milled rice, fruits, and vegetables, with little flesh foods or milk; these peoples were of smaller size and inferior strength, and were short-lived, as well. The peoples of tribes farther north, who used unmilled millet or wheat along with goats' milk and butter, had splendid physiques and enough stamina to make good soldiers. In remote sections of the Himalaya Mountains races were found whose frugal diet was made up mostly of apricots (sun-dried for winter use), vegetables, and goats' milk, with meat eaten only on feast days; these peoples were unusually strong, healthy, and long-lived.

The long-lived Balkan peoples eat little meat, but use whole-grain cereals, cheeses, and the fermented milk known as koumiss. Studies of African tribes have shown that, of two tribes living not far apart, one may have relatively large-sized and healthy bodies, while the other may be puny and disease-ridden due to defective diet[3] (though genetic differences may also exist). Two such tribes studied were the Masai, who tend herds and live mainly on meat and milk, and the Akikuyu, who eat chiefly corn and sweet potatoes, along with other cereals and vegetables. A full-grown man of the former tribe averaged 5 inches taller and 23 pounds heavier than one from the latter tribe, and his muscular strength was 50 percent greater. The diet of many poorer classes in Central and South American countries provides too little protein, and what is provided often comes almost entirely from beans and corn. On such a diet, young children, after weaning, often develop severe deficiency symptoms, and those who manage to survive make less than normal growth (Fig. 1–2).

It has become increasingly clear that diet is correlated not only with physical stamina, but also with mental alertness and emotional stability. In extensive studies on undernutrition, Keys and coworkers,[4] in classic studies on human volunteers in World War II, showed that changes in behavior and work capacity result from prolonged underfeeding. Today, hundreds of research studies are being conducted in many countries on animals and man which demonstrate that inadequate nutrition can result in lowered intelligence, poor mental health, abnormal behavior, and actual damage to nerve and brain tissue.[5, 6]

Malnutrition Still Widespread Throughout the World

In spite of years of accumulated knowledge of the importance of ade-

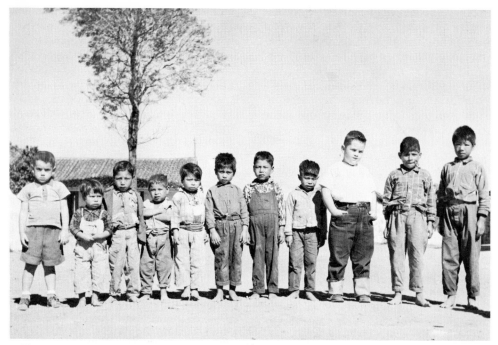

Figure 1–2. A group of Guatemalan boys, showing stunted growth caused by the inadequate native diet, as compared with two boys of the same racial stock who had superior type diet and are of normal weight and height for their age. The boy at left (normal) is 4½ years old, while the four boys next to him range from 5 to 7 years of age. The boy third from right is nearly 7 years old and is of normal height; the three smaller boys beside him are 7–8 and the two boys to his right (approx. same height) are 11 and 12 years old. (Courtesy Dr. Miguel A. Guzmán, Institute of Nutrition for Central America and Panama.)

quate food and of good nutrition for the health of people, hunger and malnutrition exist throughout the world—even in the so-called "developed" countries.

In the United States, typical of many highly industrialized countries, the nutritional situation is no better today than it was 10 or 20 years ago (and it may be even worse).[7-11] At least 30 percent of the United States population shows some evidence of malnutrition in the form of inadequate intake of food and nutrients (especially iron, calcium, vitamin A, vitamin C, and riboflavin), or in the form of anemias, obesity, or diseases closely associated with poor nutrition, such as the circulatory diseases (heart disease, hypertension, stroke, etc.), diabetes, severe dental and periodontal disease, and alcoholism.

Especially vulnerable to malnutrition are young children, adolescents, young pregnant women, families of the poor, handicapped persons, and people over 65 years of age.

Our situation in the United States is not much different from most other industrialized countries, such as Canada, the European countries, and Japan. However, the prevalence of hunger and malnutrition is still much more widespread in most of the non-industrialized and the developing countries—especially those in the tropical areas of South and Central America and the West Indies, in Africa, in India, and in many other Asian countries, including the numerous islands from the Philippines to New Guinea and the East Indies. In some of these countries hunger unfortunately is widespread, and many effects of malnutrition are common, including blindness from vitamin A deficiency and poor growth due to protein-calorie deficiencies of babies and children (Chaps. 5, 9). Many national and international groups, such as the World Health Organization (WHO) and the Food and Agricultural Organization (FAO) of the United Nations, are attempting to solve the world malnutrition problem, but the task is immense (see list of supplementary readings).

Basic Causes of Hunger and Malnutrition

Why does so much malnutrition exist in the supposedly enlightened world of the 1970's? The lack of nutrition education is only one of six major causes of malnutrition, which are, on a broad basis:

1. Lack of adequate food, poor food distribution programs, and overpopulation;

2. Social and cultural differences in food habits, including severe food faddism;

3. Widespread ease of availability and use of highly processed and often nutritionally inadequate foods;

4. Lack of adequate nutrition education in schools and the home;

5. Poor or misdirected motivation to eat properly, and complacency; and

6. Inadequate recognition by local, state, and national leaders of the importance of good nutrition.

You can, no doubt, think of still other reasons for the presence of hunger and malnutrition in your own community.* Having sufficient good food is a basic need of all individuals — probably more basic than any other human need. More human effort, on a world basis, goes toward the production, processing, marketing, and consumption of food than toward any other human need (for further discussion of the world food problem, see Chapter 17).

Our food habits often stem from prejudices acquired in childhood, either from parental examples or from childish whims that are indulged. Education that explains *why* foods selected should include those needed to supply all the essentials for an adequate diet will provide motivation to change old food habits for new ones. This is especially true when food habits in the home are based on cultural or religious practice. Deep-rooted food habits, if bad, can often be overcome by suggestions that larger amounts of certain liked or permitted foods should be taken or that new foods may be cooked in well liked or familiar ways. Diet fads and advertising literature that sponsors them may also induce a person to take unbalanced diets which furnish too little of certain nutritive essentials, and the advertising "boosting" of some types of food may persuade one to use such foods too largely and depend too little on other needed foods.

Complacency, or indifference, is also a strong factor working against change of food habits. Unless a person has a vision of the greater vitality to be attained by improving his food habits, he is apt to believe that he is well enough off as he is. There must be education as to why certain foods are essential for health. Remote goals, including longevity, can strongly influence choice of foods in the diet. With teenagers, a more immediate objective, such as the physical prowess, athletic ability, and

---

*President Richard Nixon, in a message to the 91st Congress, on May 7, 1969, stated: ". . . there can be no doubt that hunger and malnutrition exist in America, and that some millions may be affected. That hunger and malnutrition should persist in a land such as ours is embarrassing and intolerable. But it is an exceedingly complex problem, not at all susceptible to fast or easy solutions. Millions of Americans are simply too poor to feed their families properly. For them, there first must be sufficient food income. . . . People must be educated in the choosing of proper foods. All of us, poor and non-poor alike, must be reminded that a proper diet is a basic determinant of good health." (House of Representatives Document 91-115.)

good looks that are associated with buoyant health, may prove more effective in stimulating interest in good food habits. Young college women, as prospective mothers, should be vitally concerned in good diets to safeguard their own health and that of their children; instead, they are often careless in eating habits or follow reducing fads in order to retain slender figures.

One of the aims of nutrition should be to prolong the vitality of the prime of life into later years. There is still much room for dietary improvement, provided nutritional teaching can convince people that alteration of their dietary habits is worth while.

Functions of Food and Essential Nutrients

We have defined nutrition earlier as the science of food as it relates to optimal health and performance — that is, providing adequately for the body's *growth, maintenance, repair,* and *reproduction.* Except for the *water* we drink and *oxygen* taken in from the air we breathe, the needs of the body must be met by the intake of foods. To nourish the body, foods must contain substances that *function* in one or more of *three* ways:

1. Furnish body fuel, substances whose oxidation in the body sets free *energy* needed for its activities;
2. Provide materials for the *building* or *maintenance* of body *tissues;* and
3. Supply substances that act to *regulate body processes.*

An individual food may fulfill all three of these functions or only one, but all three functions must be served by the diet as a whole in order to maintain the body in health. Most foods can fulfill more than one function because they are *mixtures* of a number of chemical substances. Any chemical substance found in foods that functions in one or more of the three ways named above is known as a *nutrient.*

Six general classes, or *kinds of nutrients,* which are necessary to the body are:

1. Carbohydrates
2. Fats
3. Proteins
4. Vitamins
5. Minerals
6. Water

Carbohydrates, fats, and proteins are often spoken of as the fuel or *energy nutrients,* since they are the only substances that the body can use to supply energy for work and heat. They belong to the great division of chemical substances known as *organic* compounds, which contain carbon and are combustible. The mineral elements and water are sometimes called *inorganic nutrients,* since they do not contain carbon.

Proteins, minerals, and water all enter into the composition of body tissues, and hence are necessary for *building* new *tissues* or repair of those already built. *Vitamins* are chemically diverse organic substances which occur in minute quantities in foods but are essential for normal growth and health. Certain ones may be built into or stored in the tissues, but their chief function is to serve in regulating body processes. Mineral salts and vitamins act as *body regulators* by promoting oxidative processes, normal functioning of nerves and muscles, and vitality of tissues, and are of assistance in many other bodily functions. Water also serves as an important regulating substance in the body. It holds substances in solution in the digestive juices, blood, and tissues, and aids in regulation of body temperature, excretion, circulation, and many other body processes. Vegetable fiber (cellulose) acts along with water to promote intestinal elimination.

The three energy nutrients — carbohydrates, fats, and proteins — can be used by the body more or less interchangeably to supply *energy,* depending on which is more abundant in the diet. These three classes of substances are by far the most abundant nutrients in

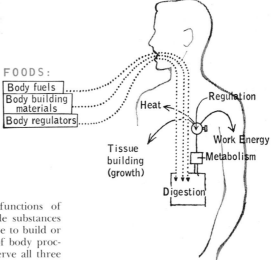

FOODS:
Body fuels
Body building materials
Body regulators

Figure 1-3. Diagram summarizing the functions of foods. To qualify as a food, it must provide substances that act as body fuel to provide energy, serve to build or maintain body tissues, or act as regulators of body processes. Many foods contain substances that serve all three purposes.

our food—minerals and vitamins being present in relatively small, or even trace, amounts.

For building tissues, different proteins are *not interchangeable*, since the "building stones," called amino acids, which compose them vary in kind and relative amounts. Some 8 or 10 of these amino acids cannot be made in the body and must be supplied in the diet. Also, the fats eaten must supply some of the substances known as essential fatty acids. Some 12 to 15 different mineral elements must be supplied, in either major or minor amounts, and at least 14 different vitamins are known to be needed, although not all of these have been proved to be essential for man. Hence, there are actually some 40 to 45 different nutrients essential for normal nutrition. The exact number will differ with various authorities, according to whether certain ones, chiefly mineral elements and vitamins, are considered to have been proved essential for man.

General Composition of Foods and Units of Measurement

It is important that the nutrition student have a basic understanding of the major differences in the composition of the six classes of nutrients in common foods of distinctly different origins. Table 1-1 shows the composition on a fresh and dried basis of corn (maize), a typical food of plant origin, compared with a typical animal body on the same basis. A column is included for hamburger, a typical animal food. It should become obvious, after study of this table, that a *major characteristic of animals which eat largely vegetable material is the conversion within the body of plant carbohydrates to body fats (after energy needs)*. Along with making this conversion, the animal body accumulates minerals and protein. Only small amounts of carbohydrates are present in animal tissues (see Chapter 3). Knowing the figures in Table 1-1, one can estimate, in a rough, general way, the composition of almost all foods, plant or animal.

The detailed composition of many common foods is given in Table 2 of the Appendix for further comparison. In order to understand food composition tables and to have a clear idea of the *amounts* of foods which we actually need and eat, one must first be at home with the various *units of weight and measurement* commonly used in nutrition. Most countries of the world now use the metric system, which is by far the

Table 1–1.   Some Typical Composition Figures of Plant vs. Animal Foods

Classes of Nutrients	Corn (Maize) Fresh	Corn (Maize) Dried	Typical Animal Body (Live Basis)	Typical Animal Body (Dried)	Hamburger (Fresh)
	%	%	%	%	%
Water	75.0	12.0	60.0	12.0	50.0
Total carbohydrates	21.0*	73.4*	trace	0.1	trace
Crude fats	1.1	4.0	19.0	41.7	25.0
Crude proteins†	2.5	9.0	17.0	37.0	24.0
Minerals	0.4	1.4	4.0	9.0	1.0
Vitamins‡	trace	0.2	trace	0.2	trace
Total	100.0	100.0	100.0	100.0	100.0

*Primarily starch and sugars.
†Including small amounts of other compounds containing nitrogen.
‡Including various miscellaneous compounds.

most useful way to describe and measure vitamins and trace minerals. A kilogram (metric system) equals 2.2 pounds (visualize, roughly, by thinking of slightly more than 2 pounds of butter or margarine, flour or sugar, or a quart – or liter – of milk). Other very useful conversion figures are shown in Table 1–2. We suggest that your understanding of nutrition will be much more complete if you learn these relationships now.

How Composition of Foods is Studied

What nutrients and how much of each are present in our various everyday foods is usually determined either
1. by chemical analysis, or
2. by biological assay.
CHEMICAL ANALYSIS. This provides useful data as to the approximate distribution of carbohydrates, fats, proteins, minerals, vitamins, and water in any given food. Methods commonly used for determining the relative amounts of the nutrients are briefly discussed in the following outline.

Water is determined by weighing a sample of the food before and after drying to constant weight.

Ash (mineral matter) is ascertained by completely burning the combustible portion and weighing the noncombustible residue.

Protein is computed by multiplying the nitrogen content of a food (chemically determined) by 6.25, since proteins are known to consist of about 16 percent (one-sixth) nitrogen by weight. This is the classic "Kjehldahl method." Slight errors result both because other nitrogen-containing substances that may be present in the food are included as proteins and because proteins vary somewhat in the amount of nitrogen they contain. This measure, $N \times 6.25$, is often referred to as "crude protein" for this reason.

Fats are determined by extracting a dried sample of the food with ether. With the true fats (weighed after evaporating to dryness the ether extract) will be included small amounts of other ether-soluble substances such as resins, waxes, and coloring matter (pigments). This measure is often called "crude fat," or "ether-extract."

Carbohydrates are usually determined by difference; that is, the remainder of the weight not accounted for under one of the above heads is assumed to be carbohydrate in nature and is listed as such. Although this residue undoubtedly does consist largely of carbohydrates, it will also include organic acids (in fruits and vegetables), indigestible carbohydrates (cell-

Table 1-2.   Common Units Used in Nutrition and in Measurement of Foods*

Metric units†	1 kilogram (kg)	= 1000 grams	
	1 gram (gm)‡	= 1000 milligrams	
	1 milligram (mg)§	= 1000 micrograms (mcg. μg. or γ)	

	Metric		*U.S. Avoirdupois*
Weight	1 kilogram = 1000 gm		= 2.2 pounds
	0.1 kilogram = 100 gm		= 3.52 ounces
	0.454 kilogram = 454 gm		= 1.0 pound
	0.028 kilogram = 28.4 gm		= 1.0 ounce

Volume, liquid	3.785 liters		= 1 gallon = 4 quarts¶
	1.000 liter = 1000 ml		= 1.06 quarts
	0.946 liter = 946 ml		= 1 quart = 2 pints
	0.473 liter = 473 ml		= 1 pint = 2 cups
	0.227 liter = 227 ml		= 1 cup = 16 tablespoons (tbsp)
	0.014 liter = 14.2 ml		= 1 tablespoon = 3 teaspoons (tsp)
	4.7 ml		= 1 teaspoon

Weight per volume of water**	1 liter = 1 kg	
	1 milliliter = 1 gm	= 1 cubic centimeter (cc)
	1 quart = 946 gm	
	1 cup†† = 227 gm	= 8 ounces = ½ pound

Length	1.609 kilometers = 1 mile	
	1 kilometer = 0.621 mile	
	0.305 meter = 1 foot	
	1 meter = 3.281 feet	
	25.4 millimeters = 1 inch	
	1 millimeter = 0.039 inch	

*Many of these are approximations only. See Table 5 of the Appendix for more conversion values. (We should use the metric system whenever possible to avoid the confusion of the above table, which must be used when we work with two systems.)

†Kilo means × 1000; milli, × $\frac{1}{1000}$; micro, × $\frac{1}{1,000,000}$. Therefore, kilogram means gram × 1000, milligram means gram × $\frac{1}{1000}$, milliliter means liter × $\frac{1}{1000}$.

‡Visualize a gram of food as about the size of a common pencil eraser, or one lima bean (broad bean).
§A milligram of powdered sugar would be about the size of a pinhead—easily seen with the naked eye.
¶British Imperial Gallon = 4.545 liters.
**Other liquids may be lighter (e.g., salad oil) or heavier (e.g., corn syrup) than water.
††A cup is not an official unit of measurement. The values given here are approximations only to help one visualize sizes and weights. The weight of a "cup" depends on what is being measured, of course.

ulose and hemicelluloses), which have no food value, and various other undetermined substances not carbohydrates.

In some cases, the crude *fiber* is determined separately, subtracted from the total carbohydrates, and the remainder listed as *utilizable carbohydrates*. More accurate figures may be obtained by direct analyses for determining the carbohydrates through their reducing powers.

Vitamins must be determined individually. Most of the vitamins may be deter- mined by chemical methods (by specific color reactions, by chromatography, or by complicated laboratory equipment using various chemical or physical properties of the vitamins studied). A few vitamins are still measured by biological tests using bacteria or one or more animal species.

Tables of food composition, obtained by the above methods, can never be absolutely accurate for several reasons. First, certain errors are inherent in the methods used or in the manner of calculating results (as pointed out in describing the methods above). Then, even in the hands of skilled chemists, small errors occur which are magnified on calculating the composition from the basis of a small sample to a percentage basis for the food as a whole. Lastly, and probably of most importance, foods may vary considerably in composition either in samples from different sections of the country or from soils of different compositions (which may affect trace mineral levels); in different parts of the same sample of food; or especially in cooked foods where moisture and fat content are frequently variable. When a large number of samples of some raw food material, such as flour, milk, or eggs, have been analyzed, *average* values are obtained from which individual specimens probably will not differ much in composition. With cooked foods, fruits, and vegetables, or whenever only a few samples have been analyzed, variations will be larger and figures less accurate.

BIOLOGICAL ASSAY OF FOODS. This

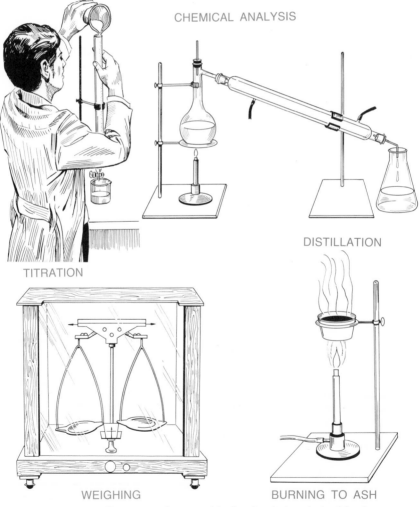

CHEMICAL ANALYSIS

TITRATION

DISTILLATION

WEIGHING

BURNING TO ASH

Figure 1–4. Some procedures used in the chemical analysis of foods.

method involves actual feeding experiments on laboratory animals (usually rats, mice, guinea pigs, or chickens) under controlled conditions. White rats, whose heredity and previous diet history are known, are considered the best "standardized" animals and hence are likely to give the most accurate results. Moreover, the chemistry of their body tissues is, for the most part, reasonably similar to that of man. Also their life cycle is short enough so that one can watch the effects of some special diet on several generations. Such animals are fed a simple diet of known composition which is planned so as to provide plenty of all the essential nutrients *except one*. A certain food is added to this basal diet in known amounts to serve as the sole source of the nutrient in which it is lacking and for which the special food is being tested.

By such experiments, the existence of *vitamins* in natural articles of food was established. Likewise it was discovered that numerous different vitamins are necessary in the diet for the well-being of both man and animals, and the relative amounts of each vitamin supplied by different foods have been more or less accurately determined. Laboratory feeding experiments also give information, not obtainable by chemical analyses, as to how *efficient* the *protein* content of different foods is for growth or maintaining weight, and how well *assimilated* and utilized the *mineral* content of certain foods may be. Biological assay shows us how effective different foods really are in supplying the needs of the body for each nutrient.

All of the vitamins may now be determined by **physical** methods (measurement of absorption spectra, chromatography, fluorescence, turbidity, etc.),

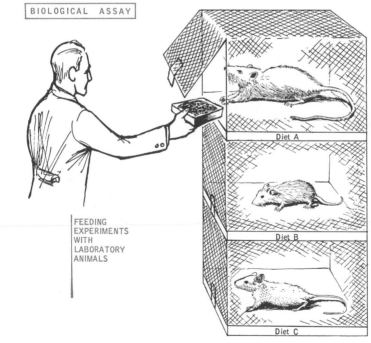

BIOLOGICAL ASSAY

FEEDING
EXPERIMENTS
WITH
LABORATORY
ANIMALS

Diet A

Diet B

Diet C

Figure 1–5. Biological assay is used to show how efficient different foods are in supplying body needs for proteins, various mineral elements, or vitamins. The rat is the favorite animal for feeding experiments, and the effectiveness of the diet in supplying body needs is gauged by relative growth and health of animals. In this drawing, the animal fed Diet A obviously got the most complete and adequate diet, while the other two rats either made less growth or show varying degrees of deficiency of one or more essential nutrients.

A Guide to Good Eating

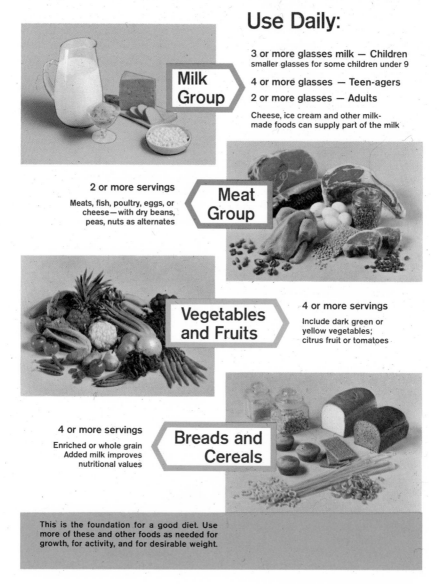

Use Daily:

Milk Group

3 or more glasses milk — Children
smaller glasses for some children under 9

4 or more glasses — Teen-agers

2 or more glasses — Adults

Cheese, ice cream and other milk-
made foods can supply part of the milk

Meat Group

2 or more servings

Meats, fish, poultry, eggs, or
cheese—with dry beans,
peas, nuts as alternates

Vegetables and Fruits

4 or more servings

Include dark green or
yellow vegetables;
citrus fruit or tomatoes

Breads and Cereals

4 or more servings

Enriched or whole grain
Added milk improves
nutritional values

This is the foundation for a good diet. Use
more of these and other foods as needed for
growth, for activity, and for desirable weight.

Figure 1–6. The specified number of servings from each food group together provide a well balanced diet, adequate in all nutrients, except that extra fuel foods will usually be needed. (Courtesy of National Dairy Council, Chicago.)

by *chemical* methods (chiefly by color reactions), or by *microbiological assay* (influence on growth of bacteria). However, feeding tests with animals retain their usefulness and in some cases are indispensable.

Learning About Foods—Food Groups

A simple and convenient way to study the different common foods is to *group them in several classes*, according to the nutrients they supply most abundantly. Thus, there have been in the past the "seven food groups," the "five food groups," and more recently the well-known "four food groups" (see Figure 1–6). Foods grouped together in this way are similar in general chemical make-up and hence contribute the same types of nutrients to the diet.

The basis of good nutrition is eating a *variety* of foods from different food groups. No single food group supplies all the essential nutrients in proper proportions to maintain health, but a food plan that includes a suggested number of servings from different groups furnishes at least a major portion of the proteins, minerals, and vitamins needed for an adequate diet. Additional foods may be required to meet the energy needs, and these may be supplied by extra portions of the foods listed in groups of "sweets" (sugars, candies, cakes, jams, etc.) and "fatty foods" (butter, margarine, salad oils, etc.), which often are not included in the food plans given in Figure 1–6. These foods are useful either entirely or chiefly for their fuel value, for pure sugar and fats contribute little except energy value to the diet. (Fats, however, may carry vitamins A and E and essential fatty acids.) Usually appetite determines how much of these foods should be eaten, although it is by no means an infallible guide.

The "Four Food Groups"

For a very simple daily food guide, the United States Department of Agriculture suggests planning the basic diet around *four* food groups, along with the number of servings from each group that should be included (Figure 1–6).[12] These four food groups, together with the main contributions in nutrients that each group makes to the diet, are listed in Table 1–3.

The daily "four food groups" guide has, actually, six groups, if we include two subgroups in the vegetable-fruit group. Nevertheless, this guide has the advantages of simplicity and enough freedom of choice to fit individual preferences and different economic levels. However, it is by no means "foolproof." A basic diet, selected in accordance with

Table 1–3. Daily Food Plan Based on Four Food Groups

Group	Role in Diet
Grain products—bread, flour, cereals, baked goods (whole grain or enriched preferred).	Inexpensive sources of energy and proteins. Whole-grain or enriched products carry more iron and B vitamins.
Meat group—meats, poultry, fish, shellfish, and eggs. Dried beans, peas, and nuts as alternates.	Valuable sources of protein; also furnish certain minerals (e.g., iron) and B vitamins.
Milk group—milk, cheese, ice cream.	Valuable sources of protein, calcium, other minerals, and vitamins.
Vegetable-fruit group—all fruits and vegetables, including potatoes.	Chiefly important as carriers of minerals, vitamins, and fiber (cellulose).
Leafy, green, and yellow vegetables.	High in iron, vitamin A, and folacin.
Citrus fruits, tomatoes, raw cabbage, etc.	Rich in vitamin C.

the rules laid down, may range in essential nutrients from barely adequate (or even inadequate) to one that supplies an extra margin of these nutrients beyond body requirements, depending largely on the *choice of foods* within the four food groups and the *size of the servings* eaten. The choice of foods in turn may be influenced both by lack of nutritional knowledge and by the economic status of the family.

Although the foods within a group belong together because they furnish, in general, the same kinds or types of nutrients, these nutrients may be present in quite different quantities or proportion in different foods within the same group. For instance, if only highly milled grain products are eaten (instead of whole-grain or enriched ones, as specified), less than adequate amounts of certain minerals and B vitamins may be provided. Within the "meat group," the alternates suggested for flesh foods (dry beans, peas, and nuts) must be taken in fairly large amounts to furnish as much protein as an average serving of meat. Also, the proteins in vegetable foods are not fully equivalent to those in animal foods. Milk products differ also.

Finally, the "vegetable and fruit group" is widely diversified as to composition. It could well be (and sometimes is) divided into several subgroups—the starchy vegetables (potatoes, peas, beans, etc.); those that are either leafy, green, or yellow; citrus fruits and others that are relatively rich in vitamin C; and succulent fruits and vegetables high in water content (peaches, melons, celery, summer squash, etc.). To make sure of an adequate intake of certain nutrients (chiefly iron, folacin, and vitamins A and C), the rules specify serving leafy, green, or yellow vegetables at least every other day, and serving citrus fruits or other fruit or vegetables important for vitamin C daily.

The "four food groups" guide is probably the best teaching device we have, at present, for young students,

homemakers, and others just learning about good nutrition practices. However, in addition to the several limitations discussed in the previous paragraphs, nutrition educators know that students become bored hearing year after year about the plan. They begin to want to know *why* certain foods are important to us and to know more about food sources of individual nutrients. Also, the caloric (energy) content of foods and their taste and appeal often seem more important than their nutrient content.

There are two other major disadvantages of the "four food groups" guide. One is that many cultural, religious, and social groups of people here in the United States and in most other parts of the world do not, or cannot, have all the foods in this particular plan readily available to them. For instance, milk products are not universally used or even tolerated. Second, today many manufactured foods are available in the market which do not conveniently fit into one of the four food groups (for instance, pizza, hamburger "with the works," imitation cream products, or complete "meal replacements"). (Also see Chap. 18.)

Alternate Food Plans

It is now clear that there are many ways possible to learn about good food choices. This is a rapidly developing field today. The final selection of food by groups of people depends upon the types of foods readily available and utilized by the target group, and their level of understanding about nutrition. In the United States we can expect the emergence in the next few years of new and often better guides for teaching about good nutrition. There no doubt will soon be better and more specific guides established for the feeding of infants and children, for different ethnic groups (for instance, Spanish-American and Chinese food guides are now widely available in the United

States and elsewhere), for high school and college students, for pregnant women, for partial and complete vegetarians, for oldsters living alone, and for people living in, or from, different countries and cultures.

There is no magic or secret way to good nutrition, nor is it easy. Some degree of nutrition knowledge is essential if an individual is going to ensure good health and physical fitness through good and economical nutrition practices, when so many negative forces are all around us today.

Chapter 17 has a more detailed discussion of "food groups and their place in the diet," and Chapter 18 discusses the planning of adequate diets for normal adults.

History of Nutrition

The history of nutrition is fascinating, but the authors believe the subject is enjoyed more when studied in connection with the individual nutrients throughout the book. Nutrition begins with the beginning of mankind on this earth, and many references to food and nutrition exist in man's earliest writings. Early man had to seek the facts for himself, largely by trial and error, as he chose his food from available plants, berries, nuts, roots, grains, fruit, and from the plentiful supply of animal life all around him. All of man's history has been greatly influenced by the distribution, availability, and search for foods and spices.

It was not until the development of modern science in the eighteenth and nineteenth centuries that there began to be an appreciation of the essential nature of certain nutrients. Among the first nutrients to be recognized as essential were protein, oxygen, calcium, iodine, and a scurvy-preventing factor (later identified as vitamin C). Most of the early pioneers in nutrition and the more recent discoverers of the various nutrients will be mentioned later in this book. Students interested particularly in nutrition history will find references on this subject listed at the end of this chapter, and will enjoy reading about the lives and discoveries of such early nutrition pioneers as Lavoisier, Priestley, Liebig, Bernard, Mulder, Spallanzani, Magendie, Davy, E. Fischer, Abderhalden, Beaumont, Voit, Lusk, Rubner, Chittenden, Lind, Lunin, Takeki, Eijkman, Hopkins, Mellamby, Babcock, Hart, Wills, McCollum, Osborne, Mendel, Funk, Elvehjem, Goldberger, Jansen, R. R. Williams, Steenbock, Mitchell, Evans, Forbes, Morgan, Armsby, Burr, Deuel, Rose, Kuhn, Murlin, Sherman, Roberts, and many others to whom we owe so much.

Likewise, others living today (though retired) have pioneered in nutrition discoveries which have greatly influenced the course of nutrition history and the health of all of us. Interested students will want to learn more about such nutrition pioneers as King, György, Best, R. J. Williams, Folkers, Lepkovsky, Sebrell, Emerson, Zilva, Szent-Györgyi, Rose, Kleiber, Macy-Hoobler, Cowgill, Steibling, Kon, Norris, Waddell, Dam, and Almquist, along with many others still active today. (See references at the end of this chapter and later chapters for more information about these persons.)

As far as we know, the first professor of (human) nutrition in the United States was Professor M. Jaffa, in 1908, at the University of California, Berkeley.[13] In 1912 he became chairman of the Department of Nutrition at the Berkeley College of Agriculture. (This may also have been the first department of nutrition in America.) Since then nutrition departments or divisions have prospered in most all general colleges and universities of the country and are widely scattered throughout the world, in departments of home economics, animal science, or biochemistry. In the past few years separate nutrition departments or graduate training groups have been formed in at least a dozen universities of the United States. Unfortunately, though, there is as yet little nutrition training in American medical schools.

Approximately 10,000 research papers are published each year in the world's literature on food and nutrition. It is evident by now that the science of nutrition is well established throughout the world and new important discoveries are being made almost every day. Almost every major country has a nutrition society and publishes its own scientific journal. Recently the International Union of Nutritional Sciences (IUNS) has become considerably more active and is in the process of setting up international standards for nutrition research, nomenclature, and training.

A list of resource materials to the broader aspects of nutritional sciences may be found at the end of this chapter.

QUESTIONS AND PROBLEMS

1. What is meant by nutrition, a nutrient, an adequate diet?

2. Why do some peoples prosper physically on diets consisting of only a few types of food, while others show physical degeneration on the limited types of diet that they take?

3. How is it possible to improve an apparently adequate diet and what benefits may be expected as a result of doing this? Name the chief motives for making changes in food habits indicated as nutritionally desirable, and some of the factors that stand in the way of changing food habits.

4. What are the three uses of food in the body? Name the six kinds of essential nutrients found in foods. Which of these can serve as body fuel and why? Which are used in the building and repair of tissues? Which are necessary to regulate body processes?

5. Name the four general groups of foods suggested as a basis around which to plan an adequate diet and the main nutrients contributed by each of these food groups to the diet. How many average servings are recommended from each group daily? Why are green and yellow vegetables and citrus fruits singled out for more frequent use than other fruits and vegetables? Using foods from *each* of the four main food groups in the number of servings specified in Figure 1–6, plan a day's diet. What other foods will be needed to round out the diet and satisfy energy needs?

6. Explain what is meant by the biological assay of foods. What information can be obtained by biological assay and how does it supplement facts obtained by chemical analysis? Describe how a food may be assayed for its content of a certain vitamin.

7. Make a record for 3 or 4 days of the kinds of foods (including beverages) and the number of servings in each of the four food groups consumed each day. Compare the amounts of each class of food actually consumed against those recommended in Figure 1–6. What foods did you eat in larger or smaller quantities than recommended as the basis for an adequate diet? Did you supplement your diet with additional fuel foods? How could you improve your dietary habits?

8. As a special project, write a report on some aspect of the history of nutrition or on one of the nutrition pioneers.

REFERENCES

1. Jacobziner, H.: Physical fitness in New York City schools. Gen. Prac., 29:112, 1964.
2. McCarrison, R.: Faulty food in relation to gastro-intestinal disorder. J. Amer. Med. Assoc., 78:1, 1922.
3. Orr, J. B., and Gilks, J. L.: Studies on nutrition: the physique and health of two African tribes. British Medical Research Council, Special Report No. 155, 1931.
4. Keys, A., et al.: *The Biology of Human Starvation.* Minneapolis, University of Minnesota Press, 1950.
5. Scrimshaw, N. S., and Gordon, E. (eds.): *Malnutrition, Learning and Behavior.* Cambridge, Mass., MIT Press, 1968.
6. Kallen D. J.: Nutrition and society. J. Amer. Med. Assoc., 215:94, 1971.
7. Schaefer, A. E., and Johnson, O. C.: Are we

well fed? The search for the answer. Nutr. Today, *4*(No. 1):2, 1969.

8. U.S. Department of Agriculture: Food intake and nutritive value of diets of men, women, and children in the United States, Spring 1965: A preliminary report. ARS 62-18. Beltsville, Md., Agricultural Research Service, U.S. Department of Agriculture., 1969, 97 pp. (for other reports in this series see supplementary reading list).

9. Kelsay, J. L.: A compendium of nutritional status studies and dietary evaluation studies conducted in the United States, 1957–1967. J. Nutr., *99*, Suppl. 1:123, 1969.

10. Davis, T. R. A., Gershoff, S. N., and Gamble, D. F.: Review of studies of vitamin and mineral nutrition in the United States (1950–1968). J. Nutr. Educ., *1*(No. 2 – suppl.): 41, 1969.

11. Briggs, G. M.: Hunger and malnutrition. J. Nutr. Educ., *1*(No. 3):4, 1970.

12. Page, L., and Phippard, E. F.: *Essentials of an Adequate Diet.* Home Economics Research Report No. 3., Washington, D.C., U.S. Department of Agriculture. Government Printing Office, 1957.

13. As cited in the University of California Bulletin of 1908.

SUPPLEMENTARY READING

American Medical Association, and American Association for Health: Exercise and fitness. J. Amer. Med. Assoc., *188*:133, 1964.

Anonymous: Fortified foods: The next revolution. Chem. Eng. News, Aug. 10, 1970, p. 36.

Aykroyd, W. R.: *Conquest of Deficiency Diseases.* Geneva, World Health Organization, 1970.

Bailey, M. A.: Nutrition education and the Spanish speaking American. J. Nutr. Educ., *2*:50, 1970.

Berg, A.: Nutrition as a national priority. Amer. J. Clin. Nutr., *23*:1396, 1970.

Blackburn, M. L.: Who turns the child "off" to nutrition? J. Nutr. Educ., *2*:45, 1970.

Bradfield, R. B., and Brun, T.: Nutritional status of California Mexican-Americans: A review. Amer. J. Clin. Nutr., *23*:798, 1970.

Brennan, R. E., Anderson, L., Joslyn, M. A., and Briggs, G. M.: A bookshelf on foods and nutrition. Amer. J. Public Health, *58*:621, 1968.

Calloway, D. H.: Malnutrition: Poverty or education. J. Nutr. Educ., *1*:No. 4, 9, 1970.

Correa, H., and Cummins, G.: Contribution of nutrition to national growth. Amer. J. Clin. Nutr., *23*:560, 1970.

Duzen, J. V., Carter, J. P., Secondi, J., and Federspiel, C.: Protein and calorie malnutrition among preschool Navajo Indian children. Amer. J. Clin. Nutr., *22*:1362, 1969.

Dwyer, J. T., Feldman, J. J., and Mayer, J.: Nutrition literacy of high school students. J. Nutr. Educ., *2*:59, 1970.

Emerson, G. A.: Nutritional status, U.S.A. J. Nutr., *91*, Suppl. 1:51, 1967.

Erhard, D.: Nutrition education for the "now" generation. J. Nutr. Educ., *2*:135, 1971.

Filer, L. J. Jr.: The U.S.A. today – is it free of public health nutrition problems? Amer. J. Public Health, *59*:327, 1969.

Food and Agriculture Organization: *Nutrition and Working Efficiency.* Pamphlet. Rome, FAO, 1962.

Goldsmith, G. A.: More food for more people. Amer. J. Public Health, *59*:694, 1969.

Handler, P.: Science, food, and man's future. Rev. Nutrition Research (Borden), *31*, No. 1:2, 1971.

Harper, A. E.: Nutrition: Where are we? Where are we going? Amer. J. Clin. Nutr., *22*:87, 1969.

Heinzelmann, F., and Bagley, R. W.: Response to physical activity programs and their effects on health behavior. Public Health Rpts., *85*:905, 1970.

Huth, M. J.: Malnutrition in developing countries. J. Home Econ., *61*:269, 1969.

Klevay, L. M.: Teaching the recommended dietary allowances. Amer. J. Clin. Nutr., *23*:1639, 1970.

Mann, G. V.: Nutrition education – U.S.A. Food and Nutrition News, *41*:1, Nov. 1969.

May, J. M., and Lemons, H.: The ecology of malnutrition. J. Amer. Med. Assoc., *207*: 2401, 1969.

McGanity, W. J.: Nutrition survey in Texas. Texas Medicine, *65*:40, 1969.

Owen, G. M., Garry, P. J., Kram, K. M., Nelsen, C. E., and Montalvo, J. M.: Nutritional status of Mississippi preschool children. Amer. J. Clin. Nutr., *22*:1444, 1969.

Pangborn, R. M., and Bruhn, C. M.: Concepts of food habits of "other" ethnic groups. J. Nutr. Educ., *2*:106, 1971.

Parrish, J. B.: Implications of changing food habits for nutrition educators. J. Nutr. Educ., *2*:140, 1971.

President's Council on Physical Fitness: *Fitness for Leadership.* Pamphlet. Washington, D.C., U.S. Government Printing Office, 1964.

Rasmussen, C. L.: Man and his food: 2000 A.D.: Economics, supply, and morality. Food Technol., *23*(No. 5):56, 1969.

Sanjur, D., and Scoma, A. D.: Food habits of low-income children in northern New York. J. Nutr. Educ., *2*:85, 1971.

Schaefer, A. E.: Malnutrition in the U.S.A.? Nutrition News, *32*:13, 1969.

Sebrell, W. H. Jr.: Recommended dietary allowances – 1968 revision. J. Amer. Diet. Assoc., *54*:103, 1969.

Smith, R. L.: "Health" books: Reader beware. Today's Health, *47*(No. 4):30, April, 1969.

Stewart, M. S.: *Hunger in America,* Public Affairs Pamphlet No. 457, 381 Park Ave. South, New York, 1970.

Stitt, K.: Nutritional value of diets today and fifty years ago. J. Amer. Dietet. Assoc., *36*:433, 1960.

U.S. Department of Agriculture: Dietary levels of households in the United States, Spring, 1965, Report No. 6, Washington, D.C., 1969 (also see other reports of this series).

U.S. Department of Agriculture: Nutritive value of foods. Home and Garden Bulletin, No. 72 (revised) 1971.

Watt, B. K., and Murphy, W. W.: Tables of food composition: Scope and needed research. Food Technology, *24*:674, 1970.

Wilson, C. S.: Food beliefs affect nutritional status of Malay fisherfolk. J. Nutr. Educ., *2*:96, 1971.

Zee, P., Walters, T., and Mitchell, C.: Nutrition and poverty in preschool children. J. Amer. Med. Assoc., *213*:739, 1970.

NUTRITION HISTORY REFERENCES: GENERAL

Atwater, W. O.: *Chemistry and Economy of Food.* U.S. Department of Agriculture, Bulletin No. 21, 1895.

Chittenden, R. H.: *The Nutrition of Man.* New York, F. A. Stokes Co., 1907.

Goldblith, S. A., and Joslyn, M. A.: *An Anthology of Food Science, Vol. 2, Milestones in Nutrition.* Westport, Connecticut, Avi Publishing Co., Inc., 1964.

Lusk, G.: *Clio Medica X, Nutrition.* New York, Paul B. Hoeber, Inc., 1933 (reprint edition, New York, Hafner Publishing Co., 1964).

Maynard, L. A.: *Animal Nutrition.* New York, McGraw-Hill Book Co., 1951 (also see earlier and more recent editions of this textbook, especially the first, 1937, edition).

McCollum, E. V.: *A History of Nutrition.* Boston, Houghton Mifflin Co., 1957.

McCollum, E. V., Orent-Keiles, E., and Day, H. G.: *The Newer Knowledge of Nutrition.* 5th Ed. New York, Macmillan Co., 1939 (also see earlier editions, especially the first edition by McCollum in 1918).

Todhunter, E. N.: Development of knowledge in nutrition. J. Amer. Dietet. Assoc., *41*:328, 1962.

Todhunter, E. N.: *The Story of Nutrition.* In *Food, the Yearbook of Agriculture,* Washington, D.C., U.S. Department of Agriculture, U.S. Government Printing Office, Ch. 2, 1959, p. 7.

GENERAL NUTRITION RESOURCES

Journals

American Journal of Clinical Nutrition, published monthly by the American Society for Clinical Nutrition Inc., 9650 Rockville Pike, Bethesda, Maryland 20014.

American Journal of Public Health, published monthly by the American Public Health Association Inc., 1740 Broadway, New York, N.Y. 10019.

British Journal of Nutrition (with the *Proceedings of the Nutrition Society*), published quarterly and semiannually respectively for the Nutrition Society by the Cambridge University Press, Bentley House, 200 Euston Road, London NW 1, or 32 East 57th St., New York, N.Y. 10022.

Cereal Science Today, published monthly by the American Association of Cereals Chemists, St. Paul, Minnesota 55104.

CERES, FAO Review, published bimonthly by the Food and Agriculture Organization of the United Nations. Available in major cities of the world, including Rome (Via delle Terme de Caracalla, 00100) and New York (UNIPUB, Inc., 650 First Ave., P.O. Box 433).

Ecology of Food and Nutrition, published quarterly by Gordon and Breach Science Publishers Ltd., 440 Park Avenue South, New York, N.Y. 10016.

Family Health, published monthly by Family Health Magazine, P.O. Box 2900, Boulder, Colorado 80302.

Federation Proceedings, published bimonthly by the Federation of American Societies for Experimental Biology, 9650 Rockville Pike, Bethesda, Maryland 20014 (containing review articles and abstracts of the American Institute of Nutrition, etc.).

Food Technology, published monthly by the Institute of Food Technologists, Suite 2120, 221 N. LaSalle St., Chicago, Illinois 60601.

Indian Journal of Nutrition and Dietetics, published bimonthly by the SRI Avinashilingam Home Science College, Coimbatore-11, India.

Journal of the American Dietetic Association, published monthly by the American Dietetic Association, 620 North Michigan Ave., Chicago, Illinois 60611.

Journal of the American Medical Association, published weekly by the American Medical Association, 535 North Dearborn, St., Chicago, Illinois 60610.

Journal of Home Economics, published 10 issues a year by the American Home Economics Association, 1600 20th St., Washington, D.C. 20009.

Journal of Nutrition, published monthly by the American Institute of Nutrition, 9650 Rockville Pike, Bethesda, Maryland 20014.

Journal of Nutrition Education, published quarterly by the Society for Nutrition Education, P.O. Box 931, Berkeley, California 94701.

Nutrition Abstracts and Reviews, published quarterly by the Commonwealth Bureau of Animal Nutrition, Rowett Research Institute, Bucksburn, Aberdeen, AB 2 9SB, Scotland.

Nutrition Reviews, published monthly by the Nutrition Foundation, 99 Park Ave., New York.

Nutrition Today, published bimonthly by Enloe, Stalvey, and Associates, 1140 Connecticut Ave., N.W., Washington D.C. 20036.

Today's Health, published monthly by the American Medical Association, 535 North Dearborn St., Chicago, Illinois 60610.

War on Hunger, published monthly by the Agency for International Development, Department of State, Washington D.C. 20523.

General Books on Nutrition

Beaton, G. H., and McHenry, E. W. (eds.): *Nutrition: A Comprehensive Treatise.* New York, Academic Press, Vol. 1: 1964, Vol. 2: 1964, Vol. 3: 1966.

Davidson, S., and Passmore, R.: *Human Nutrition and Dietetics.* Baltimore, Williams and Wilkins Co., 1969.

Fomon, S. J.: *Infant Nutrition.* Philadelphia, W. B. Saunders Co., 1967.

Halpern, S. L. (ed.): *Current Concepts in Clinical Nutrition.* Medical Clinics of North America, Vol. 54 (No. 6). Philadelphia, W. B. Saunders Co., 1970.

Heald, F. P.: *Adolescent Nutrition and Growth.* New York, Appleton-Century-Crofts (Meredith), 1969.

Lowenberg, M. E., Todhunter, E. N., Wilson, E. D., Feeney, M. C., and Savage, J. R.: *Food and Man.* New York, John Wiley and Sons, 1968.

National Research Council: *Recommended Dietary Allowances,* Publ. 1694, 2101 Constitution Ave., Washington D.C., 1968.

Pike, R. L., and Brown, M. L.: *Nutrition: An Integrated Approach.* New York, John Wiley and Sons, 1967.

Report of the White House Conference on Food, Nutrition and Health, December 2–4, 1969. Superintendent of Documents, Washington D.C. 20402, 1970.

Robinson, C. H.: *Basic Nutrition and Diet Therapy.* New York, Macmillan Co., 1970.

U.S. Department of Agriculture: *Food for Us All, Yearbook of Agriculture,* Washington D.C., U.S. Govt. Printing Office, 1969. (Also see the 1959 yearbook, *Food.*)

Williams, R. J.: *Biochemical Individuality.* New York, John Wiley and Sons, 1958.

Williams, S. R.: *Nutrition and Diet Therapy.* St. Louis, C. V. Mosby Co., 1969.

Wohl, M. G., and Goodhart, R. S.: *Modern Nutri-* *tion in Health and Disease.* Philadelphia, Lea and Febiger, 1964.

Public and Private Agencies Which Provide Nutrition Information*

American Dietetic Association, 620 North Michigan Ave., Chicago, Illinois 60611.

American Heart Association, 44 East 23rd St., New York, N.Y. 10010.

American Home Economics Association, 1600 20th Street, N.W., Washington D.C. 20009.

Cereal Institute Inc., Education Department, 135 So. LaSalle St., Chicago, Illinois 60603.

Food and Agriculture Organization, Rome or New York (UNIPUB, Inc., 650 First Ave., P.O. Box 433). (Publishes various nutrition education materials and booklets.)

National Academy of Sciences, Food and Nutrition Board, 2101 Constitution Ave., Washington D.C.

National Dairy Council, 111 North Canal St., Chicago, Illinois 60606. (Publishes a bimonthly "Dairy Council Digest" and quarterly "Nutrition News.")

National Live Stock and Meat Board, 36 South Wabash Ave., Chicago, Illinois 60603. (Publishes a monthly "Food and Nutrition News.")

Nutrition Foundation, Inc., 99 Park Ave., New York, N.Y. 10016.

Poultry and Egg National Board, 8 So. Michigan Ave., Chicago, Illinois 60603.

Public Affairs Committee, Inc., 381 Park Ave., South, New York, N.Y. 10016.

Society for Nutrition Education, P.O. Box 931, Berkeley, California 94701. (Has a national clearing house of nutrition education information.)

U.S. Department of Agriculture (Cooperative Extension Service; Food and Nutrition Service; Consumer Marketing Service; Agricultural Research Service; Office of Information; or National Library of Agriculture), Washington D.C. 20250.

U.S. Department of Health, Education, and Welfare, Washington D.C. (Children's Bureau; National Institutes of Health; Office of Child Development.)

Nutrition Reviews

A year-long study of nutrition of Jordanian children (by Pharaon, H. M., and Wilson, C. S.). 25:289, 1967.

Protein supplementation of a school lunch in India. 26:10, 1968.

*See a more complete listing of such agencies in *Journal of Nutrition Education,* 1(No. 1):24, 1969. Many state and county agencies and universities also supply nutrition information.

Features of kwashiorkor and nutritional marasmus in Jamaica. *26*:38, 1968.

Seasonal hunger in underdeveloped countries. *26*:142, 1968.

Malnutrition and hunger in the U.S.A. (by Stare, F. J.). *26*:227, 1968.

Sociological techniques in nutrition studies. *26*:297, 1968.

Heights and weights of Jamaicans. *27*:14, 1969.

Childhood malnutrition in Iran. *27*:69, 1969.

Low calorie intakes of Jamaican adults. *27*:73, 1969.

Dietary iodine and goiter in Ceylon. *27*:108, 1969.

The green revolution. *27*:133, 1969.

Malnutrition and mental behavior (by Monckeberg, F.). *27*:191, 1969.

Nutritional status — U.S.A. *27*:196, 1969.

A report on the White House conference on food, nutrition and health, December 2–4, 1969 (by Mayer, J.). *27*:247, 1969.

Nutritional status — Japan (by Innami, S., and Mickelsen, O.). *27*:275, 1969.

Environment and growth. *27*:282, 1969.

Food technology and society (by Pyke, M.). *28*:31, 1970.

Agricultural planning and nutrient availability. *28*:143, 1970.

Priority of nutrition in national development (by Berg, A.). *28*:199, 1970.

Mothercraft centers (by King, K.). *28*:307, 1970.

Nutrition in the 1970's (by Darby, W. J.). *30*:27, 1972.

Nutrition perspectives in the seventies (by Pearson, P. B.). *30*:31, 1972.

two

Energy Needs

The necessity for foods to supply energy in sufficient amounts to perform the work of the living organism is easily recognized, for without sufficient energy-bearing foods a person burns up his own tissues and grows thin. The nutrients that provide energy—fat, carbohydrate, and protein—together with water account for almost all the weight of the daily diet.

Energy is defined as the *power to do work.* The body needs energy because it has certain indispensable work to perform. Internal work is carried out to maintain life processes, even during sleep, in the uncounted numbers of chemical and physical activities of the cells and organs. Muscular work is required to sit and stand erect and to move the body or objects. Energy is also needed to form new tissues during growth and pregnancy or after an injury, to produce milk, and sometimes for heating the body.

ENERGY FOR WORK FROM BURNING BODY FUELS

The body gets energy for its internal and external work in a manner superficially similar to that in which an internal combustion engine sets free energy from fuel. In an automobile engine, gasoline vapor is mixed with air, ignited by a spark, and burned (oxidized) with a resultant release of energy in the form of work and heat. In the body, the three chief energy nutrients (carbohydrates, fats, and proteins) are oxidized in the cells, by means of oxygen brought to the tissues by the blood, and energy is liberated as heat and work. The energy set free as a result of oxidation was stored up in the fuel in both cases in the form of chemical energy. During the process of combustion, carbon and hydrogen in the fuel or energy nutrient are oxidized to carbon dioxide and water, products that contain less chemical energy than the substances which gave rise to them.* Since no energy is ever created or lost, the extra energy appears as heat and work.

---

*Every substance carries a definite amount of chemical energy in each atom or molecule; in fact, this is what characterizes the substance and makes it what it is. Because no two substances have the same amount of chemical energy, every chemical change involves an energy change. Some chemical changes set energy free, while others (those in which the products hold more energy than the original substances) require extra energy to make them take place.

23

The body is like a combustion engine in these respects:

1. Energy for work is released by *oxidation* or burning of fuel.
2. *Heat* is a *by-product* of the transformations by which energy is released.
3. Both conform to the *law of the conservation of energy*.

Fuel is oxidized in the machine and, to some extent, in the body for the purpose of setting free *mechanical energy* to be utilized in doing work. However, in both cases, more of the energy set free is in the form of *heat* than of mechanical energy. The relative proportion of fuel energy that is converted into mechanical energy is called the *mechanical efficiency* of an engine. A steam locomotive can convert only about 10 percent of its fuel energy into mechanical pull on a train of cars, whereas the mechanical efficiency of a good gasoline engine is 20 percent and that of a Diesel engine is nearly 40 percent. The average mechanical efficiency of the body may be said to be about 20 percent, approximately that of a good automobile engine. This means that to do a given amount of work about five times as much body fuel must be oxidized as would be represented by the work alone, since only about one-fifth of the energy of the fuel is transformed into work energy while about four-fifths of it appears as heat. It is no wonder that we experience the feeling of heat while doing strenuous work and that even the internal work of the body generates enough heat so that temperature regulation of the body is called into play.

The law of the conservation of energy holds true for the human body. This means that all energy used in the body must come from the burning of energy-yielding foods or of body tissues, and that all energy supplied in food is sooner or later recovered in some form. If a person eats an insufficient amount of food to cover the cost of energy expended, he is forced to burn up some of his body tissues and loses weight, because the body cannot create energy out of nothing. On the other hand, if his intake of food is in excess of his energy needs, the extra energy is stored in the form of tissues (usually fat) and he gains weight.

The analogy between the body and the combustion engine does have its limitations. In a number of respects the living organism differs radically from the nonvital machine, and in practically all instances these differences represent advantages to the body in adjusting to its environment and varied needs. In the body, the three kinds of energy nutrients can be used (within limits) interchangeably as fuel, whereas the gasoline engine can use only one kind of fuel. In the body, oxidation is a controlled process during which energy is released slowly in a number of steps rather than in a single instantaneous combustion. (These complex processes are described in Chapter 14.)

The internal work of the body never stops. The body needs materials and energy for repairing wear and tear on its tissues, and for the continuous upkeep of the other vital internal activities for which there is no counterpart in the machine. But we all know that the

---

Energy Transformations in Oxidation of Fuel

Chemical   =   Chemical   + Mechanical   + Thermal

Food
   or   + Oxygen   =   End-products   + Work   + Heat
Fuel

life processes do not stop, nor does one even need to discontinue external work, if he stops eating for a few days. Fortunately, we possess a safety device which renders it almost impossible for the body to run out of fuel. Whenever there is a greater amount of energy in the food intake than is required to supply the current needs of the body, most of this excess energy is saved and stored up in the tissues.

The form in which extra fuel is usually stored in animals is in fatty tissue, and the body can work over an excess of carbohydrates, fats, and proteins in the diet and build them into fats for storage. The body can store only a very limited amount of carbohydrate as animal starch, or glycogen, in the liver and muscles. This it uses as a short-term supply to maintain the sugar level of the blood and to support other cellular processes, rather like "cash in the pocket." Fat in the tissues is also drawn on for muscular work, and excess fat in adipose tissue acts as the body's "savings account" to be drawn on when less energy is taken in the diet than is used by the body.

Although the body possesses little ability to store extra protein, the muscle and glandular tissues are rich in protein, some of which can be used for fuel if necessary. As they form part of the most vital structures of the body, protein tissues are not drawn on for energy until the carbohydrate store is exhausted. With continued lack of food the body burns up its *reserve* fuel in the following order: first the limited amount of carbohydrate stored (glycogen), then the fatty tissues and some protein. Thus, under ordinary conditions of living, we have a wide margin of safety as to fuel stored in the body.

ENERGY MEASUREMENT

Naturally, one is interested to know how much energy he needs for the internal and external work of his body. This has been measured by methods

called direct and indirect calorimetry. *Direct calorimetry* measures the amount of heat given off as a by-product of energy metabolism. This method was elucidated in 1761 by the Scottish physician Joseph Black, who measured the heat resulting from chemical combustion by melting ice under controlled conditions. During the period 1782 to 1784, the French scientists Lavoisier and Laplace used this principle to demonstrate that animal metabolism is a kind of combustion in which heat is given off, oxygen is used, and carbon dioxide is produced. With much further refinement, the exact relationships of oxygen usage and heat production were quantified, enabling measurement of energy metabolism indirectly from oxygen utilization, that is, by *indirect calorimetry*.

Proof of these relationships in man was quite a feat. Such experiments had actually been undertaken by Lavoisier (c. 1784), but his research was literally cut short when he was sent to the guillotine by the French Revolutionary tribunal. More than a century passed before Atwater, Benedict, and Rosa constructed the first human respiration calorimeter at Wesleyan University in Connecticut (between 1897 and 1905). Several more of these costly instruments were built later in Washington, New York, and Boston. This device, a few of which are still in use, is called a respiration calorimeter because in it can be measured not only the respiratory exchange (amounts of oxygen used and carbon dioxide produced) but also the amount of heat given off by the human subject. The calorimeter portion of the apparatus consists primarily of a copper box large enough to hold a man comfortably, encased and insulated to prevent any loss of heat through the walls. The heat generated by the subject is carried away by water circulating through a coil of pipe near the roof of the chamber, so that the inner temperature is maintained constant. The heat that is transferred to the water and the heat required to vaporize water in the subject's breath (and perspiration) together represent the total heat production of his body in a given time *(direct calorimetry).*

At the same time, by devices included in the closed circuit of air which the subject breathes, the quantity of oxygen consumed and carbon dioxide given out are measured. From these values, the amount of energy that would have been set free by oxidations within the body can be calculated *(indirect calorimetry).* By many very careful determinations in the respiration calorimeter, it has been established that values obtained by the two methods differ by only a fraction of 1 percent.

We now find it practicable to measure metabolism by means of a relatively simple apparatus that determines only the respiratory exchange. The use of a portable, easily operated respiration apparatus has made it possible to measure the metabolism of patients in bed, of students in the classroom, and of people in many parts of the world. Early apparatus used to measure resting metabolism (Fig. 2–1) recorded the amount of oxygen consumed by the person when rebreathing in a closed circuit of oxygen-rich air for 6 to 10 minutes, then calculating the heat that would have been produced by this amount of oxidation in the body under the standardized conditions of the test. Energy cost of work is now commonly measured by any of several devices (Figs. 2–2, 2–3, and 2–4) that collect part or all of the air exhaled by a subject during a given time period. By determining the amount of oxygen and carbon dioxide present in the exhaled air and in the atmosphere, the amount of oxygen used and carbon dioxide produced can be computed and, from these values, the amount of energy expended and the nature of the fuels burned. (The significance of the ratio of oxygen used to carbon dioxide produced, the respiratory quotient, will be discussed in Chapter 21.)

Energy metabolism and requirements are customarily expressed in terms of

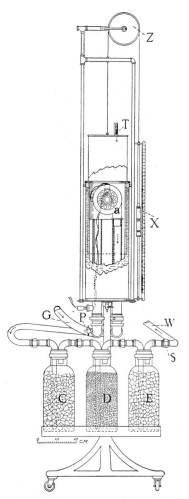

Figure 2–1. Spirometer and absorbing system of portable respiration apparatus developed by F. G. Benedict. G, Large caliber pipe conducting expired air to spirometer; a, air impeller; C, first water absorber; D, carbon dioxide absorber; E, second water absorber; S, point at which rate of ventilation may be tested by disconnecting coupling; W, pipe conducting purified air to subject; P, petcock for introducing oxygen; T, thermometer for obtaining records of temperature of spirometer. The spirometer bell is counterpoised by the weight, X, attached to silk thread passing over aluminum wheel, Z. Scale on which pointer indicates height of spirometer bell is shown at right of X. (Reprinted from the Boston Medical and Surgical Journal, 1918.)

calories, a heat unit. One calorie is the amount of energy (heat) required to raise the temperature of one gram of water one degree centigrade, and is

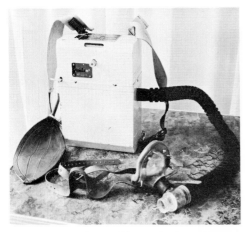

Figure 2–2. A portable respiration apparatus (Kofranyi-Michaelis apparatus) for measuring energy expended in various physical activities. It consists of a lightweight box, which contains a meter that records the volume of expired air. Samples of the expired air are automatically taken at intervals and stored in a small bag attached to the meter. Analysis of the gas in this bag for carbon dioxide and oxygen content gives the necessary data for calculating energy expenditure.

equivalent to 4.184 Joules. (Joule is the energy unit accepted by all scientists. One Joule, a work unit, is 10^7 ergs.) Adoption of the calorie by nutritionists followed quite naturally from the original methods of measuring energy metabolism. However, the magnitude of human energy metabolism made it awkward to record the calories measured, so the convention of the large Calorie was accepted. The nutritionists' Calorie is 1000 calories and is abbreviated Cal or, more properly, kcal to indicate that it is 1000 times (k) as large. Total energy needs vary widely, but for adults 1800 to 3600 kcal (7500 to 15,000 kJoule or kJ) per day would be typical.

BASAL METABOLISM

The word *metabolism* is a general term used to cover all the chemical changes that go on in the tissues of the body. Under energy metabolism we include the chemical changes by which

fat, carbohydrate, and protein (and alcohol) are broken down and gradually oxidized to release energy or by which they may be synthesized into compounds in which unneeded energy may be stored. Technically we also include the physical changes by which energy is transformed from one kind to another in the body—for example, chemical energy in food and oxygen is set free as work and heat when food is oxidized in the body. Since metabolism includes only chemical changes in tissue cells, it does not include those that occur in digestion of foods.

In a living organism, cells have to be continually active to maintain the life processes, and energy is necessary to maintain these vital processes of the various organs and tissues. The nervous system never stops working, and the activity of the brain alone accounts for about one-fifth of the energy expended by the body at rest. The liver and kidneys constantly work at a high rate; other activities go on at a somewhat lower rate during rest—for example, the beating of the heart, the work of the lungs and of the chest and diaphragm in breathing, the peristaltic movements of the stomach and intestines, and the work of digestive glands in forming their secretions. Even when

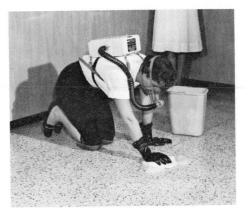

Figure 2–3. Respirometer shown in Figure 2–2, held in position by belt so that arms are free for scrubbing floor, while measurement of energy expended in task is made. (Courtesy of Ohio State University.)

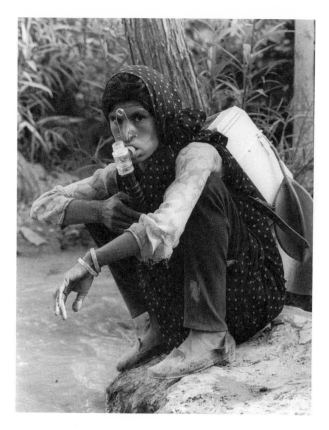

Figure 2–4. Respiratory gases are being collected in a field study of the energy cost of village work in Iran. (Courtesy of C. G. Brun and T. Brun, Department of Nutritional Sciences, University of California, Berkeley.)

a person is apparently completely in repose, the tone of the skeletal muscles is maintained.

This internal work of the body is known as *basal metabolism* because upon it are superimposed the other energy needs of the body—the extra amount of energy needed because of intake of food and muscular work, and at times for adjustment to climate and for the formation of new tissues. Basal metabolism represents the amount of energy required to maintain life at rest—that is, for the internal work of the body. It is defined as the amount of energy expended by the body when lying quietly in a comfortable environmental temperature, relaxed but awake and without food (12 to 15 hours after the last meal). Energy expenditure measured under the same conditions but at different intervals after eating is called resting metabolism. Basal metabolism

of adults amounts to about 1200 to 1800 kcal (5000 to 7500 kJ) per day. The basal energy needs are comparatively *constant* in amount for the same individual, but vary slightly at different times and perhaps more widely in different persons.

Factors That Influence Basal Metabolism

The *main* factors that determine the basal metabolic energy requirement are:

1. Body size.
2. Age.
3. Sex.
4. Secretions of endocrine glands.

Total basal metabolic expenditure varies as a function of body size, but not precisely with weight. When expressed as calories per unit of metabolic body size (square meter body surface area* or the three-fourths power of body weight), *basal metabolic rate* of persons of the same sex and age is found to be remarkably uniform, irrespective of wide differences in body build and body composition. In fact, basal metabolism of warm-blooded animals ranging in size from mice to elephants is said to be nearly the same when referred to surface area or to the three-fourths power of body weight. The basal metabolic rate is higher in young people than in older individuals; it increases for some months after birth, then decreases (at first fairly rapidly, but later more gradually) up to and through adolescence. In adults, there is a still slower decline in basal metabolic rate with increasing age. Metabolic rate is also higher in males than in females (Fig. 2–5).

Why these relationships exist is not certain. The close correlation between internal work and surface area, or the three-fourths power of body weight, is explained by some as due to a mathematical relationship these measurements may have to the active cellular mass of the body. Basal metabolism reflects the activity of all body functions carried on in the resting state (including maintenance of body temperature), and these functions reside in the soft, lean tissues.

Attempts have been made to relate basal energy output directly to the amount of lean body mass. (Cell mass can only be measured by indirect methods, of course, so absolute correspondence cannot be proved.) This concept has a certain plausibility when one considers that men have more lean body mass in proportion to fat than do women of the same age, and men have higher basal metabolic rate (BMR) than do women. Also the percentage of body fat rises with age in both sexes, and metabolic rate declines with age. However, other facts do not fit the theory so neatly. Adipose tissue is an active tissue, having about the same rate of oxidation per unit of protein as does kidney tissue, one of the more active tissues of the body. (Of course, adipose tissue, when filled with fat, has only one-third to one-fourth as much protein as does kidney tissue.) *Total* basal energy expenditure does increase with increasing lean body mass, but the increase is not linear, because the body tissues do not increase in size proportionately. (See Table 2–1.) In the adult, skeletal muscle is the largest component of the non-bone lean mass and muscle has a relatively low resting rate of metabolism; the brain, a very active tissue, increases little in weight from infancy to adulthood. Other tissues, such as the liver and kidneys, increase less in size than does the muscle mass during the growth years and comprise about the same percentage of body weight in muscularly well developed adults as in those who are less fit. For purposes of nutritional planning it is sufficient to remember that the total basal energy requirement is greater in persons of larger size than in smaller persons of the same age and sex; and that the *rate* of basal metabolism is higher in men than in women and decreases with age. Basal metabolism of healthy men requires about 1600 to 1800 kcal (6500 to 7500 kJ) daily; basal expenditure of women is about 1200 to 1450 kcal (5000 to 6000 kJ).

The secretions of the endocrine glands are the primary regulators of the rate of metabolism of the cells.[†]

---

*Because of the difficulty of actually measuring the body surface area, it is usually computed from the body weight and height by means of a mathematical equation;[1] or from a nomogram constructed from DuBois' chart by Boothby and Sandiford[2] (Fig. 2–5); or the metabolic size may be computed from body weight alone according to formulas of Brody[3] or Kleiber.[4]

[†]The endocrine glands manufacture substances (called hormones) that are absorbed directly into the blood stream and carried to all parts of the body. These glands are more fully discussed in Chapter 15.

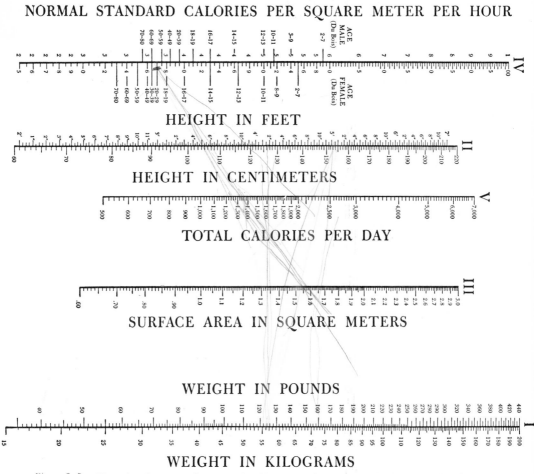

Figure 2–5. Place the chart on a flat, smooth table. Use only a ruler with a true straight edge. Do not draw lines on the chart but merely indicate their positions by the straight edge of the ruler. Locate the various points by means of needles (pin stuck through the eraser of a lead pencil). Locate the patient's normal weight on Scale I and his height on Scale II. The ruler joining these two points intersects Scale III at the patient's surface area. Locate the age and sex of the patient on Scale IV. A ruler joining this point with the patient's surface area on Scale III crosses Scale V at the *basal* energy requirement. To convert Calories (kcal) to kJ, multiply by 4.184. (Nomogram of Boothby and Sandiford,[2] adapted by the Mayo Clinic and reprinted with their permission.)

The overall rate of cellular oxidation is under the control of the **thyroid** gland. Thyroxine, the iodine-containing hormone secreted by the thyroid, has a very potent influence in speeding up all the oxidative processes of the body. When the thyroid gland is overactive, it forms too much of this substance and basal metabolism becomes much more rapid than normal. In abnormal conditions, when the thyroid gland is underactive, the amount of thyroxine formed is too small to keep the basal metabolic rate up to what it should be. Thyroxine is so potent that 1 milligram of it is sufficient to increase the energy metabolism 2 to 3 percent. It is remarkable that the amount of

Table 2–1. *Percentage of Basal Metabolic Rate (BMR) Due to Five Major Organs and the Rest of the Body in an Infant Whose BMR is 540 kcal per Day and an Adult Whose BMR is 1780 kcal per Day**

| | 10 kg (22 lb) Infant | | | 70 kg (154 lb) man | | |
| | *Organ Weight* | *Organ Metabolism* | | *Organ Weight* | *Organ Metabolism* | |
Organ	(KG)	KCAL/DAY	% OF BMR	(KG)	KCAL/DAY	% OF BMR
Brain	0.92	240	45	1.4	365	21
Heart	0.05	30	6	0.3	180	10
Kidney	0.07	28	5	0.3	120	7
Liver	0.30	105	19	1.6	560	32
Lung	0.12	24	4	0.8	160	9
Total of above	1.46	427	79	4.4	1385	79
All other	8.64	113	21	65.6	395	21

*In the infant the organs comprise 15 percent of body weight and account for 79 percent of BMR. These organs still account for 79 percent of BMR in an adult of normal weight and leanness but make up only 6 percent of body weight. Thus, BMR does not increase linearly with lean body mass or with total body weight. (Adapted from Holliday et al.[5])

this potent substance secreted by the thyroid gland is regulated to such a nicety that the basal metabolism (energy output for internal processes) is kept at a constant and normal rate.

Because the iodine-containing secretion of the thyroid gland (the hormone *thyroxine*) constitutes the most important single factor influencing the rate of tissue oxidation, or basal metabolism, determination of the *level of thyroid hormone* in the blood stream has been used to detect the *relative rate of basal metabolism.* Thyroxine (tetraiodothyronine) is circulated in the blood in temporary union with blood proteins so that what the chemical test measures is the *protein-bound iodine content of the blood*, which in turn serves as an index of relative activity of the thyroid in releasing its hormone into the blood—hence, the approximate basal metabolic rate. Because this test (PBI, for "protein-bound iodine") is much simpler for both patient and technician, and because many doctors feel it is more dependable, for clinical purposes, it has largely replaced the measurement of oxygen consumption by respiration apparatus. However, some clinics run both types of tests to compare results of the two methods, and the respiratory method is still used in scientific experiments.

The internal secretion produced by the **adrenals,** two small glands situated just above the kidneys, also exerts an influence on basal metabolism, although not so markedly as does the thyroid secretion. Stimulation of the adrenal glands (such as happens in fright, excitement, and other emotions) causes a temporary rise in the metabolic rate, while it has been shown that cats have a fall of about 25 percent in basal metabolism after an operation to remove these glands. The **pituitary** gland also has an indirect influence on metabolism. (See Chapter 15.)

The sex difference in metabolism is brought about by the activity of the male and female hormones. The difference is primarily due to the effect these hormones have on body composition, since women have more fatty tissues than do men.

Supplementary Factors Affecting Basal Metabolism

Several factors may affect the accuracy of determination of basal metabolic rate, which is why the standardized conditions of measurement include the stipulation that the subject must be awake, but physically and mentally relaxed, in a postabsorptive state (12 to 15 hours after eating), in a comfortable environment, and free from fever.

SLEEP. Individual sleep patterns vary; some rest quietly for about an hour and are restless for the remainder of the night, while others rest completely all night. It is not surprising, then, that energy expenditures during a period of sleep may be about the same as in the basal (resting quietly but awake) state, or more or less than that. During the hours of sleep, the internal processes gradually slow down, reaching a minimum that is 10 percent below basal rate after about 5 to 6 hours.

MUSCLE TONUS. Most people do not realize that the muscles are *never completely relaxed,* for maintenance of a certain amount of tension (muscular tone or tonus) is necessary even in sleep. The amount of energy required for muscular tension varies considerably with the degree of tenseness or relaxation of the individual, but this amount of energy is of significance because the total amount of muscle tissue is so great. The greatest degree of relaxation will be found on first waking and muscular tension will increase as the day advances. For this reason, it is best to make tests for determining basal metabolism early in the morning.

EMOTIONS AND MENTAL STATES. Emotions and mental states act on basal metabolism through their effect on the endocrine glands and on muscular tension. It has been mentioned previously that stimulation of the adrenal glands, such as takes place under emotional stress, results in an increased rate of body processes. One marked effect of mental strain seems to be in increasing muscular tonus, and the tenseness of the muscles during suspense, anxiety, or excitement, or even during mental work is a familiar phenomenon. In measuring metabolism, relaxation is aided by reassurance that the test will not cause discomfort. Even so, a second test will often give lower figures than the first (and therefore more truly represent "basal" metabolism).

EXERCISE. Of course when we are talking of *basal* metabolism, or the energy required for internal processes only, exercise is ruled out, since basal metabolism always means metabolism at rest. However, the after effects of severe muscular work persist for a long while after the work has ceased, and the metabolic rate during the night that follows a day in which much exercise was taken is higher than after an inactive day. The oxidative recovery processes keep going on in the body for hours after severe muscular effort and for shorter periods after less strenuous work.

FOOD. The immediate influence of food is ruled out in measuring basal metabolism, which is always taken 12 to 15 hours after a meal, but the after-effects of food sometimes linger on into the resting period, as is the case with exercise. The products of the digestion of protein seem to stimulate metabolism, so that following a day when a great deal of protein has been eaten the basal metabolism is usually somewhat higher than it is after a day when the diet had been mainly carbohydrates and fats.

FASTING. In *prolonged* fasting or semistarvation the body seems able to adjust to a slightly lower level of metabolism, thus conserving its energy when a very limited supply of fuel is available. The internal processes are somewhat slowed down, and the basal energy requirement is lower after a long fast or in an adult whose food supply has been insufficient for his needs for some time. This adjustment of the body to run with greater economy of energy does not occur in a short period of food deprivation.

During World War I, a group of 12 young male students volunteered for a prolonged period of underfeeding as to calories. Benedict found that, when they had sustained an average weight loss of 12 percent, there was an average lowering of basal metabolism per unit of body weight by 18 to 20 percent.[6] Similar experiments in undernutrition, made at the time of World War II to simulate conditions in occupied countries, showed an average 18 percent reduction in the metabolic rate (together with a lowered expenditure of energy for exercise) on a daily energy intake of 1500 kcal.[7] In undernourished children, however, there is sometimes normal basal metabolism per unit of weight and an increased rate during recovery.

FEVER. In fevers, or when heat loss from the surface of the body is prevented, the temperature of the body itself will rise. Because the rate or intensity of the internal processes is speeded up, there is a rise in temperature, and the basal metabolism will be increased in this event. It has been calculated that the increase in energy expenditure is about 7 percent for every degree Fahrenheit rise in body temperature[1]—that is, a fever of 4° F (39° C, 102.6° F) would call for 490 kcal added to the basal metabolism of an average-sized man.

MUSCULAR WORK

No person could live for long on the basal level of energy requirement. The ordinary activities of life necessitate moving about, which involves muscular work. Even holding the body in sitting or standing posture requires some muscular work, as do the minor movements that all of us are constantly making even when sitting at rest or during sleep. Some persons take active exercise or must do muscular work in earning their living. What is more, everyone must eat, and the taking of food in itself raises the energy output.

Muscular work is *by far the most important* of those factors which raise the energy requirement of adults above the "basal" amount needed at rest. Whenever muscular work is done, energy is used, and the amount required is proportional to the work done. Smaller quantities of energy are needed for maintaining the body in sitting or standing position, while active work, such as walking, climbing stairs, and pushing

or lifting objects, requires a great deal larger energy expenditure. The heavier the person moving about or the greater number or size of muscles involved, the larger the amount of energy that is required. Thus walking, even at moderate pace, requires more energy than typing rapidly.

If the energy metabolism of a man sitting still is estimated at 85 to 100 kcal per hour, the metabolism of the same man *when working* may range from 150 to 600 kcal per hour, according to the amount and kind of work done. To get an idea of how much larger the increase in energy need resulting from external work is than that resulting from any other factor, there is a 100 to 500 percent increase in metabolism from active work, or two to five times the basal energy expenditure.

Of course such an active energy output cannot be kept up for very long at a time, so that the total increase in energy requirement for the day (working eight hours) may not be more than 50 to 100 percent over the maintenance requirement even for active workers. In an inactive (sedentary) man or woman the distribution of the energy used during the day is usually about two-thirds for the internal work of the body and one-third for visible muscular movements. For example, a small woman might spend a total of 1800 kcal (7500 kJ) with 1200 kcal due to basal metabolism and only 600 kcal above that for body movement. As soon as more exercise is taken, however, the energy required for external work mounts rapidly, while that needed for body processes continues as before. (Fig. 2–6). Thus the proportion of the energy used for visible work may come to be as much as a half to three-fourths of the whole, and the total amount of energy needed will be increased until it may be more than doubled. A young college man during football training might have a basal metabolic rate of 1800 kcal per day but use a total of 4000 kcal (17,000 kJ) or more per day due to his vigorous activity, for instance.

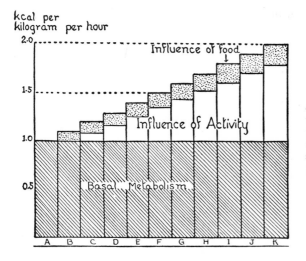

Figure 2-6. Theoretical distribution of energy expenditure and its increase with varying degrees of muscular activity, which ranges from lying still (with food, *B*) through sitting at ease (*E*) and standing relaxed (*F*) to walking at 1 mile per hour on level (*K*).

It is difficult to generalize concerning energy needs at various occupations or trades, since not only do the workers vary in body weight and rate of working, but under modern conditions jobs in the same industry often involve widely different amounts of physical exertion. In an automobile factory, a 68 kg (150 lb) man who sits and operates a machine (which does the real work) may require no more than 2500 kcal per day while an 80 kg (175 lb) man whose job calls for much walking and some lifting obviously uses much more energy—3700 kcal or even more. Both men belong to the same union and are classed as factory or industrial workers. Furthermore, the way one employs his leisure time affects his total energy need. A sedentary worker, such as an office clerk, by working "out-of-hours" at home (carpentry, painting, gardening, or going in for some active sport) may raise his energy requirement to that of a man whose working day involves more physical exertion.

EFFECTS OF FOOD

DuBois[1] compared the effect of food on metabolism to a tax, deducted at the source, which thus reduces the amount of a man's income; we do not derive the full fuel value of the foods taken in because a small portion of this fuel goes to cover the energy "cost" of their metabolism. This energy deduction in metabolizing fuel foods is due to the costs of digestion and absorption and to the fact that the products of its digestion, after they are absorbed, stimulate metabolism in the tissues. In the case of the digestion products of the fats, energy metabolism seems to be increased mainly because a larger amount of oxidizable material is brought to the tissues by the blood. Carbohydrates seem to act in a different way—that is, heat is produced by the chemical reactions required for their metabolism in the tissues. Proteins may act in a similar manner, although it is thought by some that the heat by-product of metabolism of amino acids is related to rearrangement of amino acids and to the splitting off of nitrogen as ammonia and formation of urea as the end product of nitrogen metabolism. The stimulating effect of the fuel nutrients on energy production (different for each of the three classes) is called their *specific dynamic action*, which for convenience is often referred to as SDA.[9, 10]

The rise in metabolism after eating carbohydrate food is only 6 percent of the total fuel value of the food eaten (i.e., energy expenditure increases by 6 kcal for each 100 kcal of carbohydrate consumed), and the increase caused by fat is not very different in magnitude. The rise in metabolism after taking 100 calories of protein is much greater, however, amounting to about 30 percent. If the diet contains a great deal of meat, the day's increase in metabolism may amount to 18 percent, or even more. However, on the ordinary mixed diet, the usual allowance to cover the stimulating effects of the food itself is about 10 percent of the total intake. Thus, in order to have his energy intake equal to output so that weight is maintained, a boy whose energy needs for internal work plus muscular work amount to 2200 kcal would probably require about 220 extra kcal to cover the effects of the food.

Although any major influence of specific dynamic action of food is ruled out in measuring basal metabolism, it should be remembered that measurements of the energy cost of physical activities are made in individuals who have eaten normal mixed meals and hence reflect the sum of all processes going on at the same time — work, basal metabolism, and specific dynamic action. As we have pointed out in our preceding discussion, "basal metabolism" is arbitrarily defined as energy expended under precise conditions of measurement, conditions that exist only briefly and infrequently. Sleep states are not uniform, there are variable effects from preceding exercise, and many people eat small meals or snacks at irregular times. For these reasons, it is customary to estimate energy requirement from oxygen utilization of persons resting quietly at various times of the day and carrying out representative or actual work tasks. Using those values, there need be no extra allowance for SDA of healthy people eating mixed diets.

CLIMATE AND HEAT REGULATION

Cold-blooded animals such as fish and frogs have no ability to regulate their body temperature, which accordingly rises and falls as the temperature of their environment changes. Man (and the other warm-blooded animals) possesses a heat-regulating apparatus which keeps the body temperature almost constant at a point which is usually considerably higher than that of his surroundings (37° C, 98.6° F). Small variations of body temperature are normal; the normal range in health is about 2° F, but variations ordinarily do not exceed 1° F.

Temperature regulation is ordinarily accomplished in the body without effect on the basal metabolism or total energy needs. Excessive heat loss in a cool environment is prevented by insulation (clothing, shelter) and the heat produced as a by-product of body processes and muscular work is more than sufficient under these circumstances. *Heat regulation thus is usually a problem of getting rid of the surplus heat produced.* About 80 percent of this excess heat is dissipated by loss at the body surface, or through the skin. Some is lost through the lungs by evaporation of moisture in the expired air, and a small amount is lost in the excreta (for diagram indicating the various ways of effecting heat balance see Fig. 2–7).

Heat is lost from the skin by (1) *radiation* or *conduction* and (2) by *evaporation* of moisture (invisible or visible perspiration). The relative ease with which heat can be got rid of from the skin by one or the other of these two paths depends on the surrounding conditions. Low temperature of the air favors heat loss by radiation and conduction, whereas high temperature of the air cuts down heat loss by this means and favors loss by evaporation. Low humidity aids evaporation and high humidity reduces the opportunity for loss of heat through this channel. Wind or circulating currents of air favor heat loss by both con-

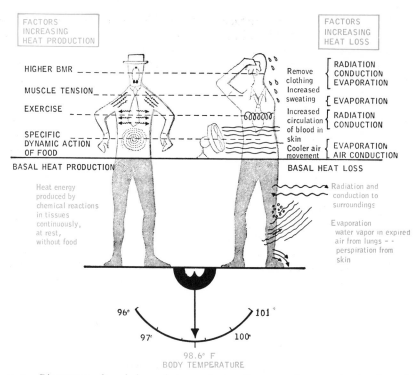

Figure 2-7. Diagram to show balance between factors that cause heat production in and heat loss from the body, thus effecting normal regulation of body temperature.

duction and evaporation. A further aid in temperature regulation is the variable amount of blood sent to the surface under different conditions of heat and cold; the skin becomes flushed on a hot day and blanched or bluish on exposure to cold.

Under only two conditions do changes in the temperature of the environment have any effect on metabolism. First, if the body surface is insufficiently protected from heat loss and the temperature of the air is sufficiently low, extra fuel must be burned to keep body temperature up to normal. In such a case, there is likely to be shivering (involuntary muscular activity) and increased oxidative processes in the tissues (chemical heat regulation) to generate the extra heat needed, so that the rate of metabolism increases. Conversely, under conditions of extreme heat, some energy is required for body cooling owing to increased work of the heart and circulatory system and the secretion of sweat.

The main factors which affect the rate at which heat is lost from the body surface are the amount of body surface; the presence or absence of a layer of fat under the skin; and insulation provided from clothing and shelter.

BODY SURFACE. A child has a larger amount of body surface in relation to its total size than an adult has, the tiny infant having the largest relative amount of surface for its size. *Shape* of the body also influences the amount of surface. A tall, thin person possesses about 1½ times as much surface area as a short, fat person of the same body weight. Since heat loss is through the surface, the body with a large amount of surface must generate more heat to maintain its normal temperature under conditions of cold than one with a relatively smaller surface exposure. Surface area is a less important factor in adults than in infants and children, in whom there is a larger proportion of surface to volume.

SUBCUTANEOUS FAT. A layer of fatty tissue, directly under the skin, is normally present in well-nourished individuals. The extent and thickness of this layer of subcutaneous fat vary considerably in different individuals, according to sex, general build, and dietary habits. Fat is a very poor conductor of heat, or a good insulator, so that persons with a well developed layer of fat under the skin lose heat to the exterior much less readily than do those who have little subcutaneous fat. Thin people radiate about 50 percent more heat per pound than fat people. This may be an advantage in winter but may not be in hot weather when, because the heat is held within by this layer of insulation, fat people are likely to experience discomfort, especially if they generate any extra heat within their bodies by exercise.

CLOTHING. In summer, we leave some of the body freely exposed and wear loose clothing of porous weave and light color which allows heat to escape readily. In cold weather we resort to covering the body with several layers of clothing usually of thicker, less porous material and dark in color, and we use blankets at night. Winter clothing usually helps considerably in conserving body heat. Exposure to cold water also involves great heat loss, and even the heat generated by vigorous swimming may be insufficient to maintain body temperature, unless additional fuel is burned for warmth. Scuba divers have learned to wear protective suits, and distance swimmers often apply grease to the body as insulation, but prolonged chilling will increase energy needs.

SHELTER. Even primitive housing conditions protect somewhat from extremes of temperature and from exposure to the elements, but civilized man has now equipped his houses with heating devices so that heat can be main-

tained in them throughout the winter season. In fact with modern conditions of heating houses in the United States, the body is very seldom called on to burn any of its fuel for the purpose of maintaining its normal temperature. Air conditioning, which permits homes and public buildings to be kept at constant temperatures both winter and summer, is a further factor in ruling out a direct influence of the seasons on body temperature.

Net Effects of Climate

In cold climates, a small extra energy expenditure (2 to 5 percent) may be incurred by reason of the extra weight and hobbling effect of cold weather clothing. If the body is inadequately clothed, body cooling will occur and energy needs will increase because of shivering.

People who live *and perform necessary physical work* at a temperature range of 30 to 40°C (86 to 104°F) may require an extra calorie allowance to compensate for the energy expenditure at such *high temperatures* (increased metabolic rate, lower mechanical efficiency, and efforts to rid the body of excess heat, such as profuse sweating).[11] Under these conditions, an increase in energy allowances of at least 0.5 percent for every degree of temperature rise between 30° and 40° C is recommended. However, the average individual probably reduces physical activity at high environmental temperatures sufficiently to counterbalance the needs for increased energy just outlined, so that no adjustment in energy allowance is necessary. In fact, total energy expenditure may even be reduced in extremely hot climates.

OTHER FACTORS AFFECTING NEED

Mental Work

Because the brain is always active, *complex mental work does not affect the energy requirement appreciably* except as it may be accompanied by muscular tenseness. Although the metabolism of nervous tissue is increased slightly by activity, the amount of energy required is sufficiently small that the influence of this activity is insignificant. Benedict and Benedict, who found that the effort of complicated mental arithmetic increased metabolism 3 to 4 percent during the short periods it was carried on, compare the relative effects of mental and muscular work as follows: "The professor absorbed in intense mental effort for an hour has an extra demand for food or for calories during the entire hour not greater than the extra need of the maid who dusts off his desk for five minutes."[12]

Growth, Pregnancy, and Lactation

Most adults desire to have the fuel intake just about balance the energy requirement so that the body weight will be maintained constant. With children, on the other hand, it is important to provide energy *over and above* that required for the internal work of the body and for muscular activity, in order that additional material may be available for increasing the body weight in *growth*. Rapidly growing infants have been shown to be storing 12 to 15 percent of the energy value of the food taken. This extra energy is stored in the form of newly built tissues. As growth rate diminishes, although the total food requirement is more because of the increased size, the allowance needed per unit of body weight becomes smaller. Adults recovering from a wasting illness also require extra energy for building new tissue. In pregnancy there is also need for energy to build new tissue (growth of fetus and increased size of uterus, mammary glands, etc.), and in lactation to provide for the energy value of the milk secreted. Information concerning the special energy needs of children and pregnant or nursing women is contained in Chapters 19 and 20.

ESTIMATION OF ENERGY REQUIREMENTS

General: Based on Proportionate Energy Costs at Varying Degrees of Activity

The total allowance for energy requirement must cover amounts needed for internal work (basal metabolism) and external work, and the lesser factors of energy "cost" of the food intake, temperature regulation, growth, and lactation.

Basal metabolism determinations on healthy adults have shown average values with the following ranges:

Men
1600–1800 kcal (6500–7500 kJ)
Women
1200–1450 kcal (5000–6000 kJ)

Resting metabolism of healthy adults throughout the day is about 10 percent above the basal level and ranges from 0.8 to 1.4 kcal per hour per kilogram of body weight (Table 2–2). Depending on body composition, the value for men is about 10 to 20 percent higher than for women. A man of average body build and weight (70 kg or 154 lb) exhibits an approximate resting metabolism of $1.2 \times 24 \times 70$, or 2016 kcal. The resting metabolism of an average woman (128 lb or 58 kg) is about 1320 kcal per day.*

A quick and approximate estimation of one's energy requirement may be made, based on resting metabolism (which is based on body weight) and

---

*These values are only approximations. Technically, there should be a small deduction in the day's basal metabolism to allow for the slightly lower metabolic rate during sleep. However, this correction amounts to only 0.1 kcal/kg/hr, or for 8 hours sleep for a 70 kg man, about 56 kcal. Also, the correction for sleep varies with the soundness of sleep and amount of body movement during sleep. Hence, it is ignored in the rough estimation of energy requirement.

*Table 2–2. Resting Energy Metabolism of Adults
According to Body Weight and Composition**

Men	Women	Body fat, %	50	55	60	65	70	75	80
						Weight in kg†			
						kcal per minute			
Thin		5	0.99	1.06	1.12	1.19	1.26	1.32	1.39
Average		10	0.94	1.01	1.08	1.14	1.21	1.28	1.34
Plump	Thin	15	0.89	0.96	1.03	1.09	1.16	1.23	1.30
Fat	Average	20	0.84	0.91	0.98	1.05	1.11	1.18	1.25
	Plump	25	0.80	0.86	0.93	1.00	1.07	1.13	1.20
	Fat	30	—	0.81	0.88	0.95	1.02	1.08	1.15
						kJ per minute			
Average		10	3.93	4.23	4.52	4.77	5.07	5.36	5.61
	Average	20	3.52	3.81	4.10	4.40	4.65	4.94	5.23

*These values are slightly higher than basal because the subject is not in the strictly postabsorptive condition (12 hours or more from the last meal). (Adapted from Durnin and Passmore.[13])
†To convert to pounds multiply by 2.2.

the degree of physical activity as the two variables. The increase above resting is proportional to the degree of activity as follows: for very light (sedentary) activity, add 30 percent of the resting; for light activity, 50 percent; for moderate activity, 75 percent; for strenuous activity, 100 percent or more. A brief description of what is meant by these varying degrees of activity follows:

Very light:
Sitting most of day, studying, talking; about 2 hours of walking or standing.
Light activity:
Typing, teaching, shop work, laboratory work; some walking.
Moderate activity:
Walking, housework, gardening, carpentry, light industry; little sitting.
Strenuous activity:
Unskilled labor, forestry work, skating, outdoor games, dancing; little sitting.
Very strenuous activity:
Tennis, swimming, basketball, football, running, lumbering; little sitting.

It should be emphasized that the method of estimating energy needs just discussed gives only a rough approximation and that results vary considerably from the average, because the amounts of energy required for differ-

ent occupations included under one level of activity, the vigor with which one works, and the amounts of time devoted to the different activities vary. Because it is not possible to include more than two variables in such a table, the two that have the most influence in determining energy requirement (body weight and level of physical activity) have been used and the relatively minor factor of influence of climate ignored. Moreover, the age group is limited to young adults; if the older age groups were included, the decreasing rate of basal metabolism and vigor of effort due to increasing age would need to be taken into account.

Any young adult may calculate his or her energy requirement by calculating the basal metabolism, then adding the appropriate percent of the basal metabolism for the level of activity selected by the individual as most typical of his or her daily routine.

As an example, we may calculate the daily energy requirement of a young woman, 20 years of age, weight 125 lb, and with light physical activity, based on the method outlined at the beginning of this section (p. 38) and using a factor for physical activity. Her weight in pounds (divided by 2.2) converts to 56.8 kg; her resting metabolism (56.8 ×

0.95 × 24 hr) is 1295 kcal; a 50 percent allowance for light exercise results in 647 kcal; her daily requirement totals:

Resting metabolism	1295 kcal
Energy cost of light exercise	648
Total	1943 kcal (8100 kJ)

Individual: Energy Costs of Activities Estimated

The only way to get a more exact idea of one's individual need for energy is to keep a detailed record of the time spent at different types of activity throughout a representative day and compute the energy used in each activity by means of figures such as are listed in Table 2–3. Values for the energy cost of all kinds of specific tasks (sedentary occupations, walking at different speeds, standing jobs such as ironing or dishwashing, and sports such as tennis or horseback riding) have been determined by numerous research workers.[13, 14] In Table 2–3, these figures are grouped at certain

Table 2–3.   *Gross Energy Costs for Different Activities of Average Young Adults**
(inclusive of basal metabolism and influence of food)

	kcal/min†		kcal/min†
Sleep (basal)	1.0–1.2	Work tasks	
Dressing, washing, etc.	3.0–4.0	Sweeping floors	1.7
Light indoor activities		General laboratory work	2.3
Lying at ease	1.4–1.5	Machine sewing	2.8
Sitting at ease	1.5–1.6	Scrubbing, kneeling	3.4
Standing at ease	1.7–1.9	Garage mechanic	4.1
Sitting, writing	1.9–2.2	Ironing	4.2
Sitting, playing cards, or		Typing, 40 words/minute	
musical instruments‡	2.0–2.6	Manual typewriter	1.5
Transportation		Electric typewriter	1.3
Walking, 140–145 lbs		Gardening, weeding	4.4–5.6
2 mph, level	3.1	digging	8.6
with 22 lb load	3.3	Ploughing with tractor	4.2
2 mph, up 10% incline	5.6	Light industry§	2.2–3.0
with 22 lb load	6.4	Carpentry tasks	2.4–9.1
2 mph up 20% incline	7.9	Coal mining tasks	5.3–8.0
with 22 lb load	9.5	Recreation involving moderate	
Driving a car	2.8	exercise	
Piloting aircraft	1.6	Playing with children	3.5
Canoeing, 2.5 mph	3.0	Dancing, waltz	5.7
4.0 mph	7.0	rhumba	7.0
Horseback riding, walk	3.0	twist	10.0
trot	8.0	Archery	5.2
Cycling, 5.5 mph	4.5	Tennis	7.0
9.4 mph	7.0	Recreation involving hard exercise	
Stair climbing		Swimming, surface	5.0–11.0
Weight, 140 lb	6.2	underwater with fins	
180 lb	8.6	and suits	8.0–18.0
Walking on loose snow,		Football	8.9
level, 2.5 mph, 180 lb		Cross-country running	10.6
man, with 44 lb pack	20.2	Climbing, light load and slope	10.7
		heavy load and slope	13.2
		Skiing, hard snow	
		Level, 3.7 mph	9.9
		Uphill, max. speed	18.6

*Adapted from Passmore, R., and Durnin, J. V. G. A.[13, 14]
†One kcal = 4.184 kJ.
‡Playing piano strenuously or instruments such as woodwinds, stringed instruments, or drums—4.0–4.2.
§Industry such as printing, radio mechanics, shoe repairing.

levels of activity, ranging from sleeping, through sitting tasks, to those that require moderate or more severe physical exertion. As the exertion increases, the energy cost increases gradually from about 1.0 to 1.2 kcal per minute (sleeping) to an average of 9 to 18 kcal per minute for tasks or sports that involve strenuous muscular activity (swimming, rowing, track events, etc).

In calculating the energy cost of the day's activities, the time accounted for must, of course, add up to 24 hours and the total calories for activity must then be multiplied by the time spent at each activity. In some activities body weight is also an important factor and must be considered. For example, a 140 lb man spends 6.2 kcal per minute in stair climbing but a 180 lb man must lift an additional 40 lb and uses 8.6 kcal per minute (Table 2–4).

Two examples of such computation of individual energy requirements are given in Table 2–5. Both are for students — one, a young man most of whose day is spent in sedentary occupations (meals, classes, study, watching movies or television); the other, a young man whose day is spent fairly similarly except that he takes about 1½ hours of moderately strenuous exercise, which markedly increases his energy requirement. Both spend three hours in the

classroom; we have assumed that one man drives in a car between home and campus, both walk some about the campus, and that the second walks to and from home. In spite of similar schedules as students, the energy cost of one's activities is one-fourth greater than the other's — 2710 kcal (11,300 kJ) versus 3400 kcal (14,200 kJ).

The student may also find Table 2–2 of interest for comparison of various activities as to their relative energy costs, some of which are rarely listed in the usual tables of activities. For instance, sitting playing cards and driving a car are about on a par as to energy cost, although there is a difference in energy required for driving a car rapidly on a main throughway or at a moderate speed on a country road or suburban street. Walking on the level (180 lb man at 2 miles per hour) takes about three times more energy than sitting at ease. Modern athletic-type dancing is about on a level with other active sports, such as rapid swimming, football, skiing (on level), or cross-country running. It should be noted that, for some of the activities, there is a wide range in energy costs, depending on the conditions under which they are performed (speed, on level or on incline, etc). Even for sleep there is a 20 percent variation. Often a me-

Table 2–4. *Energy Cost of Walking as Affected by Body Weight and Speed of Movement**

		Body Weight					
Speed/hr		*kg:* 46	55	64	73	82	91
mi	*km*	*lb:* 100	120	140	160	180	200
		kcal per minute†					
2	3.7	2.2	2.6	2.9	3.2	3.5	3.8
3	5.6	3.1	3.6	4.0	4.4	4.8	5.3
4	7.4	4.1	4.7	5.2	5.8	6.4	7.0

*Adapted from Passmore and Durnin.[14] Work is defined as the overcoming of force. In walking, man is using his biological machinery to move his body mass against the force of gravity, and the work done is equal to force × distance. If a mass of 1 gm is accelerated at a speed of 1 cm per second per second, then 1 erg has been expended. One Joule is 10^7 ergs and 1 kcal is 4.184 kJoules. A woman weighing 55 kg and walking over level ground at a rate of 3.7 km per hour actually expends energy at the rate of 2.6 kcal per minute (equal to 10.9 kJoule or 1×10^{11} ergs). However, only part of this cost is reflected in mechanical work because the body operates with only 20 per cent efficiency and internal processes continue during work.

†To convert to kJ, multiply by 4.184.

Table 2–5.   Calculation of Total Energy Requirements of Two
Male Students of 70 Kg Body Weight*

Activity	Approximate Energy Cost kcal/min	Student A — Active		Student B — Sedentary	
		Time	kcal	Time	kcal
Sleep (basal)	1.0–1.2	450 min	490	480 min	530
Dressing, washing, shaving	3.5	15 min	50	20 min	70
Eating breakfast	2.5	20 min	50	30 min	75
Walking to campus	5.0	20 min	100		
Driving to campus	2.8			10 min	30
Sitting in classrooms	1.5	180 min	270	180 min	270
Walking to and from classes, etc.	5.0	40 min	200	40 min	200
Eating lunch	2.5	30 min	75	45 min	115
Studying in library	2.2	180 min	395	180 min	390
Walking between locations	5.0	30 min	150	20 min	100
Playing tennis	7.0	40 min	280		
Playing cards	2.4			50 min	120
Walking home	5.0	20 min	100		
Driving home	2.5			10 min	30
Eating dinner	2.5	40 min	100	45 min	115
Ironing shirt	4.2	15 min	65		
Driving to and from date	2.8	20 min	55		
Dancing, active	10.0	40 min	400		
Eating snack	2.5	30 min	75	30 min	75
Sitting and talking to date	1.5	120 min	180		
Bull session, watching television	1.5			150 min	225
Studying	2.2	120 min	260	120 min	260
Undressing, showering, etc.	3.5	30 min	105	30 min	105
TOTAL			3400		2710

*Factors inclusive of basal metabolism, influence of food, and energy costs of various activities per min, (as given in Table 2–3) were used.

dian value is used, so perfect accuracy cannot be expected.

The rate of energy expenditure is less for women than for men because of the smaller body weight involved. Not only is basal metabolism less at lower body weight, but in all activities that require moving the body about (walking, climbing stairs, active exercise, etc), the expenditure required increases as the body mass to be moved increases in size. This means that, when the rates of energy expenditure for various activities are given as a combined amount (a single factor that includes basal metabolism, influence of food, and cost of the specific activity), this factor should vary slightly according to sex and body weight. However, the differences are small enough that they are either ignored or covered by a range in the activity, as given in the table.

RECOMMENDED ALLOWANCES VERSUS ACTUAL NEEDS

In the United States, recommended dietary allowances have been formulated for some years by a special committee (Food and Nutrition Board) of the National Research Council, and these dietary allowances are revised approximately every five years.[15] They include allowances for most of the essential nutrients (for full table see Appendix, Table 1) for adults, children, and pregnant women. An attempt was made by this committee to base the energy allowances on those for the "reference" man and woman used by the Food and Agricultural Organization of the United Nations (FAO) for international tables,[16] but these proved unrealistic for the American population. The specified height and weight of the reference man and woman are less and the presupposed degree of physical activity is greater than the average in the United States, where the automobile is used so freely and adequate exercise is probably the exception rather than the rule. In the last two revisions of the Food and Nutrition Board's Recommended Allowances, the allowances for energy have accordingly been scaled downward.

From Table 2–6 we see that the Food and Nutrition Board has taken as a reference American man and woman individuals 25 years of age, weighing 70 kg (154 lb) and 58 kg (128 lb) respectively. It is suggested that during the age range of 18 to 25 years the caloric intake should gradually be adjusted downward from the high allowances for growing boys (14 to 18 years, 3000 kcal). The downward adjustments (to cover decreased activity and basal metabolism) with increasing age are suggested to be 5, 8, and 10 percent below that of the reference individual (at 25 years) for each decade between 35 to 55 years, 55 to 75 years, and 75 years and beyond respectively. Discussion of allowances for other age groups than young adults will be found in Chapters 18, 19, and 20.

In Table 2–6 are the daily energy allowances for men and women of various *body weights*, as suggested by the Food and Nutrition Board in the pamphlet accompanying their 1968 recommendations. It should be emphasized that these caloric allowances are based on the assumption that one's weight is desirable (suitable for height) and that the weight attained at 25 years of age should not be allowed to increase in later life. Overweight persons should use the energy allowance given for their proper or ideal weight for height,

rather than for their actual weight (which has obviously been too high).

The energy allowances for different weights (in Table 2–6) are also based on the assumption of an average or standard physical activity in all cases. Because physical activity is the most important single factor in altering energy requirements, adjustments need to be made for those who take more or less exercise than that assumed as standard. For these allowances the Canadian standards[17] are illustrative (Table 2–6). The Canadian levels are stipulated according to body weight and activity and indicate a range from 1900 kcal per day for a sedentary woman to 3000 kcal for a moderately active person. A moderately active woman would do heavy household chores or work as a commercial cook or laundress and have recreational interest in participant sports. Very heavy work at 4100 kcal per day would involve intensive training for marathon races. The FAO requirements[16] are also stipulated according to occupational activity category.

Because of differences in physical activity, there may be wide variations of energy needs within the same age group. For instance, take the example of two men, both 45 years of age and weighing 70 kg; one is a business executive and the other a day laborer. The first may consider himself active, but his activity is more of the mind than of the muscles, so that he may require no more than 2100 to 2200 kcal daily. The man who works 8 hours a day at a job that involves muscular activity probably requires at least 3300 kcal a day, often more.

The FAO[16] in discussing the effects of climate notes that the impact will vary according to occupation and conditions of clothing and shelter. The agricultural worker in the open has some ability to protect himself against cold, if he is not too poor to purchase clothing, but little opportunity to escape heat. The rich businessman may avoid

Table 2–6. *Variation in Energy Allowances for Healthy Adults According to Climate, Weight, and Physical Activity**

Conditions			kcal per day†	
			MEN	WOMEN

International Standards from FAO[16]

	Weight			
Moderately active occupations Mean annual temperature 10° C	55 kg (RF)‡		2530 (10.5 MJ)†	2200‡ (9.4 MJ)†
(50° F)	65 kg (RM)		3000‡ (12.5 MJ)	2600 (11.0 MJ)

United States[15]

	Weight, kg (lb)			
Light activity Comfortable environment (20° C)	50 (110)		2200	1800
	55 (121)		2350	1950
	58 (128) (RF)		–	2000‡
	60 (132)		2500	2050
	65 (143)		2650	2200
	70 (154) (RM)		2800‡	2300
	80 (176)		3050	–
	90 (198)		3350	–

Canada[17]

Allowances for the 25th, 50th and 75th percentile weights of Canadians aged 25–29 years, 1953

Activity	Weight, kg (lb)				
Sedentary	Men	Women	Percentile		
	65 (144)	50 (111)	25	2150	1750
	72 (158)	56 (124)	50	2300	1900
	80 (176)	62 (136)	75	2500	2050
Light activity			25	2650	2200
			50	2850	2400
			75	3100	2550
Moderate activity			25	3400	2800
			50	3650	3000
			75	3950	3250
Heavy manual work or athletic training			50	4250	3550
Very heavy work or sports			50	4900	4100

*U.S. allowances for "light activity" include 8 hours at rest, 8 hours of sitting activities, 5 hours of standing activities, 2 hours of purposeful walking, and 2 hours of intermittent activity of higher energy cost, and apply to the life style of most U.S. citizens. Canadian standards recognize a very wide range of occupations. Note that the U.S. "light activity" level of women has the same calorie allowance as the Canadian category of maintenance of "sedentary" life, but the values for men are in agreement. The FAO standard for moderately active occupations is comparable to "light activity" by Canadian standards.

†To convert to kJoules multiply by 4.184. For convenience, the larger unit megajoule (MJ, 10^3kJ) is used.

‡RF and RM indicate the reference or usual weight of female and male populations.

both. Considering all factors, the FAO concludes that there is no valid basis for adjusting resting and exercise energy requirements according to the climate. If physical activity is restricted by environmental factors, allowances should be selected according to activity level.

It should be evident that the energy allowances set by the Food and Nutrition Board are estimates intended for general use and based on the energy needs of so-called average men and women living and working in a comfortable environment (definite weight and arbitrary degree of muscular activity). For persons who vary much from this norm, the energy requirement really needs to be calculated individually to achieve any degree of accuracy. The recommended allowances for most other nutrients are purposely set higher than the actual needs (about 30 to 50 percent above), but in respect to energy, the intake should be in balance with the output in order to avoid a loss or gain in body weight. Many persons do not reduce their energy intake sufficiently to compensate for the slightly lower basal metabolism and the far greater influence of decreased activity in later life. Even a relatively small excess of energy foods over the amount needed leads to an accretion of weight over a period of years. (See Chapter 23.)

ENERGY VALUE OF FOODS

How Fuel Value of Foods is Determined

The energy value of foods depends primarily upon their chemical composition, i.e., upon the relative amounts of the three primary energy nutrients—carbohydrates, fats, and proteins—and alcohol that they contain. Energy value of a food may be determined by either of the following methods:

1. Complete combustion in a calorimeter.
2. Calculation from its content of the energy nutrients.

The energy value of either a pure nutrient or a natural food may be determined by direct calorimetry, i.e., by complete oxidation in a calorimeter like the one shown in Figure 2–8, in which the calories released are measured by the rise in temperature of a known volume of water.

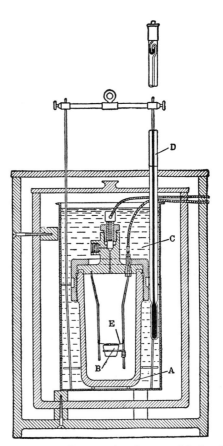

Figure 2–8. Cross-section diagram of the bomb calorimeter used for determination of the fuel value of foods. A weighed sample of the food is placed in the dish *B* in the inner chamber, which is charged with oxygen and sealed tight. The burning is set off by an electric spark (passed between the wires) and the heat liberated is measured by the rise in temperature of a known volume of the surrounding water; the outer sections are for insulation to prevent loss of heat to exterior. (Courtesy of Emerson Apparatus Co., Boston, Mass.)

The average heats of combustion of the *pure energy nutrients*, determined by numerous experiments, are, in kcal per gram: carbohydrate, 4.1; fat, 9.45; protein, 5.65; and alcohol, 7.1. Fats and alcohol have a higher fuel value because their molecules contain such large amounts of carbon and hydrogen, along with relatively little oxygen; much extra oxygen is required for their burning, and much heat is released. Carbohydrates have enough oxygen in their molecules to combine with all of the hydrogen, so only enough oxygen is required for burning to combine with the carbon and less than half as much heat is liberated. Proteins are intermediate between fats and carbohydrates in energy value, when they are completely oxidized in the calorimeter.

The potential energy value of a food may be computed by multiplying the number of grams of each energy nutrient in a given quantity by the caloric values per gram of carbohydrate, fat, protein, and alcohol. But the energy values which the body can derive from these substances are not identical with those obtained when they are completely oxidized in the calorimeter. There is a small loss entailed due to incomplete digestion and absorption from the intestine. A further deduction must be made in the case of proteins, because these substances are not as completely oxidized in the body as in the bomb calorimeter; the nitrogen-containing products excreted in the urine represent latent heat that amounts, on the average, to 1.3 kcal for each gram of protein burned in the body. When the necessary corrections for these factors are made, the *physiological fuel values* per gram for the three fuel nutrients are as follows:

	Bomb calorimeter value, kcal	Physiological energy value	
		kcal	kJ
Carbohydrate	4.1 −2% loss in digestion = 4.02	4.0	17
Fat	9.45 −5% loss in digestion = 8.98	9.0	38
Protein	5.65 −8% loss in digestion = 5.20		
	−17% loss in urinary end products = 4.32	4.0	17
Alcohol	7.1 −small loss in urine and breath = 7.0	7.0	29

Calculating the Energy Value of Foods

The above general factors—4, 9, 4 kcal for protein, fat, and carbohydrate,

respectively—are sufficiently accurate for practical estimates of the fuel value of any food whose composition is known. For example, the fuel value of milk is calculated as follows:

Milk contains 4.9 gm carbohydrate, 3.5 gm protein, and 3.7 gm fat for every 100 gm.

Each gram of carbohydrate and of protein has a value of 4 kcal, and each gram of fat furnishes 9 kcal.

100 gm of whole milk will have a caloric value of

carbohydrate	4.9 × 4 =	19.6
protein	3.5 × 4 =	14.0
fat	3.7 × 9 =	33.3
total		66.9 kcal

A glassful of milk (8 oz) weighs 244 gm, and hence has a caloric value of 66.9 × 2.44, or 163 kcal.

During the time of food shortages in World War II, use of the more specific factors derived from tests of individual foods was proposed for calculating the caloric values of food supplies, chiefly grains, available in different countries.

For the usual mixture of foods in the American diet, differences between the two methods of calculating are not large. Differences are significant in the case of foods which contain considerable undigestible matter, however. Comparison of the values for white and whole-wheat breads obtained by the two sets of factors are given below as an example.

	kcal per 100 gm computed using:	
	General factors	Specific factors
Bread, white, enriched	270	275
Bread, whole wheat	257	240
Beef, pot roast	366	375
Potato, peeled, boiled	69	65

The energy values of foods listed in the most recent tables of food composition issued by the government[18] and in Appendix Table 2 are based on these more specific but more complicated factors.

Foods of High and Low
Energy Value

Foods *vary widely in their energy value.* Some are such concentrated sources of fuel that it takes only a small volume of them to yield a considerable amount of energy, or a large number of calories. Others contain so much of non-energy-producing substances, such as water and fiber, and have so low a content of the energy nutrients that they yield only a small number of calories for a comparatively large volume of food.

In general, the foods with *high energy value* are those that are either *rich in fat* or *low in water* content. Thus, all the fatty foods (such as butter, nuts, cream cheese, mayonnaise, bacon) are relatively high in calorie value, as are foods low in moisture content (dried fruits, cookies, candy bars, and the like).

Foods of *low energy value* include most fresh fruits and vegetables, especially green leafy vegetables, since these foods have a high content of both water and fiber. Lean meats, cereal foods, and starchy vegetables are intermediate in energy value.

The ***100-kcal portions*** of different foods have been used as an aid in visualizing and remembering which foods are high or low in fuel value (Fig. 2–9). It takes only a small amount of a high-calorie food to furnish 100 kcal, while a relatively large mass of low-calorie food must be taken to give the same calorie value, as should be readily apparent from Table 2–7. It does serve to dramatize the contrasts in concentration of calories between high- and low-energy foods to realize that 1 tablespoonful of any clear fat or 2 chocolate creams furnish the same amount of food energy as 1/2 cantaloupe or 4 cups of shredded cabbage, even though it is difficult to indicate the quantity of 100-kcal portions in terms of average servings or household measures with any degree of accuracy.

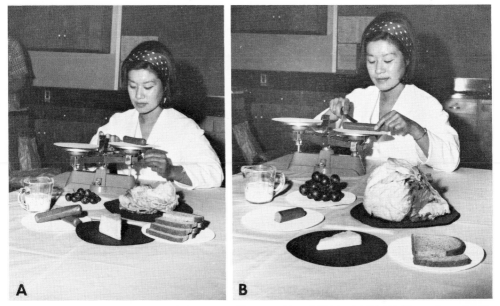

Figure 2–9. A comparison is made between 100 gram (**A**) and 100 kcal (420 kJ) (**B**) portions of milk, grapes, lettuce, bread, cheese, and meat in order to visualize foods of high- or low-energy content in relation to bulk. (Courtesy of University of California, Berkeley.)

Table 2–7.   100 kcal (420 kJ) Portions of Some Foods

Food	Quantity
High Energy Value	
Chocolate creams	2 medium-sized
Brazil nuts	4 medium-sized
Almonds	16 medium-sized
Figs	2 large
Dates	4–4½
Cheese, American	1½ in. cube
Peanut butter	1 tbsp
Butter or margarine	1 tbsp
Mayonnaise, or any clear fat	1 tbsp
Cream, thick	1 tbsp, 2 tbsp whipped
Sugar, white or brown	1¾ tbsp
Sweet alcoholic liquors	1 oz
Whiskies, rum	1–1½ oz
Intermediate Energy Value	
Eggs	1¼ med., 1 large
Lean meats, cooked, med. done	2 ounces (lean portion 1 small loin lamb chop)
Bread, white	1½ avg. slices
Breakfast cereals:	
Cooked meals	¾–1 cup
Ready-to-eat, Flakes	¾–1 cup
Puffed, rice or wheat	2 cups
Potato, white, baked	1 medium-sized
Banana	1 medium
Apple	1 large
Milk, whole	⅝ cup
Milk, skim	1⅛ cup
Cola, root beer	1 cup
Beer	1 cup
Dry Table Wine	½ cup
Low Energy Value	
Strawberries, fresh	1 pint
Grapefruit	1 large
Peaches, fresh	2 medium
Tomatoes, raw	4 medium
Cantaloupe	½ melon, 6 in. diam.
Celery	14 large stalks
Asparagus	30 medium stalks
Cabbage, shredded	4 cups
Lettuce (iceberg type)	2 large, firm heads

More exact tables of the energy value of foods are required for a fairly accurate check on the number of calories furnished by a day's diet. These have been provided for a wide variety of foods in a recent government bulletin[18] on a 100 gm basis. The energy values of **average servings** (based on weight in grams) of the more common foods are listed in the table on Nutritive Values of Foods in Table 2A of the Appendix and are also to be found in another government bulletin.[19]

WEIGHT CONTROL

Stationary Weight an Index of Energy Balance

Although it is sometimes of interest to make a check on about how much energy one is taking daily, this is usually not necessary because body weight constitutes an unerring index of whether the food is furnishing energy equal to, in excess of, or below the energy requirements of the body. When energy intake just about balances outgo, the body neither gains nor loses in weight. Minor weight variations (1 kg or 2 lb) from day to day are of little significance and often may be due to fluctuations in water content of the body. But if the body weight keeps about the same over a considerable period, we can know that the energy value of the food intake is adjusted so that it is practically equal to the energy requirements.

After an adult has attained full growth, it is advantageous to maintain body weight at about a certain norm for the height; either overweight or underweight represents disadvantages which usually make for lesser efficiency and poorer health, as we will see in Chapter 23.

QUESTIONS AND PROBLEMS

1. What is the unit used for expressing quantitatively the energy values of foods and energy needs of the body? Define the large calorie and give abbreviations for it. Why is the calorie, a heat unit, used for expressing energy values? What is the factor for converting calories to Joules? Pounds to kilograms?

2. Define basal metabolism. Describe briefly the methods by which it may be determined. How closely do results obtained by the methods compare? Name four main factors that have an influence in determining basal metabolism, explaining how and why each has the effect that it does.

3. Name the categories of energy needs that together make up the *total* energy requirement of a normal adult. What factor has by far the greatest effect quantitatively in raising energy expenditure above the level of basal

metabolism? Why does mental work have such an insignificant effect on the total energy expended? Under what special circumstances will an adult need an extra allowance of energy for building new tissues?

4. The amount of energy required for muscular work is proportional to the amount and severity of the work done, as illustrated by the following problem: If a man lying quietly requires 77 kcal per hour and his energy need sitting in a chair is 30 percent higher, how much energy per hour will he need sitting at rest? If typewriting rapidly increases the energy need by 82 percent over that lying down, how many calories will he use per hour sitting and typing?

5. Violent muscular exertion causes a great rise in energy expenditure over that at the resting level, but when continued for only a short time it does not markedly increase the total day's energy requirements, as illustrated by the following problem: Suppose that a man is sitting in the station quietly; he suddenly realizes his train is about to leave and makes a run for it; after the run that lasted two minutes, he relaxes in a seat on the train. If he uses 100 kcal per hour sitting at rest, and 570 kcal per hour while making his dash for the train, how much energy would he use in the two minute run?

6. Make a record of your own activities for a sample day, classifying them as nearly as possible under the headings of activities given in Table 2–3. Group the sitting activities, those that involve standing or walking about the room, those that require light or moderate exercise, and select the nearest comparable figure in Table 2–3 for calories per minute for each, and multiply by the time involved. Add energy required for all activities for 24 hours.

7. What is the energy allowance given in the revised 1968 recommended allowances of the Food and Nutrition Board for your weight (without clothing) and the age group nearest your

own age (see Table 2–6). Would you classify your degree of physical activity as sedentary or standard? How does your individual energy requirement, as computed in question 6, compare with the general recommendation for your age, weight, and the standard of activity? If your specific requirement differs much from the average, explain what factors cause it to differ (e.g., variations from average in size and degree of muscular activity).

8. How may the energy value of foods be determined? Why is the physiological energy value of the nutrients somewhat less than their value as determined in the bomb calorimeter? What types of food are high in energy value? Low in energy value?

9. Give the general calorie value *per gram* of pure protein, carbohydrate, and fat. Calculate the energy value of 100 gm of each of the foods whose composition is given below (by multiplying the grams of protein, fat, and carbohydrate each by the proper caloric value per gram, and adding these figures).

	Protein, gm	Fat, gm	Carbo-hydrate, gm
100 gm of white bread contains	8.7	3.2	50.5
100 gm of butter or margarine contains	0.6	81.0	0.4
100 gm of raw cabbage contains	1.3	0.2	5.4

REFERENCES

1. DuBois, E. F.: *Basal Metabolism in Health and Disease.* 3rd Ed. Philadelphia, Lea & Febiger, 1936.
2. Boothby, W. M., et al.: Studies of the energy of metabolism of normal individuals. A standard for basal metabolism with a nomogram for clinical application. Amer. J. Physiol., *116*:468, 1936.
3. Brody, S.: *Bioenergetics and Growth.* New York, Reinhold, 1945.
4. Kleiber, M.: *The Fire of Life.* New York, John Wiley & Sons, Inc., 1961.
5. Holliday, M. A., Potter, D., Jarrah, A., and Bearg, S.: The relation of metabolic rate to body weight and organ size. Pediat. Res., *1*:185, 1967.
6. Benedict, F. G., et al.: Human vitality and efficiency under prolonged restricted diet. Carnegie Institute of Washington, Pub. No. 280, 1919.
7. Keys, A.: Human starvation and its consequences. J. Amer. Dietet. Assoc., *22*:582, 1946.
8. Montgomery, R. D.: Changes in the basal metabolic rate of the malnourished infant and their relation to body composition. J. Clin. Invest., *41*:1653, 1963.
9. Griffith, W. H., and Dyer, H. M.: Present knowledge of specific dynamic action. Chapter VII in *Present Knowledge in Nutrition*, 3rd Ed. Nutrition Foundation, 1967.
10. Buskirk, E. R., Iampietro, P. F., and Welch, B. E.: Variations in resting metabolism with changes in food, exercise and climate. Metab. Clin. Exptl., *6*:144, 1957.
11. Consolazio, C. F., et al.: Energy requirements in extreme heat. J. Nutr., *73*:126, 1961.
12. Benedict, F. G., and Benedict, C. G.: The energy requirement of intense mental effort. Science, *71*:567, 1930.
13. Durnin, J. V. G. A., and Passmore, R.: *Energy, Work, and Leisure.* London, Heinemann Educational Books, Ltd., 1967.
14. Passmore, R., and Durnin, J. V. G. A.: Human energy expenditure. Physiol. Rev., *35*:801, 1955.
15. Food and Nutrition Board: *Recommended Dietary Allowances.* Pub. 1694, 7th Ed. Washington, D.C., National Research Council, National Academy of Sciences, 1968.
16. FAO—WHO, Energy and Protein Requirements, in press, 1972.
17. Canadian Council on Nutrition: Dietary standard for Canada. Canad. Bull. Nutrition, *6*:1, 1964.
18. Watt, B. K., and Merrill, A. L.: *Composition of Foods—Raw, Processed, Prepared.* U.S. Department of Agriculture Handbook No. 8. Washington, D.C., Government Printing Office, 1963.
19. U.S. Department of Agriculture: *Nutritive Value of Foods.* Home and Garden Bulletin No. 72. Washington, D.C., Government Printing Office, 1964 (revised, 1971).

SUPPLEMENTARY READING

Adams, W. C.: Influence of age, sex, and body weight on the energy expenditure of bicycle riding. J. Appl. Physiol., *22*:539, 1967.
Ashworth, A.: Metabolic rates during recovery from protein-calorie malnutrition: the need for a new concept of specific dynamic action. Nature, *223*:407, 1969.
Benedict, F. G.: Basal metabolism: The modern measure of vital activity. Sci. Monthly, *27*:5, 1928.
Blaxter, K. L. (ed.): *Energy Metabolism.* European

Association for Animal Production Publ. No. 11. New York, Academic Press, 1966.

Bradfield, R. B., ed.: Symposium: Assessment of typical daily energy expenditure. Amer. J. Clin. Nutr., 24:1111 and 1405, 1971.

Brozek, J.: Body composition. Science, 134:920, 1961.

Bullard, R. W., and Rapp, G. M.: Problems of body heat loss in water immersion. Aerospace Med., 41:1269, 1970.

Buskirk, E. R., et al.: Human energy expenditure studies. I. Interaction of cold environment and specific dynamic effect. II. Sleep. Amer. J. Clin. Nutr., 8:602, 1960.

Buskirk, E. R., Thomson, R. H., and Whedon, G. D.: Metabolic response to cold air in men and women in relation to total body fat content. J. Appl. Physiol., 18:603, 1963.

Chatfield, C.: *Food Composition Tables for International Use.* Food and Agriculture Organization Studies 3 and 11. Rome, FAO, 1949, 1951.

Crampton, E. W., Farmer, F. A., McKirdy, H. B., Lloyd, L. E., Donefer, E., and Schad, D. J.: A statistical study of apparent digestibility coefficients of the energy-yielding components of a nutritionally adequate mixed diet consumed by 103 young human adults. J. Nutr., 72:177, 1960.

Dodds, S. C.: Calorie balance in man. Proc. Nutr. Society, 20:52, 1961.

Durnin, J. V. G. A.: The use of surface and body weight as standards of references in studies of human energy expenditure. Brit. J. Nutr., 13:68, 1959.

Durnin, J. V. G. A., and Brockway, J. M.: Determination of the total daily energy expenditure in man by indirect calorimetry: Assessment of the accuracy of a modern technique. Brit. J. Nutr., 13:41, 1959.

Easty, D. L.: Food intake in Antarctica. Brit. J. Nutr., 21:7, 1967.

Elliot, D. E., and Patton, M. B.: *Manual of Techniques Used in Determining Human Energy Expenditures.* Research Circular 121. Ohio Agricultural Experimental Station, Wooster, Ohio, 1963.

FAO: Nutrition and working efficiency. FFHC Basic Study No. 5, 1962.

Gold, A. J., Zornitzer, A., and Samueloff, S.: Influence of season and heat on energy expenditure during rest and exercise. J. Appl. Physiol., 27:9, 1969.

Grisola, S., and Kennedy, J.: On specific dynamic action, turnover and protein synthesis. Perspect. Biol. Med., 9:578, 1966.

Groen, J. J.: An indirect method for approximating caloric expenditure for physical activity. A recommendation for dietary surveys. J. Amer. Dietet. Assoc., 52:313, 1968.

Hunscher, H. A.: Pertinent factors in interpreting metabolic data. J. Amer. Dietet. Assoc., 39:209, 1961.

Issekutz, B., Jr., Birkhead, N. C., and Rodahl, K.: Effect of diet on work metabolism. J. Nutr., 79:109, 1963.

Johnson, R. E.: Caloric requirements under adverse environmental conditions. Fed. Proc., 22:1431, 1963.

Kleiber, M.: Joules vs calories in nutrition. J. Nutr., 102:309, 1972.

Konishi, F.: Food energy equivalents of various activities. J. Amer. Dietet. Assoc., 46:186, 1965.

Kraut, H. A., and Muller, E. A.: Caloric intake and industrial output. Science, 104:495, 1946.

Leverton, R. M., et al.: Source of calories in the recorded self-chosen diets of women. J. Home Econ., 51:33, 1959.

McCance, R. A., and Widdowson, E. M.: The chemical composition of foods. Spec. Report Series No. 297. London, Medical Research Council, 1960.

Miller, D. S., and Payne, P. R.: Weight maintenance and food intake. J. Nutr., 78:255, 1962.

NAS/NRC: Biological Energy Interrelationships and Glossary of Energy Terms. Publ. 1411, 1966.

Parks, J. R.: Rats and exercise, men and work. Amer. J. Physiol., 216:666, 1969.

Pilcher, H. L., et al.: Comparison of analyzed and calculated energy values of food intakes of adult women. Metabolism, 10:46, 1961.

Rice, E. E.: The effect of processing operations on the energy available from foods. Food Technol., 21:259, 1967.

Richardson, M., and McCracken, E. C.: Energy expenditures of women performing selected activities. U.S.D.A. Home Econ. Res. Rept. No. 11, 1960.

Richardson, M., and McCracken, E. C.: Work-surface levels and human energy expenditure. J. Amer. Dietet. Assoc., 48:192, 1966.

Rochelle, R. H., and Horvath, S. M.: Metabolic responses to food and acute cold stress. J. Appl. Physiol., 27:710, 1969.

Shipman, W. G., Oken, D., and Heath, H. A.: Muscle tension and effort at self-control during anxiety. Arch. Gen. Psychiatry, 23:359, 1970.

Stolwijk, J. A. J.: Thermal loads in lunar ambulation. Aerospace Med., 41:1266, 1970.

Swindells, Y. E.: The influence of activity and size of meals on caloric response in women. Brit. J. Nutr., 27:65, 1972.

Thompson, A. M., and Billewicz, W. Z.: Height, weight and food intake in man. Brit. J. Nutr., 15:241, 1961.

U.S. Department of Agriculture, Agricultural Research Service: *An Evaluation of Basal Metabolic Data for Children and Youth in the United States.* Home Economics Research Report 14. Washington, D.C., U.S. Government Printing Office, 1961.

U.S. Department of Agriculture, Agricultural

Research Service: *Evaluation of Basal Metabolic Data for Infants in the United States.* Home Economics Research Report 18. Washington, D.C., U.S. Government Printing Office, 1962.

Weaver, E. K., and Elliot, D. E.: Factors affecting energy expended in home-making tasks. J. Amer. Dietet. Assoc., *39*:205, 1961.

Webb, P.: Body heat loss in undersea gaseous environments. Aerospace Med., *41*:1282, 1970.

Nutrition Reviews

The neglected field of heat loss (by DuBois, E. F.). *1*:385, 1943.

Measure of energy content of foodstuffs. *16*:51, 1958.

Diet and work metabolism. *21*:211, 1963.

Are all food calories equal? *22*:177, 1964.

Fasting metabolic rate of cattle. *24*:315, 1966.

Variability in basal metabolic rate (BMR). *25*:13, 1967.

Energy of recovery from undernutrition. *25*:112, 1967.

Present knowledge of calories (by Johnson, O. C.). *25*:257, 1967.

Energy cost of simulated space activities. *25*:301, 1967.

Calories and activity in infants. *26*:239, 1968.

Components of energy expenditure in the rat. *27*:25, 1969.

Malnutrition and metabolic rates. *28*:279, 1970.

Assessing the energy value of the human diet. *29*:131, 1971.

three

Carbohydrates

The three major classes of energy nutrients—carbohydrates, fats, and proteins—are by far the most abundant nutrients in foods. Most natural foods contain all three nutrients but in widely varying proportions. In order to have a clear idea of the nature of and the differences between these three classes of nutrients, we will begin with definitions of each, devote the rest of this chapter to discussion of carbohydrates, and treat fats and proteins in the two following chapters.

All *carbohydrates* are either sugars or more complex compounds, such as starch, which are formed by the union of many sugar groups. The class name is suggested by the fact that they are made up of the elements carbon, hydrogen, and oxygen, with the hydrogen and oxygen present in the same two-to-one proportion as in water—hence the word hydrate.

Fats are also composed of carbon, hydrogen, and oxygen, but with these elements present in different relative amounts from those in carbohydrates. All true fats are alike in chemical nature and physical properties; they have a greasy feel, are insoluble in water, but are soluble in such solvents as ether and gasoline. Every molecule of a true fat yields on digestion one molecule of glycerol (an alcohol)* and three molecules of fatty acids.

Proteins consist of carbon, hydrogen, and oxygen, again in different proportions, and in addition they always contain the element *nitrogen*. Most proteins also contain some *sulfur*, and others contain phosphorus, iron, iodine, or other trace minerals, in addition to the elements common to all proteins. The "building stones" of proteins are amino acids, and on digestion each molecule of protein breaks down to yield many molecules of various kinds of amino acids. Proteins characteristically have a "gluey" consistency and are precipitated or coagulate on heating.

Chemical Nature of Simple Sugars

Simple sugars form the basis for all carbohydrates and all of these compounds that occur commonly in food

*Alcohol is the class name of chemical compounds containing a particular configuration of oxygen and hydrogen (—OH, a hydroxyl group). The alcohol in spirituous beverages is ethyl alcohol, or ethanol.

53

or in the body are either hexoses (6-carbon sugars) or multiples of hexose sugar groups. So it is a good thing to learn how carbon, hydrogen, and oxygen atoms are linked up in a molecule of a typical hexose sugar, *glucose.* The student should understand that every molecule of a given substance is exactly alike, with the same number of atoms of each element, linked to each other in precisely the same arrangement; any variation from this pattern makes it a different substance.

Each molecule of glucose consists of 6 carbon, 6 oxygen, and 12 hydrogen atoms; in other words, its formula is written as $C_6H_{12}O_6$. The carbon atoms each have four bonds, with which they can link up to other atoms or groups of atoms called radicals; in glucose, the six carbons use one or two of these bonds to unite with each other in a chain or in an irregular-shaped ring. The bonds not used for linking up with other carbons are free to hold onto hydrogen atoms (which have only one bond), a hydrogen-oxygen combination known as the hydroxyl radical (one bond), or a separate oxygen atom (two bonds). In this way, in the glucose molecule, a chain of 6 carbon atoms holds in combination 6 oxygen and 12 hydrogen atoms.

The other simple hexose sugars—*fructose* and *galactose*—both have the same formula ($C_6H_{12}O_6$), but the hydrogen and oxygen atoms are held in slightly different arrangements about the 6-carbon chain, which makes them different substances.

Kinds of Carbohydrates and Their Occurrence

Carbohydrates are subdivided into three groups, according to the relative complexity and size of their molecules. These three classes are known as *simple sugars,* or *monosaccharides* (one sugar group per molecule); *disaccharides* (two sugar groups per molecule); and *polysaccharides* (many sugar groups per molecule). The linkage of sugar groups to form di- and polysaccharides is shown in Figure 3–1.

The carbohydrates most important in the diet and the groups to which they belong are as follows:

Glucose, fructose, and *galactose*—monosaccharides, or simple sugars;
Sucrose, maltose, and *lactose*—disaccharides, or double sugars;
Starch, dextrins, glycogen, cellulose, and *hemicelluloses*—polysaccharides.

These divisions are of interest to the student of nutrition because the more complex carbohydrates must all be broken down by digestion into the simple sugar groups of which they are composed before they can be absorbed and used by the body. The di- and polysaccharides are split into monosaccharides by hydrolysis, a reaction with water (*hydro-,* water; *-lysis,* breaking down).

All the food carbohydrates except lactose (milk sugar) are formed in the vegetable kingdom. Because the **sugars** are very soluble in water, they are the form in which plants transport carbohydrate from one part to another in the sap or tuck it away for temporary use in the juices of the fruits. Hence, glucose, fructose, and sucrose are found chiefly in plant juices and in fruits. The sweet taste of green corn and peas is due to the presence of sugar that will be converted to starch as the immature seed ripens; in some fruits (e.g., bananas) starch is present in the unripe fruit and turns to sugar on ripening. Carrots, beets, onions, winter squash, turnips, and sweet potatoes are vegetables that contain appreciable amounts of sugars (as well as green peas and unripe corn).

Our sugar supply for table use and cooking is *sucrose,* a disaccharide made up of glucose and fructose. It comes chiefly from juices of the sugar cane or sugar beet, and over one-third of our supply is derived from the latter source. The sugar obtained from the sap of the sugar maple tree is also su-

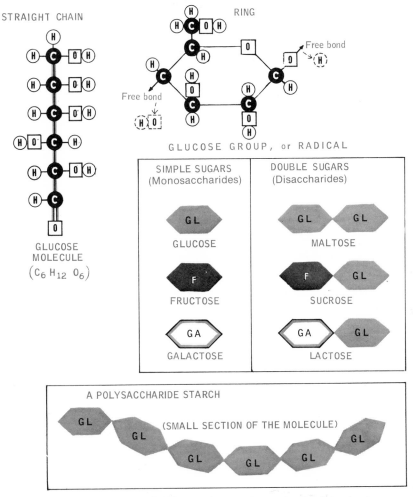

STRAIGHT CHAIN

RING

GLUCOSE
MOLECULE
$(C_6 H_{12} O_6)$

GLUCOSE GROUP, or RADICAL

SIMPLE SUGARS (Monosaccharides)	DOUBLE SUGARS (Disaccharides)
GLUCOSE	MALTOSE
FRUCTOSE	SUCROSE
GALACTOSE	LACTOSE

A POLYSACCHARIDE STARCH

(SMALL SECTION OF THE MOLECULE)

Figure 3–1. Diagram showing arrangement of the atoms in a molecule of the simple sugar — glucose — and in the glucose radical; also included is diagrammatic representation of the molecules of disaccharides and a few links in the long chain of glucose radicals that make up the large molecules of starch. The glucose group, or radical, is represented as having one free bond at each end of the ring owing to the loss of a hydrogen atom and a hydroxyl radical (OH) in the process of linking up with another sugar group. When broken apart by hydrolysis (either by digestion or boiling in dilute acid), these component parts of water (H and OH) are taken up again, and glucose molecules are split off.

crose. Fructose and glucose occur in honey in about 50–50 proportion.

The sugar *maltose* is formed as an intermediate product during the digestion of starch in the body and is also found in germinated grains such as "malt," and in products prepared from partly digested starch such as corn syrups, malted breakfast foods, and malted milk. The sugar made by hydrolyzing corn starch completely is the simple sugar, glucose. *Lactose* occurs in the milk of most mammals, and serves as a source of energy for the young; on digestion it is broken down into glucose and galactose.

Starch is the carbohydrate found in the seeds, tubers, and roots, where it functions as an energy store for future use of the plant. Starch is formed by union of many molecules of glucose. It has been estimated that the number

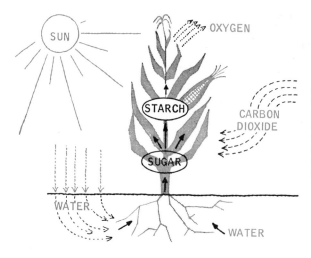

Figure 3–2. Synthesis of sugar from carbon dioxide and water through the agency of sunlight and the green pigment—chlorophyll—a process known as photosynthesis. Sugar circulates in the plant sap, but excess not needed for immediate use is made into starch, which is stored in the maturing kernels of the ear of corn.

of sugar groups in the starch molecule may average around 300 to 400. Starch occurs in two types of molecules, one (amylose) consisting of long unbranched chains (wavy or kinked so as to form a three-dimensional spiral), the other type (amylopectin) in highly branched chains. Such large molecules have no sweet taste and are not soluble in water. In the plant, starch is laid down in "granules" coated with a cellulose-like substance, and different plants have granules of characteristic size and shape, so that the source of a starch can be determined by microscopic examination. When subjected to moist heat (as in cooking), starch granules absorb water, swell, and are ruptured. After such treatment, starch forms a colloidal dispersion in water, and it is more easily digested in this state. Before starch can be used as a source of energy, either in the plant or in the body, it must first be broken down into the simple sugar groups of which it is composed, each starch molecule yielding many molecules of glucose. *Dextrins* and *maltose* are intermediate products formed in the process of breaking down starch to glucose; dextrins are more soluble than starch and their molecules may average about one-fifth the size of those of starch. Our chief food sources of starch are grains and all products made from them (breads, breakfast cereals, macaroni, cakes, and other pastries), legumes (beans and peas), and certain tuber and root vegetables (such as potatoes and sweet potatoes).

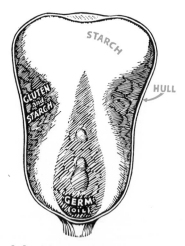

Figure 3–3. Diagram showing the structure of the corn kernel. Starch is the principal component, the kernel containing about 60 percent of this substance. In the starch manufacturing industry, the gluten (protein) and the hulls are made into feed for livestock. The germ contains a high percentage of oil, which after purification is used for salad oils and vegetable shortenings. (Courtesy of the Corn Industries Research Foundation.)

Cellulose is also a polysaccharide of glucose, more resistant than starch to digestion or hydrolysis outside the body, and also to attempts at solution. Starch is insoluble in water, but heating it in water causes a colloidal dispersion (starch paste) to be formed. Cellulose is only softened by cooking processes and is not digested by man, so that it is not an energy source.[2] (It is used by bacteria and thus serves as an energy source for ruminants.) Cellulose and the closely related hemicelluloses make up the structural or fibrous part of plants (leaves, stems, roots, and seed and fruit coverings) and also the cell walls. Since most of this material taken in plant foods remains undigested, it serves to give bulk to the food residues in the intestine. Further discussion of cellulose and the function of fiber in the diet is found in Chapter 14.

Glycogen is sometimes called "animal starch" because it is the polysaccharide stored in animal tissues instead of starch. Glycogen molecules are large and seem to vary in size. They are similar in many respects to those of the branched form of starch (amylopectin), but they have shorter chains of glucose units and hence a more complicated branched structure. Glycogen is therefore well adapted to being broken into smaller units or to being rebuilt as needed from smaller units in the body tissues. When it is needed for use it is converted to glucose and then oxidized to yield energy. Carbohydrate is an immediate source of fuel for animals. For this purpose animals use glucose, which is the only sugar found in substantial amounts in the blood or tissue fluids. Only limited amounts of glycogen can be stored in the liver and muscle tissues, and this is used up rapidly during fasting or muscular work. Since animals have limited ability to store carbohydrate, there is little of it present in our animal foods, such as muscle meats. Liver usually contains about 1.5 to 5 percent glycogen, while shellfish (including oysters) have 0.5 to 5 percent.

Carbohydrate-Rich Foods

Some typical foods of relatively high-carbohydrate content, together with the approximate amount of carbohydrate each contains, are shown in Figures 3–4 and 3–5. A few highly refined substances—such artifically prepared foods as refined sugar and corn starch—are pure carbohydrate (99.5 and 88 percent respectively, the rest of the weight being due to small amounts of water); but even those foods relatively rich in either sugar or starch contain in their natural state other substances besides carbohydrates. Although highly milled dry rice and patent flour are more than four-fifths starch and have a total carbohydrate (starch) content of 81 and 76 percent respectively, they also contain protein in amounts of 6.5 to 10.5 percent. Whole-grain cereals have somewhat more protein and less starch. Dry peas and beans have over 20 percent of protein along with approximately 60 percent of starch; soybeans differ from other legumes in that they contain less starch and more protein and fat. The legumes and whole grains also contain some indigestible fiber, and certain minerals and vitamins.* Starchy roots of the taro and cassava (manioc), which are staple foods in parts of Africa and the islands of the South Pacific, have very little protein, minerals, or vitamins.

Foods of high sugar content (65 to 99 percent) include table sugars, honey, syrups, candies, cakes, jams, jellies,

---

*Figures for the carbohydrate content of foods used here and elsewhere in the book are for *total* carbohydrate, as given by the U.S. Department of Agriculture.[1] These figures are apt to be slightly higher than the actual amount of carbohydrates available to the body, because they are usually determined by difference (assuming that the remainder of the weight other than that accounted for by protein, fat, ash, and water is due to carbohydrate). Total carbohydrate (by difference) includes, besides utilizable carbohydrate, relatively small amounts of fiber (unutilizable carbohydrate) as well as organic acids and other noncarbohydrate substances.

TYPICAL CARBOHYDRATE-RICH FOODS AS SERVED

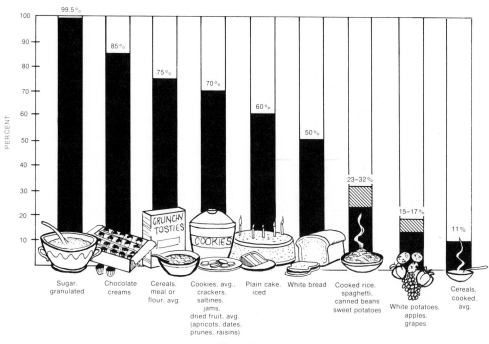

Figure 3–4.

Table 3–1.   Fiber in Foods*

	Fiber (in grams)
Apple, 1 small	1.0
Banana, 1 medium	0.5
Beans, lima, ¼ cup	1.8
Beets, diced, ½ cup	0.8
Beet greens, cooked, ½ cup	1.3
String beans, cooked, ¾ cup	1.0
Carrots, cubed, ¾ cup	1.0
Peas, green, fresh, ¾ cup	2.0
Bread, whole wheat, 3 slices	1.0
Bread, white, 4 slices	0.2
Shredded wheat biscuit, 1	0.7
Oatmeal, cooked, ¾ cup	0.2
Cream of Wheat, cooked, ½ cup	trace
Raspberries, red, ¾ cup	3.0
Prunes, 6 medium + 2 tbsp juice	0.8
Strawberries, fresh, ⅔ cup	1.4

*Calculated from figures in *Composition of Foods,* Agriculture Handbook No. 8, Agriculture Research Service, U.S.D.A., 1963.

preserves, and dried fruits (dates, figs, raisins, prunes, apricots); others containing appreciable amounts are fresh fruits (9 to 23 percent) and soft drinks (8 percent). Taken in considerable quantities, these last two sources may contribute appreciable amounts of energy (calories).

The grains (wheat, corn, rice, rye, barley) and dry products made from them (dry breakfast cereals, crackers, breads, etc.) are rich in starch (50 to 85 percent); cereal puddings, potatoes, cooked legumes, and cereals are of higher, but variable, water content, so they range in carbohydrate from about 10 to 20 percent. Cooked rice, spaghetti, macaroni, and sweet potatoes are 23 to 32 percent carbohydrate, with white potatoes (boiled or baked in skin)

TYPICAL CARBOHYDRATE-RICH FOODS, DRY BASIS

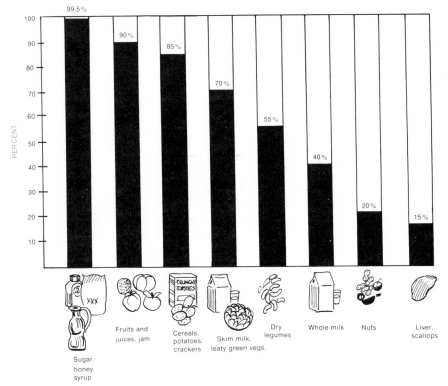

Figure 3–5.

about 17 to 22 percent. Cooked breakfast cereals (e.g., oatmeal and Cream of Wheat) vary with water content but average about 11 percent starch.

Place of Carbohydrate-Rich Foods in Diet

There are no definite requirements for carbohydrate, nor can we state that any special level of carbohydrate intake is most conducive to health. The relative prominence of carbohydrate-rich foods varies widely with individuals and in different parts of the world, depending chiefly on the availability and relative cost of fat- and protein-rich foods (animal products such as meats and dairy products) and the amount of money that can be spent for food. Such foods as grains, starchy roots or tubers, and dried peas or beans are usually the

cheapest foods for energy value. In Japan, for example, carbohydrates (rice) contribute four-fifths the total energy intake, while in the United States (where fats are used more liberally) only one-half (or less) the energy intake comes from carbohydrates.

There need be no health hazard in subsisting chiefly on carbohydrate-rich foods, *provided* those foods are not lacking in proteins, minerals, and vitamins or the diet includes some rich source of these nutrients. On the other hand, there is no clear evidence that more than a very small amount of carbohydrate need be present in the diet if substances from which the body can make sugar are sufficient. (See Chapters 14 and 23.)

In summary, the main contributions to the diet by carbohydrate-rich foods (sugars and starchy foods) are to:

1. Provide an economical energy supply.

2. Furnish some proteins, minerals, and vitamins (whole grains, legumes, and potatoes).

3. Add flavor (sugars) to foods and beverages.

QUESTIONS AND PROBLEMS

1. Define carbohydrates, fats, and proteins. Which vital element is supplied in utilizable form only by proteins? Why are these three classes of foods called "the most abundant nutrients"? Why are they referred to as the fuel foodstuffs or energy nutrients?

2. Explain the chemical basis for the division of carbohydrates into mono-, di, and polysaccharides. How do the mono- and disaccharides (sugars) differ in properties (taste, solubility, etc.) from polysaccharides (starch, cellulose, etc.)? How are these differences in properties related to the size of the molecules?

3. Name three common monosaccharides and some foods in which they are found. Consult the diagram of the molecular structure of glucose in Figure 3–1. How many carbon atoms are there in each molecule; how many hydrogen atoms; how many oxygen atoms? Why are they called carbo*hydrates*? Why are the monosaccharides that occur most commonly in nature called hexoses? What is the hexose sugar that occurs in blood and body tissues?

4. When two molecules of a monosaccharide link up to form a disaccharide (as two glucose molecules to form one molecule of maltose), what substance is split off at the point of linkage? Does the same thing happen when many molecules of glucose unite to form the polysaccharide starch? What happens when these linkages are broken during digestion or hydrolysis outside the body? Why is this breakdown called hydrolysis?

5. What is the chemical name of common table sugar and from what sources in nature is it made? Is maple sugar the same or a different substance? Is sugar a relatively expensive or inexpensive source of food energy? Does it carry any other nutrients? What are the disadvantages of using sugar too liberally? Name four common foods of high sugar content.

6. What types or classes of food have a high content of starch? Into what monosaccharide is starch broken down in digestion? Does this process take place gradually or all at once? Why? What polysaccharide found in foods is of no use to the body and why is this so? Plants store starch in seeds or tubers; what polysaccharide is stored in the body, chiefly in the liver?

7. Make a list of the foods you have consumed in one day, including sugar added at the table and any between-meal snacks. Using the table in the Appendix on Nutritive Values of Foods in Average Servings, calculate your total intake of carbohydrate for the day. At 4 kcal per gram, how much energy did you obtain in the form of carbohydrate? Since the figures for total carbohydrate include small amounts of indigestible carbohydrate in the form of fiber, how would this affect the total energy actually obtained? Of what use is the fiber in vegetable foods?

8. What are the chief uses of carbohydrate-rich foods in the diet? In what countries and under what economic conditions is the consumption of carbohydrates high? What are the disadvantages of diets that are made up chiefly of carbohydrate-rich foods? Why is it important that whole-grain or enriched bread and cereal be used when grain products make up a large proportion of the diet?

REFERENCES

1. U.S. Department of Agriculture Handbook 8. Revised December, 1963.
2. Mangold, E.: The digestion and utilisation of crude fibre. Nutr. Abstr. Rev., 3:647, 1934.

SUPPLEMENTARY READING

Anonymous: Lactose intolerance. Dairy Council Digest, *42*:31, 1971.

Anonymous: Nutritional significance of lactose. Dairy Council Dig., *33*:5, 1962.

Anonymous: Sugar in fruits. J. Amer. Dietet. Assoc., *59*:227, 1971.

Antar, M. A., and Ohlson, M. A.: Effect of simple and complex carbohydrates upon total lipids, nonphospholipids, and different fractions of phospholipids of serum in young men and women. J. Nutr., *85*:329, 1965.

Booher, L. E., Behan, I., and McMeans, E.: Biologic utilizations of unmodified and modified food starches. J. Nutr., *45*:75, 1951.

Burton, B. J.: Carbohydrates. In *The Heinz Handbook of Nutrition*. New York, McGraw-Hill, 1965, Chap. 8.

Carbohydrate digestion and absorption. Dairy Council Dig., *40*:30, 1959.

Corn Industries Research Foundation: *Cornstarch*. Pamphlet. Washington, D.C., Corn Industries Research Foundation, 1964.

Duncan, D. L.: The physiological effect of lactose. Nutr. Abst. Rev., *25*:309, 1955.

Grande, F., Anderson, J. T., and Keys, A.: Effect of carbohydrates of leguminous seeds, wheat and potatoes on serum cholesterol concentration in man. J. Nutr., *86*:313, 1965.

Gray, G. M.: Carbohydrate digestion and absorption. Gastroent., *58*:96, 1970.

Hardinge, H. G., Swarner, J. B., and Crooks, H.: Carbohydrates in food. J. Amer. Dietet. Assoc., *46*:197, 1965.

Harper, A. E.: Carbohydrates. In *Food*. Yearbook of Agriculture, Washington, D.C., U.S. Department of Agriculture, Government Printing Office, 1959, p. 88.

Hodges, R. E., and Krehl, W. A.: The role of carbohydrates in lipid metabolism. Amer. J. Clin. Nutr., *17*:334, 1965.

Macdonald, I.: Physiological role of dietary carbohydrates. World Rev. Nutr. Dietet., *8*: 143, 1967.

Macdonald, I. (ed.): Symposium on dietary carbohydrates in man. Amer. J. Clin. Nutr., *20*:65, 1967.

Olsen, W. A.: Carbohydrate digestion and absorption: Clinically significant abnormalities. Postgrad. Med., April 1972, p. 149.

Passmore, R., and Swindells, Y. E.: Observations on the respiratory quotient and weight gain of man after eating large quantities of carbohydrates. Brit. Med. J., *17*:331, 1963.

Rao, M. N., and Sunderavalli, O. E.: Extraneous cellulose: Effect on protein utilization. J. Amer. Dietet. Assoc., *57*:517, 1970.

Rees, D. A.: Shapely polysaccharides. Biochem. J., *126*:257, 1972.

Nutrition Reviews

Present knowledge of carbohydrates. *24*:65, 1966.

Galactose utilization in young and adult rats. *24*: 80, 1966.

Effect of pectin on cholesterol absorption. *24*: 209, 1966.

Starch digestion in ruminants. *25*:55, 1967.

Effect of fructose and glycerol upon alimentary hyperglyceridemia. *25*:78, 1967.

Dietary carbohydrates and serum lipids of man. *25*:102, 1967.

Dietary sucrose restriction and blood lipid levels. *25*:172, 1967.

Propionate utilization in glucose synthesis in sheep. *25*:347, 1967.

Absorption and effect of ingested mannoheptulose. *27*:206, 1969.

Body composition and high carbohydrate diets at high altitude. *27*:283, 1969.

Squirrel monkey and carbohydrate metabolism. *28*:15, 1970.

Galactose toxicity and cellular growth of fetal brain. *28*:55, 1970.

Fructose utilization by the baby pig. *28*:132, 1970.

Change in lipoprotein composition with dietary carbohydrate. *28*:153, 1970.

four

Fats and Other Lipids

Discovery and Background

Fats are a part of every meal and are familiar to everyone—butter, margarine, vegetable oils, lard, and suet being common examples. In America, the average person consumes about one-fourth of a pound of fat (about 110 gm) per day in one form or another, a practice not without its nutritional hazards.

The story of fats goes back to man's earliest history when fats, oils, and tallows were first used for food, for soap manufacture, for lubrication of axles of the earliest wheels, as a fuel for light and heat, and for cosmetics and medicine. Many Biblical passages refer to fats and oils.

The name of the first individual to notice fats in nature will never be known. McCollum[1] has reviewed the early history of studies on fats. These go back to records surviving from the early Egyptians, and include the classic discoveries of the French chemist M. E. Chevreul, who in 1823 first discovered the chemical nature of fats. The word "margarine" comes from Chevreul's "margaric acid."

In the late 1800's, physiologists provided proof that excess dietary carbohydrates were readily converted to fats in the body and stored as adipose tissue, a fact experienced and suspected by laymen centuries earlier. In 1929 Burr and Burr[2] demonstrated the essential nature of certain fatty acids in the diet, a subject discussed later in this chapter.

Composition and Occurrence of Fats

Fats are formed by chemical combination of three *fatty acids* with an organic alcohol called *glycerol* (commonly known as "glycerin"), as shown in Figure 4-1. The fatty acids contain large amounts of carbon and hydrogen, along with a relatively small amount of oxygen, and hence fats have very high fuel value. Fatty acids exist rarely in the free form in nature. The combined form (with glycerol) represents the chief form in which animals store extra energy for future use, just as plants store energy in the form of starch. Some plants store fats in fruits, seeds, seed germs, or nuts, which we see as the vegetable oils (from the olive, coconut, peanut, soybean, corn germ, cottonseed, etc.) used for food.

Many food fats are of animal origin—butter, lard, fatty meats and fish, egg

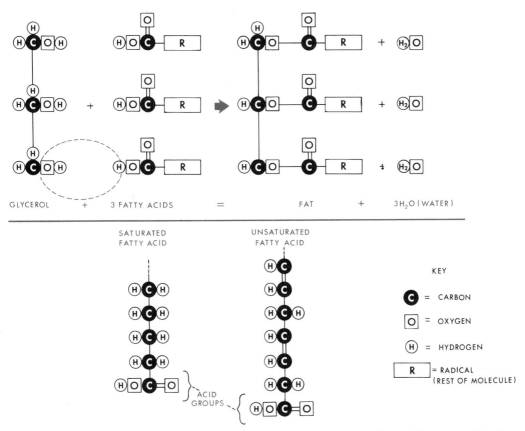

Figure 4–1. Diagrams showing molecular structure of glycerol, fatty acids, and fats. Fatty acid molecules have a chain of carbon atoms with hydrogen attached and at one end of the chain, an organic acid group (COOH). In the fatty acids that occur most commonly in food fats, there are either 15 or 17 carbon atoms in the chain attached to the organic acid group. Saturated fatty acids have only single bonds between carbon atoms in the chain. Unsaturated fatty acids have one or several double bonds between carbons and can add on more hydrogen when these double bonds are broken and reduced to single bonds; hence, they are unsaturated in respect to hydrogen.

yolk, cream, and full-milk cheeses. An interesting fact is that fishes store fat instead of glycogen in their livers, the source of the fish-liver oils that are widely used medicinally for their valuable content of fat-soluble vitamins.

The *physical properties* of fats are important, sometimes affecting their nutritive value. That fats are insoluble in and lighter than water is easily apparent from the fact that the fat in milk is separate from the fluid portion and rises to the top on standing (the specific gravity of common fats ranges between 0.92 and 0.94). Most fresh whole milk now sold has been *homogenized*—that is, put through a process that breaks up the fat into such fine particles that it remains evenly distributed in the fluid.

Fats that are in small droplets in a fluid (emulsified), as in milk and egg yolk, are more quickly digested because the tiny droplets can be surrounded and attacked by digestive juices (see Fig. 4–2). Fats that are fluid at body temperature are generally more easily digested than those that have higher melting points.

Every fat has its characteristic melting point. Fats known as *oils* are liquid at room temperatures. Butter, lard, and other solid cooking fats melt with only a little heating. Mutton suet, on the other hand, has the highest melting

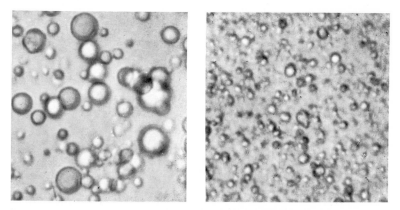

Figure 4-2. **Left,** Fat globules in milk magnified 1000 times. **Right,** The same in evaporated milk, broken up so fine that the cream does not rise. (Courtesy of Evaporated Milk Association, Chicago.)

point among the meat fats, most of which are solid at room temperatures.

The difference in consistency of various fats at room temperatures (that is, the difference in melting points) is due to differences in the kinds and amounts of fatty acids that enter into their composition. *Palmitic* and *stearic* acids, which enter largely into the composition of solid fats, have a type formula of $C_nH_{2n}O_2$; they are said to be *saturated* because they cannot take up any more hydrogen. Some fatty acids are *unsaturated* with respect to hydrogen — that is, they have type formulas like $C_nH_{2n-2}O_2$ (oleic acid) and $C_nH_{2n-4}O_2$ (linoleic acid). The more highly unsaturated fatty acids (linoleic, linolenic, and arachidonic acids) have two, three, and four double bonds (respectively) per molecule; hence, they are said to be *polyunsaturated.* These have great nutritional importance. The more detailed structure of fats and of saturated and unsaturated fatty acids is shown in Figure 4-1 and in Table 12 of the Appendix.

When a fat is composed largely of unsaturated fatty acids, the fat will have a relatively low melting point and be commonly encountered in liquid state as an oil. Oleic acid (with only one double bond) is found in relatively large amounts in oils, along with variable

amounts of polyunsaturated fatty acids. By suitable chemical treatment, the double bonds in the molecules of unsaturated fatty acids may be reduced to single ones, setting free bonds that enable the compound to take up more hydrogen atoms; by this process oils may be converted to a semisolid or solid state. It is by *hydrogenation* and other chemical modifications that vegetable oils are converted into a semisolid state for use as cooking fats (lard substitutes) and margarines.

Uses of Fats in Food

Some fats are used as spreads; others are used in cookery. Fats incorporated and naturally present in foods give prized *flavor* and *satiety* value. The flavor varies somewhat with the kind of fat used, individual preference being largely based on habit and economic conditions. Since certain fats have become scarcer and more costly, the attitude of American consumers has altered to larger acceptance of formerly less used but cheaper fats — for example, corn or cottonseed oil instead of olive oil, and margarine instead of butter, at least in part. Because margarines are now improved nutritionally by the addition of vitamin A (to the level found in average butter), usually have vitamin D added, and are permitted to be sold in colored form, their consumption has greatly increased.

The *satiety value* of fats depends on the fact that fats slow digestion and the emptying time of the stomach; meals that contain considerable fat remain longer in the stomach and so prevent the early recurrence of the "hunger pangs" that occur when it is empty. When food is scarce or when one is on a "reducing diet," small or moderate amounts of fat are a help in preventing hunger. But when too much fat is taken, especially when it is intimately mixed with starch or protein, the meal may stay so long in the stomach as to cause discomfort.

The high-energy value of fats (9 kcal per gm) means that relatively small quantities of fat-rich foods decidedly raise the energy value of the diet. Fats are useful when it is desirable to have a higher intake of food energy without adding unduly to the bulk of the diet. A diet very low in fat often either supplies less energy than the body needs, thereby causing weight loss, or it is much more bulky than the customary American or European diet. If one overeats in regard to fats, the diet very likely provides food energy in excess of body needs, and causes undesirable weight gains. Excess energy value of the diet, whether taken in the form of fat, carbohydrate, or protein, is converted into body fat and stored in fatty tissues in various parts of the body.

Fat deposits in the human body may be either advantageous or disadvantageous, according to whether they are moderate or excessive. Some deposition of fat, usually under the skin or about the abdominal organs, serves a useful purpose as a *reserve store of fuel* to be drawn on in time of need. Moderate deposits of fatty tissue also serve to *support organs* and protect them from injury and to *prevent undue loss of heat* from the body surface, since fat is a poor conductor of heat. But an overfed

person goes on storing fat which he may never need to burn as body fuel; such excessive fat deposits cause undesirable weight gains and place undue strain on the heart and other vital organs. Insurance figures show that overweight persons have a much lower life expectancy than those who maintain normal weight for their height and age.

Uses of Fat in the Diet

Fats and fat-rich foods are useful in the diet for five main purposes:
1. As a source of essential fatty acid. (This is the sole essential use of fat—the others below are very useful, though not essential.)
2. As carriers of fat-soluble vitamins A, D, E, and K.
3. As a concentrated source of energy.
4. For making foods appetizing.
5. For satiety value.

Fatty Foods

Some typical fat-rich foods are listed in Figure 4–3. The principal foods that are almost pure fat are butter, lard, margarine, vegetable oils, and cooking fats. These foods are generally used in moderate amounts at a time by being spread on or mixed into other foods low in fat content. Mayonnaise is about 80 percent fat, but other types of salad dressings range between 40 and 60 percent. Foods whose fat content ranges from 20 to 70 percent include cream and full milk cheeses, fat meats and poultry, chocolate, nuts, and peanut butter. These foods are also generally used in moderation. Olives and avocados are among the few fruits fairly rich in fats (16 to 20 percent).

It must be remembered, however, that foods such as butter, margarines, salad oils, and cooking fats are "visible" fats, and we are conscious of how much of them we use. However, we often fail to recognize that approximately

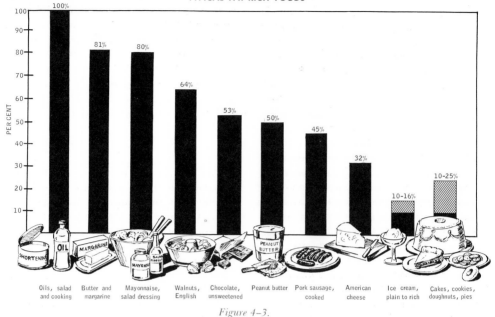

Figure 4–3.

half of our total fat intake comes from the "hidden fat" in meats, nuts, whole milk, cream, ice cream, cheese, nuts, and pastries. Thus, even though all visible fat is trimmed off meats, the separated lean meat (cooked) still contains 4 to 15 percent "hidden" fat. It often contains more in the case of choice cuts, in which the flesh is "marbled" with fat.

Linoleic Acid, a Dietary Essential

The body tissues possess a marked ability to build (synthesize) complex compounds by combining relatively simple ones. It is well known that excess carbohydrate or protein can be transformed into fat for deposition in fatty tissues. For this purpose, the long carbon chains of saturated fatty acids (and also oleic acid with one double bond) are built by combining simple (2-carbon) acetate radicals. However, the body is not able to synthesize *linoleic acid*, a very

important polyunsaturated fatty acid which contains two double bonds (see formula in Appendix, Table 12). Linoleic acid, therefore, is an *essential fatty acid*, since it has to be obtained in the diet for growth and well-being of all species of higher animals, including man. Arachidonic acid, with four double bonds and 20 carbon atoms, used to be included as an essential fatty acid, but since it is found in nature only in animal foods (and then only in less than adequate levels), and since it can be readily made in the body from linoleic acid, it is not actually essential in the diet. In the past the term "vitamin F" was sometimes used for the essential fatty acids. Though the dietary need for linoleic acid is somewhat similar to the need for vitamins, it is not actually a vitamin and the use of the term "vitamin F" for this purpose is a misnomer.

The discovery of the need for linoleic acid began in 1929, when Burr and Burr demonstrated that rats fed on fat-free diets (adequate as to other nutrients) failed to grow or lost weight, developed a scaly condition of the skin and tail, and developed kidney damage that eventually led to their death.[2] These conditions could be prevented or alleviated by giving linoleic acid.[3] Hansen and coworkers were the first to diagnose symptoms in infants of poor growth and eczematous skin lesions due to a deficiency of essential fatty acids (Fig. 4–4).[4, 5]

Other workers in this field[6, 7] concur and place the minimum requirement for infants at 1.4 to 4.5 percent of the calories furnished as linoleic acid, the higher requirement being for premature babies. Human milk and commercially prepared formulas provide a generous allowance of linoleic acid, but formulas based on cow's milk just barely meet the minimum requirement. Hansen and associates have done extensive work in this field and have definitely established that adults as well as infants require essential fatty acids.[8]

There is no set allowance for essential fatty acids, but the Food and Nutrition Board[9] states that linoleic acid intake equivalent to nearly 2 percent of the total calories in the diet should be sufficient for adults (e.g., about 6 gm per day in a diet of 2700 kcal) and 3 percent of calories for infants. The average American diet seems to at least meet this requirement.[10]

Metabolic Functions of Fat

The disadvantage of having separate chapters on lipids, proteins, and carbohydrates is that the student may not appreciate how closely related these various compounds are within the body itself. They are intimately and dynamically related within each body cell and in all body functions. To separate certain compounds as being more important than others, metabolically, would be very difficult, and even to study them separately can be misleading unless this close relationship is clearly understood.

The various lipids play extremely important roles, metabolically, in many

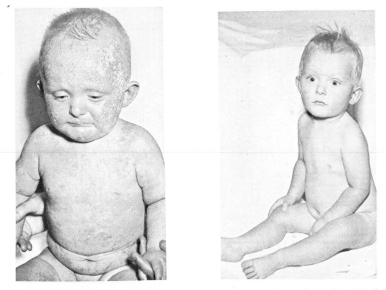

Figure 4–4. Certain fatty acids, found in fats of low melting point, must be furnished in the food. Skin troubles result when these essential fatty acids are lacking. **Left,** Six month old infant with very resistant eczema since 2½ months of age. **Right,** The same child 6 months later, after a source of linoleic acid had been included in the diet. (Courtesy of Dr. A. E. Hansen.)

enzyme reactions, in cell membrane structure, in the synthesis and regulation of certain hormones, in the maintenance of the proper structure of blood vessels, and in energy metabolism, digestion, tissue structure, nerve impulse transmission, memory storage, and others. In recent years, for instance, we have learned of the importance of *prostaglandins*, a class of vital hormone-like compounds made in various tissues of the body from arachidonic acid (and other derivatives of linoleic acid) and important in the regulation of such diverse reactions as gastric secretion, pancreatic functions, release of pituitary hormones, and in smooth muscle metabolism.[11, 12] Clearly, fats can no longer be considered just as a source of energy for body heat and work.

Sources of Linoleic Acid

Table 4–1 summarizes the content of saturated and unsaturated fatty acids and linoleic acid in several common foods.[13] One can readily see that most of the fats of animal origin are relatively high in saturated fatty acids, and though the unsaturated fatty acids are also high, this is mostly attributable to oleic acid. The polyunsaturated fatty acid content (as measured by linoleic acid) in most fats of animal origin is only moderate. The amount in eggs, poultry, and red meats can be influenced to a limited extent by the kinds and amount of dietary fatty acids (though this is not a practical means of greatly increasing linoleic acid consumption).

Vegetable fats, on the other hand, generally have a much lower content of saturated fatty acids, with a relatively high content of unsaturated fatty acid and linoleic acid. Corn, cottonseed, soybean, and wheat-germ oil are especially rich in linoleic acid, while margarines, vegetable shortenings, and peanut oil are good sources of linoleic acid.

Table 4–1. Distribution of Saturated and Unsaturated Fatty Acids in Some Common Food Fats*

		Edible Portion of Food		
	% Fat	% of Total Fat†		
		SATURATED	OLEIC	LINOLEIC ACID
Animal fats				
Beef	5–37	43–48	43	0.5–3
Butter	81	57	33	3
Egg	11.5	35	44	8.7
Fish (tuna)	4.1	24.4	24.4	0.5
Lamb	21.3	56.5	38	4.7
Milk (whole, pasteurized)	3.7	57	33	3
Pork	52	36.5	42	9.6
Vegetable fats				
Coconut oil	100	85	6	0.5
Corn oil	100	10	28	53
Cottonseed oil	100	25	21	50
Margarine, regular	81	22.2	58	17.3
Margarine, special	81	23.4	38.3	36
Peanut oil	100	18	47	29
Shortening, hydrogenated vegetable oils	100	23	65	7
Soybean oil	100	15	20	52

*Figures adapted from U.S. Department of Agriculture, Handbook 8.[13] Also see Waltking, A. E.: Nutr. Rep. Int'l., 6:17, 1972.

†Figures do not add up to 100 because there are additional unsaturated fatty acids and other fats.

From a nutritional point of view it is often important to know the kind, and fatty acid composition, of the fat one is consuming. It is hoped that improved labeling of manufactured food products will provide more information about this matter in the future.

Lipids Other Than True Fats

The term *lipid* is applied to any substance that has physical properties similar to fats—that is, oily or greasy in consistency and soluble in fat solvents. In addition to true fats and fatty acids, lipids include some substances chemically related to fats plus some others that are totally unrelated. *Phospholipids*, for example, are composed of glyceryl esters of only two fatty acids plus a non-lipid component instead of the usual third fatty acid in a true fat. The phospholipid *lecithin*, which is prominent in egg yolk, is formed by the union of one molecule of glycerol, two molecules of fatty acid, and one molecule each of phosphoric acid and choline, a nitrogenous base. All phospholipids contain phosphoric acid radicals but differ in that other non-fat compounds may take the place of choline or a fatty acid group. Groups may also be attached to a substance other than glycerol in other types of lipids. A third class of lipids consists of the *sterols*, which are complex alcohols of high molecular weight. *Cholesterol* is the most prominent member of this group found in the body, while ergosterol and sitosterol are common sterols found in plants.

Phospholipids and sterols are widely distributed in small amounts in foods and are normal constituents of body tissues. They are concentrated especially in the liver and in lesser amounts in the blood and other tissues. Cholesterol, a normal body constituent, gives rise to an intermediate substance (7-dehydrocholesterol) from which vitamin D is formed by ultraviolet light

when it penetrates the skin. Certain hormones formed in the adrenal cortex and sex glands are also sterols, closely related chemically to cholesterol which serves as a precursor in their synthesis. The bile acids, likewise derivatives of cholesterol, are formed in the liver and excreted by way of the bile into the intestine, from which some may be reabsorbed and used over again, others being excreted in the feces. The same pathway (bile, intestine, feces) serves for the excretion of cholesterol and other related sterols.

Cholesterol is thus seen to be a substance normal in, and useful to, the body. Approximately 2 gm is synthesized, and metabolized, each day within the body of normal adults. The level of cholesterol in the blood is normally kept constant by a balance between the sum of it taken in the diet plus that manufactured in the body, and the amount used up in the body plus that excreted through the intestine along with the bile. This explains why it is so difficult, and in many cases impossible, to lower the cholesterol level in the blood by restricting cholesterol in the diet (see also Chapter 23).

Waxes are included among the lipids and are normally present in very small amounts in many foods usually of vegetable origin. Comb honey is an example of a rich source of dietary wax.

Place of Fat-Rich Foods in the Diet

The amount of fat in the diet may be varied widely, as is the case for carbohydrate intake (p. 59), according to personal tastes, money spent for food, and availability of fat-rich foods. Only about 10 percent of the energy in the average diets of Asiatic peoples is furnished by fats because overpopulation requires that land be used for production of carbohydrate-rich foods, which furnish energy at the least cost, instead of for the production of more expensive meat and dairy products. Among people of moderate means in most European countries, fat intake may account for 10 to 25 percent of their total energy intake. In countries such as Holland, Denmark, New Zealand, Canada, and the United States, meat fats, dairy products, and vegetable oils (or shortenings and spreads made from them) are available at prices most people can afford. Under such conditions, 40 to 45 percent of the energy content of the diet may come from fat-rich foods (which is the United States average intake of fat calories).

Many nutritionists believe that a reduction to a level at which fats furnish only about 25 percent of the calories would be less inclined to result in overweight. Those inclined to overweight or prone to coronary disease are well advised to keep to a lower level of fat intake, at which a normal variety of fats should provide sufficient unsaturated fatty acids.

Perhaps one should also be warned that diets too low in fat are not desirable either. When the diet is very low in fats or practically fat-free either from unavailability of fatty foods, from restriction for weight reduction, or for other therapeutic purposes, the average person cannot or does not increase his consumption of carbohydrates and proteins sufficiently to furnish equivalent energy and so will lose weight and may have less vigor. Also, because essential fatty acids and most fat-soluble vitamins gain entrance to the body through fat intake, a low-fat diet may result in less than adequate amounts of these essential nutrients. Although precursors of vitamin A are found in green and yellow vegetables, it is difficult to eat enough of these foods to supply body needs for this vitamin when the diet is fat-free. Reducing diets that are low in fat probably need to be supplemented with vitamin A in capsule form, and such diets may be more difficult to stick to because of between-meal hunger (see Chapter 23).

QUESTIONS AND PROBLEMS

1. What physical properties are characteristic of fats? What substances does any true fat yield on hydrolysis (in digestion or outside the body)? Consult the diagrams in Figure 4–1 as to the chemical elements and structure of glycerol and fatty acids. How many molecules of fatty acid does a molecule of glycerol link up with to form one molecule of fat? Do the fatty acids most commonly found in fats consist of long or short chains of carbon atoms? Is the proportion of carbon to the amount of hydrogen and oxygen greater or less in a molecule of fatty acid than in a molecule of glucose? How does this account for the fact that, when fats are burned or oxidized in body tissues, they yield more than twice as much energy as carbohydrates do?

2. What is the difference between a saturated and an unsaturated fatty acid (consult Fig. 4–1)? What is the difference between a *mono*unsaturated and a *poly*unsaturated fatty acid? Is oleic acid a polyunsaturated fatty acid? What is the name of the polyunsaturated fatty acid found most abundantly in fatty foods? How do the kinds of fatty acids (saturated or unsaturated) that predominate determine the consistency (solid, semisolid, or liquid) of foods that are almost pure fat? Name two fatty foods that are solid, two that are semisolid, and two that are liquid.

3. What is meant by an essential fatty acid? What symptoms sometimes occur in infants because of insufficient essential fatty acids in their foods? Does essential fatty acid deficiency ever occur in adults on normal diets? Why? If one wished to increase the intake of polyunsaturated fatty acids, what foods should be included in moderate amounts in the diet?

4. How can unsaturated fatty acids be made to take on more hydrogen—that is, be converted into saturated ones? Does butter carry any unsaturated fatty acids? When a fluid fat such as

corn or cottonseed oil is converted to a semisolid by hydrogenation to make cooking fats or margarine, are all the unsaturated fatty acids converted to saturated ones? Consult Table 4–1 and compare the content of unsaturated fatty acids in butter, ordinary margarines, and special margarines.

5. Define lipids, true fats, phospholipids, and sterols. In what body tissues are phospholipids most abundant? What sterol is found in animal tissues and blood? Can it be formed in the body, and if so, where? Is the level of cholesterol in the blood closely related to the amount of it ingested? Does the intake of total calories, the proportion of the caloric intake furnished by fats, or the ratio of saturated to polyunsaturated fats in the diet influence blood cholesterol level? If so, with what results?

6. What are the chief uses of fats in the body? Of fatty foods in the diet? What percentage of the total caloric (fuel) intake is furnished by fats in the average American diet? What are the disadvantages of too high a level of fat in the diet or of very low fat intake? What special foods would you avoid or take in smaller amounts in order to decrease the relative amount of fat in the diet?

REFERENCES

1. McCollum, E. V.: *A History of Nutrition.* Boston, Houghton Mifflin Co., 1957, Chapter 3.
2. Burr, G. O., and Burr, M. M.: A new deficiency disease produced by the rigid exclusion of fat from the diet. J. Biol. Chem., *82*:345, 1929.
3. Burr, G. O., and Burr, M. M.: On the nature and role of the fatty acids essential in nutrition. J. Biol. Chem., *86*:587, 1930.
4. Hansen, A. E.: Serum lipids in eczema and other pathological conditions. Amer. J. Dis. Child., *53*:933, 1937.
5. Hansen, A. E., et al.: Role of linoleic acid in infant nutrition. Pediatrics, *31*:171, 1963.
6. Hughes, G., Kelly, J., and Stewart, A.: Linoleic acid—an essential nutrient: its content in infant formulas and pre-cooked cereals. Clin. Pediat., 2:555, 1963.
7. Holman, R. T., et al.: The essential fatty acid requirement of infants and assessment of their dietary intake of linoleate. Amer. J. Clin. Med., *14*:70, 1964.
8. Wiese, H. F., Gibbs, R. H., and Hansen, A. E.: Essential fatty acids in human nutrition, I and II. J. Nutr., *52*:355 and 367, 1954; and Wiese, H. F., Hansen, A. E., and Adams, D. J. D.: Essential fatty acids in human nutrition. J. Nutr., *66*:345, 1955.
9. Food and Nutrition Board: *Recommended Dietary Allowances.* Washington D.C., National Academy of Sciences, Publ. 1694 (7th Ed.), p. 10, 1968.
10. Food and Nutrition Board: *Dietary Fat and Human Health.* Washington D.C., National Academy of Sciences, Publ. 1147, 1966.
11. von Euler, U. S., and Eliasson, R.: *Prostaglandins.* New York, Academic Press, 1967.
12. Pickles, V. R.: Prostaglandins. Nature, *224*: 221, 1969.
13. Watt, B. K., and Merrill, A. L.: *Composition of Foods.* U.S. Department of Agriculture, Handbook 8, p. 122, 1963.

SUPPLEMENTARY READING

Albin, I. A., Seik, T. J., Sather, L. A., and Lindsay, R. C.: Flavor preferences for butter and margarine. J. Dairy Sci., *52*:394, 1969.

Albutt, E. C., and Chance, G. W.: Plasma and adipose tissue fatty acids of diabetic children on long-term corn oil diets. J. Clin. Invest., *48*:139, 1969.

Ali, S. S., and Kuksis, A.: Excretion of phospholipids by men on fat-free diet. Canad. J. Biochem., *45*:689, 1967.

Antonis, A., et al.: The influence of seasonal variation, diet and physical activity on serum lipids in young men in Antarctica. Amer. J. Clin. Nutr., *16*:428, 1965.

Birkbeck, J. A.: The fatty acid composition of depot fat in childhood: II. A comparison of superficial and deep fat. Lipids, *6*:212, 1971.

Bogert, L. J.: Fats and related substances. In *Fundamentals of Chemistry.* 9th Ed., Philadelphia, W. B. Saunders, 1963, Chap. 23, p. 386.

Call, D. L., and Sanchez, A. M.: Trends in fat disappearance in the United States 1909–65. J. Nutr., *93*: (Suppl. 1, Part II), 1967.

Casdorph, H. R.: Fats in the diet. Geriatrics, *20*:168, 1965.

Caster, W. O.: Studies of butterfat as related to human nutrition. Food Product Development, May 23, 1969.

Council on Foods and Nutrition of the American Medical Association: How essential are fatty acids? J. Amer. Med. Assoc., *178*: 930, 1961.

Dayton, S., Hashimoto, S., Dixon, W., and Pearce, M. L.: Composition of lipids in human serum and adipose tissue during prolonged feeding of a diet high in unsaturated fat. J. Lipid Res., 7:103, 1966.

Evans, D. W., Turner, S. M., and Ghosh, P.: Feasibility of long-term plasma-cholesterol reduction by diet. Lancet, 1:172, 1972.

Feeley, R. M., Staton, A. L., and Moyer, E. Z.: Fat metabolism in pre-adolescent children on all-vegetable diets. J. Amer. Dietet. Assoc., 47:396, 1965.

Griffith, W. H.: The fatty acid story—lessons and expectations. J. Nutr., 91 (Supp. 1):17, 1967.

Holman, R. T., et al.: The essential fatty acid requirement of infants and assessment of their dietary intake of linoleate. Amer. J. Clin. Med., 14:70, 1964.

Hughes, G., et al.: Linoleic acid—an essential nutrient and its content in infant formulas and precooked cereals. Clin. Pediat., 2:555, 1963.

Insull, W., Jr., Lang, P. D., and Hsi, B. P.: Adipose tissue fatty acid differences in American men between 1962 and 1966. Amer. J. Clin. Nutr., 23:17, 1970.

Jagannathan, S. N.: Fatty acid composition of adipose tissue in Indian adults: Sex difference and influence of pregnancy. Ind. J. Biochem., 6:222, 1969.

Kilgore, L., and Bailey, M.: Degradation of linoleic acid during potato frying. J. Amer. Dietet. Assoc., 56:130, 1970.

Kritchevsky, D., Tepper, S. A., DiTullo, N. W., and Holmes, W. L.: The sterols of seafood. J. Food Sci., 32:64, 1967.

McKay, D. G., Kaunitz, H., Csavossy, I., and Johnson, R. E.: Electron microscope studies of the absorption of lipids. III. Long chain saturated triglycerides. Metabolism, 16:137, 1967.

Mellati, A. M., Beck, J. C., Dupre, J., and Rubinstein, D.: Conversion of glucose to lipid by human adipose tissue in vitro. Metabolism, 19:988, 1970.

Melnick, D.: Development of organoleptically and nutritionally improved margarine products. J. Home Econ., 60:793, 1968.

Mikasta, S. C.: Margarine: 100 years of technological and legal progress. J. Amer. Oil Chem. Soc., 48:169A, 1971.

Murphy, E. W., Page, L., and Koons, P. C.: Lipid components of type A school lunches. J. Amer. Dietet. Assoc., 56:504, 1970.

Nelson, G. J.: The phospholipid composition of plasma in various mammalian species. Lipids, 2:323, 1967.

Nichaman, M. Z., Sweeley, C. C., and Olson, R. E.: Plasma fatty acids in normolipemic and hyperlipemic subjects during fasting and after linoleate feeding. Amer. J. Clin. Nutr., 20:1057, 1967.

Okey, R. (ed.): Basic problems of lipid metabolism of importance to man. California Agricultural Experiment Station, Bulletin 840, 1968.

Pfeiffer, C. J.: Absorption of fat. Postgraduate Medicine, December, A-83, 1967.

Pikaar, N. A., and Fernandes, J.: Influence of different types of dietary fat on the fatty acid composition of some serum lipid fractions in infants and children. Amer. J. Clin. Nutr., 19:194, 1966.

Rao, K. S. J., and Prasad, P. S. K.: Serum triglycerides and nonesterified fatty acids in kwashiorkor. Amer. J. Clin. Nutr., 19:205, 1966.

Scheig, R.: What is dietary fat? Amer. J. Clin. Nutr., 22:651, 1969.

Schlierf, C., Falor, W. H., Wood, P. D., Lee, Y., and Kinsell, L. W.: Composition of human chyle chylomicrons following single fat feedings. Amer. J. Clin. Nutr., 22:79, 1969.

Slotbloom, A. J., and Bonsen, P. P. M.: Recent developments in the chemistry of phospholipids. Chem. Phys. Lipids, 5:301, 1970.

Stroink, J. B. A.: Composition and consumption of dietary fats in U.S.A., U.K. and common market countries in 1961. Nutr. Dieta, 9:56, 1967.

Trulson, M. F., et al.: Comparisons of siblings in Boston and Ireland. J. Amer. Dietet. Assoc., 45:225, 1964.

Underwood, B. A., Hashim, S. A., and Sebrell, W. H.: Fatty acid absorption and metabolism in protein-calorie malnutrition. I. Effect of fat-free and fat-containing diets on fecal fatty acids. Amer. J. Clin. Nutr., 20:226, 1967.

Wiese, H. F., et al.: Skin lipids of puppies as affected by kind and amount of dietary fat. J. Nutrition, 89:113, 1966.

Wilcox, E., Hawthorne, B. E., and Okey, R.: Cholesterol. California Agricultural Experiment Station, Bulletin 785, 1962.

Yudkin, I.: Dietary fat and dietary sugar in relation to ischemic heart disease and diabetes. Lancet, 2:4, 1964.

Zilversmit, D. B.: Formation and transport of chylomicrons. Fed. Proc., 26:1599, 1967.

Nutrition Reviews

Unsaturated fatty acid isomers in nutrition (by Aaes-Jørgensen, E.). 24:1, 1966.

Present knowledge of fat (by Mead, J. F.). 24:33, 1966.

Dietary fat in essential hyperlipemia. 24:103, 1966.

Citrate cleavage and lipogenesis. 24:153, 1966.

Nutritional evaluation of inter-esterified fats. 24:201, 1966.

Present knowledge of intravenous fat emulsions (by Jones, R. J.). 24:225, 1966.

Mineral oil in human tissues. 25:46, 1967.

Metabolism of polyunsaturated fatty acids. 25:90, 1967.

five

Protein

We have seen that carbohydrates and fats are widely distributed in both plants and animals and that they are made up of carbon, hydrogen, and oxygen, in varying proportions and combinations. Proteins are larger and more complex molecules than those of either fats or carbohydrates, and they are the only class of energy nutrients that contain *nitrogen* (in addition to carbon, hydrogen, and oxygen). Most also contain sulfur, and many contain phosphorus, iron, or other minerals. Proteins are present in all living tissues—plant or animal—and they are essential to life, because proteins are a vital part of the nucleus and protoplasm of every cell. Protein makes up more than half of all the organic matter in the human body.

Various tissues each contain proteins that are peculiar to themselves and that are present in varying amounts according to the types of tissues. The outer layers of skin, the hair, and the nails consist almost entirely of an insoluble protein called *keratin*. The most active and abundant tissues of the body—the muscles and glandular organs—are high in protein content. Muscles contain

about 70 percent water, but even on a moist basis, lean muscle, heart, and liver contain 17 to 21 percent protein, by far their most abundant solid constituent. Connective tissues consist mainly of proteins with quite different properties from muscle. Blood carries the important iron-containing protein *hemoglobin* in red cells and several proteins in the fluid (plasma) portion. Even fatty tissue, which acts chiefly as a storage depot for excess fat, has some protein, though a small amount.

The large molecules of the proteins are made up of great numbers of relatively simple units, the nitrogen-containing compounds called ***amino acids***. These basic units all contain at least one organic acid radical (COOH) and one amino radical (NH_2) (Fig. 5–1). A few amino acid molecules contain two acid or two amino groups. Some 22 different amino acids are known to be present fairly commonly in proteins that occur in nature. The number of different amino acids in the molecules of individual proteins varies from 8 to 18, according to the size and complexity of the molecules of different proteins. These amino acids are joined together in an intricate pattern characteristic of each individual protein. Because not

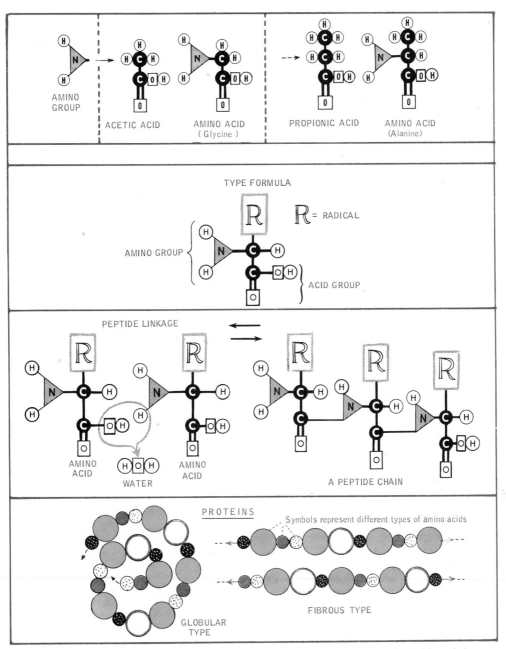

Figure 5–1. Diagrammatic representation of the arrangement of atoms in amino acids and the way they link up to form proteins (peptide linkage). The nitrogen is present in amino groups attached to $\left[\begin{array}{c} \textbf{N} \; (NH_2) \end{array} \right]$ the carbon atom next to the acid group (COOH); the rest of the amino acid molecule may be represented by R (radical), which may be relatively simple (as in glycine and alanine shown above) or very complex. Amino acids are linked by the acid group of one joining with the amino group of another, splitting off water. When many different amino acids are linked together in long chains, coiled or straight, they form the large protein molecules, small sections of which are represented in the diagram at bottom of this drawing.

only the kinds of amino acids may vary but also the relative quantities of each, the number of individual proteins that are possible is almost infinite. The molecules of protein are so large that their molecular weight varies from several thousand up to several million.

The manner in which the amino acids link together to form proteins is important in that it is common to all proteins. This is called *peptide linkage* (Fig. 5–1). Since each amino acid carries a terminal acid group (COOH) and an amino group (NH_2) attached to the carbon atom next to the acid group, the basic amino group of one molecule can react with the acid group of another, linking up by the loss of one hydrogen atom and one OH radical, with the formation of a molecule of water. When proteins are broken down, as happens in digestion, by reaction with water (hydrolysis) the components of water (H and OH) lost when the peptide link was formed are restored to the individual amino acids, the peptide linkage is broken, and the protein molecule is broken down into the amino acids (building blocks) from which it was originally formed. Proteins must first be resolved into their constituent amino acids by digestion before they can be absorbed into the blood, and when they are thus carried to the tissues, each tissue utilizes the specific amino acids required to build its own characteristic proteins.

Conjugated Proteins: The Biological Importance of Nucleoproteins

The preceding discussion applies chiefly to **simple proteins**—those that yield only amino acids on hydrolysis. These are of course prominent both in foods and in the body. Proteins that are soluble in water or in dilute salt solution (albumins and globulins) predominate in animal fluids such as blood, while other globulins, such as myosin in muscles, are prominent in the tissues. Readily soluble proteins such as the albumins are present in egg white and

milk; less readily soluble proteins are found in grains (glutenin and gliadin in wheat, zein in corn).

Conjugated proteins are even more complicated molecules than simple proteins. They are *compounds of proteins with some nonprotein substance.* Hence, they yield on hydrolysis, in addition to amino acids, some other substance or substances. Protein molecules may be conjugated with *fat* (lipoproteins in the blood) or *carbohydrate* (glycoproteins, such as are found in the mucus secreted into the digestive tract). Other important conjugated proteins are formed by linkage with *phosphoric acid* (phosphoproteins); with the lipid *lecithin* (fibrin in clotted blood, vitellin in egg yolk); with an *iron-containing* compound (heme) to form the oxygen-carrying substance *hemoglobin* in the blood; and with *nucleic acid* to form nucleoproteins, which are essential components of cell nuclei and protoplasm.

By intensive study of the *nucleoproteins,* scientists have made extremely important discoveries concerning the life processes of body cells. Nucleoproteins may be broken down into proteins and nucleic acids, complex compounds that in turn may be broken down to yield phosphoric acid, a five-carbon sugar, and cyclic nitrogenous bases (purines and pyrimidines). The sugar is either ribose or deoxyribose; accordingly, the two types of nucleic acid are known as *ribonucleic acid* (RNA) and *deoxyribonucleic acid* (DNA).

DNA is found in all cell nuclei and is different for each species (even slightly so for individuals within a species). These differences consist of minor rearrangements or sequences among the nitrogenous bases, which constitute a *code* containing all the information on the heritable characteristics of cells, tissues, organs, and individuals. Only four nitrogenous bases are found in DNA; these are adenine, guanine, thymine, and cytosine. The heredity or genetic code can be thought of as a string of about 10,000 words in which the bases occur in specific frequencies and patterns (ATGC, CGTA, etc.). The DNA structure is a long, fibrous molecule with two spiral "backbones," consisting of linked sugar and phosphate groups twined about a common axis, forming a double helix (Fig. 5–2). The nitrogenous bases are attached in these spirals so as to extend inward and approach each other in pairs that are joined by a weak hydrogen bond. Of the four bases, adenine can form a pair only with thymine; guanine, only with cytosine. The code by which DNA directs the formation and life processes of various cells consists in variations in the kinds and sequences of these pairs.

Ribonucleic acid (RNA) is the messenger that transmits the coded information of DNA. RNA is similar to DNA in structure but differs in two respects — the sugar in the spiral chains is ribose (instead of deoxyribose), and among the nitrogenous bases, uracil is substituted for thymine. The RNA, formed in the cell nuclei under the direction of DNA, migrates to the surface of granules (ribosomes) in the fluid portion of the cell (cytoplasm). (See Chapter 14.) Another type of RNA — *transfer RNA* — picks up certain amino acids from the cytoplasm and transfers these amino acids to the messenger RNA, where they are lined up in proper order to form specific enzymes or cell proteins (Fig. 5–3).

What we know of the composition and structure of DNA and RNA molecules has been proved, but the concepts of how they bring about their effects in the cells are chiefly theoretical and are still being revised.

Nitrogen Cycle in Nature

Considering all forms of life, it is the element nitrogen that is indispensable for life, rather than protein, for plants can use the simple nitrogen-containing inorganic compounds in the soil (chiefly nitrates) to build their own special kinds of protein. The carbon, hydrogen, and oxygen are furnished by water and carbon dioxide in the air. Some bacteria can even utilize gaseous nitrogen from the air. Animals, however, cannot utilize these simpler sources of nitrogen for the synthesis of proteins, but must get their amino groups pre-formed, directly from plant foods, from single celled organisms, or from the proteins in the milk, eggs, or body tissues of other animals. The animal converts the amino acids, which enter the tissues as products of protein digestion, into the special proteins and other nitrogen-containing compounds needed for maintenance of tissues and life processes. The final end products of protein metabolism in the animal's tissues are the

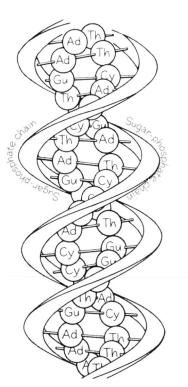

Figure 5–2. Diagram of structure of DNA, showing the double coils of sugar and phosphate groups, with the purines and pyrimidines (adenine, thymine, guanine, and cytosine) joined in pairs by hydrogen bonds, thus holding the molecule in a rigid structure. (From Carpenter: *Microbiology.* Philadelphia, W. B. Saunders.)

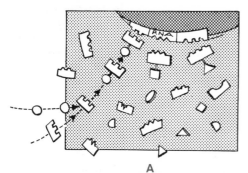

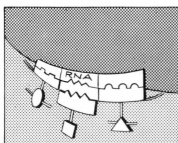

A

B

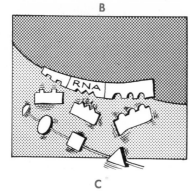

C

Figure 5–3. Schematic representation of the manner in which RNA functions to bring about synthesis of enzymes and other proteins in the cell. The RNA is made by DNA in the cell nucleus, and then migrates to ribosomes (small dense particles of cytoplasm outside the nucleus) to whose surface it becomes attached. These three diagrams represent the later stages of protein formation.

A, RNA attached to ribosome (*dark surface*) attracts small sections of another kind of RNA (transfer RNA), each link of which fits into a specific section of the original RNA. The sections of transfer RNA, in turn, each attract some specific amino acid from the cytoplasm.

B, The sections of transfer RNA, each carrying a certain amino acid, migrate to the RNA on the surface of the ribosome (messenger RNA), where they attach themselves in a regular order. The amino acids that the sections of transfer RNA carry are thus brought close together and lined up in a definite order.

C, The amino acids link together and separate from the transfer RNA as a protein chain, thus forming a molecule of some specific protein. The transfer RNA sections are freed from the RNA attached to the ribosome and ready for use in further protein synthesis.

Only a small part of the large molecules of RNA and protein can be shown in the diagrams. The hormone insulin (a relatively simple protein) was the first protein for which the order and arrangement of amino acids is known. In its molecule there are 51 amino acid residues. Myoglobin (a muscle component) consists of an ordered sequence of 153 amino acids and hemoglobin of more than 600 amino acids.

simpler compounds that plants can use to build into amino acids and protein. This completes the "nitrogen cycle," if the excreta of animals and the products of the decay of both plants and animals, which contain nitrates and ammonium compounds, are returned to the soil.

Amino Acids, Essential and Nonessential

Certain amino acids are known to be *essential*—that is, they must be provided pre-formed in the food. In reality, all amino acids are essential for the build-ing and upkeep of body tissues, but more than half the number needed can be made in the body if insufficient amounts are furnished in food. Hence, an amino acid is referred to as *nutritionally essential* or *indispensable* only if it cannot be synthesized in the body out of materials ordinarily available at a speed that will supply the demands for normal growth. Rose and co-workers at the University of Illinois found that ten different amino acids must be supplied in adequate amounts in the food to support normal growth in young rats, whereas his evidence indicated that only eight of these were essential for maintenance of nitrogen equilibrium in fully grown young men.[1]

The type formula of amino acids is given as

$$\underset{\underset{\displaystyle H}{|}}{\overset{\overset{\displaystyle NH_2}{|}}{R-C-COOH.}}$$

In the nonessential amino acid alanine, the radical represented by R is simply CH_3. The body can make this amino acid readily in any amount needed because the carbon chain is a common metabolic product to which the amino group from some donor amino acid can be added. Phenylalanine in whose molecule R represents a ring, or cyclic group (Fig. 5–4), cannot be made in the body but must be supplied pre-formed in the food. The phenyl radical in phenylalanine consists of six carbon atoms joined in a hexagonal ring with hydrogens attached (C_6H_5). The R in tryptophan is more complex—a closed cyclic structure of carbon atoms with one nitrogen.* Neither of these carbon skeletons can be formed in the human body, so these amino acids cannot be manufactured even though donor amino groups are available.

The nonessential amino acids tyrosine and cystine are an intermediate class, between amino acids that can easily be formed from a number of precursors and those that cannot be made at all. Tyrosine can be made only from the essential amino acid phenylalanine, by addition of one OH group, and the reverse reaction (removal of the OH from tyrosine to form phenylalanine) does not take place. Part of the need for phenylalanine in the body is to form tyrosine if the latter is not included in the diet. Thus, the presence of tyrosine will reduce the amount of phenylalanine required in the diet. The nonessential sulfur-containing amino acid cystine can be formed from the essential amino acid methionine, and the reaction is not reversible. The cystine needed in the body (to make hair protein, for example) may be supplied in the diet as cystine, or it will be made from methionine if no cystine is eaten. Thus, cystine will spare the need for methionine. Other nonessential amino acids (such as alanine and glycine) can be assembled from carbon chains derived from the metabolism of carbohydrates, fats, or proteins, and amino groups taken from amino acids or other amino-containing compounds. Proteins of the human body include both the essential and nonessential amino acids in their structure, but the nonessential ones can be manufactured, provided the necessary precursors are available.

---

*For those who wish to know more about the chemical differences among amino acids, the structural formulas of the amino acids commonly found in foods or tissues are given in Table 13 of the Appendix (pp. 580–582).

Functions of Protein in the Body

The principal uses for protein in the body are as follows:

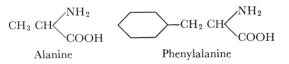

Alanine   Phenylalanine

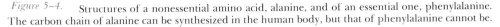

Figure 5–4. Structures of a nonessential amino acid, alanine, and of an essential one, phenylalanine. The carbon chain of alanine can be synthesized in the human body, but that of phenylalanine cannot be.

1. For *building new tissues* in growing children, during pregnancy, in athletic training, and after injury.

2. For *upkeep of tissues* already built and replacement of regular losses.

3. As *regulatory substances* for internal water and acid-base balances.

4. As a *precursor* for enzymes, antibodies, some hormones, and one of the B vitamins.

5. For *milk* formation.

6. For *energy*.

BUILDING NEW TISSUES. Since protein is vital to body tissues, and we cannot form protein from simple nitrogen compounds as plants do, amino acids must be supplied in the diet for building new tissues. Proteins provide the amino acids from which the bases of the information code (adenine, etc., in DNA and RNA) are made as well as the substance of the cells.

The *amount* needed for these purposes naturally depends on the extent or rapidity of these processes. For instance, in the rapidly growing infant as much as one-third of the dietary protein may be retained for building new tissue. As growth becomes less rapid, the percentage of the protein intake retained in the body for tissue building becomes less, but a plentiful supply of high quality protein is necessary throughout the growth period to secure the best possible growth and development. In the later months of pregnancy an extra quota of protein is also needed. Likewise, an athlete in training may require some extra protein for building muscle tissue, because his muscles strengthen and enlarge as a result of exercise.

Excessive destruction of body protein occurs in various periods of stress. Obviously, after severe hemorrhages, extra protein is needed for regeneration of hemoglobin and other blood proteins. Also after extensive burns, there is excessive loss of protein from the burn surface, as well as need for protein to rebuild damaged skin and muscle tissues. A slow but prolonged loss of nitrogen from extra breakdown

of body protein follows bone fractures, and a similar but brief protein loss occurs even after simple surgical operations. Selye's pioneering studies demonstrated that this catabolic reaction of the body to trauma is due to increased output of hormones from the pituitary and adrenal glands.[2] Increased quantities of protein or amino acids are properly given during convalescence, when the metabolic processes become anabolic, to replenish the body protein. If the patient cannot take nourishment by mouth, he is given intravenous solutions of amino acids (protein hydrolysates), with glucose or emulsified fat added to provide energy and to spare protein.

MAINTENANCE OF TISSUES. Although the adult does not build new tissues as a child does, there are some tissues that never stop growing, even in the aged. Skin, hair, and nails are obvious examples. The lining of the intestinal tract is renewed about every day and a half; much of this cellular protein is absorbed but some cells are lost in the fecal matter. Blood cells have a limited life span of 120 days and if replacement protein is not adequate for formation of new cells, anemia develops. In fact, all the body proteins are constantly being degraded and resynthesized (turned over) at varying rates. So the continuous need for protein to provide for maintenance of tissues already built should not be thought of as due exclusively to death of tissue cells. Functional proteins in and outside of cells continuously turn over in carrying out life processes.

Proteins in the cells are in a state of dynamic equilibrium with the amino acid mixtures (resulting from digestion of protein in foods and catabolism of body proteins) brought to them by the blood and extracellular fluids (Fig. 5–5). The cells transfer some amino acids to the surrounding fluid and take up others from it for utilization in the tissues. This constant flux was discovered by administering amino acids tagged with nitrogen-15, an isotope of ordinary nitrogen. A good deal of this heavy ni-

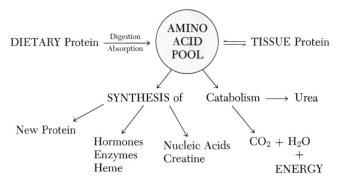

Figure 5–5. Amino acids from food and body tissues enter a common pool which is drawn upon for synthesis of protein and other compounds or from which amino acids are degraded for energy needs. (From Routh, Eyman and Burton: *Essentials of General, Organic and Biochemistry.* Philadelphia, W. B. Saunders.)

trogen failed to appear in the urine as would have been expected if tissues were static, proving that the labeled amino acids must have been rather freely taken up by tissue cells.[3] Thus, a supply of protein is needed for upkeep of the tissues and is indispensable to life.

REGULATORY FUNCTIONS. Proteins in tissue cells and in body fluids, such as the blood, also serve as regulatory substances. Because of their contribution to osmotic pressure, proteins exert an important influence on the exchange of water between tissue cells and the surrounding body fluids, and upon the *water balance* of the body as a whole. For instance, after a prolonged low level of protein intake, the protein content of the blood serum may be less than normal; under such conditions, extra water is retained in the tissues, which become puffy and swollen, making supply of nutrients to the cells and removal of cellular waste products less efficient. This condition is known as starvation, low-protein, or nutritional *edema,* to differentiate it from water accumulation due to disease processes. The ingestion of extra protein sufficient to raise the level of serum protein to normal is followed by excretion of the excess water by the kidneys and disappearance of the edema. Such retention of extra water in the tissues is often

seen in persons who have suffered prolonged undernutrition, and it is a common symptom of protein-deficiency disease in children. A plump-looking malnourished baby is often revealed to be pitifully thin when the refeeding regimen restores normal water distribution and edema disappears.

A second regulatory function of proteins is in maintenance of *acid-base balance* of the blood and tissues. The reaction of blood and tissues is normally maintained very slightly alkaline (pH 7.4) by balance between several different factors, one of which is their protein content. Through the basic amino (NH_2) groups and the organic acid (COOH) radicals present in all amino acids, proteins are able to unite with either acidic or alkaline substances, as these may be taken in or arise in the body from metabolic processes. When these substances are bound by protein, they have little effect on the level of tissue acidity. Considerable amounts of acids formed in metabolism may thus be discharged into the blood stream without any free acid being present to make the reaction of the blood more acid. Hemoglobin and oxyhemoglobin in red cells of the blood also help maintain acid-base equilibrium by forming loose chemical combination with carbon dioxide from cellular metabolism. (Carbon dioxide in water

forms a weak acid, carbonic acid.) Ultimately, carbon dioxide is excreted in
expired air.

PRECURSORS OF ENZYMES, ANTIBODIES,
HORMONES, AND A VITAMIN. Smaller
amounts of protein, or of certain amino
acids, are needed for making enzymes*
that are essential for digestion and
metabolic processes in the tissues; for
making such potent hormones† as those
of the thyroid gland (thyroxine), adrenal glands (epinephrine or "adrena-
line"), and pancreas (insulin); and for
building the antibodies that help ward
off infectious diseases. It has also been
shown that the amino acid tryptophan
can act as a precursor of niacin, one of
the B-complex vitamins. Another amino
acid—methionine—is related indirectly
to two other B vitamins, for less of these
vitamins is needed when plenty of
methionine is supplied by the diet.
(See Chapter 7.)

MILK FORMATION. The proteins of
human milk are built by the mammary
glands. During lactation a woman needs
as much extra protein in the diet as
she secretes in her milk plus the amount
required for conversion of dietary amino
acids to milk protein. This will be discussed in Chapter 19.

PROVIDING ENERGY. If more protein
is eaten than is needed for the essential
functions listed above, this extra protein is oxidized to supply energy or is
converted to body fat if the total energy
intake is excessive. If the energy intake
is inadequate, i.e., if the diet does not
supply carbohydrates and fats in suffi-

cient quantity to meet the energy needs
of the body, proteins are burned for
energy, because *energy needs have a
higher priority than does maintenance of
some of the tissue proteins.* In this event,
building or repair processes will suffer.

Nitrogen, which is indispensable as
long as protein is used for tissue building, becomes a liability when it is necessary to use protein for energy. Amino
(NH_2) groups are split off from the
constituent amino acids and formed
into simple nitrogen-containing substances (chiefly urea) that are excreted
by the kidneys. The non-nitrogenous
fragments of amino acids, the carbon
chains, are then oxidized in the same
way that carbohydrates and fats are
metabolized. Since energy is more
economically supplied by carbohydrates
and fats, the consumption of protein
greatly in excess of body need for amino
acids is usually disadvantageous. On
the other hand, it is certainly unwise
to take a low-calorie diet that is likewise
low in protein, since the body may then
be forced to burn for energy protein
needed for tissue building or upkeep.
When caloric inadequacy is superimposed on limited protein supply, as it
often is among poor peoples all over
the world, protein deficiency disease
becomes rampant.

THE PROTEIN REQUIREMENT

Proteins were referred to as "al-
buminous matter" until 1838, when
Mulder coined the word *protein* from
a Greek root which means *to come first.*
Their prime importance in living organisms was appreciated by the German
scientist Liebig, who had, however, the
erroneous idea that muscle protein was
the source of energy for muscular work.
(The idea that proteins have some connection with muscular work still persists
in the popular mind, in spite of proof
that most energy for such work comes
from carbohydrate and fat.) With the
idea that working men need the most
protein, Voit in 1881 studied the diets
of German workers and, based on their

---

*Enzymes are substances formed in living cells
that speed up, or catalyze, specific chemical reactions without themselves entering into the reaction. All chemical changes that occur during the
digestion of food and in the tissues of the body
are brought about through the agency of enzymes,
which are themselves proteins (for their formation
in cells through the agency of RNA, see p. 77).

†Hormones are chemical compounds secreted
by the endocrine glands into the blood stream and
thus distributed throughout the body. They act
to regulate and coordinate body processes or the
activity of certain tissues; for example, thyroxine
regulates oxidative processes by which body fuel
is burned and energy set free (see p. 31).

usual consumption of protein, suggested 118 gm of protein daily as a desirable allowance for this nutrient. In 1902, the American pioneer in nutrition, Atwater, recommended an allowance of 125 gm of protein, based on studies of protein consumption among men.[4] We know now that these figures are far above the actual *need* for protein but instead reflect the consumption of meats that was customary in the groups surveyed.

Chittenden of Yale was the first to maintain (1904) that such a high intake of protein is not only unnecessary for maintenance of body tissues but might even be disadvantageous to health. For months he studied a volunteer group of athletes and soldiers (men who performed considerable muscular work) given a low-protein diet. He found that 44 to 53 gm of protein daily sufficed to keep them in excellent health, with their physical abilities in no way lessened.[5] Chittenden kept his own protein intake to about 35 gm a day for years and maintained that, as compared with his previous history, he was freer from minor ailments and more vigorous on such a diet. Since he lived to be over 80 years old, he apparently suffered little or no damage thereby. Over 40 years later, Chittenden's findings were confirmed by other investigators, who found that men and women could exist without apparent harm on intakes of protein from vegetable foods at a level of 25 to 40 gm a day.[6]

On the other hand, it is no longer widely believed that harm might come from more liberal consumption of protein. It was supposed that the metabolism of such an excess of nitrogen, above the amount needed for tissue maintenance, might overburden the liver (responsible for the conversion of nitrogen into urea) and the kidneys (which must excrete this urea). The Kroghs found that the Eskimos of Greenland, who subsisted almost entirely on a carnivorous diet, had an average protein intake of 280 gm a day, were healthy, had excellent physical

endurance, and were free from gout and liver and kidney disease.[7] The explorer Stefansson, who had used a nearly all-meat diet in the Arctic for long periods and found it quite satisfactory, with his associate Andersen lived for a year under observation by DuBois while they ate a diet exclusively of meats and animal fats (daily intake: 100 to 140 gm of protein, 200 to 300 gm of fat and only 7 to 12 gm of carbohydrate). They showed no high blood pressure, gout, or liver or kidney damage during or after the test.[8] There is laboratory evidence that an exceptionally large intake of protein—600 gm per day or about 80 to 85 percent of total caloric intake from protein—is undesirable,[9] but no ordinary diet of natural foods would provide anything like that amount of protein. There is no indication of harm from consumption of 300 gm of protein daily if enough drinking water is available to take care of the extra urinary wastes (Chapter 14).

There appears to be a wide range of protein intake to which adults can adapt and be maintained in good health. The consensus now is that a liberal margin over the minimum requirement is good insurance against times of stress, but that superabundant supplies provide no added advantage. Minimal intakes for maintenance of health are of chief interest in parts of the world where protein-rich foods are very scarce or people cannot afford the cost of them. A safe level of intake, or *recommended allowance*, lies between the very low and very high levels of protein intake cited here.

Nitrogen Balance

Nitrogen balance experiments serve to show whether the amount of protein metabolized in the body is equal to, greater than, or less than the amount taken in the food. Because nitrogen makes up (on the average) 16 percent of protein, we determine the nitrogen content of foods and multiply these figures by the factor 6.25 (100 ÷ 16) to give the corresponding values in grams of protein. The nitrogen of the urine represents a measure of how much protein has been broken down and oxidized in the body during a day, since nitrogen-containing end products of protein metabolism leave the body mainly in the urine.* The amount of nitrogen in the feces, consisting of unabsorbed dietary protein, bacteria, and intestinal residues, must also be deducted from intake in estimating balance.† When intake and outgo are practically equal, the body is said to be in *nitrogen* (or protein) *equilibrium*. A *positive* nitrogen balance—intake is greater than output—indicates that new tissue is being built with consequent retention of nitrogen in the body. If output is greater than intake (*negative* balance), some body protein must have been oxidized in addition to that provided in the food.

An interesting fact about nitrogen balance is that it is usually unrelated to the actual need for protein, because the body can establish nitrogen equilibrium at any level of protein intake that is above *the minimum requirement*. We have noted that protein consumption varies widely in different parts of the world according to foods available. The extremes cited were the low-protein, mainly vegetarian diets common in tropical and less affluent societies (50 gm daily, or less) and the traditional diets of polar regions (about 300 gm daily). Where a variety of protein-rich foods is abundant, protein consumption is usually determined by personal preferences, cultural habits, and the money available for food. Most people seem to prefer a diet in which 12 to 15 percent of calories are from protein. The amount of protein used as an energy source when the energy intake is adequate depends upon the protein intake, and adults will be in nitrogen balance with quite different amounts in the excreta, depending on the amount habitually eaten.

There is little provision for storing protein in the body. Ordinarily a positive nitrogen balance, which indicates protein storage in tissues, is found only in conditions such as growth and pregnancy, when new tissues are being formed. Sometimes, after prolonged undernutrition or serious illness, the protein content of tissues becomes depleted, and on giving plenty of protein, retention of nitrogen continues until the normal protein content of the tissues is restored. Also, on changing from a high level of protein consumption to a diet lower in protein, there is always a few days' lag during which nitrogen balance is negative. Likewise there is a delay in adjusting the balance between the amount metabolized and the intake on changing to a higher protein level, and balance is positive for the first several days. Under these conditions the body nitrogen pool‡ is decreased or increased, reflecting gradual adjustment to a changed protein intake.

It is certain that, when energy intake exceeds body needs (whether from carbohydrate, fat, or protein, or combinations of these energy nutrients), most of the excess is converted to fat and stored in the adipose tissues. Whether or not the body can build true protein reserves is uncertain, but on a liberal protein intake, such tissues as the liver and muscles may have a slightly higher content

---

*A small percentage of nitrogen in urine is present in uric acid and creatinine—products of the metabolism of the nitrogen-containing purines and pyrimidines (from nucleoproteins) and creatine. Probably 90 to 95 percent is urea and ammonium salts—end products of protein metabolism.

†Small quantities of nitrogen are also lost in perspiration, menstruum and seminal emissions, nail parings, and hair clippings. Except under conditions in which perspiration is excessive or when unusual accuracy is required, these nitrogen losses, amounting to less than 1 gm daily, are usually disregarded.

‡The word "pool" refers to the total amount of a substance present in the body. "Pool" is a concept, rather than a delineated location, mass or compartment.

of protein, amino acids, or other nitrogenous products. This might constitute a reserve that could be drawn on in time of protein lack or extra need. From studies involving tagging of body proteins by feeding amino acids containing isotopic nitrogen or carbon, scientists have shown that part of the protein in cells is more labile — that is, more readily drawn on for metabolic uses in body tissues — while the remainder is more firmly fixed as cellular constituents that cannot be withdrawn without damage to cells. In protein deficiency the liver is the most susceptible to depletion of cellular protein, the muscles are relatively easy to deplete, and the brain the most difficult. Opinion is divided concerning the functional importance of this labile protein. Some investigators have reported no benefit from a previous high protein intake in rats subsequently deprived of protein, but others reported that pretreatment with protein was beneficial to chicks. The weight of evidence supports the view that liberal protein intakes favor better condition of tissues and perhaps also greater resistance to infections and toxic substances.[10]

Negative nitrogen balance inevitably occurs when the protein intake is reduced below the amount required for maintenance of body tissues — the minimum requirement. However, negative nitrogen balance may occur at levels of protein intake that are above the minimum requirement, if the body is forced to burn protein because the diet furnishes too little carbohydrate and fat to meet the energy requirement. Carbohydrates and fats are both spoken of as being *protein sparers*, for the presence of a liberal quantity of these foodstuffs in the diet does away with the necessity of using protein for energy. It is especially important that the diet supply sufficient carbohydrate and fatty foods to meet energy needs whenever new tissues are being formed, as in childhood, pregnancy, or recovery from wasting illness. Children can make their best growth only when their food supplies both a liberal quantity of protein, which furnishes all the amino acids needed for tissue building, and, in addition, an amount of fat and carbohydrate entirely adequate to cover their energy needs.

Protein requirement is increased, or tissue proteins are not maintained if only the normal minimum amount is eaten, when the diet is devoid of carbohydrate — even if large amounts of fatty acids are available.[11] Under these conditions, the carbon chains of some of the amino acids are used to supply essential amounts of glucose to the tissues, a function that fatty acids cannot fulfill. (These relationships will be described more fully in Chapter 14.)

Minimum Requirements for Essential Amino Acids

Rose[1] determined how much of each essential amino acid was needed to meet the minimum requirement by feeding the nitrogen in the form of a well balanced mixture of all the known *amino acids in pure form* (instead of in proteins) in an otherwise adequate diet (plenty of energy supplied by pure carbohydrate and fat and all needed minerals and vitamins added) (Fig. 5–6). In following periods, the different amino acids were left out of the mixed solution, one at a time, and the effect on nitrogen balance was observed. If the amino acid omitted could be made in the body, no notable results followed; but if the amino acid was one that must be furnished in the food, negative nitrogen balance (denoting inability to build enough protein for tissue maintenance) developed in the young men. Histidine and arginine, which were essential for rat growth, did not seem to be essential for maintenance of nitrogen balance in young men. Subsequently, histidine was shown to be essential in the diet of infants,[12] and there is some evidence from studies[13] of longer duration than those of Rose that it is needed by adults as well. The tenth amino acid, arginine,

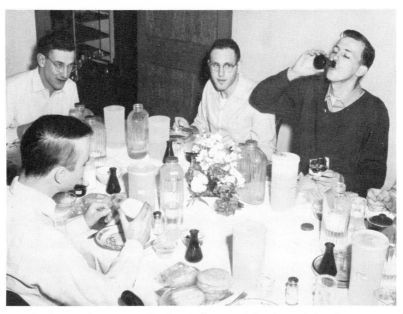

Figure 5-6. Students, volunteers on Dr. Rose's diet squad for determining the amounts of essential amino acids required, consuming their experimental diet. The basal diet consisted of pure foodstuffs (sugar, starch, fat). Nitrogen was furnished by a mixed solution of purified amino acids in known amounts (in liquid containers on table). All needed minerals and vitamins were also supplied in known amounts. Although monotonous, the diet kept the young men in excellent health. (Courtesy of Dr. W. C. Rose, University of Illinois.)

can be synthesized by man, although some doubt remains if it can be manufactured at a sufficiently rapid rate to meet needs under all conditions.

Sufficient data have been accumulated so that the minimum human requirements for eight amino acids essential to the diet can now be stated with fair accuracy. These are listed in Table 5–1. Rose suggested that twice the minimum necessary to prevent negative nitrogen balance would give a safe level of intake to allow for individual differences of need or extra needs at special times. The content of the average American diet in these eight amino acids (based on the average consumption of various foods or food groups) has been calculated[14] and is given in the right-hand column of Table 5–1. The intake of each of these essential amino acids is well above the safe level, so there is little danger of their shortage when the diet contains as much of animal proteins as is customary in the United States, Canada, and most European countries.

These minimum standards and safe levels are particularly helpful in evaluating diets in parts of the world where most of the protein comes from foods of vegetable origin. United Nations agencies have been actively seeking supplementary sources to provide mixtures rich in the essential amino acids, which are apt to be lacking in low protein diets of vegetable origin.

The intake level of dispensable or *"nonessential" amino acids* cannot be ignored when determining the requirements for specific essential amino acids. To meet the total protein needs a somewhat larger quantity of the nonessential amino acids is needed than of essential ones. For their synthesis, the diet must provide a sufficient amount of amino

Table 5–1. *Minimum Daily Requirements of Essential Amino Acids and Estimated Amounts in the Average American Diet*

Essential Amino Acids	Infants,* mg/kg	Minimum Daily Requirements		Safe Levels, gm/day		Average American Diet, gm
		WOMEN,† GM	MEN,† GM	WOMEN	MEN	
Histidine	34	‡	‡	‡	‡	
Isoleucine	126	0.45	0.70	0.90	1.4	5.2
Leucine	150	0.62	1.10	1.24	2.2	8.0
Lysine	103	0.50	0.80	1.00	1.6	6.1
Methionine	45§	0.55**	1.01**	1.10**	2.0**	3.4§
Phenylalanine	90¶	1.12††	1.40††	2.20††	2.8††	8.2††
Threonine	87	0.30	0.50	0.61	1.0	3.9
Tryptophan	22	0.16	0.25	0.32	0.5	1.2
Valine	105	0.65	0.80	1.30	1.6	5.5

*From Hoyt et al.[12]
†From National Research Council.[14]
‡Probably required at level of 0.55 gm/day. See text and reference 14.
§In presence of adequate cystine.
¶In presence of adequate tyrosine.
**Methionine plus cystine.
††Phenylalanine plus tyrosine.

groups and carbon chains needed to assemble the molecules of these amino acids. These building blocks are drawn from a pool to which all nonspecific amino nitrogen sources (essential and nonessential amino acids, ammonium salts, and urea) contribute. For this reason, one would not be able to determine the absolute *minimum* requirement for essential amino acids under conditions wherein a portion of them must be broken down to provide chemical groups needed for nonessential amino acids. For instance, a liberal supply of cystine will "spare" methionine so that only about one-fourth as much methionine needs to be supplied in the diet. All of the essential amino acids can be used to supply amino groups for formation of various nonessential amino acids. Hence, the minimal requirements for the various essential amino acids depend upon the adequacy of nonessential amino nitrogen sources.

Nutritional Value of Individual Proteins and Those in Mixed Diets

It should be evident from the preceding discussion that the quality of a protein—that is, its relative usefulness for tissue protein formation—depends on how well balanced a mixture of amino acids (especially the essential ones) it provides after digestion and absorption into the blood.

Some of the first information on how the amino acid make-up of a protein determines its biological value came from the pioneer experiments of Osborne and Mendel in feeding isolated proteins to rats. They worked at Yale University starting about 1911, and we owe them much. Osborne contributed the skill required to obtain proteins in pure form and to analyze them for kinds and amounts of amino acids they contained; Mendel planned and supervised the feeding experiments, so that the rats received a ration adequate in all respects except that only a single protein provided that nutrient. In one series of experiments, young rats were fed diets containing 18 percent protein in the form of either casein (a milk protein), gliadin (a wheat protein), or zein (a protein from corn). With casein as the sole protein, the rats remained healthy and made excellent growth; those fed gliadin were able to maintain their weight but did not grow much;

those whose sole source of protein was zein not only could not grow, but lost weight and died eventually if kept on this diet.

Since casein evidently supplied all the amino acids needed for growth, it was said to be a *complete* protein. Gliadin was found to contain too little of the amino acid lysine to support growth; when lysine was added to the ration, the animals grew normally. Since gliadin provided for maintenance but not growth, it was said to be a *partially incomplete* protein. Zein, on the other hand, proved to be an *incomplete*, or *inadequate*, protein which supported neither growth nor maintenance because it was quite low in lysine and tryptophan. When the diet was supplemented with suitable amounts of these two amino acids, the animals grew and thrived. These experiments showed conclusively that both lysine and tryptophan must be furnished by the food. Casein at the 18 percent level provided for normal rate of growth, but when it was fed at only 9 percent of the diet, the rats grew only half as rapidly. Casein was found to contain relatively small amounts of the sulfur-containing amino acids, and addition of methio-

nine (or cystine) to the diet led to growth at a normal rate. When a protein is low in some needed amino acid, this is said to be the *"limiting factor,"* for only as much tissue can be built as the smallest amount of necessary tissue ingredient provided.

In general, proteins of animal origin (such as those in eggs, dairy products, and meats) yield mixtures of amino acids that are well balanced, with none of the essential amino acids lacking or in very small amounts. Therefore, they are said to be of higher *biological value* than other proteins. Yet they are not all alike in efficiency for promoting growth. For example, Osborne and Mendel found lactalbumin (one of the proteins in milk) to be quite efficient for promoting growth in rats; only 8 percent of lactalbumin in the diet produced the same weight gain as 12 percent of casein (a second protein in milk) and 15 percent of edestin (found in nuts). The amounts of certain essential amino acids provided differed. Enough of any protein or mixture of proteins must be taken to furnish the minimum requirement for the amino acid that is in poorest supply or is the limiting factor.

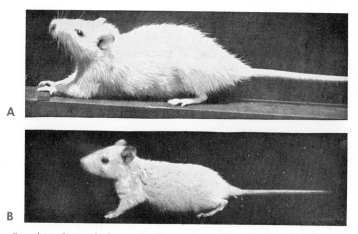

Figure 5–7.   Stunting of growth due to feeding an incomplete protein as sole source of protein in the diet. Contrast between two rats of same age kept on diets alike except for the protein, which was a complete protein (casein from milk) in the case of **A**, and an incomplete protein in the case of **B** (gliadin from wheat). (From experiments by Osborne and Mendel, Connecticut Agricultural Experiment Station; pictures reproduced by courtesy of Yale University Press.)

The mixture of proteins found in egg has been judged to be the best quality natural protein for maintenance of tissues and, hence, received a rating of 100 for comparison with other natural proteins in rat assays of protein quality.[14, 15] On this basis, the mixed proteins of milk rank about 85, those in meats and soybeans rate about 75, and those of other legumes, vegetables, and cereals are in the range of 60 to 40[15] (Table 5–2).

In 1957, the Food and Agricultural Organization (of the United Nations) published an extensive study of the amino acid content of the different foods used in various countries and proposed an "ideal or reference pattern" of amino acids (limited mostly to essential amino acids) as a measure of the relative nutritive value of the proteins furnished by various foods or combinations of foods in the human diet.[16]

This was revised by FAO–WHO in 1972 on the basis of additional evidence.[17] These organizations propose a *chemical protein score* that would depend on the most limiting amino acid in a given food or combination of foods (Table 5–3). If the most limiting amino acid (farthest below the level in the reference pattern) is 80 percent of the amount called for in the ideal pattern, then the food or combination of foods in the diet is given a score of 80.

A protein that may in itself be deficient or low in some amino acid can supplement another protein by furnishing one or more of the amino acids that may be present in insufficient amounts in the other protein. This is shown by the percentage of three amino acids in some typical proteins shown in Table 5–3. White wheat flour is an incomplete protein because it is lacking in lysine and tryptophan, yet

*Table 5–2. Quality of Some Common Food Proteins Estimated by Various Methods**

Food	Food Protein			Digestibility,† %	Rat Biological† Value, %	Net Protein† Utilization, %	NDpCal, %‡	PER§	Egg-Based Chemical Score¶
	% AS PURCHASED	% OF DRY SOLIDS	KCAL, % OF TOTAL KCAL						
Hen's egg, whole	13	48	33	99	94	94	31	3.92	100
Cow's milk, whole	3.5	27	23	97	84	82	19	3.09	60
Fish	19	72	61	98	83	81	49	3.55	70
Beef	18	45	29	99	74	73	21	2.30	69
Soybeans	38	41	39	90	73	66	26	2.32	47
Dry beans, common	22	25	22	73	58	42	9	1.48	34
Peanuts	26	27	16	87	54	48	8	1.65	43
Green leaves	1.5–4.5	23–31	18–45	85**	64**	54**	6–24	–	33
Yeast, brewer's	39	41	54	84	66	55	30	2.24	45
Wheat, whole grain	12	14	13	91	65	59	8	1.53	44
Wheat, white flour	11	12	12	99	52	51	6	0.60	32
Corn, whole grain	10	11	7	90	59	53	4	1.12	41
Rice, brown	8	9	7	96	73	70	5	–	57
Rice, polished, white	7	8	7	98	64	63	4	2.18	56
Potato, white	2	9	7	89	67	60	4	–	34
Cassava (manioc)	2	2	1	No information				–	41

*From FAO Nutrition Studies.[15]

†Determined by rat feeding studies. Digestibility is the amount of fed protein absorbed, and biological value is the portion of absorbed protein that is retained as body tissue. Net utilization is simply digestibility × biological value.

‡Net dietary protein calories as percentage of total calories. The percentage of calories from protein in the food is adjusted according to the net utilization, or quality, of the protein, i.e. (gm protein/100 gm food × NPU × 4 kcal) kcal/100 gm food.

§Protein Efficiency Ratio is the grams of weight gained per gram of protein eaten by the rat.

¶Chemical score is based on amino acid composition. The amount of the most limiting amino acid present is expressed as a percentage of the amount present in egg protein.

**Values listed are for kale; net utilization of other leaves may be higher (mustard greens, 60) or lower (cabbage, 35).

Table 5–3.   Content of Three Essential Amino Acids in Proteins and in 1957 FAO Pattern*

	Lysine	*Methionine + Cystine*	*Tryptophan*
Safe allowance, adult, gm/day	1.6	2.0	0.5
gm per 100 gm protein†			
FAO reference pattern	4.2	4.2	1.4
Hen's egg	7.0	5.8	1.5
Cow's milk	7.1	3.3	1.4
Soybean	7.0	2.8	1.4
White wheat flour	2.3	4.4	1.2
Mixtures			
⅓ milk + ⅔ flour	3.9	4.0	1.3
⅓ soybean + ⅔ flour	3.9	3.9	1.3
% of FAO pattern			
Hen's egg	167	138	107
Cow's milk	169	79	100
Soybean	167	67	100
White wheat flour	55	105	86
Mixtures			
⅓ milk + ⅔ flour	93	95	93
⅓ soybean + ⅔ flour	93	93	93

*From FAO Nutrition Studies.[16] Egg protein contains more of each of these key amino acids than the FAO pattern requires. Milk and soybean proteins are low in the sulfur-containing amino acids, while wheat protein is low in lysine but has plenty of methionine and cystine, so a mixture of these proteins is better than milk, soybeans, or wheat by itself. Note, however, that 70 gm of any of these proteins or protein mixtures provides the recommended allowance for an adult of each of the amino acids, and the *minimum* required amount is provided by 35 gm of protein.

†Computed from amino acid content reported per gm of nitrogen, adjusted to the following percentages of nitrogen in the proteins: egg, 16.0; milk, 15.7; soybean, 17.5; rice, 16.8; and white flour, 17.54.[15]

it furnishes sulfur-containing amino acids that will supplement the low content of these amino acids in milk and soybeans. These foods contain other amino acids in addition to the ones shown in Table 5–3, and they may supplement each other in numerous respects as to the amino acids they contribute. Milk has a better balanced amino acid make-up and carries all amino acids needed for tissue building; therefore it is said to be of higher *biological value.* An example of the supplementary value of milk for wheat is shown in the rat growth curves in Figure 5–8.

Imbalance of amino acids in the diet may sometimes have deleterious effects—for example, an excess of a certain amino acid may reduce the utilization of, or increase the need for, another amino acid.[18] For fear of such effects,

most nutritionists recommend supplementing a protein low in one or more amino acids with some other food protein known to be rich in those amino acids, rather than simply eating much more of the former protein. The poorer proteins are usually low in more than one amino acid, so it is more expedient to supplement with proteins than with pure amino acids. If the mixed proteins in the diet are of too low a value (probably below a protein score of 60), it is wise to supplement by addition of some protein of higher value (as animal protein foods).

In the American diet, with at least 50 percent of the protein from foods of animal origin, there is little danger of the need to increase quantity of protein intake because of low nutritional value of the combination of proteins in the diet. The vegetable proteins,

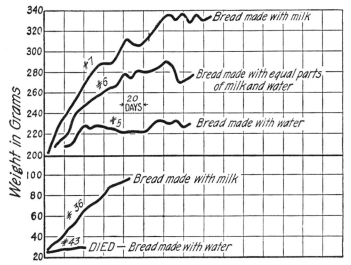

Figure 5–8. Contrasting effects on rat growth of bread made with water and with milk. Milk proteins supplement those of grains in promoting growth. (Courtesy of Dr. H. C. Sherman and the *Journal of Biological Chemistry.*)

although they may be low or even lacking in some essential amino acids, contribute other amino acids that supplement those furnished by animal proteins so that the amino acid mixture provided is sufficiently high in quality to more than come up to so-called "safe levels" for all essential amino acids (Table 5–1).

Another factor that must be considered in practical dietaries is the amount of protein in a food relative to the amount of calories supplied. Foods such as the cereal grains have fairly high energy value, but most of this comes from starch rather than protein (Table 5–2). They may be thought of as "dilute" protein foods, and in order to meet the required amount of *protein,* so much of them must be taken that they provide *energy in excess of body needs.* This is why protein malnutrition is most commonly seen where foods of relatively low protein content form the basis of the diet (such as cassava in Africa and rice in the Orient). It is possible to provide an adequate diet from relatively dilute protein sources (such as rice or potatoes), if supplemented with smaller amounts of some food such as milk that is an excellent source of protein of high biological value.

Even when the diet contains only high quality sources, protein may be inadequate. The total amount of protein or *amino nitrogen* may be the limiting factor rather than lack of any essential amino acid – that is, it is possible to run out of total amino acids before reaching a limiting amount of essential amino acids. This has been demonstrated in infants fed milk protein[19] and adults fed egg[20] as the only source of protein.

The factors of *digestion* and *absorption* are ordinarily not too important, though it should be evident that proteins which are less completely digested and absorbed than others are slightly less efficient for meeting the body's protein needs on this account. Early experiments of Atwater and Bryant showed that, in an ordinary mixed diet, the proteins from animal foods have a high "coefficient of digestibility"* (i.e.,

---

*Apparent protein digestibility is calculated as the amount of nitrogen in the feces subtracted from the amount eaten, divided by the amount eaten, times 100. For example, with 75 gm protein in diet (12 gm N) and 1.3 gm N in feces, digestibility is $(12 - 1.3) \div 12 \times 100$, or 89 percent. To determine true protein digestibility, fecal nitrogen must be corrected for the amount excreted when no protein is fed.

the net percentage digested and absorbed) of about 95 to 99, while those from cereals, fruits, and vegetables have lower values of 85 to 90, and some legumes have values as low as 75 to 80 (Table 5–2). Nitrogen loss in the feces is increased when the diet is composed chiefly of foods that are high in indigestible matter, such as cellulose and other fiber, probably because of the increased intestinal bacterial growth these carbohydrates support.

Another factor that influences the percentage of food protein that is absorbed and retained in the body is the treatment to which the food may have been subjected in cooking or processing. The protein in legumes is rendered more digestible by cooking, but high heating of cereals (as in toasted or puffed breakfast cereals) and milk (as in processing of some canned and dried products) causes adverse structural changes in the protein. Reactions occur between amino acids and carbohydrates with heating that make a portion of the amino acids (especially lysine) unavailable for their essential functions. Processing with acid and heat, as is done in the manufacture of gelatin, completely degrades one amino acid (tryptophan) and damages others. Careful home cooking and commercial processing techniques are required to preserve maximum protein quality.

The distribution of protein foods in the meals throughout the day is also thought to be important. All the essential amino acids must be present at the same time in order to build tissue protein, as well as the nonessential ones that are present in that particular protein. That is, protein formation is an all-or-none reaction and if one amino acid is missing, no protein is made. To some extent, partially complete mixtures of amino acids may be adjusted by contributions from the tissues (such as the intestinal tract), but for assured maximum utilization balanced protein mixtures should be included in the meal and taken with sufficient calories to prevent the use of protein for energy.

STANDARD PROTEIN ALLOWANCES FOR ADULTS AND HOW TO SECURE THEM IN THE DIET

How can we determine approximately how much protein must be taken daily to provide for maintenance of body tissues in the average man? Dietary studies to find out how much protein is usually eaten are of no help, for people usually consume more protein than their actual need and adjust to show nitrogen equilibrium at any level of intake above the minimum requirement. If we determine the nitrogen excretion when fasting, this figure is too high because some of the nitrogen excreted will certainly arise from the necessity to burn protein to meet the energy requirement. The way to get a true measure of the protein actually required for tissue upkeep is to determine nitrogen balance on progressively lower levels of protein intake at the same time that *plenty of carbohydrate and fat are given to meet the energy needs.* A figure slightly above the *protein level at which negative nitrogen balance appears* may be taken as about the intake required for maintenance, or the minimum requirement.

Sherman examined data obtained in this way from 47 different persons and, to make them comparable, calculated each to a common basis of 70 kg body weight.[21] Although there was quite a range of individual values, the average was about 44 gm of protein per day as maintenance requirement for a man of average weight. Sherman estimated that probably 0.5 gm of protein per kg of body weight would suffice to meet the minimum requirement (35 gm daily for a 70 kg man). A summation[6] of all data available 50 years later supports Sherman's estimate, and indicates the normal individual variability to be within ± 15 percent of that value.

Although it would be unwise to limit the protein intake over long periods to the minimum for maintenance, the establishment of such a figure (at about

0.5 gm protein per kg body weight) is useful in permitting us to gauge how much more protein should be included in the diet to provide a suitable margin to cover variations in individual needs, as well as a factor of safety to ensure the best nutritional condition during periods of stress.

We have seen in the preceding pages how many influences come into play to affect the quantity of amino acid intake that is retained in the body for tissue building or upkeep—such as the quantity of carbohydrate and fat in the diet, the quantity, quality, and digestibility of the various proteins ingested, the state of the body, and the distribution of the protein over the day's meals —to mention only a few. Since conditions may be more favorable for nitrogen assimilation at one time and much less favorable at another, it is reasonable that the diet should supply some extra protein over the minimum requirement, as a factor of safety to ensure plenty under any condition. How liberal should this extra amount be?

The protein allowance and factor of safety should be especially liberal in conditions of growth or repair of body tissues, such as childhood, pregnancy and lactation, recovery from malnutrition, or conditions in which assimilation of food is poor. A generous factor of safety may also be valuable when proteins of lower biological value make up a large portion of the intake. In setting protein allowances, national and international advisory groups have considered individual and regional variations in needs and have arrived at somewhat different conclusions concerning the magnitude of the necessary margin of safety, as we shall see presently. Other factors that are thought to have a systematic effect on protein need are dealt with separately. These are body *size* and *age*, and the conditions of *pregnancy* and lactation.

SIZE. The total amount of protein needed for tissue upkeep is dependent in part upon the amount of active tissues in the body; for this reason the protein requirement is reckoned as so much *per unit of body weight*. If the minimum requirement is placed at 0.5 gm per kg, a woman who weighs only 44 kg (97 lb) should consume a minimum of 22 gm of protein daily; a tall and muscular man weighing 80 kg (176 lb) would need to take a minimum of 40 gm, which is 5 gm more than the amount (35 gm) for a man of "average" weight (70 kg). Regardless of sex, a person of small body weight requires less, and one of larger than average weight needs more than a standard allowance based on average body weight.

AGE. The age of the individual is a factor that comes into play chiefly in the younger years when extra protein is needed for building new tissues in growth. Rapidly growing young children may need two to three times as much protein per unit of body weight as adults do, to provide for protein storage in new tissues. The high protein requirement of infants and young children is striking when considered per unit of weight, but the total amount needed by their smaller bodies is, of course, less than the amount needed by an adult. Thus the allowance for a two-year-old who weighs 13 kg (29 lb), even at 2.5 gm per kg, is only 32 gm of protein daily. The amount of extra protein needed for growth is less per kg body weight as the child is older and enters a period of less rapid growth, reaching adult level after puberty (age 12 to 16 for girls and 14 to 18 for boys). Modern theories give value to liberal (not excessive) protein supplies as one of the factors that favor prolonging vigor into later years. Dietary records of older persons sometimes disclose that they are subsisting on considerably less than optimal protein intakes (e.g., meats may be mostly eliminated because of low income or difficulty in chewing). It is now advised that, although calories should be somewhat reduced, the level of protein intake for old people should be kept about the same as in younger years of adult life.

PREGNANCY AND LACTATION. Extra

protein is needed during pregnancy primarily for the growth of the baby during the second and third trimesters and smaller amounts for the development of maternal supporting tissues and fluids. Additional dietary protein is also required for production of milk. The basis for these recommendations is given in Chapter 19.

MUSCULAR WORK NOT A FACTOR IN PROTEIN REQUIREMENT. Although muscular work is the largest single factor in determining energy needs, it has no appreciable effect on the protein requirement except during initial periods of training when muscular tissue is developing. Careful experiments by Atwater proved that muscular work sufficient nearly to double the energy metabolism showed very little effect on the protein metabolized, as measured by the nitrogen output. Although there is no basis for the popular idea that a man requires extra protein-rich foods such as meats if he is doing muscular work, he does require more carbohydrate and fat in order to provide necessary energy. Since protein is an integral part of many foods, such a working man usually increases his protein intake somewhat when he increases his total food consumption.

Standard Allowances of Protein

The daily allowances of protein recommended by various governmental agencies for adults and "teenagers" are as shown in Table 5–4.

The United States NRC[22] allowances for normal adults are based on 0.9 gm protein per kg body weight. If the minimum requirement of 0.35 to 0.5 gm per kg weight is accepted as correct, a 100 percent factor of safety is provided. Authorities agree that such an allowance gives a safety margin of 50 to 100 percent above the normal requirements for maintenance, the margin varying somewhat with individual differences in utilization and body needs. The Canadian Council on Nutrition[23] recommends somewhat less protein, 0.7 gm per kg of body weight, allowing a smaller margin of safety.

The FAO–WHO[17] has expressed protein allowances in terms of egg or milk proteins with the understanding that this will be adjusted according to the quality of local food supplies. The egg-milk allowances for men and women are 0.57 and 0.52 gm per kg respectively. If the local food supply is 70 percent as good as egg when measured by animal growth, nitrogen retention, or chemical score, the allowances would be adjusted as follows:

$$\frac{\text{arbitrary score of egg-milk}}{\text{local diet test score}} \quad \frac{100}{70} =$$

1.43, the correction factor.

Then, daily allowances are 1.43×0.57 or 0.8 gm per kg for men and 1.43×0.52 or 0.7 gm per kg for women.

Table 5–4. *Recommended Daily Allowances of Protein (in Grams) for Healthy Adults*

Country	Men		Women	
	ADOLESCENT	MATURE ADULT	ADOLESCENT	MATURE ADULT
United States[22]				
Per kg body weight	0.9	0.9	0.9	0.9
Per day, avg. weight	60 (67 kg)*	65 (70 kg)	55 (58 kg)	55 (58 kg)
Canada[23]				
Per kg body weight	0.74	0.70	0.74	0.70
Per day, avg. weight	47	48 (72 kg)	41	39 (57 kg)
United Kingdom[24]				
Percent of energy	10	10	10	10
Per day, moderately active	75 (61 kg)	75 (65 kg)	58 (56 kg)	55(55 kg)

*Value in parentheses is average or reference body weight.

The protein allowances given above are for adults of average weight. Persons who are markedly under- or overweight should have protein allowances based on the normal weight for their height, rather than on actual body weight.

The allowances for pregnant and lactating women and for children who are growing and maturing provide more protein per kg body weight. A woman in the second and third trimesters of pregnancy should have an additional 6 to 10 gm protein daily, and during lactation 15 to 20 gm protein above the normal allowance may be required. Allowances for younger children (which usually range from 1.5 to 2.5 gm protein per kg body weight) are found in Chapter 20.

Using a different philosophy, a United Kingdom panel[24] has recommended that the protein intake should furnish 10 *percent of the energy intake*. In making this recommendation it was observed that the majority of persons in the United Kingdom take between 10 and 15 percent of their energy in the form of protein, that this habitual intake is without apparent harm, and that this level of protein contributes to the palatability of the diet. For persons of normal energy expenditure, an arbitrary allowance of 10 percent of energy intake clearly exceeds minimum requirements by an adequate margin for safety.

On the other hand, we know that muscular exercise is the factor of greatest magnitude in determining need for energy, while it has very little effect on the protein requirement. If a sedentary man had an energy requirement of 2400 calories, his recommended protein allowance would be calculated as follows: 2400 × 10% = 240 ÷ 4 (caloric value per gm protein) = 60 gm protein. However, if he engaged in hard physical labor, his energy need could be 4400 kcal per day and his allowance would then be 4400 × 10% ÷ 4, or 110 gm protein. If he weighed 70 kg, his allowance on a basis of 0.9 gm per kg would be 63 gm protein. With children, the calculation on percentage of energy works approximately only, because their high protein needs are accompanied by an increased caloric allowance per unit of body weight. Small or very sedentary women and old people may well be allotted too little protein on this basis, because their

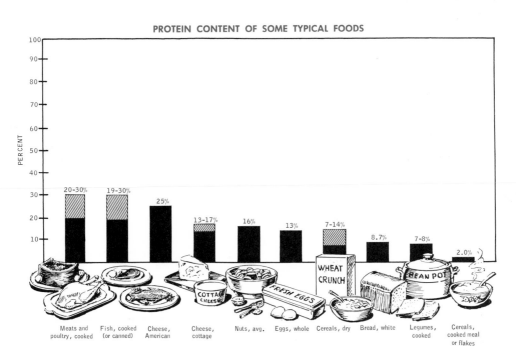

PROTEIN CONTENT OF SOME TYPICAL FOODS

Figure 5–9.

appetite and energy needs are low but their protein needs will not have decreased correspondingly.

How to Secure Protein Allowance in the Diet

For the average adult sufficient protein of excellent quality will be ensured if the daily diet includes four average servings of milk, meat, fish, poultry, eggs, or other protein-rich foods. The "other" protein-rich foods may be legumes such as peas, beans, or peanuts, other nuts, cheese, or additional servings of the foods listed.

The protein furnished by the food pattern just given will vary according to the size of the portions of meat, the way it is cooked and the choice of other protein-rich foods. One should be able to count on an average of at least 30 to 50 gm protein from this group of foods.

Grain products and the vegetables needed to make an adequate diet can usually be relied on to provide about 15 to 20 gm protein, which would make up the protein ration to 50 to 70 gm, which is about the amount usually recommended for the average adult.

To show how this rule might be worked out at three different cost levels and for persons who are either heavy or light meat eaters, foods are listed in Table 5–5 with the number of grams protein they furnish.

It can be seen that the foods in Table 5–5 provide about 65 gm protein (with about 60 to 80 percent of it of animal origin), or about the amount needed by a man of average weight. Of course, a vegetarian diet can be made entirely adequate in quality of proteins by the liberal use of legumes and cereal products, and by supplementing vegetable proteins with milk and milk products or with eggs. Meats are one of the most expensive sources of protein, but they furnish it in concentrated form; a 3½ oz (100 gm) serving of meat may be depended on to give 18 to 25 gm protein (depending on its fat and moisture content), or about one-fourth to one-third of the adult's daily ration (Table 5–6). Fish, shellfish, and poultry are usually leaner and slightly higher in protein content than the red meats. Among the least expensive foods for protein are dried legumes, cereal products, dark green leafy vegetables, and potatoes. Eggs and milk, especially dried skim milk, are usually low to moderate in cost.

Normally we include protein-rich food in each meal, partly for its satiety value. Breakfast may be an exception for those who eat a hurried or light

Table 5–5. Protein Allowance in the Diet at Different Cost Levels*

High Cost	Protein (in gm)	Moderate Cost	Protein (in gm)	Low Cost	Protein (in gm)
Milk, ½ pint	8.5	Milk, 1 pint	17.0	Milk, 1 pint (from skim	
Ice cream, ¾ cup	4.0	Hamburger patty, 3 oz	20.5	milk powder)	17.0
Roast beef, 5 oz	35.0	2 eggs	12.5	Pork and beans, canned,	
Cheese, Roquefort, ½ oz	3.5		50.0	1 cup	16.0
	51.0			Cottage cheese, ½ cup	16.0
					49.0
Whole wheat bread, 2 sl.	5.0	Whole wheat bread, 4 sl.	10.0	White bread, 4 sl.	8.0
Cereal flakes, 1 cup	1.0	1 med. potato	2.5	Oatmeal, ⅔–¾ cup	2.0
2 med. cup cakes	3.5	Apple pie, ⅙ pie	3.5	Bread pudding with	
1 med. potato	2.5		66.0	raisins, ⅔ cup	5.0
	63.0				64.0

*Vegetables should contribute another 3 to 6 gm of protein, or more if several large servings are taken. For example, 5 oz of dark leafy greens provides about 5 to 6 gm protein, but ½ cup tomatoes only 1 to 1.5 gm.

Table 5–6. *Protein Yield of Some Common Foods as Served*

Food	Serving Size	
	HOUSEHOLD MEASURE	COOKED WEIGHT, GM
Protein 20 to 25 gm per serving or nearly $1/2$ the adult daily allowance:		
Meat, fish, poultry	3–3$1/2$ oz	90–100
Soybeans	1 cup	260
Other dry beans, peas	1$1/2$ cups	400
Protein 5 to 8 gm per serving or $1/10$ the adult daily allowance:		
Milk	1 glass	200–400
Brick-type cheeses	1 oz	30
Cottage cheese	$1/4$ cup	55
Egg	1	50
Nuts	1–1$1/2$ oz	30–40
Peanut butter	2 tbsp	30
Macaroni, noodles	1 cup	150
Green peas	$3/4$ cup	120
Bean or pea soup	$3/4$ cup	185
Bacon	3 strips	25
Frankfurter	1 medium	50
Custard and cream pies	$1/6$–$1/8$ pie	140–160
Puddings, ice cream	$2/3$–1 cup	120–150
Protein 2 to 4 gm per serving or $1/20$ the adult daily allowance:		
Bread	1 slice	25
Dark green vegetables	$1/2$–$2/3$ cup	70–120
Ready-to-eat cereals	$3/4$–1 cup	25–30
Potato, white or sweet	1 medium	100
Cakes	2 inch slice	50–100
Chocolate candy bar	1 oz	30

meal in the morning. In order to promote maximum retention of nitrogen in the tissues, all the essential amino acids should be in the blood stream during the absorptive period following a meal, and energy intake should be sufficient to prevent the need for protein to be used as an energy source. Inclusion of some high quality protein in each meal is especially important in periods or conditions when storage of protein in tissues is most desirable, such as growth, pregnancy, or recovery from wasting illnesses. The distribution of protein and energy throughout the day is a much more urgent matter if the diet is borderline than if it is liberal in nutrient content.

PROTEIN-CALORIE MALNUTRITION

There are many areas of the world, particularly in the developing and overpopulated countries, where protein-rich foods, especially those of animal origin, are practically unavailable to the poorer segments of the population. It was estimated in 1970 that 300 to 500 million persons in the developing countries do not get enough to eat and as many as 1500 million do not receive a nutritionally adequate diet.[25] Protein is probably the single nutrient most commonly deficient worldwide both because protein intake itself is low and because total food consumption is so inadequate that the small amount of protein eaten is not spared to function as an essential nutrient. Even in a country as rich as the United States, studies of poor people have revealed a significant incidence of protein-calorie deficiency symptoms. Disastrous food shortages due to the military strategy of blockade cost countless lives in the Nigerian Civil War in the late 1960's;[26] crop destruction continues to be employed as a warfare measure (most recently in Indochina), although it is shown to have less effect on fighting forces than on civilian populations in areas attacked.[27] Widespread famine has been averted in modern times by improved agricultural methods and international assistance programs, but poverty and war continue to take their toll.

Those most apt to show marked symptoms as a result of too little food, too little protein, or both are young children in the years immediately after weaning. Naturally, with too low a supply of amino acids for building tissue protein and with some of the small protein supply burned for energy, there is failure to grow properly and wasting of tissues. In areas where protein-calorie deficiency is endemic, adult height is reduced below the genetic potential for growth. If food deprivation occurs in the adult after growth has ceased, as happened in concentration and war-prisoner camps in World War II, severe emaciation is the obvious result. Depending on the relative deficit of protein to energy in the diet and on other factors (such as liver function), both infants and adults may show marked edema, especially of the legs and abdomen. This symptom appears most severely when protein intake is more limited than energy supply and results primarily from a fall in the amount of protein in the blood plasma. Anemia is present due to the failure to form hemoglobin and red blood cells. When people are poor and ill-fed, other public health problems abound, so cases of protein-calorie deficiency are commonly complicated by the presence of infectious diseases and intestinal parasitism.[28] Also, because foods carry more than one nutrient, the primary deficiency may have superimposed deficiencies of vitamins and minerals. Naturally, a range of different symptoms may be seen in individuals, depending on these other dietary and environmental factors.

The picture in young children may be one of *marasmus*, appropriately named

from the Greek word meaning "to waste away," in which the muscles are atrophied and the face has a wizened "old man" look. Others in whom edema is a prominent symptom are said to have *kwashiorkor*. This name comes from the Ga tribe of the African Gold Coast and was popularized by Williams when she described the condition in Ghanaian children.[29] Some say that the word means "red boy," referring to the odd reddish-orange color of the hair as well as a skin rash characteristic of the disease (Fig. 5–10). Other interpretive meanings suggest displacement or jealousy, from the frequency with which the disease occurs in children who are deprived of breast feeding by birth of a second infant or urbanization and employment of the mother. This disease, or gradations between the two types of symptom complexes, has been known by many many names over the years ("sugar baby," dystrophie des farineux, Mehlnahrschaden, distrofia pluricarencial infantil, etc.) but is one entity caused basically by lack of protein and energy.

When children are starving, mothers are rarely well fed. Childhood malnutrition may actually result partly from malnutrition experienced earlier by the mother during pregnancy and lactation. We know that experimental deprivation of pregnant animals results in permanent stunting of the offspring,[30] and that in human populations poverty, malnutrition, and high rates of infant mortality go hand in hand.[31] Undersized mothers are likely to have babies of lower birth weight and poorer survival potential.[31]

Knowledge has advanced with continued research in the laboratory and from studies of children who, with the aid of modern medical care, can often be saved even in extreme stages of malnutrition. There is no question that brain growth is impaired by severe protein lack during pregnancy and during the first few months of life.[32] Some neurologic deficit may be expected to follow deprivation throughout the early

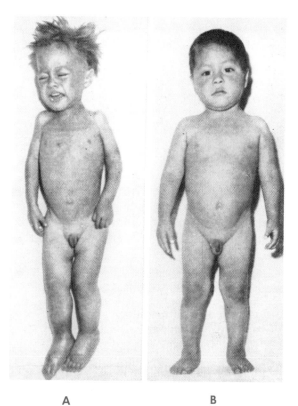

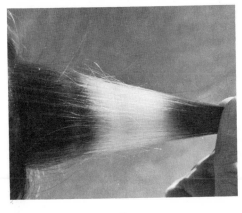

Figure 5–10. Case of kwashiorkor. **A,** Child, 2 years 8 months, on admission to hospital. **B,** Same child 19 weeks after treatment with high-protein diet (a special mixture of vegetable proteins). **C,** So-called "flag sign," often seen during recovery from kwashiorkor, when hair is changing from orange color back to black. (Courtesy of Doctors Scrimshaw and Guzmán, of the Institute of Nutrition for Central America and Panama, Guatemala City.)

years of life, until the nervous system is formed completely, but the probability is less with increasing age. This means a legacy of poor educability and achievement that may be the major cost of failure to feed mothers and babies (Fig. 5–11).

For prevention, satisfactory prenatal diets and nutritionally adequate breast or artificial infant feeding and weaning diets are essential. When milk is not available or is costly to import, other animal protein foods may be used, or an assortment of vegetable foods may be found which supplement each other as to amino acid content of proteins

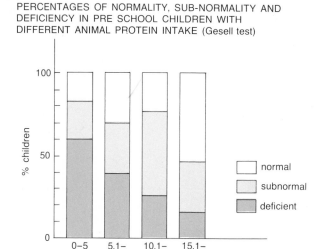

PERCENTAGES OF NORMALITY, SUB-NORMALITY AND
DEFICIENCY IN PRE SCHOOL CHILDREN WITH
DIFFERENT ANIMAL PROTEIN INTAKE (Gesell test)

Animal Protein intake (gm per day).

Figure 5–11. Frequency of mental deficiency in preschool children in a marginal population group in relation to the amount of animal proteins ingested. (Courtesy of Dr. F. Monckeberg-Barros. Reprinted from Cuadernos Médico Sociales, Colegio Médico de Chile, 9:5, 1968.)

and other essential nutrients. Addition to the diet of peanut or soybean flour, other legumes, dried yeast, or fish meal may provide such an adequate mixture of proteins; an increase in the total amount of protein intake is also usually required. Several special high-protein, low-cost infant foods have been developed by teams of nutritionists and food scientists. These take advantage of locally available foods that have supplementary amino acid compositions and conform somewhat to cultural food preferences. Examples of some of these are given in Table 5–7.

The work of the United Nations health agencies has been directed toward securing more adequate diets for peoples in underdeveloped countries. This can be done by encouraging nations to raise more of the crops that provide good quality proteins, and by improving the total and protein yield of the crops through advanced agricultural techniques and genetic improvement of grains; by educating people to use a wider variety of foods; and by raising the economic level, enabling them to purchase high-quality protein foods.

Table 5–7. Examples of Special High-protein, Low-cost Foods for Children*

Name	*Country*	*Ingredients*	*Percentage Protein†*
Incaparina	Guatemala	Corn, cottonseed flour, lysine, vitamin A, calcium	27.5
Lac-Tone	India	Peanut flour, skim milk powder, wheat and barley flour, vitamins, calcium	26.0
Pronutro	South Africa	Corn, skim milk powder, peanut, soybean, fish protein concentrate, yeast, wheat germ, vitamins, sugar, iodized salt	22.0
CSM	United States	Corn, defatted soybean flour, skim milk powder, sugar, vitamins, calcium	20.0

*From FAO.[25]
†Dry whole cow's milk contains 26 percent protein.

In countries where protein intake is low and most of it is furnished by cereal grains or legumes, some of the essential amino acids are likely to be provided in too small amounts. Lysine, tryptophan, methionine, and threonine are the ones most likely to be lacking in such diets. It has been suggested, and experiments have been made, to fortify cereal foods, such as wheat flour, rice, and corn grits, with the amino acids most apt to be low or lacking in them. Supplementation of the diet by more liberal use of some available protein-rich food or by an addition of some vegetable protein mixture is more practical because a mixture of supplementary amino acids is given thereby and, most important, there is usually some degree of energy deficit that the second food will help to correct. In the United States, reinforcement of certain foods with amino acids (such as bread and cereals with added lysine) is an unneeded expense, because most diets are already adequate. In the United States, Canada, New Zealand, Australia, and most European nations, protein malnutrition is not a major public health problem, for foods of animal origin are plentiful, and usually one-half to two-thirds of the protein intake comes from these sources.

QUESTIONS AND PROBLEMS

1. What four chemical elements are combined in proteins? Which one of these is furnished in proteins but not in carbohydrates or fats? What other elements are often or sometimes incorporated in protein molecules?

2. Define amino acids. Can animals synthesize amino acids from simple inorganic compounds of nitrogen? From what simple materials do plants build amino acids, which are later built into plant proteins? What is meant by the "nitrogen cycle" in nature?

3. Where is protein found in the body? Why is an adequate supply of protein so essential for the body welfare? Can protein be burned or oxidized in the body—that is, does protein serve as an energy nutrient as well as a substance used for tissue building and upkeep? Can a liberal supply of carbohydrate or fat in the diet "spare" protein—that is, provide conditions in which less protein needs to be used to provide energy and more is conserved for tissue maintenance?

4. What are nucleoproteins and where are they found in the body? What important biologic functions do they perform? How does DNA differ from RNA in composition and function? How do compound or conjugated proteins differ from simple proteins? What important compound protein is found in red blood corpuscles? Can you name two other proteins found either in the body or in food that are linked up or conjugated with some non-protein substance?

5. How many different amino acids have been found to occur commonly in proteins? How many are "essential" in the sense that they must be furnished pre-formed in the food? How many of these are needed for the growth of young rats? To maintain tissue proteins in human adults? Is it likely or unlikely that some arginine and histidine may also be needed by humans during periods of growth, and if so, why? Does the body need the other amino acids listed as "dispensable" to build and maintain tissues? If so, why do we not list them as "essential"? What is meant by the statement that a low supply of any essential amino acid may be a "limiting factor"?

6. Define adequate or complete proteins and inadequate or incomplete proteins. Which class of proteins is furnished by foods of animal origin? Explain how incomplete proteins may be supplemented by complete proteins in a mixed diet. Why do cereals with milk furnish a well balanced mixture of amino acids?

7. What foods or types of food contribute the largest amount of protein in the average diet? Which other types

of food contribute less, but valuable, amounts of protein? Which foods are the most expensive and which are the least expensive sources of protein?

8. How prominent a place in the diet should be given to protein-rich foods? What proportion of the calories is it usually suggested that proteins should contribute?

✗ List the foods in your diet for one day and (from the Table of Nutritive Values of Foods in the Appendix) figure out how many grams of protein you consumed and what relative proportion of the total calories this furnished. Compare this with your standard allowance for protein, and if your protein intake was as much as 20 percent lower than that recommended, make suggestions as to how to bring your protein intake up to a desirable level. Does it matter if you are eating more protein than the standard allowance? If so, why; if not, why not?

✗ Plan a day's diet for a vegetarian, which excludes meat and eggs but includes milk and/or cheese, and which furnishes 60 to 70 gm protein. Use Table 5–6 for protein substitutes for one serving of meat and one egg.

REFERENCES

1. Rose, W. C., et al.: Amino acid requirement of adult men. Nutr. Abst. Rev., 27:631, 1957.
2. Selye, H.: *The Physiology and Pathology of Exposure to Stress.* Montreal, Acta, Inc., 1950.
3. Schoenheimer, R.: *The Dynamic State of Body Constituents.* Cambridge, Harvard University Press, 1942.
4. Atwater, W. A., and Bryant, M. S.: Bulletin No. 28. Washington, D.C., U.S. Department of Agriculture, 1902.
5. Chittendon, R. H.: *Physiological Economy in Nutrition.* New York, Stokes, 1904.
6. Irwin, M. J., and Hegsted, D. M.: A conspectus of research on protein requirements of man. J. Nutrition, 101:385, 1971.
7. Krogh, A., and Krogh, M.: Meddelser om Grönland, 51:1, 1914–15.
8. McClellan, W. S., and DuBois, E. F.: Clinical calorimetry. XLV. Prolonged meat diets with a study of kidney function and ketosis. J. Biol. Chem., 87:651, 1930.
9. Calloway, D. H., and Margen, S.: Human response to diets very high in protein. Fed. Proc., 27:725, 1968 (abstract).
10. Munro, H. N., and Allison, J. B.: *Mammalian Protein Metabolism,* Vol. II. New York, Academic Press, 1964, pp. 21–24.
11. Renner, R., and Elcombe, A. L.: Factors affecting the utilization of 'carbohydrate-free' diet by the chick. II. Level of glycerol. J. Nutr., 84:327, 1964.
12. Holt, L. E., Jr., György, P., Pratt, E. L., Snyderman, S. E., and Wallace, W. M.: *Protein and Amino Acid Requirements in Early Life,* New York, N.Y.U. Press, 1960.
13. Anonymous: Evidence for liver damage in subjects fed amino acid diets lacking arginine and histidine. Nutr. Rev., 28:229, 1970.
14. Anonymous: Evaluation of Protein Nutrition. National Research Council Pub. No. 711, 1959.
15. FAO Nutritional Studies: *Amino Acid Content of Foods and Biological Data on Proteins.* No. 24, Rome, 1970.
16. FAO Nutritional Studies: *Protein Requirements.* No. 16, Rome, 1957.
17. FAO–WHO: Energy and Protein Requirements. In press.
18. Harper, A. E., et al.: Effects of ingestion of disproportionate amounts of amino acids. Physiol. Rev., 50:428, 1970.
19. Snyderman, S. E., et al.: "Unessential" nitrogen: A limiting factor for human growth. J. Nutr., 78:57, 1962.
20. Scrimshaw, N. S., Young, V. R., Schwartz, R., Piché, M. L., and Das, J. B.: Minimum dietary essential amino acid to total nitrogen ration for whole egg protein fed to young men. J. Nutr., 89:9, 1966.
21. Sherman, H. C.: Protein requirement of maintenance in man. J. Biol. Chem., 41:97, 1920.
22. Food and Nutrition Board: *Recommended Dietary Allowances,* 7th Ed. Washington, D.C., National Research Council, 1968.
23. *Dietary Standard for Canada,* Canadian Bulletin on Nutrition, Vol. 6, No. 1, 1964.
24. *Recommended Intakes of Nutrients for the United Kingdom.* Dept. Health and Soc. Sec. Rept. No. 120, 1969.
25. FAO: *Lives in Peril.* Rome, 1970.
26. Aall, C.: Relief, nutrition and health problems in the Nigerian/Biafran War. J. Trop. Pediat., 16:69, 1970.
27. Mayer, J.: Starvation as a weapon: Herbicides in Vietnam, I. Scientist & Citizen, 9:115, 1967.
28. McLaren, D. S.: A fresh look at protein-calorie malnutrition. Lancet, 2:485, 1966.
29. Williams, C. D.: Kwashiorkor: Nutritional disease of children associated with maize diet. Lancet, 2:1151, 1935.
30. Chow, B. F., and Lee, C. J.: Effect of dietary restriction of pregnant rats on body weight gain of the offspring. J. Nutr., 82:10, 1964.
31. *Maternal Nutrition and the Course of Pregnancy.*

Washington, D.C., National Academy of Sciences, 1970.

32. Scrimshaw, N. S., and Gordon, J. E.: *Malnutrition, Learning and Behavior.* Cambridge, Mass., M.I.T. Press, 1968.

SUPPLEMENTARY READING

General, History, and Reviews

Allison, J. B., and Fitzpatrick, W. H.: *Dietary Proteins in Health and Disease.* Springfield, Ill., Charles C Thomas, 1960.

Briskey, E., Cassens, R. G., and Trautman, J. C. (eds.): *The Physiology and Biochemistry of Muscle as a Food.* Madison, University of Wisconsin Press, 1970.

Lappé, F. M.: *Diet for a Small Planet.* New York, Ballantine, 1971.

Laurie, R. A.: *Proteins as Human Food.* Westport, Connecticut, Avi Pub. Co., 1970.

Orr, M. I., and Watt, B. K.: *Amino Acid Content of Food.* Home Economics Research Report 4. Washington, D.C., U.S. Department of Agriculture, 1957.

Routh, J. I., Eyman, D. P., and Burton, D. J.: *Essentials of General, Organic and Biochemistry.* Philadelphia, W. B. Saunders Co., 1969.

Scrimshaw, N. S., et al.: *The Development of INCAP Vegetable Mixture in Meeting the Protein Needs of Infants and Children.* Pub. 843. Washington, D. C., National Academy of Sciences, 1961.

Other References

Abernathy, R. P., and Ritchey, S. J.: Protein requirements of preadolescent girls. J. Home Econ., *64*:56, 1972.

Arroyave, G.: Comparative sensitivity of specific amino acid ratios versus "essential to nonessential" amino acid ratio. Amer. J. Clin. Nutr., *23*:703, 1970.

Baertl, J. M., et al.: Diet supplementation for entire communities. Growth and mortality of infants and children. Amer. J. Clin. Nutr., *23*:707, 1970.

Begum, A., Radhakrishnan, A. N., and Pereira, S. M.: Effect of amino acid composition of cereal-based diets on growth of preschool children. Amer. J. Clin. Nutr., *23*: 1175, 1970.

Bressani, R., Valiente, A. T., and Tejada, C. E.: All-vegetable protein mixtures for human feeding. VI. The value of combinations of lime-treated corn and cooked black beans. J. Food Sci., *27*:394, 1962.

Bressani, R., et al.: Supplementation of cereal proteins with amino acids. IV. Lysine supplementation of wheat flour fed to young children at different levels of protein intake in the presence and absence of other amino acids. J. Nutr., *79*:333, 1963.

Brown, L. R.: Nobel peace prize: Developer of high-yield wheat receives award. Science, *170*:518, 1970.

Bruins, H. W.: Protein-rich foods for overcoming nutritional deficiences—the industrial viewpoint. Food Tech., *18*:51, 1964.

Calloway, D. H., and Spector, H.: Nitrogen balance as related to caloric and protein intake in active young men. Amer. J. Clin. Nutr., *2*:405, 1954.

Campbell, J. A.: Evaluation of protein in foods for regulatory purposes. J. Agr. Food Chem., *8*:323, 1960.

Cohn, C., et al.: Feeding frequency and protein metabolism. Amer. J. Physiol., *205*:71, 1963.

Dalgliesh, C. E.: Time factor in protein biosynthesis. Science, *125*:271, 1957.

Gates, J. C., and Kennedy, B. M.: Protein quality of bread and bread ingredients: Effect of using nonfat dry milk and lysine. J. Amer. Dietet. Assoc., *44*:374, 1964.

Gray, G. M., and Cooper, H. L.: Protein digestion and absorption. Gastroenterology, *61*: 535, 1971.

Hatch, F. T.: Correlation of amino acid composition with certain characteristics of proteins. Nature, *206*:777, 1965.

Hegsted, D. M.: Variation in requirements of nutrients—amino acids. Fed. Proc., *22*: 1424, 1965.

Howe, E. E., Jansen, G. R., and Gilfielan, E. W.: Amino acid supplementation of cereal grains as related to the world food supply. Amer. J. Clin. Nutr., *16*:309, 1965.

Irwin, M. I., and Hegsted, D. M.: A conspectus of research on amino acid requirements of man. J. Nutr., *101*:539, 1971.

Kies, C. V., and Linkswiler, H. M.: Effect on nitrogen retention of men of altering the intake of essential amino acids with total nitrogen held constant. J. Nutr., *85*:139, 1962.

King, K. W., Sebrell, W. H., and Severinghaus, E. L.: Lysine fortification of wheat bread fed to Haitian school children. Amer. J. Clin. Nutr., *12*:36, 1963.

Le Breton, E., and Brock, J. F. (eds.): Symposium on proteins and amino acids in nutrition. Fed. Proc., *20*: supp. no. 7, 1961.

Leverton, R. M., Schlaphoff, D., and Huffstetter, M.: Blood regeneration in women blood donors. II. Effect of protein, vitamin and mineral supplements. J. Amer. Dietet. Assoc., *24*:480, 1948.

Metta, V. C.: Nutritional value of fish flour supplements. J. Amer. Dietet. Assoc., *37*:234, 1960.

Miller, D. S., and Payne, P. R.: Caloric reduction. J. Nutr., *75*:225, 1961.

Miller, D. S., and Payne, P. R.: Problems in prediction of protein value of diets: The use of food tables. J. Nutr., *74*:413, 1961.

Milner, M.: Protein food problems in developing countries. Food Tech., *16*:51, 1962.

Munro, H. N.: Role of amino acid supply in regulating ribosome function. Fed. Proc., 27: 1231, 1968.

Murti, V. V. S., and Seshadri, T. R.: Naturally occurring less common amino acids of possible nutritional interest and their simpler derivatives. Nutr. Abstr. & Rev., 37:677, 1967.

Patwardhan, V. N.: Pulses and beans in human nutrition. Amer. J. Clin. Nutr., 11:12, 1962.

Rasch, P. J., and Pierson, W. R.: Effect of protein dietary supplement on muscular strength and hypertrophy. Amer. J. Clin. Nutr., 11:530, 1962.

Rice, E. E.: Nutritive values of oilseed proteins. J. Amer. Oil Chem. Soc., 47:408, 1970.

Scrimshaw, N. S.: Nature of protein requirements: Ways they can be met in tomorrow's world. J. Amer. Dietet. Assoc., 54:94, 1969.

Swendseid, M. E., et al.: An evaluation of the FAO reference pattern in human nutrition. I. Studies with young men. J. Nutr., 75:295, 1961. II. Studies with young women. J. Nutr., 77:391, 1962.

Trusswell, A. S., and Brock, J. P.: Effects of amino acid supplements on the nutritive value of maize protein for human adults. Amer. J. Clin. Nutr., 9:715, 1961.

Waslien, C. I., Calloway, D. H., Margen, S., and Costa, F.: Uric acid levels in men fed algae and yeast as protein sources. J. Food Sci., 35:294, 1970.

Watts, J. H., et al.: An evaluation of the FAO amino acid reference pattern in human nutrition. J. Nutr., 75:295, 1961.

Watts, J. H.: Evaluation of protein in selected American diets. J. Amer. Dietet. Assoc., 46:116, 1965.

Nutrition Reviews

A new approach for evaluation of proteins. 24:49, 1966.

Reduction of nitrogen deficits in surgical patients maintained by intravenous alimentation. 24:193, 1966.

Alteration in amino acids of sorghum hybrids grown in different locations. 24:223, 1966.

Features of kwashiorkor and nutritional marasmus in Jamaica. 26:38, 1968.

Malnutrition, infection, and socio-economic status. 26:100, 1968.

Undernutrition in children and subsequent brain growth and intellectual development. 26:197, 1968.

Liver ferritin synthesis in rats depleted of protein. 26:254, 1968.

Absorption of essential amino acids in man. 26:269, 1968.

Anemia of kwashiorkor. 26:273, 1968.

Endogenous nitrogen requirement. 26:277, 1968.

Mammalian production of N_2? 26:308, 1968.

Objective measurement of hair changes in kwashiorkor. 26:330, 1968.

Nitrogen retention in man in relation to the level and pattern of essential amino acids. 27:111, 1969.

Factors causing changes in plasma amino acid patterns. 27:241, 1969.

Infant brain following severe malnutrition. 27:251, 1969.

Fatty liver in kwashiorkor. 27:261, 1969.

Malnutrition and myelination. 28:110, 1970.

Total protein turnover in animals and man. 28:115, 1970.

Recovery rates of children following protein-calorie malnutrition. 28:118, 1970.

Size and nature of the protein gap. 28:223, 1970.

Protein and calorie concentration. 29:83, 1971.

Discovery

The most dramatic chapter of nutrition deals with the discovery and study of the group of body regulators called *vitamins*. Up to the early 1900's it was generally considered that only carbohydrates, protein, mineral elements, fat, and water were needed for normal nutrition of experimental animals.[1,2] Most investigators had paid little attention to the experiments in Estonia of Lunin,[3] who in 1880 found, disconcertingly, that mice died if fed on an artificial mixture of all the then known constituents of milk. Lunin concluded, "A natural food, such as milk, must therefore contain besides these known principal ingredients small quantities of unknown substances essential to life."

In retrospect, the discovery of the nature of vitamins had to wait until the chemical nature of carbohydrates, fats, and proteins was reasonably well established (which was the situation in the early 1900's). Only then could proof be provided that "unidentified substances" existed in food which were necessary for the life of animals.

Credit for the discovery of vitamins cannot be given to any one person, but to a few foresighted chemists and physiologists, working independently in several countries, who had the curiosity and ability to study *why* diets made of purified food ingredients were not able to support life of experimental animals. It had been known for centuries that certain foods such as liver (which was advocated as a cure for night-blindness by Hippocrates), citrus fruits and fresh vegetables, and cod liver oil were able to prevent or cure specific human disorders, but science had not advanced far enough to study experimentally the reasons behind the special beneficial effect of such foods.

A few pioneers in vitamin discovery, who used chemical techniques to make concentrates of the then unknown essential substances in food, deserve mention. The Dutch physician Grijns[4] reported in 1901 that the water and alcohol extract of the outer layer of rice and other grains contained an unknown substance which prevented a deficiency disease in man and animals.

Pekelharing,[5] also Dutch, fed small amounts of whey from milk to mice and concluded it had an unknown essential substance. He stated, "My intention is to point out that there is still an unknown substance in milk which even in very small quantities is of paramount importance to nourishment. If this substance is absent, the organism loses its power properly to assimilate the well-known principal parts of food, the appetite is lost and with apparent abundance the animals die of want. Undoubtedly this substance not only occurs in milk but in all sorts of foodstuffs, both of vegetable and animal origin."

In England, from 1906 to 1912, Hopkins[6] established by careful experiments that rats sickened and died on diets of pure protein, fat, and carbohydrates to which all the presumably necessary mineral matter had been added. Less than one-third of a teaspoonful of milk per day, added to the highly purified diet, made all the difference between life and death for the experimental animals. An alcoholic extract of dried milk or of certain vegetables also enabled the animals on purified diets to live and grow, but the *ash* of milk or vegetables was ineffectual. Thus, Hopkins showed that the essential unknowns that existed in foods in the natural state were *organic* (rather than inorganic) substances that could be dissolved in alcohol. For his work in establishing the existence of the substances we now call vitamins, Hopkins later was awarded a Nobel Prize.

In 1907, Holst and Frolich[7] of Oslo developed the first experimental test in guinea pigs for what we now know to be vitamin C. This stimulated further work on the unknown substances in food. Hart and co-workers[8] at the University of Wisconsin in 1911 made independent pioneering studies, using whole grains in experiments with cattle which demonstrated the essential nature of unknown substances in corn. Hart, chairman of the then Department of Agricultural Chemistry, had a special genius for attracting good persons on his staff to work on identifying the essential substances in food.* In 1909, McCollum, then a young chemist, was hired, and in just four years (1913) McCollum and Davis[9] had proved the existence of an essential food factor in butter and egg yolk. Miss Davis was a young biologist who had just obtained her bachelor's degree from the University of California and who volunteered to do the rat work for Dr. McCollum without a salary. Later McCollum proposed the terms "fat-soluble A" and "water-soluble B" to distinguish between the essential substances in butter fat and milk whey (the water-soluble material discovered by Pekelharing, Hopkins, and others). So it was proved not only that these nutritive essentials are organic in nature but that at least one of them was soluble in water while another was insoluble in water but soluble in fats and fat solvents. Thus, it became evident that there must be two or more of these mysterious but potent "accessory food substances" carried by natural foods.

Research in the field was stimulated greatly by a young biologist, Dr. Casimir Funk, who in 1912 at the age of 28 coined the word "vitamine"[10] and who, in 1914, wrote the first book on "The Vitamines."[11] He proposed, as others had before him, that beriberi, scurvy, pellagra, and possibly rickets were caused by a lack in the diet of "special substances which are of the nature of organic bases, which we will call vitamines." This name caught the popular fancy and has persisted, despite the fact that the particular trace nutrient which suggested the name to Funk turned out to be one of the very few

---

*Other persons now famous for their discoveries in the vitamin field and whom Hart placed on the Wisconsin staff were Steenbock, Elvehjem, Lepkovsky, Snell, Woolley, Strong, and many others who will be mentioned in later chapters.

that were amines.* At the suggestion of Drummond[12] in 1920, the final "e" was dropped to avoid any chemical significance. Also, Drummond suggested that the different vitamins "be spoken of as vitamin A, B, C, etc.," thus combining the "fat-soluble A" and "water-soluble B" nomenclature of McCollum with Funk's proposal. These changes were quickly accepted.

Definition

Vitamins may be defined as organic compounds, other than any of the amino acids, fatty acids, or carbohydrates, which are *necessary in small amounts in the diet of higher animals for normal growth, maintenance of health, and reproduction.* All animals need vitamins, but not every vitamin that has been discovered is needed by all animals. All higher plants can manufacture whatever vitamins they require,† but animals must have most of their vitamins supplied in the diet. Some of the vitamin needs of animals can be supplied from microorganisms growing in the digestive tract, especially in animals with a rumen (cow, sheep, goat, for instance) or a large cecum (horse or rabbit, for instance). There are differences between the vitamin requirements of human beings and of the lower animals, but interestingly there are more similarities than differences.

The action of vitamins is not unlike that of trace elements, such as iodine and copper, in that the presence or absence of very small amounts of them in the food means the difference be-

tween normal and abnormal functioning of the body. The potent effects of very small quantities in regulating body processes also remind us somewhat of the action of the hormones (thyroxine, epinephrine, etc.) that are formed by various ductless glands. Vitamins differ from the mineral elements in that they are *organic* substances, while they differ from hormones in that they are not formed within the body but must be supplied from a source outside the body.

It is easier to describe the effects of individual vitamins than to define them as a group. This is because they have turned out to be a heterogeneous group of substances which differ widely in their chemical nature and in their physiological action. Also, a few vitamins required to be furnished in the food of man can be formed by some animals in their own bodies (and vice versa). For example, humans get scurvy on diets that provide no vitamin C, but rats make this vitamin in their bodies and do not need it in food.

Distribution in Foods

The existence of vitamins was overlooked for many years because the foods consumed by man usually provided enough of them to prevent disastrous results to health. Most foods, as supplied by nature, contain a good supply of vitamins (richer in some, poorer in others), and the foods in an ordinary mixed diet supplement each other in vitamin content. The quantities of these substances present in foods were too small to have been detected by chemists, and fortunately only small amounts of them are required to avert nutritional disaster. In occasional instances, when the choice of foods was limited for one reason or another, diseased conditions did arise (e.g., scurvy occurred on long sea voyages, in besieged cities, or in times of famine), but it was many years before it dawned on people that such mysterious diseases might be caused by the

---

*Dr. Funk was not, as some have called him, the "father of vitamins," although he can properly be credited for coining the word and for being one of the early vitamin pioneers. He was born in Poland in 1884, and moved to London in 1910 to attend the Lister Institute. Funk became an American citizen in 1920 and remained active in research in New York City (with interim positions in Europe) until his death in 1967.

†A few lower plant forms, such as bacteria and yeast, need an external source of some vitamins.

lack of something in the diet. When refined foods, such as sugar and highly
milled grains, assumed a more prominent place in the diet, ill health due to
at least borderline deficiencies of certain
vitamins became fairly frequent. Now
we have come full cycle and are adding
some vitamins (and some minerals) to
foods from which they have been removed in the course of food processing
(e.g., enriched white bread).

What foods are our chief sources of
vitamins? Animals get most of their
vitamins either directly from plants,
in which they are formed from simple
substances (carbon dioxide, water,
and mineral salts with the aid of sunlight, and the well-known photosyn-
thetic pathway), or indirectly from animals which have fed on plants. The
green leaves of the plant are its chemical
laboratories in which vitamins are made
along with many other substances.
Hence, green leafy vegetables have high
content of most vitamins, as have also
the green, growing shoots of plants.
Seeds, such as legumes, nuts, and
whole-grain cereals, also have a good
content of certain vitamins. Root vegetables and fruits usually have a lower
content of most vitamins, although
there are notable exceptions. It should
be remembered that the different vitamins are often unevenly distributed in
food, and the vitamin content of fruits
and vegetables may vary, depending on
the variety, on the soil on which they
are grown, their stage of ripeness when
picked, conditions of storage and cooking, and other factors.

The lean flesh of animals (muscle
meats) is a good source of the water-
soluble vitamins (except vitamin C),
but organs such as liver and kidneys are
much richer in their vitamin content.
Certain animals are useful to man in
that they concentrate vitamins in foods
suitable for human consumption. Thus
cows and hens put vitamins from their
food into milk and the yolks of eggs,
which in turn become valuable sources
of vitamins. Fish store certain vitamins
(A and D) in their body fat, especially

in their livers. This accounts for the
fact that *fish liver oils* are the richest
natural source of these particular vitamins.

Although facts about the general distribution of vitamins in foods are interesting and useful, there are many
exceptions in regard to individual vitamins, so that each vitamin must be
studied separately to determine what
foods are needed to furnish it in
amounts adequate for health.

Number and Naming of Vitamins

In the 1920's and early 1930's it
became clear, after much painstaking
research, that water-soluble "vitamin B"
was in reality a mixture of at least several unrelated vitamins. Thus, the term
"vitamin B complex" was devised (see
Chapter 7). It is used today to describe,
collectively, the nine water-soluble vitamins other than vitamin C. The B complex vitamins have little in common except that they are soluble in water, are
present in large amounts in liver, and,
unlike vitamin C, all contain nitrogen.

The naming of individual vitamins at
first presented a problem, since little
was known about their chemistry. As
the vitamins became differentiated, they
were designated by the letters of the
alphabet, determined either by the
order of their discovery or by the initial letter of some word suggestive of
their role in nutrition, e.g., vitamin K
from the initial letter of the Danish and
German word for coagulation (koagulation). As the fraction originally known
as vitamin B became subdivided into
many different chemical substances,
they were called vitamin B-1, B-2, etc.*
or by their chemical names. As the
chemical identity of the different vita-

*Following recent nomenclature suggestions
of the International Union of Nutritional Sciences,[13] the formerly common use of a subscript,
as in "B$_1$" is abandoned in this text (in connection
with B-vitamins only). This has obvious advantages in typing and printing.

mins was established, chemical names gradually supplanted the earlier designation for the specific chemical compounds. However, the letter system is still in common use and is recommended[13, 14] when referring to groups of closely related substances that show a common vitamin activity (for example, one speaks of the "vitamin A activity" of several active chemicals, and of a "deficiency of vitamin A" when the deficiency can be of more than one vitamin A-active substance in food). Most of the individual vitamins exist in several different chemical forms in nature, and use of the historic name to identify the group is preferred over arbitrary new chemical terms.

Isolation and Synthesis of Vitamins

These technical terms are used to describe the long and difficult labors of vitamin researchers which were necessary in order to find out what the vitamin unknowns consisted of chemically and how to make them in the laboratory. At first this seemed an impossible task, since vitamins were present in foods in such minute traces. The dry weight of a man's food intake for a day is a little over one pound, or about 500 gm, whereas the total vitamins in his food, if separated, would weigh about 200 mg or $1/150$th of an ounce (about the size of a small garden pea, or pill), or about one part per 2500 parts of dry food.

To add to the difficulty, vitamins are organic substances and hence liable to destruction by heat, oxidation, and chemical processes used in their extraction. The magnitude of the task and the interesting role of vitamins in nutrition, however, constituted a challenge to chemists, who continued their painstaking labors sometimes for many years before the goal was attained. Dr. R. R. Williams, for example, first became interested in the deficiency disease beriberi and the antiberiberi factor in 1910, while with the Philippine Bu-

reau of Science. He continued his research in his free time while head of the American Telephone Laboratories in New York City and more than 20 years later isolated vitamin B-1, and determined its chemical structure. In 1936 he announced its synthesis and gave it the chemical name of thiamin, a sulfur-containing amine. Other scientists in all parts of the world participated in the effort to transform vitamins from unknown mysterious substances found only as traces in foods into known, *pure chemical compounds* that could be made at will.

The first step was to obtain concentrated preparations of vitamins from materials where they occurred in nature in largest amounts. Vitamins A and D were extracted from fish-liver oils, and the early B complex vitamins from rice polishings, liver, and dried yeast. Vitamin C was first obtained in concentrated form from citrus fruits and red peppers. These crude extracts were further concentrated and purified until small quantities of apparently pure substances (usually crystals) were obtained. These were then tested for vitamin activity in animals or microorganisms and analyzed chemically. The final steps in determining the chemical groupings in the molecule of the pure substance and finding out how to put these groups together to make the substance in the laboratory were probably the most difficult part of the task.

All of the vitamins are now obtainable either in concentrated preparations or as pure, chemical substances, at pharmacies or various retail stores at prices that vary considerably according to the firm which puts out the preparation. All, however, may be obtained at reasonable prices.

The 14 vitamins shown in Table 6–1 have been isolated as chemical compounds or groups of compounds, the composition and structure of which are known. All of them, with the exception of vitamin B-12, can be synthesized in the laboratory. Most are white in color, but three of the vitamins are yellow

Table 6–1.   The 14 Known Vitamins*

Vitamin
Vitamin A
Vitamin B complex
Thiamin (vitamin B-1)
Riboflavin
Niacin
Vitamin B-6
Pantothenic acid
Biotin
Choline†
Folacin
Vitamin B-12
Vitamin C
Vitamin D
Vitamin E
Vitamin K

*The B-complex vitamins and vitamin C are water-soluble; vitamins A, D, E, and K are fat-soluble.

†The need of this vitamin for humans has not been proved. Choline, however, is a vitamin for various animals (see Chapter 7).

and one is red; two are oily in nature and liquid at room temperature in the pure form. Many are manufactured in ton lots by the chemical industry for fortification of foods and for vitamin tablets.

Overzealous promoters of "health foods" often speak of certain other substances as being "vitamins" for man, such as "vitamin B-15" (pangamic acid), or "vitamin B-17," but only those listed in Table 6–1 are recognized by nutritional scientists today. Other vitamins may yet be discovered, though the possibilities that any now unidentified vitamins play more than a minor role remain slim. (See end of Chapter 7.)

Vitamin Research Today

Research on vitamins is now centered on determining (1) how they bring about their characteristic effects on body tissues; (2) how much is needed of each of the individual vitamins in the various stages of life; (3) their distribution in, and addition to, individual diets and foods; (4) the effect of deficiencies on pregnancy, growth and development, behavior, metabolic and infectious diseases, and aging; and (5) possible interrelations among different vitamins and among vitamins and other nutrient substances, such as proteins, carbohydrates, and minerals, as well as drugs and hormones. Such research, although difficult and slow, offers the same challenge to the nutritionists which determination of the chemical nature of the vitamins offered in former years.

Recommended Dietary Allowances

Although the fact that we measure vitamins in such small units as milligrams or micrograms (or in a few cases as "International Units"—see Chapter 9) makes it apparent that they exist in foods in "trace" quantities, still the total amounts of them needed by the body are somewhat comparable to (or in some cases greater than) the amounts of certain required trace minerals. By actual weight, the minimum daily requirements of normal adults for the different vitamins range from less than about 0.01 mg of vitamin D (and even less vitamin B-12) to 10 to 25 mg of vitamin C. A man needs less vitamin D than iodine per day, for example. On the other hand, his need for niacin (one of the B-complex vitamins) is about 2000 times (20 mg per day) the vitamin D requirement, to demonstrate one of the variations in vitamin requirements. This level, 20 mg, is double a male's iron requirement for further comparison.

The minimum daily requirement of individual vitamins for man is not an exact figure, as one would expect, although approximations can be made. Because of differences of inheritance, of microbiological flora in the intestine, of greatly different food and eating patterns, of stresses and disease, and other factors, the minimum requirement of individuals within large populations might vary as much as two- to threefold, if not more. Therefore, national and international groups who establish standards generally allow considerable margin for recommended vitamin intakes to allow for this variation and sometimes to allow for losses in preparation and storage of food. Recommended allowances for vitamins, then, are generally only a generous yardstick and are 25 to 50 percent higher than the actual requirement of most of a population; thus intakes below an allowance do not necessarily indicate too low a vitamin intake. On the other hand, recommended allowances are not necessarily sufficient for persons depleted of vitamins because of prior dietary inadequacies, disease, or traumatic stresses.[15]

It is to be hoped that some uniformity of national standards can eventually be attained by international nutrition bodies. In the meantime, the different standards for the United States, Canada, Great Britain, India, and FAO are given in Table 1B of the Appendix, for comparison. In developing countries the standards must often be set very close to the minimum because of the impracticality of obtaining larger amounts in most persons' diets.

The *recommended dietary allowances* (RDA) in the United States are still only approximations and are revised every five years by the Food and Nutrition Board of the National Academy of Sciences as new research is available.[15] The 1968 revision is given in Table 1A of the Appendix and includes not only daily recommendations for vitamins, but also minerals and other nutrients. These values are most commonly cited in this book where international standards have not been agreed upon, not because they are necessarily "better" than those set by other countries but for uniformity.* The levels are not too unlike those of other countries, with vitamin C being a major exception.

---

*As revisions of the RDA's become available in the future (the next one is expected in 1973), we recommend that the new allowances be used to supplement this edition of the textbook. Generally the changes, if any, are not expected to be more than up to 10 percent different from the present figures, thus not invalidating current information appreciably.

General Uses of Vitamins in the Body

Although individual vitamins have special functions, which are taken up in the following chapters, as a group of body regulators they share in certain functions, such as:

1. The promotion of growth.
2. The promotion of ability to produce healthy offspring.
3. The maintenance of health, vigor, and long life through promoting:
   a. Normal nutrition, especially utilization of mineral elements, amino acids, fatty acids, and metabolism of energy sources.
   b. Normal functioning of appetite and the digestive tract.
   c. Mental alertness.
   d. Health of tissues and resistance to bacterial infections.

It is worthwhile to keep in mind the above general uses of vitamins, since they recur constantly in the study of the functions of individual vitamins (see Fig. 6–1). Also, it should be emphasized that when several vitamins participate in promoting some function of the body, lack of any one of them can inhibit this function. For example, vitamins A, B-1, B-6, C, and D (as well as other vitamins) all have a direct influence in stimulating growth. When any one of these vitamins is supplied in inadequate amounts, growth will be stunted, even though the food contains plenty of the other vitamins needed for growth. In similar manner, damage to reproductive ability, to functioning of the digestive tract, and to the health of various tissues may result from lack of any one of several vitamins that are needed for the welfare of these organs or tissues.

It should also be remembered that stunting of growth, lack of appetite, poor utilization of food, and so on may be caused by an insufficiency of nutrients other than vitamins (or by medical problems unrelated to the food intake). So some of the more general symptoms of vitamin deficiency are not specific—

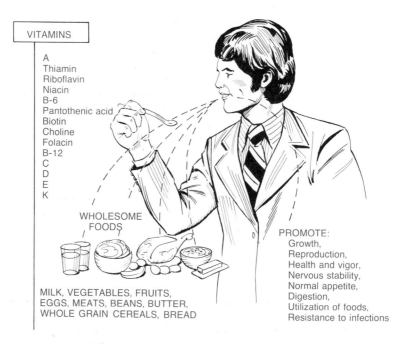

VITAMINS

A
Thiamin
Riboflavin
Niacin
B-6
Pantothenic acid
Biotin
Choline
Folacin
B-12
C
D
E
K

WHOLESOME
FOODS

PROMOTE:
Growth,
Reproduction,
Health and vigor,
Nervous stability,
Normal appetite,
Digestion,
Utilization of foods,
Resistance to infections

MILK, VEGETABLES, FRUITS,
EGGS, MEATS, BEANS, BUTTER,
WHOLE GRAIN CEREALS, BREAD

Figure 6–1. Different vitamins found in wholesome foods and their general functions in the body.

that is, not due always or solely to vitamin shortages.

Mode of Action of Vitamins

How do vitamins bring about their effects, and why are small amounts of them so indispensable for life? Before the mid 1930's the life-or-death importance of the presence or lack of these substances in trace amounts seemed mysterious, but research since then has given us at least a part of the answer to this enigma — namely, most vitamins act as an organic catalyst or as a part of a catalyst. A catalyst is a substance that speeds up a chemical reaction without itself taking part in it. Most of the hundreds of chemical reactions taking place in plant and animal tissues, which are essential to the life of the organisms, require catalysts to cause them to occur. The special types of organic catalysts that promote these reactions in living tissues are known as *enzymes* and *coenzymes,* which aid enzymes in their tasks.

Many of the vitamins occur in the body as part of enzymes or coenzymes responsible for promoting some essential chemical reaction. For instance, animal cells get much of the energy required for their life processes through oxidation of the carbohydrate, glucose. This takes place in many intermediate steps, so that energy is set free very gradually instead of all at once. Several of the B-complex vitamins have been shown to be a part of enzymes and coenzymes, each of which catalyzes only one special step in the oxidation of carbohydrate. The absence of any one of these enzymes means a failure of some indispensable link in the chain of tissue oxidations, hence the lack of a vitamin that is an essential part of such an enzyme can cripple vital oxidation processes in cells so that tissues all over the body may suffer. Since enzymes, as catalysts, are not used up in the reactions they promote, naturally only small amounts of them are needed.

Some of the vitamins occur in enzymes concerned with protein, fat, or mineral metabolism (as is described in connection with individual vitamins in the following chapters). At least two vitamins are involved in the control of oxidation and reduction (reactions of oxygen and hydrogen) within cells. Although it has not yet been established that all vitamins play their role through enzyme action, all act in some manner to promote chemical reactions that are essential for healthy tissues.

Interrelationship of Vitamins with Other Nutrients

As with the other nutrients, there is a disadvantage to studying the vitamins separately, because one tends to forget that within the body the vitamins are intimately, and very actively, involved in the metabolism and fate of all cellular substances. Most of the B vitamins have some role in energy metabolism (from carbohydrate or fat), and many are essential for proper utilization and metabolism of lipids, minerals, and/or amino acids.

Several vitamins are closely linked with calcium metabolism, while most could not function at all unless one or more phosphate radicals were attached for the coenzyme form. Additional examples of vitamin interrelationships will be given in the following chapter. For the beginning student, it is sufficient to remember that such interrelationships do exist; hence, the diet should supply a well balanced mixture of all the nutrients, including the vitamins, such as is provided by eating a wide variety of traditional foods—meat, milk, eggs, fruits (including citrus fruits), vegetables (including green leafy vegetables), whole grain cereals and bread, and butter or fortified margarine.

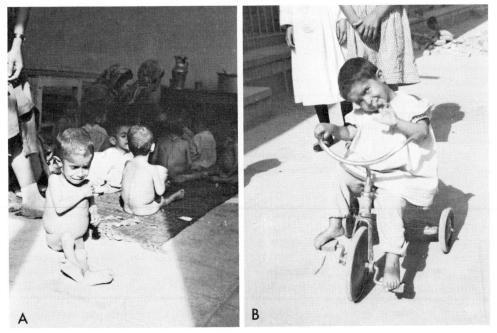

Figure 6–2. These photographs, taken by a nutritionist in one of the developing countries, illustrate the amazing progress possible for undernourished children when given proper feeding, including ample vitamins. After only 10 months on a nutritionally adequate diet, this five year old girl, once sickly and emaciated (**A**) has now the health and energy to enjoy the recreations typical of her age group (**B**). (Courtesy of Doreen Low.)

*Main Objective of Knowledge
of Vitamins*

The chief aim of the study of vitamins is to see that human beings get plenty of all of the various vitamins needed to promote positive health. This should not be lost sight of in the maze of interesting scientific facts which research on vitamins has brought to light. The need for vitamins begins before birth, since it is important that the diet of a pregnant woman should be rich in vitamins if the infant is to start life with a liberal store of these substances in its body.

Children must be liberally supplied with numerous vitamins in order to build healthy tissues and to achieve maximum growth (see Fig. 6–2). In adult life, good health and a longer life cannot be obtained without a plentiful supply of all needed vitamins. However, excessive amounts above the "optimal" confer no further benefits and may even have toxic effects. When vitamins are consumed in our ordinary foods, they are never at a toxic level of intake, but concentrates of vitamins themselves can be toxic when consumed in greater than normal amounts. Fat-soluble vitamins A and D are particularly noted for their toxicity in large doses. Large amounts of vitamins should never be taken except under the direction of a physician.

Although vitamin concentrates and pure, synthetic vitamins are very useful for the cure of conditions in which a person is unable to consume an adequate diet (illness, allergies, or emotional upsets), the objective of nutrition is to have enough of all the needed vitamins in the diet for prevention of disease and promotion of health. Moreover, when we get our vitamins from foods, we obtain in addition all the various other nutrients also essential to health.

QUESTIONS

1. Why are essential amino acids and fatty acids not classed as vitamins? Why are the "trace" elements, which are needed in very small amounts and must be supplied in food for normal body functioning, not included with the vitamins? Why are hormones, such as epinephrine and thyroxine, not called vitamins?

2. The rat and dog do not have to have vitamin C (ascorbic acid) supplied in their food, because they can make it in their own body tissues; men, monkeys, and guinea pigs cannot make this substance within their bodies, and hence must get it from foods. Could you say that ascorbic acid is a hormone for rats and a vitamin for man?

3. When was it first known that animals could not be maintained in health, or even survive, on diets of purified nutrients that provided plenty of calories, protein, and all necessary mineral elements? Approximately how long before it was recognized that natural foods provided traces of definite *organic substances* that were absent from the purified foodstuffs? When were these substances first called "vitamines"? Who first distinguished between two groups of these substances and called them "fat-soluble A" and "water-soluble B"?

4. What is meant by the following terms that are used in connection with vitamins: biological assay, International Units, U. S. Pharmacopeia units, vitamin concentrates, synthetic vitamins, a milligram, a microgram, minimum requirement, recommended allowance?

5. Why were the vitamins designated by letters of the alphabet? In general, is it better to call a vitamin by its chemical name, when it has been given one, or by a letter, and why? Are letters more convenient in some cases, for instance vitamin A instead of retinol, vitamin E instead of α-, β-, and γ-tocopherol? Why do we still speak of the group of vitamins D instead of calling them by chemical names? Can you give the chemical names for vitamins B-1, B-2, B-6 and C?

6. How can the vitamin content of foods be measured? In what types of food are fat-soluble vitamins found?

What classes of food are good purveyors of water-soluble vitamins? Name three foods that furnish considerable amounts of some water-soluble and fat-soluble vitamins together. Name five foods that carry little or no vitamins.

7. Give the general uses of vitamins in the body, i.e., functions in which several vitamins participate and to which all of them are essential. Would rats grow on a diet which furnished adequate energy, proteins, minerals, and all of the vitamins except vitamin A? Why? If it is true that vitamins A and C help to prevent infections, would you expect to raise bacterial resistance satisfactorily by taking a diet rich in one of these vitamins and poor in the other? Would taking ten times the recommended allowance of vitamin A be any more effective in raising bacterial resistance than the adequate level?

8. Explain how some vitamins have been shown to bring about their effects in the body by acting as catalysts. Why may lack of a vitamin, which forms part of an enzyme responsible for bringing about some reaction vital to metabolism of tissue cells, result in widespread tissue damage?

9. Why is it important that the vitamin intake should be well balanced, i.e., include all of the essential vitamins in the approximate proportions in which they are required by the body? Why is it advantageous to get vitamins in natural foods instead of eating a vitamin-poor diet and taking vitamins in pills or capsules?

REFERENCES

1. McCollum, E. V.: *A History of Nutrition.* Boston, Houghton Mifflin Co., 1957 (Chapters 14–20, 27).
2. Goldblith, S. A., and Joslyn, M. A.: *Milestones in Nutrition.* Westport, Conn., Avi Publishing Co., 1964.
3. Lunin, N.: Dissertation, Univ. Dorpat, 1880 (see page 204 of ref. 1); Zeit. Physiol. Chemie, 5:31, 1881 (see reprint of this paper on page 99 of ref. 2).
4. Grijns, G.: Geneesk. Tijdschr. v. Ned. Ind. 1, 1901 (see page 216 of ref. 1). Also see Eykman, C.: Arch. Hygiene, 58:150, 1906.
5. Pekelharing, C. A.: Nederlandsch. Tijdschr. N. Geneesk., 2:3, 1905 (see page 207, ref. 1).
6. Hopkins, F. G.: The Analyst, 31:385, 1906; Hopkins, F. G.: J. Physiol. (London), 44: 425, 1912.
7. Holst, A., and Frölich, J.: J. Hygiene, 7:634, 1907 (see pages 217 and 255 of ref. 1).
8. Hart, E. B., McCollum, E. V., Steenbock, H., and Humphrey, G. C.: Res. Bull. 17, Wisconsin Agric. Expt. Station, 1911.
9. McCollum, E. V.: *From Kansas Farm Boy to Scientist.* Lawrence, University of Kansas Press, 1964; McCollum, E. V., and Davis, M.: J. Biol. Chem., 15:167, 1913; 19:245, 1914.
10. Funk, C.: J. State Medicine, 20:341, 1912 (see reprint of this paper on page 145 of ref. 2).
11. Funk, C.: *Die Vitamine.* Wiesbaden, 1914 (re-published in English in 1922, and the first complete treatise on the subject of vitamins). Also see Todhunter, E. N.: J. Amer. Dietet. Assoc., 52:432, 1968.
12. Drummond, J. C.: Biochem. J., 14:660, 1920 (see reprint on page 177 of ref. 2).
13. IUNS Committee on Nomenclature: J. Nutr., 101:133, 1971; Nutr. Abs. Rev., 40:395, 1970.
14. Todhunter, E. N.: *A Guide to Nutrition Terminology for Indexing and Retrieval.* Washington, D.C., U.S. Department of Health, Education and Welfare, Public Health Service, 1970.
15. Food and Nutrition Board: *Recommended Dietary Allowances,* 7th Ed. Washington, D.C., National Academy of Sciences, 1968.

SUPPLEMENTARY READING

General, History, and Reviews
(also see refs. 1, 2, 14–15)

Harrow, B.: *Casimir Funk: Pioneer in Vitamins and Hormones.* New York, Dodd, Mead & Co., 1955.
Interdepartmental Committee on Nutrition for National Defense: *Manual for Nutritional Survey.* 2nd. Ed. Washington, D.C., U.S. Government Printing Office, 1963.
Latham, M. C., McGandy, R. B., McCann, M. B., and Stare, F. J.: *Scope Manual on Nutrition.* Kalamazoo, Mich., The Upjohn Co., 1970.
Lepkovsky, S.: The water-soluble vitamins. Ann. Rev. Biochem., 9:383, 1940.
Marks, J.: *The Vitamins in Health and Disease: A Modern Reappraisal.* London, J & A Churchill Ltd., 1968.
Medical Research Council: *Vitamins, A Survey of Present Knowledge,* Special Reports Series

No. 167. London, H.M. Stationery Office, 1932.

Robinson, F. A.: *The Vitamin Co-factors of Enzyme Systems.* Oxford, Pergamon Press, 1966.

Rosenberg, H. R.: *Chemistry and Physiology of the Vitamins.* New York, Interscience Publishers, 1942.

Sebrell, W. H., Jr., and Harris, R. S. (eds.): *The Vitamins.* New York, Academic Press, 1967–72 (in 7 volumes; Vols. VI and VII edited by György, P., and Pearson, W. N. Vols. II to V in press. Also see former editions, 1954, for older references).

Seidell, A.: The chemistry of vitamins. Science, *60*:439, 1924.

U.S. Department of Agriculture: *Food,* Yearbook of Agriculture, pp. 130–167. Washington, D.C., U.S. Government Printing Office, 1959.

Watt, B. K., and Merrill, A. L.: *Composition of Foods: Raw, Processed, Prepared.* Washington, D.C., U.S. Department of Agriculture Handbook No. 8, 1963.

Other References

Bender, A. E.: Vitamin allowances. Rev. Nutr. Food Sci., *14*:8, 1969.

Campbell, J. A.: Dietary factors affecting vitamin requirements. Proc. Nutr. Soc., *23*:31, 1964.

Girdwood, R. H.: Problems in the assessment of vitamin deficiency. Proc. Nutr. Soc., *30*: 66, 1971.

Miller, D. F., and Voris, L.: Chronologic changes in the Recommended Dietary Allowances. J. Amer. Dietet. Assoc., *54*:109, 1969.

Schroeder, H. A.: Losses of vitamins and trace minerals resulting from processing and preservation of foods. Amer. J. Clin. Nutr., *24*:562, 1971.

Sebrell, W. H., Jr.: Recommended dietary allowances—1968 revision. J. Amer. Dietet. Assoc., *54*:103, 1969.

Sorrell, M. F., et al.: Absorption of vitamins from the large intestine *in vivo.* Nutr. Rep. Internat., *3*:143, 1971.

Weits, J., et al.: Nutritive value and organoleptic properties of three vegetables fresh and preserved in six different ways. Internat. J. Vit. Res., *40*:648, 1970.

For additional up-to-date vitamin references (since this is a very active research field), see current issues of:

J. Nutr.	British J. Nutr.
J. Vitaminology (Japan)	Nutr. & Metabolism
Indian J. Nutr. Diet.	J. Amer. Dietet. Assoc.
J. Amer. Med. Assoc.	Nutrition Reviews
Amer. J. Clin. Nutr.	Internat. J. Vit. Nutr. Res.
J. Nutr. Educ.	Nutr. Abst. Rev.
	and others

Biographies of Vitamin Discoverers in J. Nutr.:

Subject	Volume
Drummond, J. C.	*82*: Jan. 1964
Eijkman, C.	*42*: Sept. 1950
Elvehjem, C. A.	*101*: May 1971
Goldberger, J.	*55*: Jan. 1955
Grijns, G.	*62*: May 1957
Hart, E. B.	*51*: Sept. 1953
Hogan, A. G.	*97*: Jan. 1969
Holst, A.	*53*: May 1954
Hopkins, F. G.	*40*: Jan. 1950
Jansen, B. C. P.	*100*: May 1970
Lind, J.	*50*: May 1953
McCollum, E. V.	*100*: Jan. 1970
Mendel, L. B.	*60*: Sept. 1956
Osborne, T. B.	*59*: May 1956
Pekelharing, C. A.	*83*: May 1964

Nutrition Reviews

Availability of vitamins and minerals in tablet form. *24*:101, 1966.

The effect of ethanol ingestion on liver dehydrogenases in various vitamin deficiencies. *25*:22, 1967.

Diet preferences and specificity of hungers in rats fed diets deficient in various vitamins and minerals. *26*:25, 1968.

seven

Vitamin B Complex

As mentioned in Chapter 6, the first experimental studies of the "essential unknown substances," now the "vitamins," were made with water-soluble extracts of natural foods. It is logical, then, to start the study of individual vitamins with what we now know to be the nine B complex vitamins and, in the next chapter, vitamin C. Both the B complex and vitamin C are water soluble.

Final proof for the existence of more than one "vitamin B," as it was then called, did not come until the 1920's, when the term "vitamin B complex" originated.* The process of identification of the vitamins was very slow until the pure substances could be isolated, or at least concentrated. They then could be added to experimental diets, necessary for proving the existence of still other unknown vitamins. Much progress was made in the 1930's when a new vitamin was discovered almost every year. The last of the B vitamins to be discovered so far was vitamin B-12 in 1948.

It should be kept in mind that although all the B vitamins have distinctive properties and, hence, must be

studied separately, they are intimately interrelated in the body in cellular reactions.

THIAMIN (VITAMIN B-1)

Discovery

Thiamin was the first of the B complex vitamins to be obtained in pure form, hence the name vitamin B-1, a term proposed by the British in 1927. Various other names were used, including "antineuritic factor," "antiberiberi factor," vitamin F, "water-soluble B," and, simply "vitamin B."

It took a period of just over 50 years, from 1885 to 1936, to unravel the mystery of the nature of vitamin B-1 and to be able to synthesize it in the chemical laboratory. The first synthesis, along with the establishment of its chemical identity, was made in 1936 by R. R. Williams and co-workers, who gave it the name "thiamine"[2] (from *thio*, meaning sulfur-containing, and *amine*: the final "e" was later dropped). (See Fig. 7-1.)

The search for the cause of the disease *beriberi* in man (see page 120) and the disease *polyneuritis*, its counterpart

---

*The first use of the term "vitamin B complex" appears to be in the paper by Salmon, in 1927.[1]

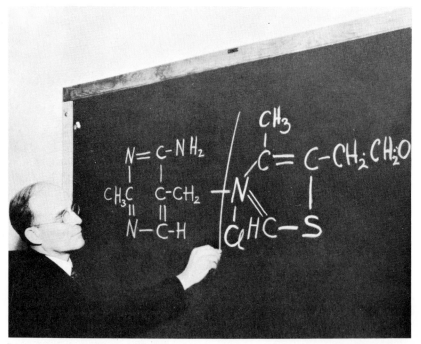

Figure 7–1.   Dr. R. R. Williams writing the structural formula of thiamin on blackboard and indicating where the molecule splits on certain chemical treatment. The important sulfur atom is seen in the right-hand part and the amino group (NH_2) in the left-hand part of the molecule. (Courtesy of the late Dr. Williams.)

in animals (fowl), was the start of the discovery of this vitamin. Beriberi had been described in Chinese medical literature before Christ. The word means "I cannot" (since persons with severe beriberi cannot move easily). Its cause was not known to be related to the diet until late in the nineteenth century. In 1880, a Dutch naval doctor, van Leent, reported that death from beriberi was greatly reduced in Indian naval crews when European-type diets were eaten instead of diets consisting primarily of rice. In 1885, Takaki (chief medical officer of the Japanese Navy) reported that beriberi had been eradicated among the sailors as a result of adding extra meat, fish, and vegetables to the regular diet. Before this time, the disease was so common that three out of every ten sailors were likely to have it, and there were many deaths.

In 1890, the young Dutch physician Eijkman, who was assigned to a prison hospital in Java, noticed that a disease similar to beriberi appeared in chickens which had been fed the leftover food from the diet of the hospital patients who had beriberi. This diet consisted of little more than polished rice. He found by careful observation, when his new hospital director forbade him the use of the leftover food, that he could cure the disease in the chickens by feeding whole rice or by returning the hull to the polished rice diet. Eijkman thought that the carbohydrate content of rice produced a toxin, thus missing the true reason for his results.

Later, his work was carried on at the same hospital by another Dutch physician, Grijns, who concluded in 1901[3] that beriberi in man and polyneuritis in chickens were caused by the *absence* in the diet of some unknown substance present in the germ or outer coat of grains, as well as in beans, but not in highly milled grains. These experiments were historically important because they led to the discovery not only of thiamin but also of other B vitamins through studies of deficiencies produced in animals. Shortly thereafter, many other workers in Java, the Philippines, and elsewhere repeated these studies, and found that the disease could be prevented also by feeding concentrates from yeast, wheat germ, and milk.

Between 1911 and 1925, the first serious attempts were made to isolate and identify the "antineuritic factor," as it was then called.[4] These were unsuccessful but helpful to later workers. One extra dividend of these early attempts was the word "vitamine," coined by Funk during his studies on the antineuritic factor (see Chapter 6).

Chemical Identification and Properties

The first pure preparation of what is now known as thiamin was isolated from rice polishings in 1926 by Jansen and Donath[5] of the Dutch East Indian Medical Service in Java in the same laboratory where Eijkman and Grijns did their pioneer work on beriberi in man and polyneuritis in fowl.* This was

---

*Of interest is the fact that instead of using pigeons and chickens for their test animals, Jansen and Donath used the native "ricebirds." They isolated 100 mg of crystals from 100 kg of rice polishings.

an important event, since it was the first time any vitamin was obtained from food in crystalline form, thus taking vitamins out of the class of "mysterious substances." However, it was ten years later before Williams was able to announce its structure and synthesis.[2]

Thiamin is a crystalline substance (Fig. 7–2), made up of carbon, hydrogen, oxygen, and sulfur (see formula in Appendix). It is readily soluble in water, slightly soluble in alcohol, and insoluble in fat solvents. Thiamin may be destroyed during storage or by heating in neutral or alkaline solutions, especially by prolonged heating. It is quite stable (not readily destroyed) in the dry state. Synthetic thiamin is usually prepared in the form of one of its salts, such as thiamin hydrochloride or thiamin mononitrate, which are more stable than the free vitamin.

Certain raw fish and seafood, particularly carp, herring, clams, and shrimp, contain the enzyme *thiaminase*, which is capable of splitting the thiamin molecule into its two major chemical groups, thus making it inactive. This effect has been seen in fox farms where the animals were fed raw fish, resulting in severe economic losses. The effect can also be produced in laboratory animals (cats, chickens, etc.) by feeding raw fish at a level of 10 to 25 percent. This action can be prevented by heating the fish first and destroying the enzyme. In most countries, humans do not normally eat sufficient raw fish or seafood to produce a vitamin B-1 deficiency, but the possibility

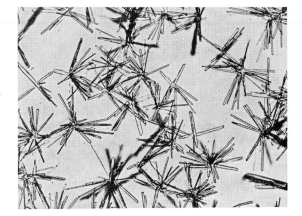

Figure 7–2. Photomicrograph of thiamin hydrochloride, crystalline form. (Courtesy of Merck & Company, Inc.)

exists that this may be a contributory factor in producing beriberi in certain populations of the world (especially in the Orient).

Other agents are known to affect thiamin levels in the body. For instance, a large amount of live yeast in the diet of man reduces the amount of thiamin absorbed from the intestine. Thiamin-splitting bacteria have been found in the intestinal tracts of people in Japan with symptoms of beriberi, but the significance of this is unknown at present.

Effects of Lack of Thiamin in Man and Animals

The *symptoms* of beriberi in humans are numbness or tingling in toes and feet, stiffness of ankles and absence of the ankle-jerk reflex, cramping pains in legs, difficulty in walking, and finally paralysis of legs with atrophy of leg muscles (see (Fig. 7–3). In later stages various nerves may be affected (giving rise to the term antineuritic vitamin used in the early literature), and disturbances of heart function are common. In the form known as *wet beriberi*, dropsical bloating or edema (especially of the legs) is a complicating factor due probably to cardiac disturbances (Fig. 7–4). Although the endemic beriberi, so prevalent in the Orient in earlier years, was probably due to a deficiency of several nutrients, there is no doubt that the primary deficiency was that of thiamin. The extensive tissue damage that occurs in beriberi, because of lack of thiamin, makes us realize how important a role this vitamin plays in normal nutrition.

EXPERIMENTAL ANIMALS. Without experimental animals to use in studying the counterpart of human deficiencies, it is likely that the discovery of many of the vitamins would have been postponed many years, and their metabolic function would be most difficult to study. For this reason and because of their possible use in classroom demonstrations, some attention is given here to vitamin deficiencies in animals, as well as human deficiencies.

In young experimental animals made deficient in thiamin, symptoms may be seen

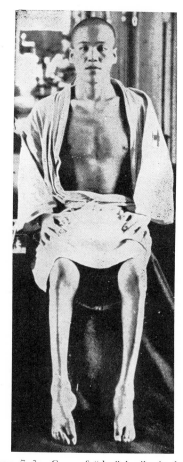

Figure 7–3. Case of "dry" beriberi, showing atrophy of the muscles due to paralysis of the legs. (Courtesy of Herzog and the *Philippine Journal of Sciences.*)

as early as three to six days after withholding the vitamin. All deficient animals show poor growth, nervous symptoms, and death in severe cases. Pigeons and fowl develop a severe and characteristic head retraction, a form of polyneuritis (Figs. 7–5 and 7–6). Swine develop generalized weakness, vomiting, and dizziness. Rats show reduced growth (Fig. 7–7), convulsions, slowing of the heart beat, and a loss of appetite. Vitamin B-1 deficiency signs, generally similar, have been produced also in the dog, monkey, guinea pig, mouse, cat, and in fact, in every animal tested except those species in which sufficient thiamin is produced by intestinal microorganisms to take care of the animal's requirement. Thiamin is also

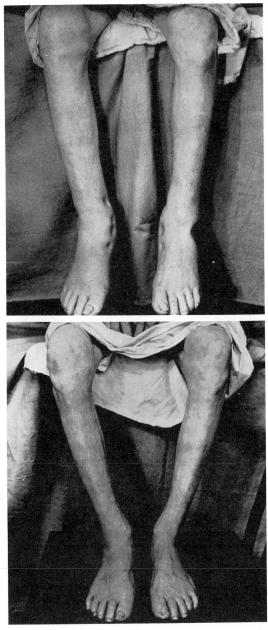

Figure 7–4. Patient before and after treatment for vitamin B-1 deficiency (so-called "wet" beriberi). **A,** Swelling of the legs and marked pitting edema in the ankle region. **B,** Ten days after initiation of thiamin therapy, during which the patient lost 40 pounds. Presumably this weight loss was due to the loss of fluid because the general nutritive state was greatly improved. (From Spies: *Rehabilitation Through Better Nutrition,* Philadelphia, W. B. Saunders, 1947.)

necessary for normal fertility and lactation in experimental animals.

Most microorganisms are able to synthesize thiamin, which is needed to promote their growth. Microorganisms in the rumen, or large stomach, of cattle, sheep, and goats (all ruminants) make sufficient thiamin, and in fact, other B complex vitamins, to take care of the animal's entire need for these vitamins. These are absorbed and utilized in the usual manner. Thus, it is not necessary to give sources of thiamin to these animals except when they are very young before the rumen is functioning. Animals

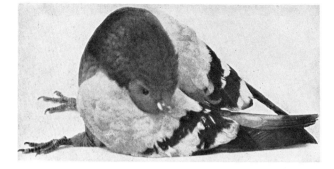

Figure 7–5. Characteristic attitude of pigeon with polyneuritis (avian beriberi) after three weeks' feeding with a diet of polished rice. The pigeon was used year after year as a class demonstration, and the extreme effect passed off within a few hours after feeding foods rich in thiamin. (From Morse: *Applied Biochemistry.* Philadelphia, W. B. Saunders, 1927.)

Figure 7–6. Pigeon shown in Figure 7–5 three hours after feeding some rich source of thiamin (rice polishings, yeast, etc.). Recovery seemed to be complete in 12 hours. (From Morse: *Applied Biochemistry.*)

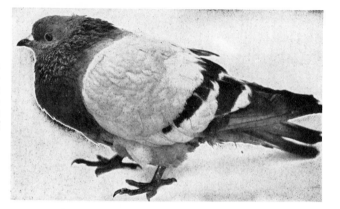

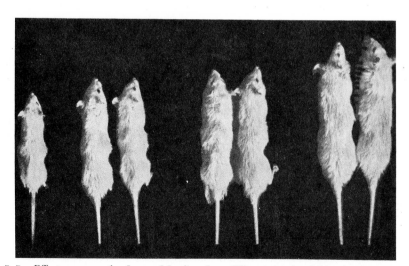

Figure 7–7. Effects on growth of rats of feeding four different levels of thiamin. (From experiments by Dr. Bertha Bisbey.)

such as rabbits and rats which routinely eat some of their feces (a practice known as "coprophagy") and thus obtain B vitamins produced by intestinal bacteria, must be kept in cages with screened bottoms in experiments for producing deficiencies, in order to reduce the chance of their eating the feces.

The composition of the diet affects the amount of intestinal synthesis by microorganisms of thiamin in man and animals. In the rat, for instance, a diet high in starch is likely to cause greater synthesis of thiamin by bacteria than a diet high in sucrose. In man some intestinal synthesis of thiamin and other B vitamins by microorganisms also takes place, but the synthesis occurs so low in the tract and in a form so poorly absorbed that it is of little use to the human body.

In most animals (including man), thiamin plays a part in promoting appetite and better functioning of the digestive tract, effects that have an indirect influence in promoting growth. The emptying time of the stomach and intestines is nearly twice as slow in thiamin-deficient animals as in normal ones. However, most authorities agree that the effect of thiamin on appetite is not restricted to this vitamin alone and is exerted only when there has been a deficiency of it in the diet, and then only to the extent of restoring normal appetite. Large quantities of thiamin do not promote a voracious appetite, and other factors may be responsible for loss of desire for food.

Thiamin has been called "the morale vitamin," because one of the earliest signs of its lack is a lowering of stamina. Studies of people who volunteered to consume a diet moderately low in thiamin demonstrated that after a very short time on such a diet (as early as 10 days) the subjects became depressed and irritable, lacking in ability to concentrate on and to take an interest in their work.[6] In three to seven weeks such symptoms as fatigue, lack of appetite, loss of weight, constipation, muscle cramps, and various pains appeared. The subjects promptly recovered normal health and morale when given larger amounts of thiamin.

Functions in the Body

In humans, after thiamin is absorbed, it is distributed widely by the blood throughout the body in all tissues and in somewhat higher concentrations in such organs as the heart, liver, and kidneys. There is limited ability of the body to store thiamin. Tissues are depleted of their normal content of the vitamin in a relatively short period if the diet is deficient, so fresh supplies are needed regularly to provide for maintenance of tissue levels. The tissues take up only as much as they need, and because it is freely soluble in water, most of the thiamin intake not required for day-to-day use is excreted in the urine, either as the intact molecule or as split halves.

Of foremost importance is the part thiamin plays in the life processes of individual cells throughout the body. A large part of the energy for the life processes of body tissues comes from the oxidation of carbohydrate, which takes place gradually through the formation of intermediate products and requires enzymes to bring about or catalyze each step of the intricate process. Many enzymes require *coenzymes* to render them active, or make them capable of bringing about a certain chemical change (Fig. 7–8). Thiamin is known to be the active part of the coenzyme *thiamin pyrophosphate*, made in tissue cells by the combining of thiamin with two phosphate groups or radicals.

This very important coenzyme is known to be necessary for at least four different enzyme systems that are needed for the complete oxidation of carbohydrate. Two of these enzymes function by splitting off carbon dioxide in the course of oxidation in the body, or in reverse reactions adding it onto some fragment of metabolism. For example, by such reactions pyruvic acid and other keto acids (intermediates in glucose oxidation) are converted step by step, with the removal of carbon dioxide (decarboxylation), to acetate radicals and eventually to carbon dioxide and water. Hence, thiamin pyrophosphate constitutes an essential link in the chain of passing along oxygen to the tissues, and it must be provided for the

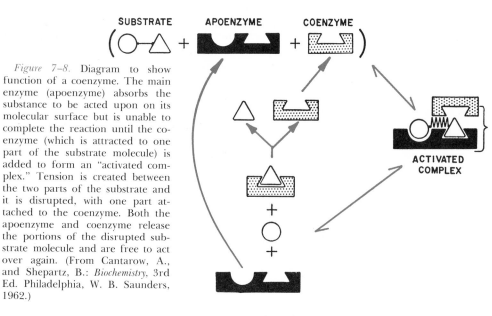

SUBSTRATE   APOENZYME   COENZYME

ACTIVATED
COMPLEX

Figure 7–8. Diagram to show function of a coenzyme. The main enzyme (apoenzyme) absorbs the substance to be acted upon on its molecular surface but is unable to complete the reaction until the coenzyme (which is attracted to one part of the substrate molecule) is added to form an "activated complex." Tension is created between the two parts of the substrate and it is disrupted, with one part attached to the coenzyme. Both the apoenzyme and coenzyme release the portions of the disrupted substrate molecule and are free to act over again. (From Cantarow, A., and Shepartz, B.: *Biochemistry,* 3rd Ed. Philadelphia, W. B. Saunders, 1962.)

complete oxidation of carbohydrate. Without a dietary source of thiamin, pyruvic acid and other intermediate compounds may build up in the blood and tissues to a toxic level, and these compounds are presumed to be an important cause of deficiency symptoms.

Thiamin pyrophosphate serves also as a coenzyme in reactions leading to the production of ribose, the important pentose sugar needed by all cells of the body (see sections on DNA and RNA, pp. 76–78). Essential cofactors in these actions of thiamin pyrophosphate are the coenzymes of several other vitamins (such as pantothenic acid and niacin), as well as magnesium, demonstrating the essential interrelationship in the body of the various vitamins and minerals.

*Requirement and Nutritional
Status*

American diets provide enough thiamin to prevent the appearance of frank beriberi in this country. However, a good many diets may provide less than optimal amounts, especially in times of body stress caused by growth, pregnancy, lactation, fevers, or surgical operations. Nervous symptoms due to a lack of thiamin are seen often in chronic alcoholic persons in this country, since their diet is often inadequate and their high intake of energy in the form of alcohol increases their requirement for thiamin.

The amount of thiamin required by adults varies according to size, degree of activity, dietary habits, and individual differences in how food is utilized. Since this vitamin takes part in the metabolism of carbohydrate, more of it is needed when the rate of carbohydrate metabolism is high. Persons who do considerable muscular work burn up more energy foods and usually obtain much of this extra energy in the form of starchy foods; hence, they need more thiamin than those who are muscularly inactive. The requirement for thiamin is usually stated in terms of the caloric intake (so much for every 1000 kcal), particularly of the nonfat calories of the diet; with more fat and a lower proportion of calories from carbohydrate, slightly less thiamin is needed. *Growing children* have higher energy needs and therefore have higher thiamin needs per unit of body weight than adults. Women during *pregnancy* have a slightly increased need for thiamin, and *nursing mothers* should have approximately 1½ times as much thiamin as under normal conditions.

The recommendations of the U.S. Food and Nutrition Board, in 1968,[7] provide a moderately liberal daily intake of thiamin for normal adults, varying according to the caloric intake recommended for the different age groups, which is greater in younger adults. For college age women the recommended intake is 1.0 mg per day and for college age men, 1.4 mg. See Table 7-1 for thiamin allowances of selected age groups (and see Table 1A in the Appendix for complete details for all age groups). These values for thiamin are slightly higher than previous recommendations of the Board on the basis of new information.

Daily allowances for adults, according to the Food and Nutrition Board, are calculated on the basis of individual calorie requirements, allowing 0.5 mg per 1000 kcal (the *minimum requirement* is approximately 0.33 mg per 1000 kcal). The Food and Nutrition Board cautions, however, that older adults who subsist on a calorie intake of less than 2000 should not have less than 1.0 mg of thiamin per day, which is recognized as about the minimum daily requirement. There is no evidence that larger intakes than the recommended allowance will be of any benefit to normal healthy adults.

Table 7-1. Recommended Allowances for Thiamin*

	Age	Allowance, mg/day
Males	12–14 years	1.4
	14–18 years	1.5
	18–35 years	1.4
	35–55 years	1.3
	55 years and over	1.2
Females	12–18 years	1.2
	18 years and over	1.0
	Pregnant	+0.1
	Lactating	+0.5

*From the Food and Nutrition Board, 1968.[7]
See Appendix Table 1C for FAO recommendations.

Dietary surveys have shown that the average intake of thiamin in the United States is not much higher than the recommended allowance, and we are indebted to the enrichment program for keeping the level as high as it is (see Chapter 17). For example, Williams and co-workers concluded in 1942 that the average American diet, prior to the introduction of enriched bread and cereal foods, provided only about 0.8 mg of thiamin per 2500 kcal which was dangerously near the minimum requirement.[8] The enrichment of bread and cereals, started during World War II, has increased by about one-third the amount of thiamin available for the average person, most all of this coming from synthetic thiamin at a negligible cost.[8] In 1969 about 1.77 mg of thiamin was available per person per day from the nation's food supply, according to the U.S. Department of Agriculture.[9] This figure is unquestionably higher than the amount actually consumed by the average person, because the U.S.D.A. figure does not take into account either waste of food or destruction of thiamin during preparation, cooking, or canning of foods.

It is apparent that many individuals must be consuming levels of thiamin very close to, or even less than, the recommended allowance. However, various recent food and nutrition surveys[10–13] have shown that in spite of intakes of excessively high amounts of carbohydrates and only borderline amounts of thiamin, few, if any, signs of thiamin deficiency are apparent in large numbers of population groups.

Food Sources of Thiamin

Few foods relatively rich in thiamin are used in quantity in our modern diets unless they are enriched with the synthetic vitamin. Although almost all natural foods contain thiamin, many of them carry only minor amounts, which may be still further reduced by cooking or processing. From available figures (see Appendix, Table 2)[14] it may be seen that the thiamin content of most fruits and vegetables, eggs, milk, and cheese does not generally exceed 0.1 mg per 100 gm. In plants it is concentrated chiefly in *seeds* (whole grains, legumes, and nuts); in animals it is abundant in the *organs* (liver, heart, kidneys). Pork flesh is much higher in thiamin content than other meats, but *meats* and *leafy vegetables* are moderately good sources. In certain processed or refined foods, such as highly milled cereals, sugar, fats, and sulfured dried fruits, thiamin is present in traces or entirely absent (unless these foods have been enriched with added thiamin). There is none in salad oils or other fats.

Our best sources of thiamin (see Table 7–2)—*whole grains, organ meats, pork,* and *legumes*—are not used in quantity in the American diet. However, foods of more moderate thiamin content are used in sufficient amounts to provide this vitamin at a fairly safe level. Of this, about 36 percent comes from bread and cereals; 27 percent from meats, fish, poultry, eggs, legumes, and nuts; 14 percent from milk and other dairy products; and 22 percent from vegetables and fruits.[9] In low-cost diets, in which grain products and potatoes furnish a higher proportion of the diet, it is especially important that bread and cereals be of a whole-grain or enriched variety. Such foods as oatmeal and dried legumes can be an economical source of thiamin. It is significant that beriberi seldom, if ever, develops in countries where meats, dairy products, fruits, and vegetables are freely used. It should be noted that sucrose and pure fats, which supply over 35 percent of the energy intake of an average American diet, provide no thiamin or other water-soluble vitamins.

Effects of Cooking and Processing

Thiamin in food suffers little destruction on exposure to air at ordinary temperatures. Under ordinary conditions of preparation, there is not too much loss of thiamin due to heat instability. Dry heating at high temperatures, as in preparation of ready cooked cereals or in toasting bread, can cause considerable loss. Moist heat (boiling for not more than an hour) causes little destruction of this vitamin, but its solubility in water means that as much as one-third of the original thiamin content may be lost if cooking water is liberal and is discarded. Thiamin is very unstable in an alkaline medium and is largely destroyed if soda is added

Table 7–2. Examples of Good Food Sources of Thiamin*

Food Source	Thiamin, mg/100 gm	Food Source	Thiamin, mg/100 gm
Bacon, Canadian	0.83	Pecans	0.86
Beans, Pinto	0.84	Piñon nuts	1.28
Buckwheat flour (dark)	0.58	Pork	0.50
Cornflakes with added		Rice polish	1.84
nutrients	0.43	Rye, whole grain	0.43
Heart, beef	0.53	Sesame seeds	0.98
Kidneys, hog	0.58	Soybeans	1.10
Lentils	0.37	Sunflower seed	1.96
Liver, lamb	0.40	Whole wheat flour	0.55
Oatmeal (dry)	0.60	Wheat germ	2.01
Peanuts (with skins)	1.14	Yeast	
Milk chocolate with		Brewer's	15.61
peanuts	0.25	Torula	14.01
Peas	0.35		

*From Watt, B. K., and Merrill, A. L.[14] Based on fresh, raw, edible portion.

in the cooking of vegetables. Meats lose 46 to 60 percent of thiamin in roasting, 30 percent in broiling, and only 15 percent in frying. In baking bread, only 5 to 15 percent of the original thiamin content is lost, while there is no significant loss of this vitamin in cooking cereals in a double boiler. Prolonged cooking, as of dried legumes, results in relatively high losses of their thiamin content. The thiamin content of vegetables is preserved by freezing and by storage below 0° C, so that, as purchased, fresh frozen vegetables are about as rich in thiamin as the original product. Canned vegetables suffer a loss owing to solubility of the vitamin in the canning fluid drained away.

RIBOFLAVIN

Discovery

In the course of years of experimenting with the growth-promoting factor called "water-soluble B," it became evident between 1917 and 1927 that there must be at least two vitamins in yeast, liver, and the outer coats of grains.[4] It would be difficult to give any one person credit for obtaining the first experimental deficiency of what is now known as riboflavin, but mention should be made of Emmett, of Detroit, who probably provided the first evidence for the existence of a second vitamin B (1917–1920).[15] Severe heating (such as at 120° C in an autoclave for several hours) completely destroyed the anti-beriberi vitamin (thiamin) in yeast, but there remained another vitamin fraction which showed growth-promoting potency. Although this heat-stable fraction is now known to consist of several vitamins, the one first discovered and studied was called *vitamin B₂* by the British in 1927, or *vitamin G* by Americans. Both these names for riboflavin are no longer used and the terms have historic significance only.

Chemical Identification and Properties

In 1933, chemists in Germany found that rats grew faster when given a dietary source of a yellow compound called "ovoflavin," which they isolated from egg white ("flavus" means yellow). It was soon shown that the flavin pigment that had been isolated and that was essential for rats was the same as the pigment associated with the classic "yellow enzyme," isolated by Warburg in Germany in 1932, and similar to the yellow pigment isolated from heart muscle by Szent-Györgyi and co-workers in 1932, which was later shown to be an important coenzyme. This proved to be *the first demonstration of a vitamin-coenzyme relationship* and opened the door to modern nutritional biochemistry. It is of interest that as long ago as 1879 yellowish-green fluorescent pigments were isolated from whey and other biological materials, but the biological significance of such pigments (now known to be riboflavin) had not been established previously.

Other workers in Germany and Switzerland, in most cases before 1933, had isolated similar fluorescent pigments from milk, liver, plant material, and egg yolk, which were given names indicating their source as "lactoflavin" (from milk) or "hepatoflavin" (from liver). It was soon learned that all these substances were similar and the name "riboflavin" was given by Karrer of Switzerland* to the most active compound in 1935 and is in general use today. Riboflavin was first synthesized in 1935 by two independent groups led by Kuhn of Germany and Karrer. It was found to have a pentose side chain— *ribitol* (similar to the sugar, ribose)— attached to a flavin-like compound, hence the name riboflavin.

---

*Karrer died in 1971. He was also the first to synthesize carotene, to be discussed in Chapter 9, and made other important discoveries in nutrition. He was awared the Nobel Prize in 1937 for these studies.

Riboflavin is an orange-yellow solid which imparts a greenish-yellow fluorescence to solutions (see formula in Appendix). One of its most important chemical properties is its change to a colorless form on reduction (addition of hydrogen molecules), and its reoxidation (removal of hydrogen) to its orange-yellow color by exposure to oxidizing agents. It is sparingly soluble in water, but it is much more soluble in alkaline solutions. It is stable to heating in neutral or acid solutions, but it may be destroyed by heating in alkaline solution or by exposure to light. In fact, it is so sensitive to light that when someone is using a dilute solution of it in a laboratory—such as when assaying it in foods —it is routine practice to turn off the lights and pull down the shades to darken the room as much as is practical. Riboflavin may also be destroyed by sunlight striking milk kept in glass bottles (see later section).

Riboflavin (most often in combined forms) is very widely distributed in both plant and animal tissues. It is formed by all higher plants, chiefly in the green leaves, and the younger parts of the plant contain more than older parts. Seeds are rather low in riboflavin, except when sprouting. Also, most microorganisms synthesize this vitamin, and bacteria in the intestinal tract may be a considerable but variable source of it for animals, just as with thiamin. Aside from this undependable source, higher animals must obtain riboflavin from their food.

Effects of Riboflavin Deficiency in Animals and Man

The need of a dietary source of riboflavin was discovered by its effect on *growth* of rats. Experimental animals which receive little or no riboflavin show stunted growth, and when they are fed graded amounts of it, they respond with corresponding increases in growth rate. They also need riboflavin in the diet for maximum health and vigor, maximum ability to bear and suckle offspring, and for delayed senility. Riboflavin is one of the factors essential for successful *reproduction*; rats on diets deficient in this vitamin produced young with abnormal skeletons and other defects.

This vitamin is essential for general health, because it is the active constituent of several enzymes or coenzymes that are essential to oxidation processes in the various body tissues. It is essential for the health of tissues of ectodermal origin, such as the skin, eyes, and nerves.

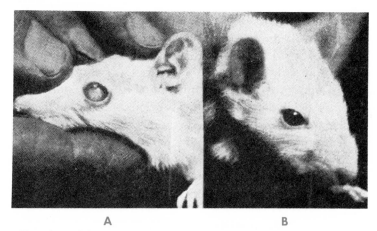

A   B

Figure 7–9. Two views of the same rat. **A,** After cataract developed in the left eye as a result of riboflavin deficiency. **B,** Several weeks after administration of riboflavin, the right eye thus being saved. Also note the marked improvement of the rat's general condition as the result of riboflavin administration. (Courtesy of Paul L. Day and the *American Journal of Public Health.*)

In experimental animals (rats), a long-continued lack of riboflavin leads to *sore mouth and nose, falling hair* and *scaly skin, eye symptoms* varying in severity from an inflamed condition of the cornea to its complete opacity in cataract (Fig. 7–9), *digestive disturbances, nervous lesions* (severe cases show paralysis of hind legs), poor utilization of food, increasing weakness, and death.

Deficient chickens show a characteristic *curled toe paralysis*, caused by degenerated nerves, in which the toes curve inward, eventually causing paralysis and death unless corrected. This formerly was very common in commercial poultry flocks, but today all poultry rations are routinely fortified with liberal amounts of riboflavin, and the condition is no longer seen. Riboflavin is needed in the diet of all monogastric animals tested, including the mouse, guinea pig, monkey, pig, dog, fox, horse, fish, and even the young calf before the rumen starts to function. Many deficiency signs similar to those seen in the rat are seen in these animals.

In man, symptoms of riboflavin deficiency are similar to those seen in animals, but they are less specific and less severe. In fact, there still is considerable disagreement as to the characteristic signs of deficiency in man; more studies are needed. Sebrell and Butler, who first produced experimental deficiency of this vitamin in human beings, reported as characteristic symptoms reddened, denuded areas on the lips, with cracks at the corners of the mouth — called *cheilosis* (Fig. 7–10).[16] These symptoms were cured when riboflavin was given. Also, other investigators have reported eye lesions in riboflavin-deficient persons, such as dimness of vision and burning of the eyes, and the possibility of cataract. Other skin abnormalities, including a greasy scaly dermatitis around the nose, and particularly on the scrotum in the male, have been seen in riboflavin deficiency. Symptoms of general debility, similar to those seen in pellagra, may also be associated with a deficient intake of riboflavin.

Ordinarily it takes several months for symptoms of riboflavin deficiency

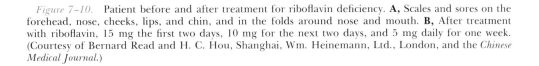

A   B

Figure 7–10. Patient before and after treatment for riboflavin deficiency. **A,** Scales and sores on the forehead, nose, cheeks, lips, and chin, and in the folds around nose and mouth. **B,** After treatment with riboflavin, 15 mg the first two days, 10 mg for the next two days, and 5 mg daily for one week. (Courtesy of Bernard Read and H. C. Hou, Shanghai, Wm. Heinemann, Ltd., London, and the *Chinese Medical Journal.*)

to appear, but Lane and co-workers[17] developed an acute deficiency in man within 10 to 25 days by using a riboflavin *antagonist** (*galactoflavin*, in which galactose has been substituted for ribitol in the vitamin) in a semi-synthetic riboflavin-free diet. The resulting symptoms seen in the six test subjects were: first, sore throat or mouth, followed by reddening and swelling of the mucous membrane of the mouth and throat; cheilosis; *glossitis* (a condition in which the tongue becomes shiny and develops a red-purple color); scaly, greasy dermatitis of the face, ears, and other parts of the body; and anemia. Anemia was a "new" symptom, so it appears that riboflavin deficiency interferes with the production of red blood cells in man, as has been reported in animals. All these symptoms were rapidly and completely reversed after administration of riboflavin.

---

*A *nutritional antagonist* is a compound whose structure is so similar to a specific nutrient that it can substitute for the nutrient in certain enzyme systems for which the specific nutrient is necessary, thus leading to at least partial inactivity of these systems. Hence, an effect similar to a deficiency is produced in a short time. True nutritional antagonism, or inhibition, can always be overcome by high enough levels of the nutrient in question.

The Role of Riboflavin in the Body

Free riboflavin, such as is found in some foods, must be phosphorylated in the intestinal tract before it can be absorbed. Once it enters the blood, it is distributed to all cells of the body. The chief function of this vitamin is the role it plays in *oxidation-reduction reactions in the tissues.* Riboflavin is contained in a number of different enzymes (called *flavoproteins*) and several coenzymes whose function is to take on hydrogen and pass it on to another substance in the long chain of oxidation-reductions by which hydrogen is finally combined with oxygen to form water (Fig. 7–11). In this way, riboflavin-containing enzymes assist in the metabolism of carbohydrate, of amino acids, and of fats. During this process, energy is released gradually and made available to the cell.

Riboflavin's *biochemical role* centers chiefly around two important coenzymes in which most of the riboflavin in the body exists— *riboflavin monophosphate* (also called, less correctly, flavin mononucleotide) and the more common but elaborate *flavin adenine dinucleotide* (or "FAD," composed of riboflavin monophosphate with additional phosphate and sugar groups plus adenine, a purine). These coenzymes are attached with various degrees of tenacity to a number of

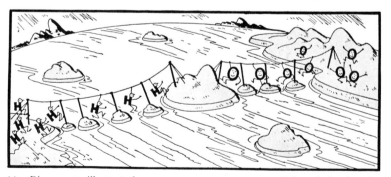

Figure 7–11. Diagram to illustrate how enzymes or coenzymes, which contain vitamins, may act as stepping stones for oxygen or hydrogen atoms in bringing about oxidation-reduction reactions in living tissues. Thiamin, riboflavin, and niacin form part of enzymes and coenzymes that function in this manner. The hydrogen and oxygen atoms, separated by an otherwise formidable barrier, are enabled by the use of stepping stones (enzymes) and the handrails (coenzymes) to move toward each other and ultimately unite to form molecules of water (H_2O). (From W. O. Kermack and P. Eggleton: *The Stuff We're Made of,* Edward Arnold & Co., London.)

highly important enzymes in the body, the flavoproteins, which catalyze oxidation-reduction reactions. Most of these enzymes act as *hydrogen carriers*, passing this element along from one substance to another until its atoms are finally united with oxygen atoms (by special enzymes) to form molecules of water. It is of interest that several of these enzymes contain a metal—for example, molybdenum or iron—demonstrating again the important interrelationships between vitamins and minerals.

Because riboflavin is essential to numerous chemical changes in tissues, it is natural that deprivation of this vitamin causes damage to many different types of tissues and that sufficient intake of it is necessary to promote the welfare of the body as a whole.

Riboflavin is found in almost all tissues, principally in the form of its coenzymes. There does not appear to be any specialized mechanism for storage of riboflavin, although muscle tissues may retain considerable amounts even in riboflavin deficiency. Unused riboflavin is excreted in the urine.

Requirement and Nutritional Status

We have learned that riboflavin is necessary in the body for energy formation, protein metabolism and many cellular reactions dealing with growth or repair of the body. Therefore, for practical purposes the amount of riboflavin needed is related to body size, metabolic rate, and rate of growth. Because of this, the Food and Nutrition Board,[7] in 1968, based its new recommended allowances of riboflavin on a person's "metabolic body size"* (rather than on caloric intake, as was formerly done). On this new basis the recommended allowance for most adults has slightly increased. The allowance for college age women is now 1.5 mg per day, and for men, 1.6 mg. For other allowances see Table 7-3, and

---

*A person's "metabolic body size" is represented as each kilogram of body weight taken to the 0.75 power.[7] This ignores rate of growth, however.

*Table 7-3. Recommended Allowances for Riboflavin**

	Age	Allowance, mg/day
Males	12–14 years	1.4
	14–18 years	1.5
	18–22 years	1.6
	22 years and over	1.7
Females	12–16 years	1.4
	16 years and over	1.5
	Pregnant	1.8
	Lactating	2.0

*From the Food and Nutrition Board, 1968.[7]
See Appendix Table 1C for FAO recommendations.

Table 1A in the Appendix for complete values. The allowance does not decrease with age and increases during pregnancy and lactation. A minimum of about 1.2 mg per day in adults is necessary to maintain adequate body stores and normal urinary output. Thus, the recommended allowances are only about 40 percent over the minimum requirement, which does not allow too great a leeway for "dietary indiscretions" of individuals—at least not over long periods.

Surprisingly large incidences of *riboflavin deficiency* in children and adults have been uncovered in the United States in recent years[10–13] after several decades of relative freedom from instances of deficiency. Riboflavin deficiency once was fairly common in the United States, especially in the South, and wherever milk, the best dietary source, was not consumed. After 1941, the start of the enrichment program (see page 398), cases of severe deficiency of riboflavin in man became very rare. Concentrates of riboflavin, from synthetic or fermentation sources, used in current enrichment programs in the United States contribute an average of 0.33 mg of riboflavin per person per day, which is about one-fourth of the requirement, a very significant amount.†

---

†The cost of riboflavin from such sources is only about 5 cents per 1000 mg (1 gm)—more than a year's requirement for one person. Synthetic riboflavin is almost as inexpensive.

However, not all states have required enrichment programs, and the riboflavin intake of many persons in these and other states is still well below recommended allowances and even below minimum requirements.[10-13] Riboflavin deficiencies also exist in other countries throughout the world. It is important, therefore, that many more efforts be devoted in all countries to increasing intakes of riboflavin (and other key nutrients to be studied later, such as vitamin D, folacin, vitamin A, calcium, and iron). To accomplish this, new programs in nutrition education, distribution of free and low cost foods to the poor, and enrichment of foods will be needed.

One of the major reasons for the low consumption of riboflavin in this country, and elsewhere, is that many persons in this country, perhaps 15 to 25 percent, do not use milk in any form, or they use it very sparingly (or equivalent sources, of which there are very few). Since milk supplies about 45 percent of all the riboflavin consumed by persons in the United States, it is clear that people not consuming milk must eat liberal quantities of liver, eggs, leafy vegetables, or legumes (or vitamin supple-

ments) to maintain an adequate intake (see next section).

Because infants generally consume a large amount of breast milk or cow's milk, their average consumption is well above the recommended allowance.[18] Only when milk is not consumed is it necessary to be concerned about an infant's riboflavin intake, and most commercial milk substitutes supply liberal amounts. (See Chapter 20.)

Riboflavin in Foods

Table 7-4 shows that *liver, milk, cheese, eggs, leafy vegetables, enriched bread, lean meat,* and *legumes* are the foods that are among the richest in riboflavin. Dried yeast is a still richer source. Both thiamin and riboflavin are almost universally distributed in foods; only such foods as pure sugars and fats are entirely lacking in them. Riboflavin is more plentifully supplied in most foods than thiamin, and this is notably true of organ meats, leafy vegetables, eggs, and milk. Milk has about four times as much riboflavin as thiamin (see Fig. 7-12). On the other hand, the whole-grain cereals, which are among

Table 7-4. Examples of Good Food Sources of Riboflavin*

Food Source	Riboflavin, mg/100 gm	Food Source	Riboflavin, mg/100 mg
Beans		Meat, lean	0.20
White	0.22	Milk, fluid	
Red	0.20	Whole	0.17
Pinto	0.21	Skim	0.18
Mung	0.21	2% fat, added solids	0.21
Soy	0.31	Pepper, chili, dried	1.33
Beet greens	0.23	Soybean flour	0.31
Cashew nuts	0.25	Spinach	0.20
Cheese, cheddar	0.46	Spleen, beef	0.37
Chicken, dark meat	0.20	Split peas	0.29
Cocoa powder	0.46	Sunflower seeds	0.23
Collards	0.31	Water chestnut	0.20
Egg, white	0.30	Wheat germ, crude	0.68
Heart, calf	1.05	Yeast	
Kale	0.26	Brewer's	4.28
Kidneys, beef	2.55	Torula	5.06
Liver, beef	3.26		

*From Watt, B. K., and Merrill, A. L.[14] Based on fresh, raw, edible portion.

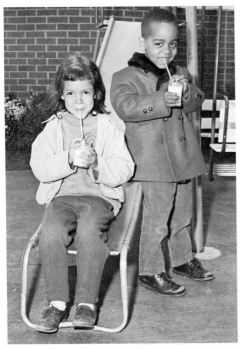

Figure 7–12. Milk supplies about 45 percent of all the riboflavin in the food supply of the United States. (Courtesy of U.S. Department of Agriculture.)

the richest sources of thiamin, have only a moderate content of riboflavin. Even when enriched with riboflavin to the level of whole grains, bread and cereals still contribute only about one-seventh the riboflavin in the average American diet.[9] Legumes, nuts, and muscle meats are good sources of both thiamin and riboflavin. Pork, which has five to seven times the thiamin content of other meats, does not differ from other meats in riboflavin content. Eggs are richer in riboflavin than are muscle meats. Vegetables—other than leafy ones and legumes—and fruits contribute less, but still appreciable amounts of, riboflavin.

The riboflavin content of different foodstuffs is not equally available on ingestion. However, cooking and drying (e.g., yeast) can increase the availability of riboflavin in most instances. Fortunately, riboflavin is stable enough on heating that little of it is destroyed in ordinary cooking processes, although some may be lost by solution in water in which foods are cooked or canned. Losses also can occur from *exposure to light* if the cooking is done in open vessels. The use of sodium bicarbonate in the cooking of vegetables can also destroy riboflavin. Average losses of riboflavin in cooking are 15 to 20 percent in meats, 10 to 20 percent in vegetables, and 10 percent in baking bread.

Because of the importance of milk as a dietary source of riboflavin, the possible destruction of this vitamin on exposure of milk to light has been emphasized. Exposure to ordinary daylight may cause considerable losses, and milk in a glass bottle left standing on the doorstep in direct sunlight may lose 50 to 70 percent of its riboflavin potency in two hours.[19] The use of paper cartons cuts down losses by exposure to sunlight or display lighting in foodstores, but even so, it is best to keep milk as much as possible in a cool, dark place, such as the refrigerator. Only minor losses of riboflavin occur in pasteurization of milk.

NIACIN

Discovery

Not until 1937 was this substance established as a member of the group of B vitamins and identified as the long-sought *"pellagra-preventing factor."* The history of its discovery over a search period lasting over 20 years is as interesting as a detective story. Goldberger had demonstrated as early as 1915 that pellagra was directly due to faulty diet, and later that this disease could be prevented or its symptoms relieved by giving liver, yeast, lean meats, or other foods rich in B complex vitamins.[4, 20] Pellagra had occurred in certain parts of Europe for over 200 years, with special prevalence in areas where corn formed a large part of the diet. One of its most typical symptoms is a reddish skin rash which later makes the skin dark and rough, from which it took the name of pellagra, in 1771, from the Italian "pelle agra" meaning painful (or rough) skin. Although a few early physicians were convinced that pellagra was caused by dietary deficiencies, the theory was advanced that it might be due to an infectious agent, or to some toxic substance present in corn, or developed in corn on spoilage. About 1907, pellagra became prevalent in the southern part of the United States, and cases increased in number so rapidly that in 1915 over 10,000 persons died of it. In 1917–1918 there were 200,000 cases of pellagra in this country—not limited to the South, but found throughout the whole country.

This was of great concern to the United States Public Health Service, which instituted special studies of the disease under the direction of Goldberger. At first, opinion was divided as to whether pellagra was due to poor sanitation or diet, but later, when Goldberger had induced the disease solely by feeding a "poor" diet to volunteer convicts and had prevented its incidence in various institutions by improvement of the diet, it was established as a dietary deficiency disease.* Although Goldberger proved that the preventive factor was a heat-stable substance present in yeast after thiamin had been destroyed by autoclaving, the exact nature of the substance remained a mystery until Elvehjem and coworkers, of the University of Wisconsin, showed in 1937 that blacktongue—an analogous disease in dogs—could be cured by giving *nicotinic acid* or the closely related *nicotinic acid amide* (nicotinamide), which they isolated from liver.[21] Administration of these substances was soon shown by several investigators to cure the most striking and characteristic symptoms of pellagra in humans.[22] Even before these discoveries, preventive dietary measures had been instituted in the southern states which resulted in marked decrease in pellagra incidence until, by 1945, acute cases were seldom seen.

Another chapter in the story of pellagra prevention was completed in 1945–1950 when it was discovered that the amino acid tryptophan was converted, in part, to nicotinic acid in the body of man and animals and that sufficient amounts could overcome pellagra in the absence of dietary nicotinic acid (see later section).

Chemical Identification and Properties

Nicotinic acid was originally discovered and named in 1867 by Huber (a German chemist). He made it by chemical treatment of nicotine—of the tobacco plant, from which it got its name.† It sat on laboratory shelves untested for many years while thousands of persons were dying from pellagra. No one knew then that there was a relationship, of course. Nicotinic acid and the related compound—nicotinamide—are white compounds, soluble in water and stable to both heating and oxidation, as well as to acids and alkalis. Little is lost in cooking unless the cooking water is discarded. Chemically, these nitrogen-containing compounds are among the simplest of the vitamins (see formulas in the Appendix); one contains an organic acid group ($-COOH$) and the other has an amino group ($-NH_2$) substituted in the acid group.

Nicotinic acid had been "rediscovered" many times as a compound present in foods and tissues even before its pellagra-preventive activity was known.

---

*Goldberger proved in 1916 that pellagra was not an infectious disease when he and a group of 15 volunteers, in a heroic and crucial experiment, inoculated themselves with blood, swabbed their throats with saliva, and swallowed the excreta of patients severely ill with pellagra. Although some of the volunteers felt a bit squeamish, none became ill with pellagra for six months afterward.[4]

---

†Nicotine itself has no vitamin activity.

For instance, both Funk in England and Suzuki in Japan isolated (and recognized) nicotinic acid from yeast and rice bran in 1912 during their search for the antiberiberi vitamin.[4] In 1935, workers in Germany made the important discovery that nicotinic acid is a part of certain coenzymes needed in energy metabolism. Also, previous to the work of Elvehjem and his associates, quite a few workers had added nicotinic acid to purified diets for rats or fowl and had obtained variable evidences of growth stimulation, but such studies were not conclusive.

Goldberger and his co-workers concentrated the active factor from yeast in their studies of dogs with *blacktongue* (animal pellagra) and used the term "P−P factor" (pellagra-preventive) for the substance in their concentrate. Both this term and the term vitamin B-5, once used for this vitamin, are no longer used.*

The name *niacin* was adopted in 1971 by the American Institute of Nutrition[23] and international agencies for all forms of the vitamin (and the term "niacin activity" for combined activity of nicotinic acid and its derivatives). The word "niacin" was coined in 1948 to be used for "nicotinic acid" with the idea of avoiding any possible implication that these normal nutrients are related in activity to nicotine, the alkaloid in tobacco. Niacin may be present in foods or tissues in free or combined forms. The amide form is preferred for therapeutic doses, because it does not cause the unpleasant skin reactions (feeling of heat, flushing, or even a red rash) and dizziness often associated with administration of very large amounts of the acid.

Symptoms Due to Lack of Niacin

The tissues that show damage as a result of niacin deficiency are chiefly

the skin, the gastrointestinal tract, and the nervous tissues.

The most striking and characteristic *symptoms of pellagra* are a reddish skin rash (especially on the face, hands, and feet when exposed to sunlight), which later makes the skin dark and rough (see Figs. 7–13 and 7–14). There are also a sore mouth and tongue, and inflamed membranes in the digestive tract, with bloody diarrhea in the later stages. There may also be distressing nervous and mental disturbances, such as irritability, anxiety, depression, and in advanced cases, delirium, hallucinations, confusion, disorientation, and stupor. Many mental institutions in this country had large numbers of such persons before the cure was discovered. Physicians sometimes refer to pellagra symptoms as "the three D's — dermatitis, diarrhea, and depression or dementia." Other general effects seen in pellagra are loss of weight, anemia (which may be associated with deficiencies of other B vitamins), and dehydration, from diarrhea. The skin rash always appears on both sides of the body at the same time — that is, *bilaterally symmetrical.*

Less acute symptoms of niacin deficiency may be difficult to recognize. Changes in the tongue are among the earliest signs of niacin lack and may be used to detect it. *Latent* or mild pellagra has been reported in infants and children, in whom the usual pellagra symptoms were lacking; weakness and failure to grow properly, however, responded favorably to treatment with niacin.[24] Hence, we see that this vitamin is necessary for *growth* and for *health of tissues,*

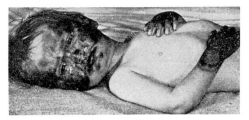

Figure 7–13. Pellagra in a child, showing typical red rash on face and hands. (Courtesy of Dr. John A. McIntosh.)

---

*Recently this vitamin has been called, wrongly, "vitamin B-3" in certain health food literature. There is no historic basis for this terminology, and its use is to be deplored.

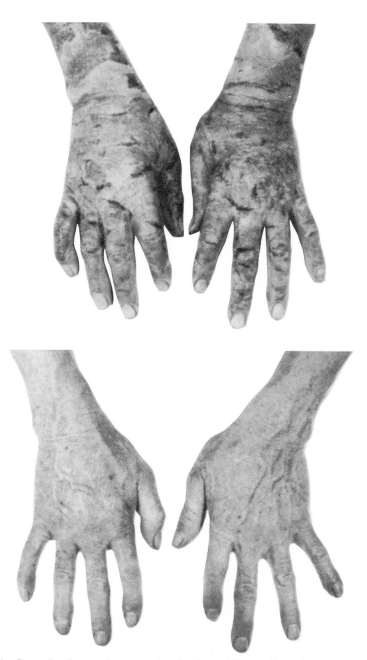

Figure 7–14. Cure of pellagrous lesions on hands of an adult by a diet rich in B vitamins, especially niacin. **A,** Hands of pellagra patient. **B,** Same patient after two weeks of corrective diet. (From Spies: *Rehabilitation Through Better Nutrition,* Philadelphia, W. B. Saunders, 1947.)

and it also promotes appetite, proper functioning of the digestive tract, and good utilization of foodstuffs in the body.

All experimental animals, except ruminants, need niacin or its equivalent in tryptophan. Deficiency symptoms are often similar to those seen in humans with pellagra, although any mental symptoms are absent or hard to detect. Dogs show a deep reddening or darkening of the tongue and mouth as well as skin rash, bloody diarrhea, wasting, and eventually death. Deficiencies have been produced in the rat, fowl, monkey, rabbit, cat, pig, guinea pig, fish, and many other monogastric animals.

The Pellagra Problem

The wide occurrence (and subsequent conquest) of pellagra in the southern United States affords an interesting example of the relation of nutritional welfare to economic conditions, and also of a dietary deficiency disease that is not due to simple deficiency of one vitamin. The South was a "one crop" region, depending almost entirely on cultivation of cotton and its manufacture into cloth. The cash income of ordinary people was low, especially around the turn of the century, so that they often ate the cheapest foods obtainable and became habituated to a poor diet. Many poor sharecroppers and mill hands lived almost exclusively on corn meal and grits, soda biscuits, corn syrup or molasses, and fatty salt pork—a diet that is deficient both as to quality and quantity of protein and in its content of several vitamins and minerals. When pellagra developed because of such diets, although most of the symptoms were due to lack of niacin, the disease was complicated by lack of other B complex vitamins, especially thiamin and riboflavin. Not only the corn products, but any flour and rice used, were degerminated and highly milled; most of the natural content of thiamin, riboflavin, and niacin was removed with the germ and outer coats of the grains. There was almost no lean meat, milk, or eggs to contribute high-quality protein and B vitamins. Riboflavin deficiency is so often associated with niacin deficiency in such diets that it is said to have a bearing on the occurrence and persistence of pellagra. Pellagra is now considered to be a complex dietary deficiency, the major symptoms of which are due to niacin deficiency. Its complete cure requires all-around improvement of the diet, especially of its protein content and intake of all the B complex vitamins (see discussion on tryptophan and its relation to pellagra, p. 139).

The campaign to stamp out pellagra thus centered on introducing into the diet certain foods established as effective in preventing the disease. Lean meats, milk, eggs, canned salmon, peanuts, peas, and vegetables were shown to be good foods to add to the diet for preventing pellagra.[25] At the same time, Wheeler and Sebrell commented,[26] "In looking for cases of pellagra, the home surrounded by evidence of a good garden, or a cow or two, a few pigs and some poultry may as well be passed up, for the chances are less than one in a thousand that pellagra will be found. On the other hand, the home surrounded only by last year's cotton patch will always bear watching."

Because many families did not have money to buy the needed foods, the campaign was centered on urging them to make home gardens, and to keep a cow and some chickens. In some areas, the Red Cross would lend the family a cow until the health, and with it the earning power, of the people improved sufficiently to enable them to buy the animal. While the educational campaign went on, public health authorities in some states supplied free dried brewer's yeast, which has a higher content of niacin and most other B vitamins than any other food.

The success of this education program was demonstrated by a dietary survey[27] made in two adjacent communities in the Kentucky mountains, one of which had a high incidence of pellagra while the other had almost none. Corn products were eaten in about the same amounts in both districts, but the people in the one which had been freed from pellagra had been influenced by the Frontier Nursing Service to understand the importance of certain foods for health, so that they had planted gardens and were keeping cows and chickens (which was not true in the other district).

This campaign to educate the people in change of food habits and increase income levels to make possible the purchase of needed foods was gradually successful. There was a decrease in mortality from pellagra in southern states from 22.4 to 5.1 per 100,000 between 1929 and 1940.[28] Since the discovery of the benefits of treatment with niacin, public institutions are no longer crowded with hopeless cases of this disease. Although the number of acute cases and of deaths from this disease is now very low, much remains to be done toward permanent improvement of the nutritive qualities of the diet of people in these areas in order to avoid low-grade niacin deficiency and to promote health by making the diet otherwise adequate.

Niacin's Role in the Body

The chief function of niacin in the body is to form the active portion of *coenzymes that play an essential role in tissue oxidations (hydrogen transport)*, and it thus is necessary for the health of all tissue cells. Nicotinamide, in both free and combined form, is carried in the blood and found in all tissues, but most richly in liver, kidney, heart, brain, and muscles.

Niacin's biochemical role revolves around its presence in two important coenzymes essential to all life. These two coenzymes (named from their initials, NAD and NADP*), are known collectively as the *pyridine nucleotides*, and they play several different roles in cellular metabolism. Their most important function is to help bring about the action of enzymes known as *dehydrogenases*, which are essential in the course of oxidation-reduction reactions. For instance, the enzyme *lactic dehydrogenase* in tissues oxidizes lactic acid to pyruvic acid only in the presence of NAD. A second function of the pyridine nucleotides, when in the reduced form, concerns the reduction of riboflavin-containing coenzymes and enzymes. In these reactions, hydrogen is passed along the reduced pyridine nucleotides to a riboflavin-containing coenzyme and then to the cytochromes and eventually to oxygen, with the formation of water. Lack of niacin to form these coenzymes in sufficient quantities handicaps vital chemical processes and may result in injury to tissues throughout the body.

Biosynthesis of Niacin; Role of Tryptophan

Study of the metabolism of niacin and the amounts that should be furnished in the diet is complicated by two facts—it can be synthesized by bacteria in the intestinal flora, and it can be made in the tissues from the amino acid tryptophan. We know that many bacteria can synthesize this and other B vitamins. Because some diets are more favorable for this synthesis than others (a vegetable diet is more favorable for synthesis than some meat diets, for example), the variability of the amounts synthesized may sometimes determine whether or not pellagra occurs when the

---

*NAD, or nicotinamide adenine dinucleotide, was the first coenzyme ever identified (in 1935). It formerly was called "coenzyme I" or "cozymase," and later DPN (for diphosphopyridine nucleotide), terms now obsolete. It contains nicotinamide (a pyridine), two ribose groups, two phosphate groups, and adenine (a purine).

NADP, or nicotinamide adenine dinucleotide phosphate, is similar to NAD but contains an extra phosphate. It formerly was called "coenzyme II" or TPN. These two coenzymes are called NADH and NADPH when they are in the reduced form.

diet contains borderline quantities of niacin and tryptophan.

The amino acid tryptophan (see Chapter 5) has a sparing action on the amount of niacin needed in the diet because it acts as a precursor substance from which niacin can be formed in the body. This was first demonstrated in experiments with rats which were fed diets high in corn and low in niacin by Krehl and his co-workers in 1945.[29] They found that feeding either niacin *or tryptophan* overcame the deficiency. Soon after this discovery, it was shown that man could substitute tryptophan for niacin at a ratio of about 60 parts of tryptophan to one part of niacin.[30] If sufficient tryptophan is eaten (amounts generally higher than in average diets), niacin itself is no longer essential in the diet—all the niacin required is made within the body. The pathway of the conversion of tryptophan to niacin in tissues of the body has been worked out, involving a number of biochemical steps.

It had been known for many years that eating diets high in corn (maize) increased the incidence of pellagra in man, but the reason for this was a puzzle to nutritionists. Many persons believed that corn might contain a toxic factor, but following the discovery that tryptophan was an effective substitute for niacin, it was soon discovered by means of animal studies that the simultaneous presence of three conditions was responsible for the detrimental effect of corn: (1) the low amount of available niacin, (2) the low amount of tryptophan, and (3) a dietary imbalance caused by the presence of relatively large amounts of other amino acids in proportion to tryptophan in corn.[31] Other foods low and unbalanced in respect to tryptophan, such as gelatin, give the same effect as corn when fed to experimental animals (as do various mixtures of amino acids devoid of tryptophan). *All three conditions must be present at once to produce pellagra.* The relatively low content of both niacin

Table 7–5. *Relative Amount of Tryptophan and Niacin in Corn and Wheat*

	Niacin	Tryptophan
Whole wheat, per 100 gm	4.3 mg	168 mg
Whole corn, per 100 gm	2.0 gm	55 mg

and tryptophan in corn, as compared to that in wheat, is shown in Table 7–5.

The fact that the body can form niacin from tryptophan also explains why some foods have far greater pellagra-preventing potency than would be expected from their actual content of niacin.* Such foods are milk and eggs, which are low in niacin but carry proteins that are high in the amino acid tryptophan, thus furnishing the body with protection from pellagra by enabling it to build niacin within the tissues.

Requirement and Nutritional Status

It should be evident from the foregoing discussion that the actual *requirement* for niacin varies with the nature of the diet (mainly whether the protein furnishes much or little tryptophan). The Food and Nutrition Board of the United States now makes use of the term *niacin equivalent* (dietary sources of niacin plus its precursor, tryptophan). Approximately 1 mg of niacin may be expected to be formed for each 60 mg of tryptophan in the diet.† A food which provides a large

*Goldberger and other early workers studying pellagra were puzzled many times by this observation. Between 1915 and 1920, Goldberger concluded that certain protein-rich foods (low in the "P–P factor") could cure patients with pellagra, and at one time he obtained relief of symptoms by feeding tryptophan. This work was not followed up, however, when it was found that yeast and liver extracts very low in protein were even more effective.

†Thus, one niacin equivalent is defined as 1 mg of niacin or 60 mg of tryptophan (or combinations thereof).

amount of tryptophan may be an excellent source of niacin equivalents even though its pre-formed niacin content is not high. A quart of milk daily, for instance, suffices to prevent pellagra, although its content of niacin is relatively low. Its high content of tryptophan may be counted on to furnish additional niacin in the body which must be added in calculating its "niacin equivalence," as shown in Figure 7–15.[7, 30]

Niacin equivalents of foods, then, can be calculated from food composition tables which give both the niacin and the tryptophan content of foods (dividing this by 60)[32] (see next section). In the absence of information on the tryptophan content of foods, one can estimate that most proteins of animal origin (milk, eggs, and meat) contain about 1.4 percent of tryptophan and most proteins of vegetable origin (cereals and legumes) about 1 percent.[7]

On the basis of the work of many persons the recommended allowances for niacin equivalents have been established by the United States Food and Nutrition Board (1968),[7] examples of which are shown in Table 7–6 (for other age groups see complete table in Appendix). The values are very similar to previous estimations by the Board. A college woman has an allowance of from 10 to 15 mg per day of niacin equivalents, and a college man 18 to 20 mg per day. The allowances decrease somewhat with age.

*Table 7–6. Recommended Allowances for Niacin Equivalents**

	Age	Allowance, mg/day
Males	12–14 years	18
	14–18 years	20
	18–35 years	18
	35–55 years	17
	55 years and over	14
Females	12–14 years	15
	14–16 years	16
	16–18 years	15
	18 years and over	13
	Pregnant	15
	Lactating	20

*From the Food and Nutrition Board, 1968.[7]
See Appendix Table 1C for FAO recommendations.

The amounts shown in Table 7–6 are approximately 50 percent greater than the minimum requirement (about 10 mg of niacin equivalents per day). They are based primarily on the energy requirement of an average individual (as is thiamin) because of the essential role of the vitamin in energy formation from carbohydrates and fats. The Food and Nutrition Board has recommended a value of about 6.6 mg of niacin equivalent per 1000 kcal. Even if less than 2000 kcal is consumed per day, the Board states that adults need a minimum of 13 mg per day.

Because human milk contains an average of 0.17 mg of niacin and 22 mg of tryptophan per 100 ml, it can supply

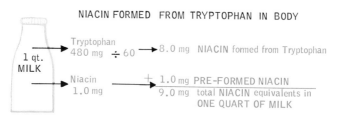

NIACIN FORMED FROM TRYPTOPHAN IN BODY

1 qt. MILK

Tryptophan 480 mg ÷ 60 → 8.0 mg NIACIN formed from Tryptophan

Niacin 1.0 mg → + 1.0 mg PRE-FORMED NIACIN
9.0 mg total NIACIN equivalents in ONE QUART OF MILK

Figure 7–15. Calculating the niacin equivalents in a quart of milk. To the niacin that is carried as such in the milk (1.0 mg per quart) should be added the amount that may be expected to be formed in the body from its tryptophan content (480 mg per quart). Assuming that approximately 1 mg of niacin is formed for each 60 mg of tryptophan (480 ÷ 60), 8 mg of niacin might be expected to arise from the tryptophan content of the milk, bringing the total niacin equivalents of a quart of milk up to 9.0 mg.

a niacin equivalent of about 4.5 mg per day if 850 ml (600 kcal) is consumed. The allowance for infants is set at 6 mg per day, and for lactating mothers an additional 7 mg of niacin equivalents per day is recommended.[7]

It should not be difficult to secure the recommended amounts of niacin equivalents from diets such as are advised for meeting other nutritive requirements. If milk, meats, whole-grain or enriched cereals, and leafy and other vegetables are used fairly freely, the diet is protected against a shortage of niacin. When such practices are not followed, the amounts of niacin provided, though above the level necessary to prevent pellagra, may be less than the recommended allowances. Most diets consumed in the United States supply from 500 to 1000 mg or more of tryptophan daily and 8 to 17 mg of pre-formed niacin for a total of 16 to 33 mg of niacin equivalents per day, according to the Food and Nutrition Board.[7] The *average* intake, therefore, is higher than the recommended allowance, even though it appears that individual diets might be borderline in their content of niacin equivalents.

Pellagra is seldom seen in the United States today. Pellagra may still be seen fairly commonly in certain countries where corn (maize) is a major part of the diet. However, in parts of Latin America and Mexico, where many persons eat large amounts of corn as one of their principal sources of energy, pellagra is seldom seen. This is because it is their common practice to soak the corn in lime, a practice which makes the niacin in corn more available to the body.

Niacin and Niacin Equivalents in Foods

Because niacin can be formed in the body if tryptophan is furnished, the amount of pre-formed niacin in foods that comprise the diet, as has been explained, is not necessarily a measure of the total quantity of this vitamin available to the body. Of greater importance are figures showing the niacin equivalents of foods[32] (see Table 7-7).

In general, animal products contain the vitamin as nicotinamide, while in plant products most of it is present as nicotinic acid. Values of niacin activity in foods, as in Table 2 of the Ap-

*Table 7-7. Niacin Equivalents of Some Representative Foods**

Food	Niacin Equivalent mg/100 gm	Food	Niacin Equivalent mg/100 gm
Almond	6.4	Lamb	8.2
Apple	0.2	Milk, cow's, pasteurized	0.9
Asparagus	1.9	Milk, human	0.5
Banana	0.9	Parsley	2.4
Bean, lima	4.7	Pork	5.4
Beef	7.3	Rice, brown	6.3
Beet root	0.7	Rice, milled, parboiled	4.9
Brussels sprouts	1.9	Sesame seed	10.2
Carrot	0.7	Soybean	11.1
Cashew nut	8.1	Spinach	1.2
Cauliflower	1.3	Sunflower seed	8.8
Chicken	10.9	Sweet potato	1.0
Chickpea	4.9	Trout	11.7
Corn, sweet	2.1	Wheat germ	8.6
Egg, whole	3.2	Wheat, whole	6.7
		Yeast, brewer's	45.0

*Calculated from niacin values in Watt, B. K., and Merrill, A. L.,[14] and tryptophan values in FAO: *Amino-Acid Content of Foods and Biological Data on Proteins*, Rome, 1970, and Orr, M. L., and Watt, B. K.: *Amino Acid Content of Foods*, Washington, D.C., U.S.D.A., 1957. Based on fresh, raw, edible portion.

pendix, are of interest in indicating what types of foods are relatively rich in this vitamin. Most foods that are good sources of thiamin and riboflavin are also high in niacin content — namely liver, lean meats, whole grains, nuts, yeast, and legumes. However, eggs, milk, and cheese are relatively low in niacin, while leafy vegetables are not much higher than other vegetables. As with thiamin and riboflavin, foods that are not rich in niacin may still furnish considerable amounts of it if they are eaten in quantity.

There is very little destruction of niacin in ordinary cooking methods, so figures for cooked foods are omitted.

As with most other vitamins, the most inexpensive source of the vitamin is the synthetic form itself (although, as pointed out elsewhere, persons should depend on traditional foods as their source of nutrients and not on pure compounds, at least for routine purposes). Nicotinic acid is available in wholesale quantities at a price of only about 8 dollars per kilogram (2.2 pounds), or only 2 cents for 2.5 gm (sufficient to supply 25 percent of the daily allowance for one person for 500 days). Obviously, the cost of enrichment of foods with niacin is negligible.

With proper nutrition education, pellagra should be a thing of the past, for niacin is so inexpensive and so readily available in our foods.

VITAMIN B-6

Lately, much greater recognition than before has been given to vitamin B-6* in human nutrition. Special impetus to this higher ranking was given in 1968 when the Food and Nutrition Board gave recognition to its importance by including it in its list of recommended dietary allowances for the first time.

*Written, very sensibly, as vitamin B-6 rather than vitamin B_6, in line with 1971 nomenclature suggestions.[23]

Identification and Properties

The jigsaw puzzle of the B complex was partially solved by György in 1934, who found that an unidentified substance, to which he gave the name *vitamin B-6*, was necessary in the diet of rats for growth and for prevention of a particular type of skin disorder.[33] This disorder, later called "rat acrodynia," had been described earlier, in 1930, by two British nutritionists, Chick and Copping.[34] Many workers were trying to identify the active compound,† though there was much confusion with the then unknown pellagra-preventive factor (niacin) which most people were seeking. By 1934 there was evidence for five B-complex vitamins, none of which had been chemically identified — hence the jigsaw puzzle analogy.

Biochemists in five different laboratories independently isolated crystals of vitamin B-6 in 1938, using the rat for the biological test, but credit for obtaining the first crystals is widely given to Lepkovsky of the University of California.[35] Vitamin B-6 was synthesized in 1939 by workers in the United States, Germany, and Japan, and it was made freely available to nutritionists, thus making it much easier for the rest of the B complex jigsaw to be assembled within the next few years.

The widely accepted name *pyridoxine* was suggested in 1939 by György and Eckardt for the first pure substance known to have vitamin B-6 activity.[36] Several years later Snell discovered the vitamin B-6 activity of two closely related substances in natural products, which he termed *pyridoxal* and *pyridoxamine*.[37] All three compounds are white solids and have about equal activity when fed to laboratory animals. The pyridoxal and pyridoxamine forms occur mainly in animal products, whereas pyridoxine is found largely in products of vegetable origin (see Appendix

†Also called Factor Y, rat antidermatitis vitamin, Factor 1, and adermin in the early years.

for structural formulas of these compounds).

Pyridoxine is much more stable to heat than the other two compounds, but they are all unusually stable to acid and alkali. All three forms may be rapidly destroyed by exposure to light, especially in neutral or alkaline solutions. Pyridoxamine and pyridoxal are considered quite labile compounds when in dilute solutions, being rapidly destroyed by exposure to air and heat. The cooking or processing of foods from animal sources may destroy up to 50 percent of their vitamin B-6 activity.[38, 39]

Effect of Vitamin B-6 Deficiency

The question of whether this vitamin is essential for humans was settled in a rather dramatic way. In 1951, babies (six weeks to six months old) in various parts of the United States, fed solely on a commercial infant food, suddenly began to develop irritability, muscular twitchings, and convulsions. Those babies who were fed the company's liquid (canned) product became seriously ill, while others fed a similar formula sold in dry, powdered form were not ill. Kline, then of the United States Food and Drug Administration, recognizing the similarity of these convulsive seizures to those seen in young rats deprived of vitamin B-6, suggested the infants might be ill because of lack of this vitamin. When vitamin B-6 was given to the affected babies, they promptly recovered. The heat used to sterilize the liquid product in cans had been high enough to destroy most of the vitamin B-6, a fact no one had noticed or would have thought important, if known. Because of the proved need for this vitamin in infants' diets,[39] this company and other manufacturers of infant foods take special precautions to make sure that it is present.

Symptoms of vitamin B-6 deficiency in man are similar in some respects to those seen in niacin and riboflavin deficiency.[7, 39–41] In addition to a diet low in this vitamin, an antagonist (see footnote, p. 130), deoxypyridoxine, is often used in experiments to develop early deficiency symptoms. A common symptom is a greasy (seborrheic) dermatitis around the eyes, in the eyebrows, and at the angles of the mouth, along with soreness of the mouth and a smooth, red tongue. An early symptom of deficiency is the excretion in the urine of large amounts of *xanthurenic acid*, an abnormal tryptophan derivative, which turns green in the presence of iron salts. Later symptoms include dizziness, nausea, vomiting, weight loss, irritability and confusion, anemia, kidney stones, and severe nervous disturbances including convulsions. All these symptoms (except kidney stones) can be corrected within several days, even within a few minutes for some symptoms, by administering vitamin B-6.

Deficiency signs in animals are similar to those seen in humans, except that the same symptoms do not occur in all species. All species need vitamin B-6 for growth. Deficient *rats* show weight loss, *acrodynia* (a dermatitis affecting the feet, ears, tail, and nose), muscular weakness, edema, peripheral neuritis, and in advanced stages, convulsions. *Dogs* and *pigs* show no skin lesions but develop anemia and later convulsions, with marked changes in nervous tissue seen at autopsy. Deficiency in *fowl* can be obtained in only four or five days, resulting in poor growth and eventually anemia, decreased clotting time, and convulsions. *Calves* show listlessness, lack of appetite, poor hair coat, and convulsions. Most farm animals are normally protected against vitamin B-6 deficiency by the high content of this vitamin in their natural feed. Cattle and sheep obtain sufficient vitamin B-6 by microbial synthesis in the rumen to avert any such deficiency.

Role of Vitamin B-6 in the Body

The three forms of vitamin B-6 are quite stable in the intestinal tract and are readily absorbed in the upper intestine. Once absorbed, all three forms are converted to *pyridoxal phosphate*—the coenzyme form—which has many important roles in metabolism, particularly in protein and amino acid metabolism. Interestingly, one of the many specific functions of pyridoxal phosphate is as a catalyst in the formation in the body of niacin from tryptophan. Vitamin B-6-deficient animals are unable to do this, which may partially explain why symptoms of vitamin B-6 deficiency in man are similar to those seen in pellagra.

Pyridoxal phosphate is essential for several highly important reactions in the body concerned with amino acid metabolism. The most important of these reactions involving pyridoxal phosphate (and to some extent pyridoxamine phosphate) are known as *transamination* and *decarboxylation*. Transamination is the shifting of an amino group (NH_2) from a donor amino acid to an acceptor acid to form another amino acid. By this type of reaction, the building of certain amino acids from non-nitrogen-carrying acids formed in metabolism is made possible. (Because of the role of vitamin B-6 in these reactions, the transaminase activity of the blood may often be a useful indicator of vitamin B-6 deficiency.)

Decarboxylation is the removal of carbon dioxide (CO_2) from an amino acid. It is necessary for the formation in the body of at least three vital physiological regulators (hormones or similar compounds) from the amino acids, histidine, tryptophan, and tyrosine, as well as for the oxidation of amino acids for energy. Pyridoxal phosphate also catalyzes the removal of SH groups from sulfur-containing amino acids.

As many as 50 specific reactions of amino acids requiring pyridoxal phosphate as a coenzyme have been discovered. It is a part of the enzyme essential in the body for the breakdown of glycogen to glucose (glycogen phosphorylase). In fact, about half the vitamin B-6 in the body is accounted for by its presence in phosphorylases of muscle, which probably explains the low blood glucose seen in deficient experimental animals. Vitamin B-6 may in some way be necessary in metabolism of polyunsaturated fatty acids, for conversion of linoleic acid to arachidonic acid.[42] Judging by the frequency of anemia and severe nervous symptoms in deficiencies, it is clearly involved in red cell regeneration and normal functioning of nervous tissues.

Vitamin B-6 deficient animals show impaired antibody responses. Thus, it must be needed by man for protection against various infections and diseases, although this remains unproved.[43]

Requirement and Nutritional Status

The United States Food and Nutrition Board, in 1968 for the first time, included vitamin B-6 in its recommended allowances.[7] For females aged 16 and older, 2.0 mg per day is recommended, with increased amounts (0.5 mg more) during pregnancy and lactation. For male adults the recommended amount is also 2.0 mg per day. The allowances are quite similar, in general, to the ones for riboflavin and thiamin, especially for growing children. See Table 7–8 for a summary of vitamin B-6 recommendations and Table 1 in the Appendix for more details.

The inclusion of vitamin B-6 in the Board's recommended allowances reflects not only new information on the human requirement for this vitamin,[39–41] but also a concern that in more than a few instances our normal diets may be borderline or low in this vitamin.[7] Unfortunately, too few studies have been made on the possible occurrence of vitamin B-6 deficiency in normal persons eating commonly available foods.

Table 7–8.   *Recommended Allowances for Vitamin B-6**

	Age	Allowance, mg/day
Males	14–18 years	1.8
	18 years and over	2.0
Females	14–16 years	1.8
	16 years and over	2.0
	Pregnant	2.5
	Lactating	2.5

*From the Food and Nutrition Board, 1968.[7]

There is good information showing increased needs of this vitamin in pregnancy and lactation, in the elderly, in alcoholics, in various pathologic and genetic disturbances, and in persons receiving certain common drugs such as isoniazid, penicillamine, and certain steroids. All such increased needs must be met by a source of vitamin B-6 in some form—often more than the amounts available in usual diets (unless foods are to be enriched with this vitamin or unless they are selected with considerable care—see next several paragraphs).

In 1961, it was estimated that most American diets furnished 2.0 to 2.7 mg of this vitamin per day, though some very poor diets supplied as little as 1.0 mg per day.[44] According to U.S.D.A. figures,[45] the overall average per capita *availability* of vitamin B-6 per day in 1969 was only about 2.15 mg, not including waste or cooking losses. Diets of foods commonly available in the United States can be devised with as little as 0.4 to 0.5 mg per day, well below the requirement. In fact, Cheslock and McCully[46] saw signs of vitamin B-6 deficiency in humans fed a diet containing cereal products, fruits, milk, vegetables, and other vitamin B-6-low foods (many of which had been processed).

Some information is available on intakes of vitamin B-6 by adults in other countries (see Sauberlich[41]). In Burma, evidence obtained in 1963 indicated an average intake of 1.7 mg per day, and it was stated that "at these intakes of vitamin B-6, a considerable number of the persons studied revealed biochemical abnormalities related to the metabolism of vitamin B-6, and excretion of the vitamin was observed to be generally quite low." In a 1964 report of Malaysia, similar observations were noted in persons on a vitamin B-6 intake of between 1.04 and 1.42 mg per day—amounts apparently inadequate. In the United Kingdom, one study estimated the daily intake to

be between 1.6 and 1.9 mg per day and another 2.3 mg.

Food Sources of Vitamin B-6

The occurrence of vitamin B-6 in foods[47] follows the general distribution of most of the other B vitamins. The best sources are meats (especially liver), some vegetables (including potatoes), wheat germ, wheat bran, and whole-grain cereals (Table 7–9; see Table 3 of the Appendix for more details). All these values are given in terms of total vitamin B-6 activity, combining the three naturally occurring forms of the vitamin. For details of the individual distribution in foods of the three forms (pyridoxine, pyridoxal, and pyridoxamine), see Table 2 of Orr.[47] All forms have about equal activity when eaten.

In the milling of white flour, more than 75 percent of the vitamin B-6 content of wheat is lost; it is not added in enrichment programs, and there are good arguments that this should be done. Synthetic pyridoxine is quite inexpensive.

Sugar and fat, of course, are devoid of this vitamin, as they are of most other vitamins (though they supply over one-third of the energy intake of the average American). Processed or refined foods are generally much lower in vitamin B-6 than the original food, often less than half. Flour, white bread, pre-cooked rice, noodles, macaroni, and spaghetti are quite low in vitamin B-6, and a diet composed solely of these or similar foods would eventually cause a vitamin B-6 deficiency (along with deficiencies of many other nutrients).

It should be obvious that vitamin B-6 is not one of the "lesser vitamins" in terms of its food distribution and its importance to good health. Not only must one choose his food with at least some degree of nutritional knowledge in order to have a sufficient amount, but well-planned food enrichment programs with vitamin B-6 will, no doubt, prove to be useful.

Table 7–9.   Examples of Good Food Sources of Vitamin B-6*

Food Source	Vitamin B-6 Activity in mg/100 gm (Edible Portion)	Food Source	Vitamin B-6 Activity in mg/100 gm (Edible Portion)
Avocados, raw	0.42	Soybeans, raw	0.81
Bananas, raw	0.51	Spinach, raw	0.28
Beans, white, raw	0.56	Sunflower seed	1.25
Beans, lima, raw	0.58	Sweet potatoes, raw	0.22
Beef, raw, lean	0.44	Trout, raw	0.69
Chicken		Tuna	
Dark meat	0.32	Raw	0.90
Light meat	0.68	Canned	0.42
Chickpeas, raw	0.54	Turnip greens, raw	0.26
Cottonseed flour	0.98	Veal, raw	0.34
Crab, cooked or canned	0.30	Walnuts	0.73
Filberts, shelled	0.54	Whole wheat flour	0.34
Halibut, raw	0.43	Wheat breakfast cereals	
Kale, raw	0.30	Bran, 100 percent	0.82
Liver		Germ, toasted	1.15
Beef, raw	0.84	Shredded	0.24
Chicken, raw	0.75	Yeast	
Peanuts, roasted, shelled	0.40	Baker's, dry, inactive	2.00
Pepper, green, raw	0.26	Brewer's, debittered	2.50
Pork, raw, boned	0.32	Torula	3.00
Prunes, dried	0.24		
Raisins, golden seedless	0.35		
Rice, brown, raw	0.55		
Salmon steak, raw	0.70		

*Adapted from Orr, M. L., 1969.[47]

PANTOTHENIC ACID

The solving of the B complex puzzle between 1933 and 1940 was aided greatly by the identification of pantothenic acid as a growth factor for yeast and later as a vitamin for animals. Though it is a dietary essential for man and plays an unusually important role in the body, pantothenic acid is so widely distributed in most foods that a deficiency has not been seen in normal populations.

The name "pantothenic acid," derived from the Greek, meaning "from everywhere," was given in 1933 by R. J. Williams, then of Oregon State, to an unknown factor in various biological materials necessary for the growth of yeast.[48] Dr. Williams, now at the University of Texas, is a brother of the late R. R. Williams, who first synthesized thiamin (page 117). He later proposed the term "pantothen" for the vitamin[49] so that the general public would not confuse the vitamin with stronger harmful chemicals.* This name has not caught on (though it would be just as useful as the term niacin for nicotinic acid).

Chemical Identification and Properties

After much painstaking research, primarily using the young chick as a test animal, workers at the Universities of California and Wisconsin, in 1939, announced that a highly active preparation of the "chick-antidermatitis factor" and Williams' pantothenic acid had iden-

*Since pantothenic acid was the third B vitamin to be clearly differentiated (1928), the name "vitamin B-3" was used for it in the 1930's by several workers.

tical growth activity.[50] In 1940, its structure was determined and it was synthesized by Williams (see formula in the Appendix).[51] Stable crystalline salts of pantothenic acid are readily available, such as synthetic sodium or calcium pantothenate.* Pantothenic acid is quite stable to heat but can be destroyed in foods by heating for long periods (two to six days)—far longer than the usual cooking or baking procedures.

Effect of Deficiency in Man and Animals

Deficiency symptoms in man, produced experimentally in volunteers by use of

---

*The D isomer of synthetic salts of pantothenate is the natural active form.

a purified diet and a specific antagonist (see footnote, p. 130), include fatigue, headache, sleep disturbances, personality changes, nausea, abdominal distress, numbness and tingling of hands and feet, muscle cramps, impaired coordination, and loss of antibody production.[52] All symptoms were cured by the administration of pantothenic acid. A well defined deficiency of pantothenic acid has not been observed in man under natural conditions.

Pantothenic acid *deficiency in experimental animals* is readily obtained by using purified diets or natural diets heated over long periods to destroy this vitamin. Deficient chickens have a characteristic dermatitis of the mouth, eyes, and feet. These animals grow poorly, and if not given pantothenic acid, death results in three or four weeks (see Fig. 7–16). In other animals, a deficiency

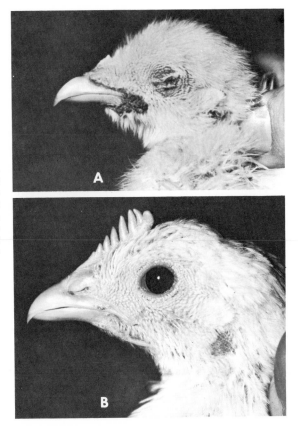

Figure 7–16. **A,** Chick after being fed a diet deficient in pantothenic acid. The eyelids, corners of the mouth, and adjacent skin are inflamed. The growth of feathers is retarded, and the feathers are rough. **B,** The same chick after three weeks on a diet containing pantothenic acid. The lesions are completely cured. (Courtesy of the Upjohn Company.)

of pantothenic acid affects many tissues, and, in general, causes poor growth and faulty reproduction. It is of interest that graying of the hair is produced in deficient rats, monkeys, dogs, and foxes; color usually can be restored by added pantothenate in the diet. In humans, this relationship between pantothenic acid intake and graying of hair is not known. (Adding extra amounts of pantothenic acid to human diets does not change the color of gray hair.) In many species, degenerative changes are found in the nervous system and especially in the adrenal glands, which may become enlarged, reddened, and hemorrhagic. The role of pantothenic acid in the activity of the adrenals was elucidated when it was shown to be part of a coenzyme *(coenzyme A)* needed for making certain hormones formed in the outer portion (cortex) of these ductless glands (cortisone and two related hormones). These hormones have important regulatory influences on metabolism and indeed are essential for life.

Biochemical Role of Pantothenic Acid

The *biochemical role* of pantothenic acid is involved primarily with coenzyme A,* one of the most important substances in body metabolism. As part of coenzyme A, pantothenic acid is essential for the intermediary metabolism of carbohydrates, fats, and proteins (for their synthesis, breakdown, and release of energy). It functions primarily by effecting the removal or acceptance of important chemical groups with two, three, four (or more) carbon atoms at a time. Coenzyme A is also needed for the formation of such important sterols as cholesterol and the adrenocortical hormones. It is also essential for the synthesis of acetylcholine (an important regulator of nerve tissue) and for making many other important compounds in the body.

---

*Coenzyme A, discovered in the 1940's, consists of a complicated molecule, *phosphopantetheine* (composed of pantothenic acid, a phosphate group, and reduced sulfur) plus two additional phosphate groups, a pentose, and adenine (a purine).

Coenzyme A is essential for so many chemical reactions in the body, such as those necessary for energy release and for building many essential complicated compounds out of simpler ones, that pantothenic acid has been said to "sit at the crossroads of metabolism." The diagram found as Figure 14–4 (p. 329) illustrates its strategic position in metabolism.

Pantothenic acid functions also as a component of the enzyme *fatty acid synthase* involved in fatty acid synthesis in the body. This enzyme contains the important unit *phosphopantetheine* (see footnote, first column) but not the complete coenzyme A molecule.

In many of these reactions of pantothenic acid, the coenzymes of riboflavin, thiamin, biotin, niacin, and pyridoxal are also involved, as well as the minerals phosphorus, sulfur, magnesium, and manganese, showing again how vitamins and minerals are interrelated.

Requirement and Nutritional Status

The dietary requirement of pantothenic acid for man is unknown, but the Food and Nutrition Board has suggested that 5 to 10 mg per day is adequate for children and adults (a recommended allowance has not been set).[7] An average intake from "adequate" diets is probably about 15 mg per day and from grossly inadequate diets about 6 mg (which is probably a borderline amount).[44] Human milk has about 2.2 mg of pantothenic acid per liter, so the daily infant requirement would be expected to be less than this. Cow's milk has about 3.4 mg per liter.

Since processing of food can, in some instances, result in appreciable losses of pantothenic acid (see next section), it is possible that unrecognized borderline deficiencies may exist in human populations, such as in multiple nutritional deficiencies associated with alcoholism.[7] Such deficiencies, if they exist, would occur only in connection with other deficiencies in man and would likely escape detection because of emphasis on other nutrients. Several recent studies in Japan show low levels of serum pantothenic acid along with other deficiencies in populations eating mainly washed rice.

Deficiencies of pantothenic acid have been seen, though rarely, in farm animals (swine) fed "natural rations." As a result, synthetic pantothenic acid is often added to commercial swine rations. How a deficiency could develop under such conditions is not clear, but this points out the need for many more studies with this vitamin in human nutrition.

*Food Sources and Effects of
Processing*

Pantothenic acid exists in all cells of living tissues and therefore is present in all natural foods (usually in combined forms). All foods in the four food groups contain pantothenic acid, but foods which are especially rich are yeast, liver, eggs, wheat and rice germ or bran, peanuts, and peas. Moderate to good amounts are contained in such foods as meat, milk, poultry, whole grains, broccoli, mushrooms, and sweet potatoes. Most vegetables and fruits and refined foods contain lesser amounts. White flour, precooked rice, and corn flakes are poor sources of the vitamin, and none is present, of course, in salad oils, shortening, sugar, and similar products. Processing and refinement of foods as well as milling of grains can result in considerable losses of pantothenic acid.[47, 53]

Losses of up to 50 percent and even more can occur in frozen vegetables and meats, contrary to common opinion. Similar losses occur in many canned food products.*

Synthetic calcium pantothenate is widely used today in vitamin supplements and to fortify a few breakfast foods, though usually only in trivial amounts. Its cost is about 6 cents per gram.

For specific pantothenic acid values of average servings of common foods, see Table 3 of the Appendix. Some examples of losses due to processing are included.

BIOTIN

Although biotin is one of the lesser known vitamins of the B complex, it is nevertheless just as important as the other vitamins to body tissues. Biotin is a white compound, stable to heat in cooking, processing, and storage. It is widely distributed in foods known to be good sources of the other B complex vitamins. Because microorganisms in the intestinal tract of man synthesize amounts about equal to, or greater than, the requirement, there is little or no concern about the amount provided in the diet.

Biotin, like pantothenic acid, was known to be a growth factor for yeast before its vitamin nature was discovered. The compound was crystallized in 1936 and given the name "biotin" since it was part of the "bios" factor needed for yeast growth. Its vitamin nature for animals was discovered by György† in 1940.[54] He had previously called it vitamin H—a term no longer used. Another early name was the "anti-egg white injury factor.") Biotin was synthesized and its structure determined in 1942 (see Appendix for its formula). It contains sulfur in the molecule, as does thiamin. Several forms of biotin are thought to exist in food.

A biotin deficiency can be produced in mice, dogs, chicks and other fowl

---

*The results of Schroeder[53] should be considered only preliminary, since the same food item was not used before and after processing.

†The same Dr. György who was involved in the discoveries of riboflavin and vitamin B-6 (see Fig. 18–1).

merely by leaving biotin out of the experimental diet. In rats and monkeys (in which there is a higher degree of intestinal synthesis of biotin), a deficiency can be induced by giving an antibiotic or a sulfa drug, which lowers the number of intestinal microorganisms, or by raising the animal in "germ-free" conditions in which no microorganisms exist.

In all mammals, including man, the addition of 15 to 30 percent, or more, of raw, dried egg white to a biotin-low diet will induce symptoms of biotin deficiency. This action has been accounted for by discovery in raw egg white of a special protein called *avidin*, which

combines with biotin in the intestinal tract, thus rendering the biotin unabsorbable. This so-called "egg white injury" can be overcome by feeding some biotin-rich food (such as egg yolk, liver, or yeast).[55] Cooking egg white, even briefly, destroys the biotin-binding action of avidin.

Effect of Biotin Deficiency and Role in the Body

The fact that biotin is a dietary essential for man was shown in 1942 by use of a diet low in biotin supplemented with dried uncooked egg white.[56] This

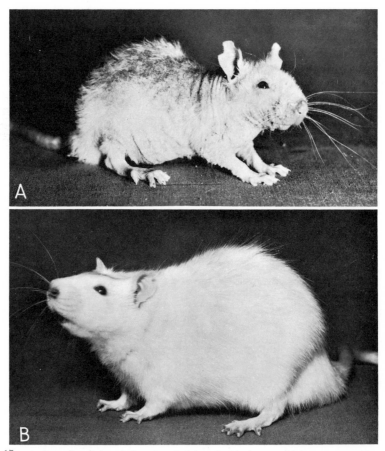

Figure 7–17. **A,** Rat after being fed a diet deficient in biotin, to which raw egg white was added. Growth has been retarded, and there is a generalized inflammation of the skin. **B,** The same rat after three months on a diet containing adequate amounts of biotin. Growth is normal, and the skin lesions are completely healed. (Courtesy of the Upjohn Company.)

resulted in pathologic changes in the skin and tongue, loss of appetite, nausea and a low-grade anemia, lassitude, intense depression, sleeplessness, and muscle pain. Injections of biotin brought marked improvement of symptoms in three to four days.

Biotin deficiency in animals has been quite widely studied with the use of experimental diets. Deficient rats grow poorly and develop a general dermatitis, muscular incoordination, and hair loss, which occurs, first, around the eye, giving rise to a typical *spectacle-eye* condition (see Fig. 7–17). Deficient fowl develop dermatitis first on the feet (extending to the beak and eyes) and eventually they become weak, show poor growth, and die. In monkeys a deficiency results in poor growth and in a reduction of the amount and color of hair. Deficiencies also have been produced in dogs, pigs, calves, and other animals.

Most biotin in the body is combined in various enzymes by means of chemical union with the amino acid lysine. When thus bound to an enzyme, biotin plays an important role in essential *carboxylation* reactions, in which carbon dioxide (CO_2) is transferred from the enzyme complex to other compounds. These reactions are reversible and are closely involved with those of pantothenic acid (coenzyme A).

Reactions requiring biotin are very important in the synthesis of fatty acids, in the production of energy from glucose, and in the formation of nucleic acid, glycogen, and several amino acids.

Requirement

There is no known figure for the requirement of biotin for man. Experimental animals require only small amounts per kilogram of diet (about 0.1 to 0.15 mg), which would be equivalent to about 0.1 mg per day for man. The Food and Nutrition Board of the United States estimates that the average American diet supplies about 0.15 to 0.30 mg of biotin per day, which is sufficient to take care of human needs.[7]

The amount of biotin excreted in the urine and feces of normal adults is greater than the known intake.[57] Synthesis of biotin from microorganisms in the intestinal tract accounts for this difference. Hence, biotin deficiency in human populations is not likely to occur except in rare instances, such as when persons might consume large amounts of raw eggs (eight to ten per day) without extra biotin sources. However, the occasional eating of a few raw eggs, as in eggnog, does not provide sufficient avidin to produce a biotin deficiency.

CHOLINE

Choline is an important B vitamin necessary in the diet of many young animals,[7] though its need by man at any stage of life has not been established. Choline (generally combined with other compounds) has several catalytic and metabolic functions in the body. Also it is an essential component of several phospholipids vital in lipid metabolism (notably lecithin and sphingomyelin, which together make up 70 to 80 percent of the phospholipids in the animal body).

Identification and Properties

Choline was isolated from bile in 1862 by a German chemist ("chole" is the Greek word for bile). Its vitamin nature was not appreciated fully until the early 1940's, after studies by Sure and György and Goldblatt,[58] who showed that it is essential for growth of rats and who confirmed early studies that it prevented the accumulation of fat in the liver ("fatty livers") in animals fed choline-low diets.

In 1930 *lecithin* (a phospholipid which contains choline) was shown to prevent fatty livers in dogs. Feeding components of lecithin, Best* and his co-workers[59]

*Dr. Best enjoys the distinction of having been a co-worker with Dr. Banting in experiments leading to the discovery of insulin in the 1920's.

at Toronto University, between 1932 and 1935, showed that choline, and less efficiently, betaine* (a closely related substance) prevented the occurrence of fatty livers in rats fed diets low in protein and high in fat, cholesterol, or sucrose. Best's work was done before any other B complex vitamin was available in pure form, and he considered choline as only an accessory food factor. By 1942, the vitamin nature of choline was fully confirmed by many other workers, who used the rat, chicken, and turkey as experimental animals.[60]

Choline, a relatively simple molecule, contains three methyl groups (CH_3--) and is strongly alkaline in its free form (see formula in Appendix). It is a water-soluble white syrup which takes up water rapidly on exposure to air (hygroscopic) and readily forms more stable crystalline salts with acids such as choline chloride or choline bitartrate. In foods, it exists primarily in phospholipids or as the water-soluble sulfate or phosphate salts. It is heat-stable and remains at nearly a constant level in dried foods when stored over long periods.

Functions in Body and Deficiency Signs

Choline has many important functions in the body—as a constituent of several phospholipids (primarily lecithin) it aids in the *transport and metabolism of fats*; as a constituent of *acetylcholine* it plays a role in normal functioning of nerves; and it serves as a source of *labile methyl groups* which are essential in metabolism.

The methyl group (CH_3--) is found

---

*Betaine, which has choline activity, is widely distributed in foods of plant origin. It derives its name from the Latin word *beta*, the beet family, which contain rather large amounts—up to 4 percent in some species. Like choline, it has a nitrogenous base, which contains three methyl groups (CH_3--) in each molecule.

in many organic substances, but in most of them it is fixed and not detachable. When a methyl group is present in such a form that it can be transferred from one compound to another, it is called a labile methyl group and the process is called *transmethylation*. The body has a pool of labile methyl groups contributed from various sources, which it uses for such purposes as the formation of creatine (important in muscle metabolism) and for methylating certain substances for excretion in the urine. These methyl groups are also used in the synthesis of several hormones, such as epinephrine, and have other essential roles. Among the dietary sources of labile methyl are choline (or related substances), the amino acid methionine and in addition, the vitamins folacin and vitamin B-12.

Mention has been made of dietary factors related to choline which can replace some of its functions (or all, in some species). The primary one of these is betaine, which can fully replace choline in preventing fatty liver in some species; in others betaine only supplements choline. Betaine may be considered a *sparing agent* and a member of the "choline group," but is not fully equivalent to choline. Methionine (though less efficiently) and, to some extent, vitamin B-12 also spare choline in some animals, but not in other species. To some extent, an abundance of any one of these or other sources of labile methyl groups may be said to "spare" or at least to partially make up for a shortage of one of the others. The action of these substances in preventing fat accumulation in the liver (and in certain other tissues) is said to be a *lipotropic* activity (a term first used by Best).

A *deficiency of choline in rats* results in fatty livers in four to six weeks. In addition, depending on the type of diet and the length of time the deficient diet is fed, symptoms such as poor growth, edema, and an impaired cardiovascular system are seen, the last of which results in hemorrhagic lesions in the kidneys, heart muscles, and adrenal glands. Fatty livers also are seen in deficient dogs, mice, guinea pigs, ducks, rabbits, pigs, calves, cats, and monkeys.[7] Chickens and turkeys are quite immune to fatty livers, but develop *slipped tendon* (a bowing of the legs), which makes walking so difficult that death usually results in six to eight weeks. Borderline deficiencies of choline have occurred in farm animals fed the usual "by-product" feeds low in methionine.

Nutritional Status and "Requirement"

Experimental deficiency of choline in humans has never been obtained, though very few serious studies have been attempted. If choline is needed, one would especially expect infants and young children to show a need, since, generally, it is the young of experimental animals fed deficient diets which are affected primarily. It would not be wise, based on our knowledge of choline, to purposely give infants and children (or adults for that matter) a choline-free diet for any extended time. On the other hand, there is no need whatsoever to worry about getting enough in one's diet when the usual types of foodstuffs are consumed.

Fatty infiltration of the liver is seen very commonly, especially in chronic alcoholics or in persons on very low protein diets (e.g., in children with kwashiorkor). Choline and other lipotropic agents have been used by physicians in attempts to cure these disorders, but the results have been inconsistent and disappointing.

The Food and Nutrition Board does not suggest any human allowance for this factor because of this lack of evidence. We estimate that an average mixed diet for adults in the United States contains 500 to 900 mg per day of choline or betaine, or about 0.1 to 0.18 percent of the diet. Human milk contains about 145 mg per liter (nearly 0.1 percent of total solids). These amounts are adequate when compared with known animal requirements.

Food Sources of Choline

Choline is present in all foods in which phospholipids occur liberally, as in egg yolk, whole grains, legumes, meats of all types, and wheat germ.[55] Fresh egg yolk contains about 1.5 per cent choline (probably the richest natural source), and beef liver contains about 0.6 percent. Legumes, such as soybeans, peas, and beans, contain from 0.2 to 0.35 percent; vegetables and milk have moderate choline activity. Most other foods (including fruits) have little or no choline activity.

FOLACIN

Folacin* (folic acid and related compounds), the next to last of the B vitamins to be discovered, is essential for all vertebrates, including man, for normal growth and reproduction, for the prevention of blood disorders, for important biochemical mechanisms within each cell, and for the prevention of a variety of symptoms in different species. The name "folic acid" (the forerunner of the term "folacin") was suggested in 1941 by Mitchell, Snell, and Williams† of Texas, for a highly purified growth factor for bacteria. It is derived from the Latin word for foliage or leaf (*folium*), because it was first isolated from spinach leaves and was known to be widely distributed in green, leafy plants.

---

*According to the latest international nomenclature rules,[23] the term "folacin" (originally proposed by the American Institute of Nutrition in the 1950's) is used here as the generic description for folic acid and related compounds exhibiting the biological activity of folic acid (pteroylmonoglutamic acid). Names of other related compounds have also been changed accordingly. There is no single compound with the name "folacin."

†R. J. Williams, who also coined the word "pantothenic acid."

Identification and Properties

The first of the *folacin group* to be obtained in crystalline form was folic acid, known chemically as *pteroylmonoglutamic acid*, isolated from natural materials by two independent groups of workers in pharmaceutical laboratories in the United States in 1943 and 1944.[62] It was first synthesized in 1946 and its structure announced by a team of 16 workers from the American Cyanamid Company.[63] It is a bright yellow powder, quite soluble in slightly alkaline or acid solutions, readily destroyed by heat when in an acid solution, but reasonably stable when in neutral or alkaline solutions (especially in the absence of air).

Its eventual discovery was aided considerably by the previous work (at the Universities of Arkansas, Missouri, California, Wisconsin, Texas, Cornell, and elsewhere) of nutritionists and biochemists who were studying unidentified growth factors for the chicken, monkey, and bacteria, which now appear to have been identical with folacin. The useful term *vitamin B-10* was suggested in the early 1940's for the substance(s) in natural foods with growth activity for young chickens (fed diets which were later found to be deficient in folacin, not available at the time).[64] Vitamin B$_c$, vitamin M, factors R and U, and *L. casei* factor were other terms used, and although folacin is a recognized member of the B-complex, these terms are not used today.

This vitamin exists in several different forms in nature, making up the folacin group of compounds. These different forms have similar activity when fed to higher animals, but they have widely different activities as growth factors for microorganisms. The parent compound, folic acid (pteroylmonoglutamic acid)—which probably does not exist free in nature—is formed by the linkage of three compounds: *pteridine*, a yellow phosphorescent pigment related to the yellow pigment in butterfly wings (the Greek word for wing is

"pteron"); *para-aminobenzoic acid* (a growth factor for bacteria);* and *glutamic acid*, an amino acid commonly found in proteins of foods and body tissues. The structural formula of folic acid may be found in the Appendix.

In addition to the parent folic acid with only one glutamic acid group in the molecule, at least two *conjugated* forms of folacin exist in foods with either three or seven glutamic acid groups per molecule (*folic acid glutamates*). These conjugated forms serve as the major precursors of the vitamin in the diet. The coenzyme form, *tetrahydrofolic acid*, the most common form in the body, is also widely distributed in foods. Another form of folacin which is active metabolically and which occurs in food is *10-formyltetrahydrofolic acid*, a reduced form of folic acid. Methyl derivatives of folic acid are also found in nature.

Effects of Lack of Folacin

Although all animals require folacin, some species can meet this need by the production of the vitamin through bacterial synthesis in the intestine. Rats, dogs, and rabbits fall in this category, but chicks, monkeys, and men must have folacin supplied in the food in order to avoid deficiency symptoms.

Folacin deficiency in *man* results in a smooth, red tongue, gastrointestinal disturbances, and diarrhea; but the primary symptom is a blood disturbance called *macrocytic anemia*. In this anemia, the mature red blood cells are fewer

---

*Para-aminobenzoic acid has considerable folacin activity when fed to deficient animals in which intestinal synthesis of folacin takes place; in fact, in the rat and mouse dietary para-aminobenzoic acid can completely replace the need for a dietary source of folacin in this manner. This explains why para-aminobenzoic acid was once considered to be a vitamin in its own right. Obviously, since it does exist in the free form in some foods, it can be considered a dietary precursor of folacin, but it is not a vitamin itself (though often listed as one).

in number, larger in size, and contain less hemoglobin than normal. The young red blood cells in the bone marrow (megaloblasts) fail to mature during folacin deficiency. Administration of folacin by mouth or injection results in prompt formation and development to maturity of a very large number of new red blood cells.* Certain anemias that develop during pregnancy, infancy, and childhood respond well to treatment with folacin, as do those seen in sprue or pellagra (due to poor intestinal absoption). Anemias due primarily to dietary lack of iron and certain other causes are not relieved by it. In *pernicious anemia,* there is some initial response (with increased level of red cells) but not as marked as after giving much smaller amounts of *vitamin B-12,* while the nervous symptoms often seen in this disease cannot be cured by treatment with folacin.

Signs of folacin deficiency in animals include poor growth, faulty reproduction, anemia and other blood disorders, and abnormal biochemical changes within the body. Chicks also show poor pigmentation and structure of the feathers and slipped tendon (as in choline and niacin deficiency). If rats are prevented from forming folacin through intestinal synthesis (by being raised in germ-free conditions or by having sulfa drugs added to the diet), deficiency symptoms will develop, including marked decrease in various types of white blood cells. Normal reproduction, lactation, and antibody formation also require folacin. In deficient monkeys, there are loss of weight, anemia, and inflammation and degeneration of the gums. Folacin deficiency has also been developed in the mouse, other fowl, guinea pig, mink, dog, and fox.

Function of Folacin in the Human Body

After absorption, the various forms of folacin are converted (reduced) by the body to several active coenzyme forms, the parent form being tetra-hydrofolic acid. These coenzyme forms are distributed throughout the body but are most abundant in the liver. Probably their primary function is to serve as carriers for single-carbon groups (specifically, the formyl and hydroxy-methyl groups), which are essential for the building of purines and pyrimidines. These compounds are, in turn, needed for synthesis of nucleic acids, which are vital to all cell nuclei. This explains the important role of folacin in cell division and in animal reproduction. Folacin coenzymes also are responsible for synthesis of certain amino acids (especially glycine and serine) used in the formation of body proteins. These reactions require ascorbic acid for maintaining folic acid in its reduced form, and they also require coenzymes of vitamins B-6 and B-12, again demonstrating the interdependence of various vitamins.

The folacin coenzymes are also necessary for the *breakdown* of many, if not all, amino acids. For instance, in folacin deficiency in man and animals, the amino acid *histidine* is imperfectly utilized, resulting in increased amounts of an abnormal derivative in the urine.†

Coenzymes derived from folacin also serve as a source of carbon and hydrogen atoms in the synthesis of *methyl* groups and thus function with choline, betaine, and methionine in supplying labile methyl groups to the body (see p. 152). In most animals, folacin cannot be depended on to supply the entire requirement of methyl groups.

Requirements and Nutritional Status

Folacin deficiency in man is now known to occur under "normal" conditions, especially during the latter stages of pregnancy and lactation when the incidence is often quite marked. For this reason, and because of much newer

---

*Dr. Spies and co-workers were the first to use folacin compounds in man.[65]

†Formiminoglutamic acid ("FIGLU").

knowledge about this vitamin in man, the United States Food and Nutrition Board[7] has now set a recommended allowance for this vitamin. A total of 0.4 mg per day of folacin activity is recommended for adult men and women (see Table 7–10 and Table 1 of the Appendix). This is higher than previous estimates, but takes into account possible losses from cooking, poor absorption, and varying activity of the several forms of folacin in foods. A minimum requirement, as suggested by the Board, may be as low as 0.05 mg per day. Average American intakes are well over this last amount, although deficiencies are seen in sprue, in low birth weight infants and infants on unsupplemented milk diets, in various disease states, and in alcoholism—as well as in pregnancy. Average American intakes are estimated to be as low as 0.5 mg per day in poor diets ranging up as high as 6 mg per day in good diets, depending on the method of assay.[7, 44]

It should be noted that the recommended levels are higher than the present legal limit of 0.1 mg allowed in vitamin supplements;* but, according to the Board,[7] an intake of 0.1 mg per day of synthetic folic acid, the form

*Kept at this low level because an excess of folacin can mask certain symptoms of pernicious anemia—but not the neurological symptoms (see vitamin B-12).

*Table 7–10. Recommended Allowances for Folacin and Vitamin B-12**

	Age	Folacin Activity, mg/day	Vitamin B-12 Activity, mcg/day
Males	10-55 years	0.4	5
	55 years and over	0.4	6
Females	10-55 years	0.4	5
	55 years and over	0.4	6
	Pregnant	0.8	8
	Lactating	0.5	6

*From the Food and Nutrition Board, 1968.[7]
See Appendix Table 1C for FAO recommendations.

generally used in vitamin supplements, satisfies the "requirement for the normal adult" (though not the recommended allowance, it will be noted). This anomaly will need to be worked out in the future. It is not known to what extent synthesis by intestinal bacteria may assist in meeting the folacin requirement.

Obviously, folacin now becomes one of our most important vitamins, since average intakes are not appreciably higher, if at all, than the current recommended intake. The need for improved eating habits should be clear.

Food Sources of Folacin

Information about the folacin activity of foods for man is incomplete because of the difficulty of assaying the many different forms of folacin in terms of animal activity. However, the richest sources are liver, yeast, and leafy vegetables[55, 66] (see Table 7–11 and Table 3 of the Appendix for more details and other references). Good sources are dried legumes, green vegetables (such as asparagus, lettuce, and broccoli), nuts, fresh oranges, and whole wheat products.

Poor sources include most meats, eggs, root vegetables, most fruits, white flour and products made with highly milled cereals, most desserts, and processed milks (especially dried milks). Sugar and table fats and oils supply no folacin. Diets made up entirely of natural foods low in folacin have produced folacin deficiencies in animals and in man.[67]

The folacin content of foods is partially destroyed by heating or processing at high temperatures. Normal cooking temperatures (110° to 120° C for ten minutes) can cause losses up to 65 percent. Fresh leafy vegetables stored at room temperature for three days may lose up to 70 percent of their folacin activity.

The use of synthetic folacin in vitamin supplements or for food enrichment

Table 7–11.   *Examples of Good Food Sources of Folacin**

Food Source	Folacin Activity, mcg/100 gm†	Food Source	Folacin Activity, mcg/100 gm†
Asparagus	110	Kidney beans	180
Beet greens	60	Lima beans	130
Cereal concentrates		Liver	
Rice		Beef	295
Germ	430	Lamb	275
Polishings	190	Pork	220
Wheat		Mung beans	145
Bran	195	Mustard greens	60
Germ	305	Soybeans	225
Chocolate	100	Soyflour	425
Cowpeas	440	Spinach	75
Filbert nuts	65	Walnuts	75
Garbanzo beans	125	Yeast	
Kale	70	Brewer's	2020
		Torula	3000

*Adapted from Hardinge, M. G., and Crooks, H.[55] Also see Appendix Table 3.
†Fresh, raw basis.

has certain legal restrictions (see vitamin B-12), so it is important to depend on dietary sources for routine purposes.

As a general guide to ensure ample folacin in a daily diet, the best advice, as with all the nutrients, is to choose one's daily diet from the traditional foods in the four food groups according to energy needs. Obviously the choice of at least one serving of green leafy vegetables per day contributes significantly to meeting the daily requirement of folacin.

VITAMIN B-12

Vitamin B-12 was the last vitamin to be discovered (1948), thus completing the B-complex vitamin jigsaw. Distinguishing characteristics are its red color, the presence in its molecule of cobalt and phosphorus, and, unlike any other vitamin, the inability of higher plants to synthesize it. Its most important deficiency state is called *Addisonian pernicious anemia.*

Pernicious anemia has long been known and was given its name because it arose from some factor inherent in the body, did not respond to any known treatment, and eventually culminated in death. In 1849, Addison, an English physician, gave a detailed description of its symptoms, but no treatment could be found until, in 1926, Minot and Murphy[68] of Boston announced that feeding large amounts of liver (1/4 to 1/2 pound per day) restored a normal level of red blood cells in cases of this disease. This indicated that the disease might well be related to nutritional factors. For this discovery they shared the Nobel Prize with Whipple, who had shown a year previously that liver was of great benefit in blood regeneration in dogs rendered anemic by bleeding. Later concentrates of liver were made available, obviating the necessity of eating large amounts of this food. Biochemists began a long series of attempts to isolate the active component present in liver concentrates, which was then called the "antipernicious anemia factor."

Identification and Properties

In 1948 Rickes and co-workers, of Merck and Co., Inc., New Jersey, announced the isolation from a liver concentrate of a crystalline, red pigment, which they called "vitamin B-12."[69] In the same month, E. L. Smith[69] (in England) isolated two similar red, noncrystalline pigments from liver concentrate. In New York, West showed that injections of vitamin B-12[70] induced a dramatic beneficial response in patients with pernicious anemia. The vitamin was isolated by the Merck group with the use of a convenient test developed at the University of Maryland by Shorb and Briggs.[71] This test, which used *Lactobacillus lactis* Dorner (a bacterium), saved much work when compared with the former tests which had to be made with humans with pernicious anemia or with experimental animals.

Vitamin B-12 is the group name for several *corrinoids* (named because of their *porphyrin*-like structure).* They are nitrogenous basic substances with very large, complicated molecules. (See formula in Appendix.) The cobalt occupies the center of the molecule and may be attached either to a *cyanide* (CN) group (in which case the compound is called *cyanocobalamin*, the first one to be called vitamin B-12) or a *hydroxyl* group (OH) (which then is called *hydroxocobalamin*, probably the most common form), or to still other groups. A coenzyme form of vitamin B-12 (coenzyme B-12), contains an *adenosine*† molecule in place of the cyanide or hydroxyl group and is thought to be the most common form in foods. It was discovered by Barker and co-workers of the University of California.[72] Methylcobalamin is another form of the vitamin which also has a coenzyme role. All these forms have about equal vitamin B-12 activity when in the diet. (The presence of

cobalt in the molecule is essential for its vitamin activity.)

The structure of cyanocobalamin was first determined in 1955 by Dorothy Hodgkins and co-workers,[73] who later received the Nobel Prize. Vitamin B-12 is the most complicated of all the vitamins and the only one that chemists have not yet learned to synthesize in the laboratory. Fortunately, highly active vitamin B-12 concentrates can be produced inexpensively by the vitamin industry from cultures of certain bacteria and fungi grown in large tanks containing special media. These concentrates are universally used as the source of vitamin B-12 in vitamin supplements and in commercial rations for animals. Neither man nor animals can synthesize vitamin B-12 in their tissues, and unlike any other vitamin, higher plants are unable to synthesize it. *All the vitamin B-12 available to man and animals comes originally from that produced by bacteria and fungi,* either directly or indirectly, in foods that have taken it up from soil or animal feeds or produced by microbial synthesis in the intestine of the animal.

Effects of Lack of Vitamin B-12 in Man; Pernicious Anemia

Vitamin B-12 deficiency in man may occur in two ways: as a result of a simple *dietary lack* (possible only in strict vegetarians) or to a *faulty absorption* mechanism which, in effect, blocks the entrance of the vitamin into the body. This results in the condition known as pernicious anemia.

In an uncomplicated dietary deficiency of the vitamin, symptoms such as sore tongue, weakness, loss of weight, back pains, tingling of the extremities, apathy, and mental and other nervous abnormalities may develop. Anemia is rarely seen. On the other hand, in pernicious anemia, anemia and degeneration of the spinal cord are the major signs—though without treatment the

---

*Porphyrin-like structures are found also in the "heme" part of the hemoglobin in blood and in chlorophyll in plants. They consist basically of four nitrogen-containing rings bound together with a mineral element in the center.

†Adenosine is a nucleoside and consists of a purine (adenine) combined with a pentose sugar, ribose.

other symptoms may appear, and eventually will result in death.

The cause of pernicious anemia was partially explained when Castle, in 1928–1930,[74] described the need for an *intrinsic factor* (formed in the stomach) essential for the absorption of an "extrinsic factor"* from food which prevented the disease in normal persons. The intrinsic factor is formed in the stomach of normal persons, but not in those with pernicious anemia (in many cases the presence of an antibody to intrinsic factor prevents its normal action). The intrinsic factor has been identified as a mucoprotein which binds tightly to vitamin B-12 and facilitates its absorption.

The metabolic defect in pernicious anemia (thought to be inherited) is the inability to secrete this intrinsic factor (and usually other gastric juices), which results in inability to absorb vitamin B-12 from the intestinal tract. Hence, there is a low level of vitamin B-12 in the blood and an inability of new red blood cells to develop normally, resulting in *megaloblastic anemia*. Various neurologic symptoms may also precede or follow the anemia. As little as 1.5 mcg of vitamin B-12, injected intramuscularly each day† in a pernicious anemia patient, will result in restoration of a normal red cell count and gradual disappearance of all the other symptoms. Because the inherent defect of faulty absorption persists, pernicious anemia patients must continue to receive vitamin B-12 in a manner which by-passes the intestinal tract (namely by intramuscular injections). Because this treatment is successful, severe symptoms are seldom seen now in pernicious anemia

patients. The intrinsic factor, in purified form (bound to vitamin B-12), can be used in the treatment of the disease, as can the administration of massive amounts of vitamin B-12 in the diet, but such methods are expensive and are not always successful.

Effects of Lack of Vitamin B-12 in Animals

For years nutritionists had studied the effects on animals of what is now known as vitamin B-12 deficiency in attempting to isolate the active substance in liver. Animals such as chickens, pigs, rats, and mice all require vitamin B-12 for normal growth and reproduction, and develop other symptoms of its lack when fed diets deficient in this factor. (As yet no animal has been found to develop the counterpart of human pernicious anemia.)

In the case of chickens, deficiency symptoms which developed when diets made entirely from plant sources were used (in the 1930's and early 1940's) could be alleviated by adding to this diet animal by-products which provided what was called the "animal protein factor."[75] After vitamin B-12 was discovered, it was found to replace the need for the previously studied "animal protein factor" and "vitamin B-11" for chicks, "Factor X"‡ and "zoopherin" for rats, the "anti-thyroid factor" of mice, and the "*Lactobacillus lactis* Dorner factor" for bacteria, as well as the "anti-pernicious anemia factor" for man.

Deficiencies in rats, fowl, young calves, monkeys, pigs, and many other species are readily obtained merely by leaving the vitamin out of the diet and, at the same time preventing the animal from eating litter, soil, or its feces. Deficient animals show poor growth and reproductive disorders, and in

---

*The term "extrinsic factor" is obsolete today, and vitamin B-12 should be used in its place. Castle's so-called extrinsic factor was said to be found in meat, but it was also found in rice polishings, tomatoes, yeast, and wheat germ, none of which, we know now, contain appreciable amounts of vitamin B-12.

†Usually injections are spaced a month or so apart, so that larger amounts are routinely given.

‡In fact, it was the specific search for the unknown "Factor X" in milk by U.S.D.A. scientists in the early 1940's which led directly to the bacterial test later used by the Merck group to isolate vitamin B-12.

severe cases they die. Pigs may show nervous irritability.

Cattle and sheep, grazing on plants grown on cobalt-poor soil (see p. 284), develop symptoms of cobalt deficiency, which include loss of weight, weakness, and *anemia.* The injection of vitamin B-12 (but not of cobalt) relieves all these symptoms, proving that the cobalt lack resulted in inability of the microorganisms in the rumen to synthesize the vitamin. Because cobalt is one of the constituents of the vitamin B-12 molecule, it is obvious that it is required by all animals which are chiefly dependent on microbial synthesis in the gut for their supply of this vitamin.

Function of Vitamin B-12

Vitamin B-12 is absorbed only to the extent of 30 to 70 percent in normal persons, and none is absorbed in persons with pernicious anemia. Once in the body, it is converted (if not already in that form) to the coenzyme form. This coenzyme circulates in the blood combined with proteins (globulins, specifically), and it is stored in the liver and kidney. It is essential for the normal functioning of all body cells, particularly those of the bone marrow, the nervous system, and the gastrointestinal tract (though is no more active qualitatively than other forms of the vitamin when it is fed or injected).

The *role of vitamin B-12 in metabolism* is not completely understood, but its most important function is in the formation of nucleic acids by aiding in the synthesis of various purine and pyrimidine intermediates, similar to the function of folacin. Coenzyme B-12 also participates, often with pantothenic acid, in the rather unique but essential *isomerism* reactions, in which several carbon units are rearranged within a molecule, such as in the formation of an amino acid, aspartic acid. It also is involved in the synthesis and transfer of labile methyl groups, along with choline, folacin, and methionine (see discussion of labile methyl under *Choline,* p. 152).

Food Sources of Vitamin B-12

There is no vitamin B-12 in plant products, such as grains, vegetables, fruits, etc., except trace amounts which might be absorbed from the soil while the plant is growing, soil being one of the better sources of vitamin B-12 because of its high bacterial content. There is none present in yeast,* the traditional source of other B complex vitamins. Richest sources are liver and organ meats. Muscle meats, fish, eggs, shellfish, milk, and most milk products, except butter, are good sources, while evaporated milk and yogurt are fair sources.[47] (See Table 7–12 for examples of good sources and Table 3 of the Appendix for more values in foods.) The coenzyme form of the vitamin, which accounts for a major portion of vitamin B-12 in food, is not very stable to the

---

*However, some special yeasts containing vitamin B-12 are available. They have been grown on media very rich in the vitamin which is then absorbed in the yeast cell.

*Table 7–12. Examples of Good Food Sources of Vitamin B-12**

Food Source	Vitamin B-12, mcg per 100 gm
Clams, raw, meat only	98
Cod, dehydrated, slightly salted	10
Crab, cooked or canned	10
Eggs	
Chicken, yolk	6
Chicken, dried	10
Turkey, yolk	9
Heart	
Beef	11
Rabbit	16
Herring, Atlantic	
Raw	10
Canned	8
Kidney, raw	
Beef	31
Calf	25
Lamb	63
Liver, raw	
Beef	80
Lamb	104
Mackerel, Atlantic raw	9
Oysters, Eastern, raw	18
Sardines, Atlantic	
Raw	11
Canned, in oil or tomato sauce	10
Liverwurst	14

*Adapted from Orr, M. L., 1969.[47] Also see Appendix Table 3.

heat used in processing procedures or to light. Up to 10 percent is lost in milk during pasteurization, and 40 to 90 percent in evaporated milk.

The most inexpensive sources of vitamin B-12 are the microbial growth concentrates. (One year's supply for one normal person costs about two cents.) These concentrates have not been used to enrich man's food, for there has been no demonstrated need for this as yet on a widespread basis.

Requirements and Nutritional Status

The Food and Nutrition Board has recently set a recommended allowance for vitamin B-12.[7] They have stated that, "if absorption is normal, a dietary intake of 5 micrograms/day of vitamin B-12 is required to ensure the replacement of normal losses." This is the recommended allowance, then, for all adults, except persons over 55 who may absorb less, and except during pregnancy and lactation (see Table 7-10 and Table 1A of the Appendix). Of course, persons with pernicious anemia, who do not absorb the vitamin, will respond to 5 mcg of vitamin B-12 only if it is injected. As little as 0.1 mcg per day can give a small response when injected in anemic persons, making vitamin B-12 one of the most potent compounds known to man.

The amount of vitamin B-12 in typical American, high-cost, low-cost, and poor diets averaged 31, 16, and 2.7 mcg respectively.[44] Except for the poor diet, these amounts are more than sufficient to meet the recommended allowance.

The vitamin B-12 content of diets in many developing countries (where foods of plant origin are more common) may be considerably less, and frank vitamin B-12 deficiencies are not unknown. For instance, vitamin B-12 deficiency in infants can occur frequently in certain areas of the world where intakes of animal products by mothers are low. In studies of pregnant mothers in southern India, Baker and coworkers reported that "babies born of and suckled by vitamin B-12-deficient mothers may have lower body vitamin B-12 stores, may receive less vitamin B-12 in breast-milk feeds, and may be in danger of developing frank vitamin B-12 deficiency.[76]

Likewise, children who live exclusively on plant foods ("vegans") may show symptoms of vitamin B-12 deficiency after extended periods. Deficiency signs have also been seen in adults, especially child-bearing women, after eating vegetable and grain diets for several years—even in the absence of pernicious anemia.[77]

All such examples are due to a straightforward deficiency. Normally, the total body stores of vitamin B-12 in well-fed adults are as much as 5 to 10 mg. These reserves are sufficient to last as long as *two to three years*, or much more, even in the absence of a vitamin B-12 supply—but eventually a deficiency will occur. A diet containing 15 mcg per day will gradually replenish body stores if they have been depleted.[7]

Vitamin B-12 deficiency is occasionally seen also in persons who have special absorptive problems, as in total or subtotal removal of the stomach by surgery, those infested with parasites such as the fish tapeworm (not uncommon in some countries), or persons with tropical anemias, sprue, and other conditions where intestinal absorption is poor.

Vitamin B-12 promises to be one of the most important vitamins for mankind. It is now possible to use plant and cereal foods much more wisely in the human diet in case of future population pressures or famines, and when animal foods are in short supply.

ARE THERE OTHER B-VITAMINS?

There appear to be no other B-vitamins than the nine presented in this chapter and listed in Figure 7-18

FOOD SOURCES AND USES IN THE BODY

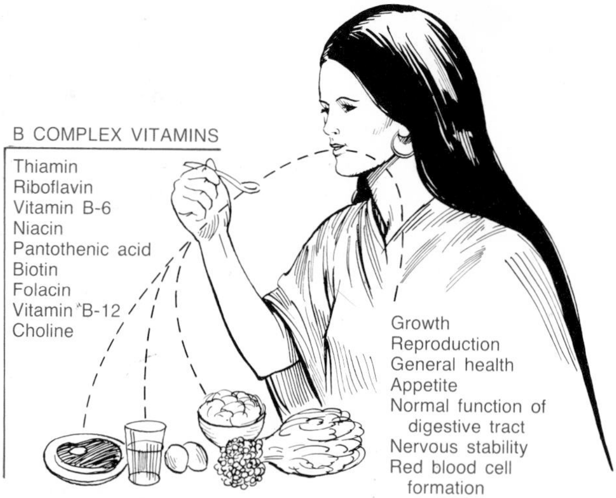

B COMPLEX VITAMINS

Thiamin
Riboflavin
Vitamin B-6
Niacin
Pantothenic acid
Biotin
Folacin
Vitamin B-12
Choline

Growth
Reproduction
General health
Appetite
Normal function of
  digestive tract
Nervous stability
Red blood cell
  formation

MEATS, MILK, EGGS, LEGUMES,
GREEN VEGETABLES,
WHOLE GRAIN BREADS & CEREALS

Figure 7–18.

(also see Chapter 6, p. 110). Occasionally, the sugar-like substance *myo-inositol* (inositol) will be listed among the B-complex vitamins (on labels, and in textbooks, catalogues, diet-ingredient lists, etc.). Myo-inositol, once thought to be a B-vitamin, is an important constituent of certain phospholipids in the body and is also present in a variety of foods. However, higher animals appear capable of synthesizing all the myo-inositol needed, and there is little evidence to confirm earlier conclusions (made with diets partially deficient in other vitamins) that myoinositol is a vitamin for either man or higher animals.[78] Nevertheless, it still remains an important "growth factor" for certain yeasts (as one of the "bios" group), for many bacteria, and for several lower organisms up to and including several species of fish. Progress on a recent study from Harvard University[79] which indicates a dietary need of inositol by the female gerbil (a small mammal used as a pet and in laboratory studies) will be watched with interest.

Another constituent of foods is *p-aminobenzoic acid*, often listed with B-vitamins in the same manner as myo-inositol. This, too, is an important "growth factor" for lower animals, but in higher animals it serves only as a "sparing factor" in the diet for folacin (see p. 154). It has no vitamin activity in animals receiving ample folacin and is no longer considered a vitamin.

There are many other natural, organic "growth factors," other than the vitamins, necessary for lower forms of life—such as lipoic acid, carnitine, nucleic acids, purines and pyrimidines, "biopterin," peptides, sterols, "hematin," and still others, but none of these fit the definition of a vitamin.

Other compounds that have growth-promoting activity in animals, or some other beneficial effect, probably exist in natural foods or may be synthesized by intestinal bacteria. These compounds are being studied in various laboratories and are conveniently termed "unidentified factors."[80] Whether any of these "unidentified factors" for animals turn out to be B-vitamins or whether they will be needed by man remains to be seen. In any event, if such unidentified vitamins actually do exist, they are of no cause for concern so long as one eats a variety of foods from the basic four food groups (which supply ample amounts of all the B-vitamins).

QUESTIONS AND PROBLEMS

1. Enumerate nine vitamins that are known as B complex vitamins. For each of the following vitamins, give its chief use (or uses) in the body and the symptoms that are characteristic results of a deficiency of it in the diet: thiamin, riboflavin, and niacin.

2. Give three specific examples of a biological relationship between a B-vitamin and an amino acid.

3. Is pellagra a clear-cut deficiency disease due to lack of niacin alone? If not, enumerate what other nutritive deficiencies are likely to occur as a result of a diet consisting mainly of corn meal and grits, white flour and rice, and fatty salt pork. What foods introduced into the diet as a result of making a home garden and keeping a cow and hens have pellagra-preventing properties? What foods could be added to further improve the diet, if money were available to buy them?

4. Either make out a day's menus for what you would consider an attractive diet, or write down your actual food intake for an average day. Specify the amounts of each food consumed. Consult the tables in this chapter and in the Appendix for content of foods in protein, thiamin, riboflavin, and vitamin B-6. Add up the total quantities of each which would be provided in the day's diet that you have planned or consumed.

5. Look up, or calculate as directed in the preceding chapter, the recommended allowance for the above three B vitamins for a person of your sex, size, and degree of activity. How does the intake of each vitamin in the calculated diet compare with the recommended allowance? What foods fairly rich in these three vitamins might be used to increase the thiamin, riboflavin, and vitamin B-6 content of the diet?

6. Give the chief nutritional functions for each of the following vitamins: folacin, vitamin B-12, vitamin B-6, and pantothenic acid. Can you give any examples of interrelations between different B complex vitamins?

7. What types of foods, used freely in the diet, ensure a sufficient intake of the whole group of B vitamins?

REFERENCES

1. Salmon, W. D.: J. Biol. Chem., *73*:483, 1927.
2. Williams, R. R., and Cline, J. K.: J. Amer. Chem. Soc., *58*:1504, 1936.
3. Grijns, G.: Geneesk. Tijdschr. v. Ned. Ind. 1, 1901 (as seen in McCollum, ref. 4).
4. McCollum, E. V.: *A History of Nutrition.* Boston, Houghton Mifflin Co., 1957.
5. Jansen, B. C. P.: Nutr. Abst. Rev., *26*:1, 1956.
6. Melnick, D., et al.: J. Nutr., *18*:593, 1939; Jolliffe, N., et al.: Amer. J. Med. Sci., *198*:198, 1939; Williams, R. D., et al.: Arch. Int. Med., *69*:721, 1942; Williams, R. D., et al.: Arch. Int. Med., *71*:38, 1943; Hulse, M. C., et al.: Ann. Int. Med., *21*: 440, 1944.
7. Food and Nutrition Board: *Recommended Dietary Allowances.* 7th Ed. Publication 1694. Washington, D.C., National Academy of Sciences, 1968; Miller, D. F., and Voris, L.: J. Amer. Dietet. Assoc., *54*:109, 1969; Sebrell, W. H., Jr.: J. Amer. Dietet. Assoc., *54*:103, 1969.
8. Lane, R. L., Johnson, E., and Williams, R. R.: J. Nutr., *23*:613, 1942.
9. U.S. Department of Agriculture: *National Food Situation.* Issue NFS-137, Washington, D.C., August 1971.
10. Kelsay, J. L.: J. Nutr., *99* (No. 1, Part II, Suppl. 1):119, 1969.
11. Davis, T. R. A., Gershoff, S. N., and Gamble, D. F.: J. Nutr. Educ., *1* (Fall, Suppl. 1):39, 1969.
12. Schaefer, A. E.: J. Amer. Dietet. Assoc., *54*: 371, 1969; Nutr. Today, *4*:2, 1969.
13. Food Consumption of Households in the United States, Spring 1965. Agr. Res. Ser., U.S. Department of Agriculture, ARS 62-17, 1968.
14. Watt, B. K., and Merrill, A. L.: *Composition of Foods: Raw, Processed, Prepared.* U.S.D.A. Handbook No. 8, Washington, D.C., 1963.
15. Emmett, A. D., and co-workers: J. Biol. Chem., *32*:409, 1917; *43*:265, 1920; *43*: 287, 1920.
16. Sebrell, W. H., and Butler, R. E.: U.S. Pub. Health Rep., *53*:2282, 1938; *54*:2121, 1939.
17. Lane, M., et al.: J. Clin. Invest., *43*:357, 1964.
18. Filer, L. J., and Martinez, G. A.: Clin. Pediat., *3*:633, 1964.

19. Ziegler, J. A.: J. Amer. Chem. Soc., *66*:1039, 1944.
20. Goldberger, J., et al.: U.S. Pub. Health Rep., *30*:3117, 1915; *31*:3159 and 3336, 1916; *33*:2038, 1918; and four reports in *35*: 1920. Goldberger was aided considerably by the early work of C. Voegtlin (J. Amer. Med. Assoc., *63*:1094, 1914).
21. Elvehjem, C. A., et al.: J. Amer. Chem. Soc., *59*;1767, 1937; J. Biol. Chem., *123*:137, 1938.
22. Fouts, P. J., et al.: Proc. Soc. Exp. Biol. Med., *37*:405, 1937; Smith, D. T., Ruffin, J. M., and Smith, S. G.: J. Amer. Med. Assoc., *109*:2054, 1937; Spies, T. D., et al.: J. Amer. Med. Assoc., *110*:622, and *111*:584, 1938; Ann. Int. Med., *12*:1830, 1939; Harris, L. J.: Chem. Ind., *56*:1134, 1937.
23. IUNS Committee on Nomenclature: J. Nutr., *101*:133, 1971.
24. Spies, T. D., et al.: J. Amer. Med. Assoc., *113*:1481, 1939.
25. Sandels, M. R., and Grady, E.: Arch. Int. Med., *50*:362, 1932; Stiebeling, H. K., and Munsell, H. E.: U.S. Department of Agriculture Technical Bulletin No. 333, 1932; Sebrell, W. H.: U.S. Pub. Health Rep., *49*:57, 1934.
26. Wheeler, G. A., and Sebrell, W. H.: J. Amer. Med. Assoc., *99*:95, 1932.
27. Kooser, J. H., and Blankenhorn, M. A.: J. Amer. Med. Assoc. *116*:912, 1941.
28. DeKleine, W.: Southern Med. J., *35*:992, 1942.
29. Krehl, W. A., Sarma, P. S., Teply, L. S., and Elvehjem, C. A.: Science, *101*:489, 1945; and J. Nutr., *31*:85, 1946.
30. Najjar, V. A., et al.: Proc. Soc. Exp. Biol. Med., *61*:371, 1946; Sarett, H. P., and Goldsmith, G. A.: J. Biol. Chem., *177*: 461, 1949; Vilter, R. W., Mueller, J. F., and Bean, W. B.: J. Lab. Clin. Med., *34*: 409, 1949; Horwitt, M. K., et al.: J. Amer. Dietet. Assoc., *34*:914, 1958; J. Nutr., Suppl., *1*, 1956; Goldsmith, G. A., et al.: Amer. J. Clin. Nutr., *6*:479, 1958; J. Nutr., *73*:172, 1961.
31. Briggs, G. M., et al.: J. Biol. Chem., *161*: 749, 1945; *165*:739, 1946; J. Nutr., *32*: 659, 1946; *45*:345, 1951; Krehl, W. A., et al.: J. Biol. Chem., *162*:403, 1946; *166*:531, 1946.
32. Paul, A. A.: Nutrition, London, *23*:131, 1969; Horwitt, M. K.: J. Amer. Dietet. Assoc., *34*:914, 1958; Horwitt, M. K., et al.: J. Nutr., *60*:Suppl. 1, p. 1, 1956.
33. György, P.: Nature, *133*:498, 1934; Amer. J. Clin. Nutr., *4*:313, 1956.
34. Chick, H., and Copping, A. M.: Biochem. J., *24*:1764, 1930.
35. Lepkovsky, S.: Science, *87*:169, 1938; J. Biol. Chem., *124*:125, 1938.
36. György, P., and Eckardt, R. E.: Nature, *144*: 512, 1939.
37. Snell, E. E.: J. Biol. Chem., *154*:313, 1944;

157:491, 1945; J. Amer. Chem. Soc., *66*: 2082, 1944; Harris, S. A., et al.: J. Biol. Chem., *154*:315, 1944; Harris, S. A., Heyl, D., and Folkers, K.: J. Amer. Chem. Soc., *66*:2088, 1944.
38. Lushbough, C. H., Weichman, J. M., and Schweigert, B. S.: J. Nutr., *67*:451, 1959; Tomarelli, R. M., Spence, E. R., and Bernhart, F. W.: J. Agric. Food Chem., *3*:338, 1955.
39. Coursin, D. B.: J. Amer. Med. Assoc., *154*: 406, 1954; May, C. D.: Pediatrics, *14*:269, 1954; Nelson, E. M.: Pub. Health Rep., *71*:445, 1956;
    Bessey, O. A., Adam, D. J., and Hansen, A. E.: Pediatrics, *20*:33, 1957.
40. Smith, S. G., and Martin, D. W.: Proc. Soc. Exp. Biol. Med., *43*:660, 1940; Mueller, J. F., and Vilter, R. W.: J. Clin. Invest., *29*:193, 1950; Snyderman, S. E., et al.: J. Clin. Nutr., *1*:200, 1953; Vilter, R. W.: Amer. J. Clin. Nutr., *4*:378, 1957; Park, Y. K., and Linkswiler, H.: J. Nutr., *100*: 110, 1970.
41. Sauberlich, H. E.: Vitamins and Hormones, *22*:807, 1964; Baker, E. M., et al.: Amer. J. Clin. Nutr., *15*:59, 1964.
42. Witten, P. W., and Holman, R. T.: Arch. Biochem. Biophys., *41*:266, 1952.
43. Axelrod, A. E., and Traketellis, A. C.: Vitamins and Hormones, *22*:581, 1964.
44. Chung, A. S. M., et al.: Folic acid, vitamin B_6, pantothenic acid and vitamin B_{12} in human dietaries. Amer. J. Clin. Nutr., *9*:573, 1961.
45. Friend, B.: *National Food Situation*. U.S.D.A., Washington, D.C., Nov. 1969, p. 28.
46. Cheslock, K. E., and McCully, M. T.: J. Nutr., *70*:507, 1960.
47. Orr, M. L.: *Pantothenic acid, Vitamin B_6 and Vitamin B_{12} in Foods.* U.S.D.A., Washington, D.C., Home Econ. Res. Rep. 36, 1969.
48. Williams, R. J., et al.: J. Amer. Chem. Soc., *55*:2912, 1933; Advanc. Enzymol., *3*:253, 1943; Nutr. Rev., *12*:65, 1954.
49. Williams, R. J.: Science, *94*:462, 1941.
50. Jukes, T. H.: J. Amer. Chem. Soc., *61*:975, 1939; Woolley, D. W., Waisman, H. A., and Elvehjem, C. A.: J. Amer. Chem. Soc., *61*:977, 1939.
51. Williams, R. J., and Major, R. T.: Science, *91*:246, 1940; Stiller, E. T., et al.: J. Amer. Chem. Soc., *62*:1785, 1940.
52. Bean, W. B., and Hodges, R. E.: Proc. Soc. Exp. Biol. Med., *86*:693, 1954; Hodges, R. E., et al.: J. Clin. Invest., *37*:1642, 1958; *38*:1421, 1959; Amer. J. Clin. Nutr., *11*: 85, 1962; *11*:187, 1962.
53. Schroeder, H. A.: Amer. J. Clin. Nutr., *24*: 562, 1971.
54. György, P., et al.: Science, *91*:243, 1940; György, P.: Science, *92*:609, 1940.
55. Hardinge, M. G., and Crooks, H.: J. Amer. Dietet. Assoc., *38*:240, 1961.
56. Sydenstricker, V. P., et al.: Science, *95*:176, 1942; J. Amer. Med. Assoc., *118*:1199,

1942; Williams, R. H.: New Eng. J. Med., *228*:247, 1943.

57. Oppel, T. W.: Amer. J. Med. Sci., *204*:856, 1942.

58. Sure, B.: J. Nutr., *19*:71, 1940; György, P., and Goldblatt, H.: J. Exp. Med., *72*:1, 1940.

59. Best, C. H., and co-workers: Amer. J. Physiol., *101*:7, 1932; J. Physiol., *75*:56 and 405, 1932; *81*:409, 1934; *83*:255, 1935; *84*:38P, 1935; Biochem. J., *29*:2651, 1935; Nutr. Rev., *11*:321, 1953; Fed. Proc., *9*:506, 1950.

60. Jukes, T. H.: J. Nutr., *20*:445, 1940; *22*:315, 1941; Griffith, W. H., and Mulford, D. J.: Nutr., *21*:633, 1941; Hegsted, D. M., et al.: J. Biol. Chem., *138*:459, 1941.

61. Mitchell, H. K., Snell, E. E., and Williams, R. J.: J. Amer. Chem. Soc., *63*:2284, 1941.

62. Pfiffner, J. J., et al.: Science, *97*:404, 1943; Campbell, C. J., et al.: J. Biol. Chem., *152*:483, 1944; Stokstad, E. L. R.: J. Biol. Chem., *149*:573, 1943; Hutchings, B. L., et al.: Science, *99*:371, 1944.

63. Angier, R. B., et al.: Science, *103*:667, 1946.

64. Briggs, G. M., et al.: J. Biol. Chem., *148*: 163, 1943; *158*:303, 1945; Lillie, R. J., and Briggs, G. M.: Poultry Sci., *26*:289, 1947; Nichol, C. A., et al.: J. Nutr., *39*: 287, 1949.

65. Spies, T. D., et al.: South. Med. J., *38*:590, 707, and 781, 1945; J. Amer. Med. Assoc., *130*:474, 1946.

66. Hurdle, A. D. F., Barton, D., and Searles, I. H.: Amer. J. Clin. Nutr., *21*:1202, 1968; Santini, R., Brewster, C., and Butterworth, C. E., Jr.: Amer. J. Clin. Nutr., *14*:205, 1964.

67. Lillie, R. J., and Briggs, G. M.: Poult. Sci., *26*:289, 1947; Herbert, V.: Ann. Rev. Med., *16*:359, 1965.

68. Minot, G. R., and Murphy, W. P.: J. Amer. Med. Assoc., *87*:470, 1926.

69. Rickes, E. L., et al.: Science, *107*:396, 1948; *108*:135, 1948; Smith, E. L.: Nature, *161*: 638; 1948; *162*:144, 1948.

70. West, R.: Science, *107*:398, 1948.

71. Shorb, M. S.: J. Biol. Chem., *169*:455, 1947; Science, *107*:397, 1948; Shorb, M. S., and Briggs, G. M.: J. Biol. Chem., *176*:1463, 1948; Shorb, M. S., and Briggs, G. M.: Univ. Maryland Agric. Exp. Station Bull. A-66, June, 1952.

72. Barker, H. A., et al.: J. Biol. Chem., *235*:181 and 480, 1960.

73. Hodgkin, D. C., et al.: Nature, *176*:325, 1955; *179*:64, 1956.

74. Castle, W. B., et al.: J. Clin. Invest., *6*:2, 1928; Amer. J. Med. Sci., *178*:748, 1929; *180*:305, 1930.

75. Bird, H. R., et al.: J. Biol. Chem., *163*:387, 393, 1946; J. Nutr., *34*:233, 1947; Nestler, R. B., et al.: Poult. Sci., *15*:67, 1936.

76. Baker, S. J., et al.: Brit. Med. J., *5293*:1658, 1962 (abstracted in J. Amer. Dietet. Assoc., *41*:352, 1962).

77. Saraya, A. K., et al.: Amer. J. Clin. Nutr., *23*:1378, 1970; *24*:622, 1971.

78. Yagi, K.: J. Vitamintol., *11*:14, 1965; Anderson, L., et al.: J. Nutr., *64*:167, 1958; Nutr. Rev., *14*:219, 1956.

79. Submitted for publication; Dept. of Nutrition, Harvard Univ., 1972.

80. Lakhanpal, R. J., et al.: J. Nutr., *89*:341, 1966; Chain, E. B.: Perspect. Biol. Med., *10*:177, 1967; Ackerman, C. J.: J. Nutr., *89*:347, 1966.

SUPPLEMENTARY READING

General B Complex Vitamins
(also see references 4, 7–14, 23, 44, 45, 47 and 55)

Beaton, G. H., and McHenry, E. W. (eds.): *Nutrition: a Comprehensive Treatise.* Vol. II. New York, Academic Press, 1964.

Bowers, J. A., and Fryer, B. A.: Thiamin and riboflavin in cooked and frozen, reheated turkey. J. Amer. Dietet. Assoc., *60*:399, 1972.

Daniel, L. J.: Inhibitors of vitamins of the B complex. Nutr. Abs. Rev., *31*:1, 1961.

Feeley, R. M., and Watt, B. K.: Nutritive values of foods distributed under USDA food assistance programs. J. Amer. Dietet. Assoc., *57*:528, 1970.

Goldblith, S. M., and Joslyn, M. A. (eds.): *Milestones in Nutrition.* Westport, Conn., Avi Publishing Co., 1964.

Goldsmith, G. A.: Vitamins of the B complex. In *Food*, U.S. Department of Agriculture Yearbook, 1959, pp. 139–149.

György, P.: Reminiscences on the discovery and significance of some of the B vitamins. J. Nutr., *91* (Suppl. 1):5, 1967.

György, P.: The water-soluble vitamins. Ann. Rev. Biochem., *11*:309, 1942.

Lipmann, F.: The biochemical function of B vitamins. Pers. Biol. Med., *13*:1, 1969.

Robinson, F. A.: *The Vitamin Co-factors of Enzyme Systems.* Oxford, Pergamon Press, 1966.

Singh, S. P., and Essary, E. O.: Vitamin content of broiler meat as affected by age, sex, thawing, and cooking. Poult. Sci., *50*:1150, 1971.

Thomas, M. H., and Calloway, D. H.: Nutritional value of dehydrated foods. J. Amer. Dietet. Assoc., *39*:105, 1961.

Thiamin
(also see references 1–14)

Ariaey-Nejad, M. R., Balaghi, M., Baker, E. M., and Sauberlich, H. E.: Thiamin metabolism in man. Amer. J. Clin. Nutr., *23*:764, 1970.

Bamji, M. S.: Transketolase activity and urinary excretion of thiamin in the assessment of thiamin-nutrition status of Indians. Amer. J. Clin. Nutr., *23*:52, 1970.

Dewhurst, W. G., and Morgan, H. G.: Importance of urine volume in assessment of thiamin deficiency. Amer. J. Clin. Nutr., *23*:379, 1970.

Henshaw, J. L., et al.: Method for evaluating thiamine adequacy in college women. J. Amer. Dietet. Assoc., *57*:436, 1970.

Jeffrey, F. E., and Abelmann, W. H.: Recovery from proved shoshin beriberi. Amer. J. Med., *50*:123, 1971.

Kahn, L. N., and Livingston, G. E.: Effect of heating methods on thiamine retention in fresh or frozen prepared foods. J. Food Sci., *35*:349, 1970.

Leichter, J., and Joslyn, M. A.: Protective effect of casein on cleavage of thiamine by sulfite. J. Agr. Food Chem., *17*:1355, 1969.

Noble, I.: Thiamine and riboflavin retention in cooked variety meats. J. Amer. Dietet. Assoc., *56*:225, 1970.

Rogers, L. E., Porter, F. S., and Sidbury, J. B., Jr.: Thiamine-responsive megaloblastic anemia. J. Pediat., *74*:494, 1969.

Sauberlich, H. E.: Biochemical alterations in thiamine deficiency — their interpretations. Amer. J. Clin. Nutr., *20*:528, 1967.

Sauberlich, H. E., Herman, Y. F., and Stevens, C. O.: Thiamin requirement of the adult human. Amer. J. Clin. Nutr., *23*:671, 1970.

Tanphaichitr, V., Vimokesant, S. L., Dhanamitta, S., and Valyasevi, A.: Clinical and biochemical studies of adult beriberi. Amer. J. Clin. Nutr., *23*:1017, 1970.

Tomasulo, P. A., Kater, R. M. H., and Iber, F. L.: Impairment of thiamine absorption in alcoholism. Amer. J. Clin. Nutr., *21*:1341, 1968.

Ziporin, A. A., et al.: Excretion of thiamine and its metabolites in the urine of young adult males receiving restricted intakes of the vitamins. J. Nutr., *85*:287, 1965; Thiamine requirement in the adult human as measured by urinary excretion of thiamine metabolites. J. Nutr., *85*:297, 1965.

Nutrition Reviews

Malfunctioning of the blood-brain barrier in thiamine deficiency. *26*:218, 1968.

Action of pyrithiamine in nerve tissue. *26*:251, 1968.

Magnesium and thiamine deficiency. *26*:347, 1968.

Early brain stem lesions in thiamine deficient rats. *27*:54, 1969.

Thiamine and oxythiamine metabolism. *27*:88, 1969.

Influence of malnutrition and alcohol on thiamine absorption. *29*:13, 1971.

Catabolites of thiamine from the rat. *29*:119, 1971.

Riboflavin
(also see references 7–19)

Beutler, E.: Glutathione reductase: Stimulation in normal subjects by riboflavin supplementation. Science, *165*:613, 1969.

Bro-Rasmussen, F.: Riboflavin requirement of animal and man, related to protein requirement or energy turnover. Amer. J. Clin. Nutr., *20*:507, 1967.

Burch, H. B., Lowry, O. H., Bradley, M. E., and Max, P. F., Jr.: Hepatic metabolites and cofactors in riboflavin deficiency and calorie restriction. Amer. J. Physiol., *219*:409, 1970.

Foy, H., Kondi, A., and Verjee, Z. H. M.: Relation of riboflavin deficiency to corticosteroid metabolism and red cell hypoplasia in baboons. J. Nutr., *102*:571, 1972.

Horwitt, M. K.: Nutritional requirements of man, with special reference to riboflavin. Amer. J. Clin. Nutr., *18*:458, 1966.

Jusko, W. J., et al.: Riboflavin absorption and excretion in the neonate. Pediatrics, *45*:945, 1970.

Jusko, W. J., Levy, G., Yaffe, S. J., and Allen, J. E.: Riboflavin absorption in children with biliary obstruction. Amer. J. Dis. Child., *121*:48, 1971.

Levy, G., and Hewitt, R. R.: Evidence in man for different specialized intestinal transport mechanisms for riboflavin and thiamin. Amer. J. Clin. Nutr., *24*:401, 1971.

Owen, E. C., and West, D. W.: Metabolites of riboflavine in milk, urine and tissues of animals in relation to alimentary symbiotic bacteria. Brit. J. Nutr., *24*:45, 1970.

Tillotson, J. A., and Baker, E. M.: An enzymatic measurement of the riboflavin status in man. Amer. J. Clin. Nutr., *25*:425, 1972.

West, D. W., and Owen, E. C.: The urinary excretion of metabolites of riboflavine by man. Brit. J. Nutr., *23*:889, 1969.

Nutrition Reviews

Ferrokinetics in riboflavin deficient baboons. *26*:345, 1968.

Riboflavin — transport and excretion. *27*:285, 1969.

Covalently bound flavin-adenine dinucleotide of succinate dehydrogenase and the influence of dietary flavin. *28*:23, 1970.

The fate of riboflavin in the mammal (by McCormick, D. B.). *30*:75, 1972.

Niacin
(also see references 7–14, 19–32)

Barboriak, J. J., and Meade, R. C.: Nicotinic acid and alcohol-induced lipemia. Atherosclerosis, *13*:199, 1971.

Bergström, J., et al.: Effect of nicotinic acid on physical working capacity and on metabolism of muscle glycogen in man. J. Appl. Physiol., *26*:170, 1969.

Copping, A. M.: Nicotinic acid. Rev. Nutr. Food Sci., *11*:10, 1968.

Dietrich, L. S.: Regulation of nicotinamide metabolism. Amer. J. Clin. Nutr., *24*:800, 1971.

Garrison, W.: The great pellagra mystery. Today's Health, February 1968, p. 59.

Goldsmith, G. A.: Niacin: Antipellagra factor, hypocholesterolemic agent. J. Amer. Med. Assoc., *194*:167, 1965.

Hankes, L. V., Leklem, J. E., Brown, R. R., and Mekel, R. C. P. M.: Tryptophan metabolism in patients with pellagra: Problem of vitamin B₆ enzyme activity and feedback control of tryptophan pyrrolase enzyme. Amer. J. Clin. Nutr., *24*:730, 1971.

Ramsay, R. A., et al.: Nicotinic acid as adjuvant therapy in newly admitted schizophrenic patients. Canad. Med. Assoc. J., *102*:939, 1970.

Srikantia, S. G., Rao, B. S. N., Raghuramulu, N., and Gopalan, C.: Pattern of nicotinamide nucleotides in the erythrocytes of pellagrins. Amer. J. Clin. Nutr., *21*:1306, 1968.

Truswell, A. S., Hansen, J. D. L., and Wannenburg, P.: Plasma tryptophan and other amino acids in pellagra. Amer. J. Clin. Nutr., *21*:1314, 1968.

Vivian, V. M., Brown, R. R., Price, J. M., and Reynolds, M. S.: Some aspects of tryptophan and niacin metabolism in young women consuming a low tryptophan diet supplemented with niacin. J. Nutr., *88*:93, 1966.

Wolf, H.: Hormonal alteration of efficiency of conversion of tryptophan to urinary metabolites of niacin in man. Amer. J. Clin. Nutr., *24*:792, 1971.

Wolf, H., Brown, R. R., Price, J. M., and Madsen, P. O.: Effect of hormones on the biosynthesis of nicotinic acid from tryptophan in man. J. Clin. Endo. Metab., *30*:380, 1970.

Nutrition Reviews

Effect of cooking on the free niacin content of foods. *23*:286, 1965.

Leucine and pellagra (by Gopalan, C.). *26*:323, 1968.

Nicotinamide deficiency and adrenocortical steroids. *26*:343, 1968.

Gastric and pancreatic function in pellagra. *27*:136, 1969.

Vitamin B-6
(also see references 7 and 33–47)

Aly, H. E., Donald, E. A., and Simpson, M. H. W.: Oral contraceptives and vitamin B₆ metabolism. Amer. J. Clin. Nutr., *24*:297, 1971.

Brin, M.: Abnormal tryptophan metabolism in pregnancy and with the oral contraceptive pill. II. Relative levels of vitamin B₆-vitamers in cord and maternal blood. Amer. J. Clin. Nutr., *24*:704, 1971.

Cinnamon, A. D., and Beaton, J. R.: Biochemical assessment of vitamin B₆ status in man. Amer. J. Clin. Nutr., *23*:696, 1970.

Donald, E. A., et al.: Vitamin B-6 requirement in young adult women. Amer. J. Clin. Nutr., *24*:1028, 1971.

Drenick, E. J., Vinyard, E., and Swendseid, M. E.: Vitamin B₆ requirements in starving obese males. Amer. J. Clin. Nutr., *22*:10, 1969.

Frimpter, G. W., Andelman, R. J., and George, W. F.: Vitamin B₆-dependency syndromes. Amer. J. Clin. Nutr., *22*:794, 1969.

Grabow, J. D., and Linkswiler, H.: Electroencephalographic and nerve-conduction studies in experimental vitamin B₆ deficiency in adults. Amer. J. Clin. Nutr., *22*:1429, 1969.

Horrigan, D. L., and Harris, J. W.: Pyridoxine-responsive anemias in man. Vitamins and Hormones, *26*:549, 1968.

Kelsall, M. A. (ed.): Vitamin B₆ in metabolism of the nervous system. Ann. N.Y. Acad. Sci., *166*:Article 1, 1969.

Luhby, A. L., et al.: Vitamin B₆ metabolism in users of oral contraceptive agents. I. Abnormal urinary xanthurenic acid excretion and its correction by pyridoxine. Amer. J. Clin. Nutr., *24*:684, 1971.

Rose, D. P., and Braidman, I. P.: Excretion of tryptophan metabolites as affected by pregnancy, contraceptive steroids, and steroid hormones. Amer. J. Clin. Nutr., *24*:673, 1971.

Woodring, M. J., and Storvick, C. A.: Effect of pyridoxine supplementation on glutamic-pyruvic transaminase and in vitro stimulation in erythrocytes of normal women. Amer. J. Clin. Nutr., *23*:1385, 1970.

Vitamin B₆: Recent nutritional and clinical data. New Jersey, Hoffmann-LaRoche Inc., 1967.

Nutrition Reviews

Vitamin B₆ and the pituitary. *24*:276, 1966.

Pyridoxine deficiency and acute porphyria. *25*:7, 1967.

Pyridoxine dependency. *25*:72, 1967.

Vitamin B₆ status of cardiac patients. *25*:116, 1967.

Tryptophan pyrrolase, kynurenine, and pyridoxine. *25*:170, 1967.

Vitamin B₆ deficiency following isoniazid therapy. *26*:306, 1968.

Metabolism of pyridoxine in the mouse. *28*:163, 1970.

Pantothenic Acid
(also see refs. 7 and 48–53)

Clifton, G., Bryant, S. R., and Skinner, C. G.: N¹-(substituted) pantothenamides, antimetabolites of pantothenic acid. Arch. Biochem. Biophys., *137*:523, 1970.

Cohenour, S. H., and Calloway, D. H.: Blood, urine, and dietary pantothenic acid levels of pregnant teenagers. Amer. J. Clin. Nutr., *25*:512, 1972.

Constable, B. J., Fidanza, A., and Wilson, P. W.: Effect of pantothenic acid on fatty acid metabolism. Acta Vitamin., *19*:121, 1965.

Fidanza, A., and Constable, B. J.: Metabolic effect of pantothenic acid. Acta Vitamin., *17*:95, 1967.

Koyanagi, T., et al.: Effect of administration of thiamine, riboflavin, ascorbic acid and vitamin A to students on their pantothenic acid contents in serum and urine. Tohoku J. Exp. Med., *98*:357, 1969.

Nishizawa, Y., and Matsuzaki, F.: The antagonistic action of homopantothenic acid against pantothenic acid. J. Vitamin., *15*:8, 1969.

Schroeder, H. A.: Losses of vitamins and trace minerals resulting from processing and preservation of foods. Amer. J. Clin. Nutr., *24*:562, 1971.

Nutrition Reviews

Relation of pantothenic acid to adrenal cortical function. *19*:79, 1961.

Pregnancy and pantothenic acid deficiency in the guinea pig. *24*:169, 1966.

Biotin
(also see references 7 and 54–57)

Arinze, J. C., and Mistry, S. P.: Activities of some biotin enzymes and certain aspects of gluconeogenesis during biotin deficiency. Comp. Biochem. Physiol., *38B*:285, 1971.

Bhagavan, H. N.: Biotin content of blood during gestation. Internat. J. Vit. Res., *39*:235, 1969.

Bhagavan, H. N., and Coursin, D. B.: Biotin content of blood in normal infants and adults. Amer. J. Clin. Nutr., *20*:903, 1967.

Caplow, M.: Biotin basicity. Biochem., *8*:2656, 1969.

Dakshinamurti, K., Tarrago-Litvak, L., and Hong, H. C.: Biotin and glucose metabolism. Canad. J. Biochem., *48*:493, 1970.

Green, N. M., and Toms, E. J.: Purification and crystallization of avidin. Biochem. J., *118*:67, 1970.

Kirk, J. E., and Sanwald, R.: Biotin content of human arterial and venous tissue. J. Atherosclerosis Res., *6*:440, 1966.

Knappe, J.: Mechanism of biotin action. Ann. Rev. Biochem., *39*:757, 1970.

Peters, J. M.: A separation of the direct toxic effects of dietary raw egg white powder from its action in producing biotin deficiency. Brit. J. Nutr., *21*:801, 1967.

Nutrition Reviews

Present knowledge of biotin (by Bridgers, W. F.). *25*:65, 1967.

Biotin and glucokinase in the diabetic rat. *28*:242, 1970.

Choline
(also see references 7 and 58–60)

Beare-Rogers, J. L.: Time sequence of liver phospholipid alterations during deprivation of dietary choline. Canad. J. Physiol. Pharmacol., *49*:171, 1971.

Beers, W. H., and Reich, E.: Structure and activity of acetylcholine. Nature, *228*:917, 1970.

Best, C. H., Ridout, J. H., and Lucas, C. C.: Alleviation of dietary cirrhosis with betaine and other lipotropic agents. Canad. J. Physiol. Pharmacol., *47*:73, 1968.

Durell, J., Garland, J. T., and Friedel, R. O.: Acetylcholine action: Biochemical aspects. Science, *165*:862, 1969.

Kwong, E., et al.: Choline biosynthesis in germ-free rats. J. Nutr., *96*:10, 1968.

Lucas, C. C., and Ridout, J. H.: Fatty livers and lipotropic phenomena. In Holman, R. T. (ed.): *Progress in the Chemistry of Fats and Other Lipids*, Vol. 10, Part 1. Oxford, Pergamon Press, 1967.

Lyman, R. L., Sheehan, G., and Tinoco, J.: Diet and $^{14}CH_3$-methionine incorporation into liver phosphatidylcholine fractions of male and female rats. Canad. J. Biochem., *49*:71, 1971.

Tani, H., Suzuki, S., Kobayashi, M., and Kotake, Y.: The physiological role of choline in guinea pigs. J. Nutr., *92*:317, 1967.

Truswell, A. S., Hansen, J. D. L., Watson, C. E., and Wannenburg, P.: Relation of serum lipids and lipoproteins to fatty liver in kwashiorkor. Amer. J. Clin. Nutr., *22*:568, 1969.

Rutherford, R. B., et al.: Production of nutritional cirrhosis in *Macacca mulatta* monkeys. Arch. Surg., *98*:720, 1969.

Rytter, D. J., and Cornatzer, W. E.: Phospholipid metabolism in cells in culture. Lipids, *7*:142, 1972.

Nutrition Reviews

Choline deficiency in baboon and rat. *23*:270, 1965.

Liver lipid fatty acids in choline deficiencies. *23*:345, 1965.

Diurnal changes in plasma and liver lipids in rats in initial stages of choline deficiency. *24*:220, 1966.

Prevention of renal necrosis in rats fed diets lacking choline. *24*:255, 1966.

Environmental temperature and choline requirement. *24*:335, 1966.

Nutritional factors in choline deficiency. *26*:51, 1968.

Choline deficiency and carnitine depletion. *26*:152, 1968.

Alleviation of dietary cirrhosis by betaine and other lipotropic agents. *27*:269, 1969.

Folacin
(also see references 7, 44, and 61–67)

Avery, B., and Ledger, W. J.: Folic acid metabolism in well-nourished pregnant women. Obst. Gynec., *35*:616, 1970.

Bernstein, L. H., Gutstein, S., Weiner, S., and Efron, G.: The absorption and malabsorption of folic acid and its polyglutamates. Amer. J. Med., *48*:570, 1970.

Burland, W. L., Simpson, K., and Lord, J.: Response of low birthweight infants to treatment with folic acid. Arch. Dis. Child., *46*:189, 1971.

Butterfield, S., and Calloway, D. H.: Folacin in wheat and selected foods. J. Amer. Dietet. Assoc., *60*:310, 1972.

Cooper, B. A., Cantlie, G. S. D., and Brunton, L.: The case for folic acid supplements during pregnancy. Amer. J. Clin. Nutr., *23*:848, 1970.

Eichner, E. R., Buergel, N., and Hillman, R. S.: Experience with an appetizing, high protein, low folate diet in man. Amer. J. Clin. Nutr., *24*:1531, 1971.

Gerson, C. D., et al.: Folic acid absorption in man: Enhancing effect of glucose. Gastroent., *61*:224, 1971.

Girdwood, R. H.: Folate depletion in old age. Amer. J. Clin. Nutr., *22*:234, 1969.

Hellström, L.: Lack of toxicity of folic acid given in pharmacological doses to healthy volunteers. Lancet, *1*:59, 1971.

Herbert, V.: Folic acid deficiency in man. Vitamins and Hormones, *26*:525, 1968.

Herbert, V., and others: Symposium: Folic acid deficiency. Amer. J. Clin. Nutr., *23*:841, 1970.

Hoppner, K.: Free and total folate activity in strained baby foods. Canad. Inst. Food Tech. J., *4*:51, 1971.

Kahn, S. B., Fein, S., Rigberg, S., and Brodsky, I.: Correlation of folate metabolism and socioeconomic status in pregnancy and in patients taking oral contraceptive. Amer. J. Obst. Gynec., *108*:931, 1970.

Meindok, H., and Dvorsky, R.: Serum folate and vitamin B_{12} levels in the elderly. J. Amer. Geriat. Soc., *18*:317, 1970.

Metz, J.: Folate deficiency conditioned by lactation. Amer. J. Clin. Nutr., *23*:843, 1970.

Osifo, B. O. A.: The effect of folic acid and iron in the prevention of nutritional anaemias in pregnancy in Nigeria. Brit. J. Nutr., *24*:689, 1970.

Rosenberg, I. H., and Godwin, H. A.: The digestion and absorption of dietary folate. Gastroent., *60*:445, 1971.

Stokstad, E. L. R., and Koch, J.: Folic acid metabolism. Physiol. Rev., *47*:83, 1967.

Streiff, R. R.: Folate deficiency and oral contraceptives. J. Amer. Med. Assoc., *214*:105, 1970.

Waslien, C. I., et al.: Folate requirements of children. I and II. Amer. J. Clin. Nutr., *25*: 147 and 152, 1972.

Nutrition Reviews

Present knowledge of folacin (by Vitale, J. J.). *24*:289, 1966.

Intestinal blind loops and folate metabolism. *25*: 43, 1967.

Folate deficiency in pregnancy. *25*:166, 1967.

Effects of folic acid antagonists on fat absorption. *25*:241, 1967.

Folic acid and pregnancy I. *25*:325, 1967.

Folic acid and pregnancy II. *26*:5, 1968.

Ethanol and hemopoiesis. *26*:300, 1968.

Anticonvulsant therapy and serum folate. *27*:78, 1969.

Drugs and folic acid utilization. *29*:34, 1971.

Alcoholism and folic acid. *30*:57, 1972.

Vitamin B-12
(also see references 7, 47, and 68–77)

Adams, J. F., Tanekl, H. I., and MacEwan, F.: Estimation of the total body vitamin B_{12} in the live subject. Clin. Sci., *39*:107, 1970.

Alperin, J. B., Haggard, M. E., and Haynie, T. P.: A study of vitamin B_{12} requirements in a patient with pernicious anemia and thyrotoxicosis: Evidence of an increased need for vitamin B_{12} in the presence of hyperthyroidism. Blood, *36*:632, 1970.

Baker, S. J.: Human vitamin B_{12} deficiency. World Rev. Nutr. Dietet., *8*:62, 1967.

Burke, G. T., Mangum, J. H., and Brodie, J. D.: Mechanism of mammalian cobalamin-dependent methionine biosynthesis. Biochem., *10*:3079, 1971.

Giannella, R. A., Broitman, S. A., and Zamcheck, N.: Competition between bacteria and intrinsic factor for vitamin B_{12}: Implications for vitamin B_{12} malabsorption in intestinal bacteria overgrowth. Gastroent., *62*:255, 1972.

Heyssel, R. M., Bozian, R. C., Darby, W. L. J., and Bell, M. C.: Vitamin B_{12} turnover in man. Amer. J. Clin. Nutr., *18*:176, 1966.

Hogenkamp, H. P. C.: Enzymatic reactions involving corrinoids. Ann. Rev. Biochem., *37*:225, 1968.

Lindenbaum, J., and Lieber, C. S.: Alcohol-induced malabsorption of vitamin B_{12} in man. Nature, *224*:806, 1969.

Rose, M. S., and Chanarin, I.: Intrinsic-factor antibody and absorption of vitamin B_{12} in pernicious anaemia. Brit. Med. J., *1*:25, 1971.

Saraya, A. K., Tandon, B. N., Ramachandran, K., and Saikia, B.: Intestinal structure and function in megaloblastic anemia in adults. Amer. J. Clin. Nutr., *24*:622, 1971.

Saraya, A. K., Tandon, B. N., and Ramachandran, K.: Study of vitamin B_{12} and folic acid deficiency in hookworm disease. Amer. J. Clin. Nutr., *24*:3, 1971.

Smith, L. *Vitamin B_{12}*, New York, Wiley, 1965.

Stadtman, T. C.: Vitamin B_{12}. Science, *171*:859, 1971.

Stewart, J. S., Roberts, P. D., and Hoffbrand, A. V.: Response of dietary vitamin B_{12} deficiency to physiological oral doses of cyanocobalamin. Lancet, *2*:542, 1970.

Sullivan, L. W.: Vitamin B_{12} metabolism and megaloblastic anemia. Seminars in Hematology, *7*:6, 1970.

Symposium on vitamin B_{12} and folate. Amer. J. Med., *48*:539, 1970.

Weissbach, H., and Taylor, R. T.: Metabolic role of vitamin B_{12}. Vitamins and Hormones, *26*:395, 1968.

Nutrition Reviews

B_{12} transport in red cell membranes. *25*:248, 1967.

Defective vitamin B_{12} metabolism in the human being: Changes in methionine and methylmalonic acid excretion. *27*:202, 1969.

Liver methylmalonate and CoA concentrations in sheep deficient in vitamin B_{12}. *27*:240, 1969.

Urinary methylmalonate and hepatic methylmalonlyl CoA mutase in vitamin B_{12} deficient rats. *29*:18, 1971.

eight

Vitamin C
(Ascorbic Acid)

Vitamin C is the very important scurvy-preventing substance found in nature primarily in citrus and other fruits and in fresh vegetables. It has a most interesting history.

Nomenclature

By the late 1910's it became clear that there were at least three distinct nutritional deficiencies in man and animals (see Chapter 6). Scurvy had been known for centuries, but as the vitamins were identified, "vitamin C"* was given, arbitrarily, third place in the vitamin alphabet (chiefly because McCollum, who started the use of alphabet letters, was working with rats which do not get scurvy!).

In 1912, the terms "scurvy vitamine" and "antiscorbutin" were first used in

the literature for the scurvy-preventing substance.[1] The first use of the letter "C" for the antiscorbutic factor (or "water-soluble C") was in 1918 and 1919 by British workers.[2] This led directly to the use in 1921 of "vitamin C" for the substance by Santos and others,[3] following Drummond's suggestion of combining the word "vitamin" with the letters then in use.[4] The shortened term "ascorbic acid" for the crystalline antiscorbutic compound was proposed in 1933 by Szent-Györgyi and Haworth,[5] after recognition by King and co-workers[6] of the vitamin nature of the compound (see page 174).

*Effects of Lack of Vitamin C
in Man and Animals*

THE SAGA OF SCURVY. Serious cases of scurvy, a disease due to prolonged lack of vitamin C, are seldom seen now, but the story of its incidence and conquest is of great interest because it led to the discovery that a disease could be caused by lack of some intangible component of the diet and to the eventual isolation of the lacking substance as a vitamin. This is one of the most fasci-

---

*Recent International Union of Nutritional Sciences Tentative Nomenclature Rules (1969–71) use the term *vitamin C* for the combined name of all compounds which exhibit the biological activity of ascorbic acid. Thus, "vitamin C activity" and "vitamin C deficiency" are preferred terms. The term "ascorbic acid" is to be used for that specific chemical compound, one of several with vitamin C activity (Ref. 13, Chap. 6).

nating stories of achievement in the development of nutrition as a science.*

Scurvy is one of the oldest diseases of mankind; early descriptions are known to exist as far back as about 1500 B.C. Symptoms of gangrene of the gums, loss of teeth, and painful legs in soldiers were described by Hippocrates (about 450 B.C.), and from records of the crusaders, it is evident that they too suffered from scurvy. In the 15th and 16th centuries, it was a scourge throughout Europe, so much so that medical men wondered if all disease might not be outgrowths of scurvy. It was particularly prevalent and severe on long voyages of sailing ships, in beseiged cities, and in times of crop failures—in short, wherever fresh foods were unavailable. When Vasco de Gama made his long voyage around the Cape of Good Hope, nearly two thirds of his crew perished from scurvy. The lives of many of the men with the explorer Cartier, when obliged to spend the winter of 1535 in Canada, were saved because they learned from the Indians that a "brew" made from the growing tips of the spruce and other trees was a cure for this malady. (It is obvious now that the "brew" contained vitamin C.)

In 1753, James Lind, a Scottish naval surgeon, published his famous report of experiments made on ships of the British Navy, proving that oranges and lemons prevented or cured the disease.[7] His classic studies generally are considered the first experiments to show that an essential food element can prevent a deficiency disease. The experiences of Lind, Cartier, and others gradually became well known, so that by the time of the historic voyage of Captain Cook (1772–1775), enough was known about the prevention of scurvy to stock the ship with fresh fruits and vegetables at every port visited, thereby keeping captain and crew well throughout the long trip. Cook[8] also

recognized that sauerkraut was antiscorbutic and supplied the ship with large quantities of it, stating that it is "not only a wholesome vegetable food, but, in my judgment, highly antiscorbutic, and spoils not by keeping." It was not until 1795, however, that citrus fruits (lime juice) were made a regulation on ships of the British Navy, providing British sailors with the nickname "limeys."

The explorers of the New World took the potato to Europe and, as potatoes (a good source of vitamin C) became a food staple there, scurvy disappeared. Epidemics of scurvy reappeared on several occasions after disastrous failures of the potato crop in certain regions, as in Norway and in Ireland. While it became generally recognized that citrus fruits and fresh vegetables were preventives against scurvy, nearly 150 years elapsed before the potency of these foods was explained as due to the presence in them of a specific substance known as a vitamin.

EFFECTS OF ACUTE LACK. The effects of an acute lack of vitamin C have been recently (1971) thoroughly studied by Hodges, Baker, Sauberlich, and others at the University of Iowa and the U.S. Army Medical Research and Nutrition Laboratory, Denver.[9] Five male prisoners volunteered to be placed on a liquid vitamin C–deficient diet for 84 to 97 days. The first symptoms of deficiency seen were *fatigue, rough skin (hyperkeratosis), pink or hemorrhagic skin follicles* (see Fig. 8–1), *hemorrhages in the eye, coiled hairs, and gum changes, followed by pains in the joints, the sicca syndrome* (including *changes in the salivary and tear glands, loss of dental fillings, dental caries, tender mouth, dryness and itching of skin, and excessive loss of hair*), *and low blood and urine ascorbic acid levels.* The skin changes were noted as early as 29 days, several weeks before the occurrence of swollen and bleeding gums, contrary to common beliefs. Giving vitamin C overcame all the symptoms eventually (after three to ten weeks).

---

*Persons interested in more detail on this subject will find a list of general references on the history of vitamin C at the end of this chapter.

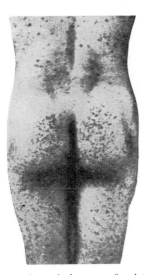

*Figure 8–1.*A typical case of adult scurvy, showing the numerous petechiae—spots where blood has effused to the skin. (From L. J. Harris: *Vitamins in Theory and Practice.* New York, Macmillan Co., 1955.)

Acute scurvy presents such a dramatic picture of degeneration in many body tissues (skin, teeth and gums, blood vessel walls, bones, cartilage, and muscle tissues) that it is not difficult to recognize. Because these severe symptoms are prevented by taking even moderate amounts of fresh or cooked fruits and vegetables, full-blown scurvy is very seldom encountered.

EFFECTS OF MODERATE LACK. A condition with less severe symptoms, known as *subacute* or *latent scurvy*, still occurs (though infrequently) among infants fed almost exclusively on heat-treated milk or cereal gruels, when sources of vitamin C are not used or are unobtainable. A deficiency shows up in persons when intake is just below the borderline of sufficiency, when there is greater need of the vitamin (as in growth), or when under conditions of physiological stress or infection.

In young children, symptoms of latent scurvy are *failure to grow* properly, weakness, restlessness, irritability, swollen joints, and tenderness of the lower extremities (see Fig. 8–2). Signs of vitamin C deficiency in older children and adults are usually listlessness, lack of endurance, fleeting pains in the legs and joints (often mistaken for rheumatism), small hemorrhages under the skin, and gums which bleed easily.

EFFECTS OF DEFICIENCY IN ANIMALS. Man, monkeys, and guinea pigs are the only common species of higher animals dependent on the vitamin C contained in their food for the prevention of scurvy.* All other common higher animals can synthesize the vitamin C they need in their bodies from glucose and galactose. This *biosynthesis* requires two specific enzymes† not present in the species which develop scurvy.[10]

Deficient guinea pigs, first studied in 1907 by workers in Norway,[11] show loss of weight (within 10 to 16 days), loss of appetite, weakness, lessening of activity, a rough hair coat, hunching with drooping head, stiffening of hind legs, obvious distress when handled, hemorrhage, beading of ribs, and death within 20 to 28 days.

Changes in teeth and gums are readily demonstrated in monkeys with scurvy, because a longer time is required to produce the deficiency, allowing the teeth changes to be produced. Other symptoms are similar to those seen in man and the guinea pig.

Scorbutic symptoms in guinea pigs, for classroom demonstration purposes, can be readily obtained merely by feeding a commercial rabbit feed (containing no added vitamin C) to young guinea pigs. The symptoms are readily cured by giving sources of vitamin C (Fig. 8–3) with no permanent harm to the animal.

Chemical Identification and Properties

In 1928, Szent-Györgyi, a Hungarian scientist now living in the United States,

---

*Food sources of vitamin C are also needed by certain species of fish, the Indian fruit bat, and over 15 bird species in India because of the same metabolic block present in primates and guinea pigs.[10] Dogs, cats, fowl, cows, horses, and other animals not mentioned do not need a dietary source of vitamin C (so you do not need to feed orange juice to your house pets unless you have guinea pigs!).

†The missing enzymes are gulonolactone oxidase and glucurono reductase.

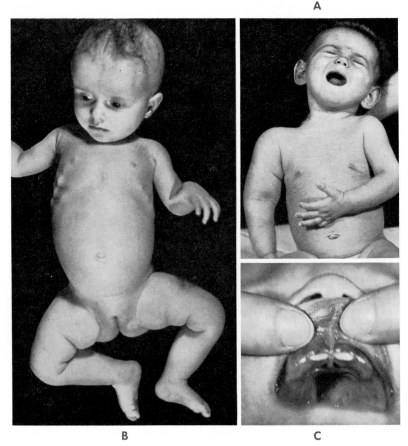

Figure 8-2.   Infant scurvy. **A,** The infant becomes irritable when handled. **B,** Characteristic position, with legs flexed at hips and knees, and thighs externally rotated. **C,** Gums are swollen and boggy. (From Cecil-Conn: *The Specialties in General Practice.* 2nd Ed. Philadelphia, W. B. Saunders Co.)

first isolated what is now known as ascorbic acid (he called it "hexuronic acid") from oranges, cabbages, and adrenal glands,[12] although it was not recognized as vitamin C and was not tried in the treatment of scurvy. In 1932, King and Waugh[6] isolated from lemon juice a crystalline material which possessed antiscorbutic activity in guinea pigs. They found their compound was identical with the substance isolated by Szent-Györgyi (who, as a result, in 1933 called it *ascorbic acid*, a shortened form of the "*antiscorbutic* factor"[5]). Shortly afterward, the structure of L-ascorbic acid was announced, and it was synthesized in the laboratory, starting with

the sugar galactose and later with glucose (Fig. 8–4).

Ascorbic acid is a relatively simple organic acid with six carbon atoms in each molecule, and has a structure fairly similar to the simple six-carbon sugars (see formula in Appendix, p. 583). It is the most unstable of all the known vitamins, as it is *easily oxidized* by the loss of two hydrogen atoms per molecule to a substance called *dehydroascorbic acid.* Both forms have vitamin C activity, although dehydroascorbic acid has only about 80 percent of the biological activity of ascorbic acid. Dehydroascorbic acid can be readily converted in the body by reduction (adding hydrogen)

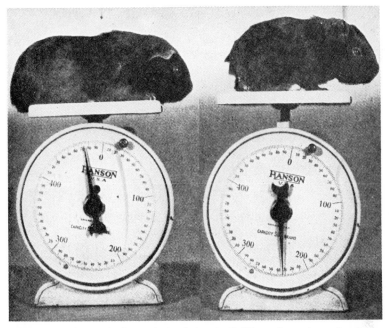

Figure 8–3. Stunting of growth due to lack of vitamin C. The guinea pig at the right, which had a vitamin C-deficient diet, was in poor condition and weighed only 234 gm. The guinea pig at the left, on the same diet plus tomato juice, weighed 473 gm. (Courtesy of Dr. F. F. Tisdall, Toronto.)

to ascorbic acid. Thus both the ascorbic acid and the dehydroascorbic acid in foods contribute to their vitamin C activity in the body. In living plant and animal tissues, this oxidation-reduction between the two substances is *reversible*. When dehydroascorbic acid is further oxidized, however, it loses its vitamin C activity, and the reaction is not revers-ible—that is, it cannot be reduced to form dehydroascorbic acid again.

The oxidation of ascorbic acid in foods is hastened by an enzyme (ascorbic acid oxidase) that is present in raw fruits and vegetables and which becomes active when leaves or fruits are damaged by drying, bruising, or cutting. In the intact plant, this enzyme is in-

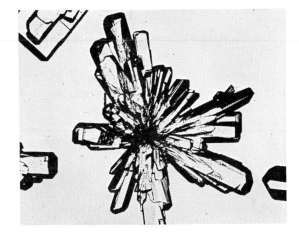

Figure 8–4. Photomicrograph showing crystalline structure of pure ascorbic acid. (Courtesy of Merck & Company.)

operative. Considerable loss of vitamin C activity occurs with the use of heat, alkalis, and catalysts such as copper (e.g., use of copper kettles). Its destruction is slowed down in foods that are acid, by refrigeration, and above all by protection from exposure to air.

Role of Vitamin C in the Body

Although the exact manner in which vitamin C functions in metabolism is yet to be explained, it is assumed that it is because of its instability, its property of being reversibly oxidized and reduced, that it plays some part vital to the welfare of cells and tissues throughout the body. As hemoglobin and other iron-containing pigments with a unique function in the body are capable of alternately taking on and giving up oxygen (reversible oxidation-reduction), so ascorbic acid is able alternately to lose and take on hydrogen. It thus can act as a "hydrogen carrier," and as such it may have an essential role in the metabolism of carbohydrates or proteins, or both. Whatever the explanation, the widespread tissue damage seen in scurvy makes it apparent that this vitamin is needed by many kinds of tissues, and hence its role would seem to be a fundamental one.

We get our clues as to many of its functions chiefly from the symptoms seen in scurvy. So many apparently unrelated tissues show damage that only some of its functions can be discussed here.

The main type of tissue showing marked damage in scorbutic animals is connective tissue. This is primarily because *collagen*, a protein important in the formation of skin, tendon, and bone, as well as supportive tissue, is not properly formed in vitamin C deficiency. Normally collagen contains the amino acid *hydroxyproline*, which is obtained by conversion from the amino acid *proline*. In vitamin C deficiency, this conversion does not take place. The

resulting impairment of connective tissue regeneration is undoubtedly the cause of many characteristic signs of scurvy, including disorganization of bone and tooth calcification and delayed healing of tissue in burns and wounds. Both animal and human studies indicate that a sufficiently low dietary intake of this vitamin results in delayed healing and less strength of the healed wound, whereas administration of vitamin C under such conditions promotes sound healing of wounds. It seems reasonable that vitamin C, which is essential for formation of substances that cement cells together, would function in the reknitting of tissues in wound healing.

Vitamin C appears to function in maintaining strength in blood vessels, a function unrelated to the maintenance of collagen in connective tissue. Small blood vessels under the skin tend to hemorrhage, especially when suction or pressure is applied. This has been used as a test for low-grade lack of vitamin C (the *capillary fragility test*). Examination of the rate of blood flow in scorbutic guinea pigs has revealed a marked sluggishness of the blood flow in vessels which are greatly dilated.

Vitamin C influences the formation of hemoglobin, the absorption of iron from the intestine, and deposition of iron in liver tissue. It also takes part in a number of reactions involving amino acids, such as tyrosine and tryptophan and the vitamin folacin.

The adrenal glands contain more vitamin C than most other tissues, and this substance appears to be concerned is some way in the secretion of hormones of the adrenal cortex. There is no evidence that this vitamin functions as a specific component of any particular enzyme system, as do many of the other vitamins, but rather its participation appears to be general and is required in the metabolism of many substances in the body. Just how or why vitamin C is concerned in so many and such varied chemical changes that are parts of normal metabolism in the tissues is not yet known, but enough is known to establish it as a very important substance for body welfare.

Vitamin C and Infections

Vitamin C also functions, in some little understood way, in *protecting the body against infections*[13] *and bacterial toxins.*[14] Menten and King fed guinea pigs graded amounts of ascorbic acid, and they found that those which received lower intakes of this vitamin suffered greater injury (loss of weight, tooth damage, etc.) from repeated doses of diphtheria toxin, even though they showed no signs of scurvy.[14] Others have shown that guinea pigs on limited vitamin C intake succumb to inoculations with different strains of bacteria which have little or no effect on animals that received liberal quantities of this vitamin. The lowered resistance to infections in infants with scurvy is notable.

Infections apparently decrease the amount of ascorbic acid in tissues and body fluids; normal recommended intakes of vitamin C are thought to be helpful in enabling the body to combat infections. There is no evidence that amounts greatly in excess of normal recommended intake confer extra benefits, except after deprivation or during periods of unusual physical stress. The possibility, recently suggested by Pauling,[15] that very large intakes of vitamin C can protect against the common cold, therefore, is without good scientific foundation.[16] In any event, the large levels of vitamin C suggested for treatment of colds are far higher than could be normally supplied by natural foods, so any possible beneficial effect (and we know of none) would be a pharmaceutical rather than nutritional effect. (There are toxicologic effects known with such high levels of vitamin C,[17] so any person taking gram levels of the substance should do so only with the advice and knowledge of a physician.)

Undocumented claims have been made over the years that smoking greatly increases vitamin C destruction in the body. Recent research shows there is some truth in this claim (but not as much as 25 mg of vitamin C per cigarette, as claimed). Heavy smokers do have lowered blood levels of vitamin C, and an apparent increased requirement, but this is well within the range of the recommended allowances.[18]

Human Metabolism and Nutritional Status

Vitamin C taken in the food is absorbed into the blood stream chiefly from the small intestine within a few hours after it is ingested. The level of vitamin C in the blood plasma is increased only temporarily, because this substance is taken up by the tissues, and any excess is excreted promptly by the kidneys or converted to carbon dioxide and exhaled through the lungs. Intravenously injected ascorbic acid is excreted within one to three hours. Although there is limited ability to store vitamin C in the body, it is present in higher concentrations in glandular tissues, especially in the adrenal glands. The amount of this substance in the body tissues depends on the quantity in the food and on the rate at which it is utilized in and excreted from the body.* About 13 to 30 mg of vitamin C

---

*Under normal conditions, higher levels of daily intake of vitamin C result in increased amounts of it both in the body and in the urine. Conversely, low levels of vitamin C in the blood and urine indicate that the daily diet provides little of this vitamin. If a vitamin C-poor diet has been long continued, the tissues become unusually low in, and are said to be "unsaturated" as to, vitamin C. When higher intakes are given to such persons, the tissues take up more vitamin C and abnormally low amounts are excreted in the urine. If high intakes of vitamin C are continued until the tissues have become "saturated" with vitamin C, urinary excretion will than rise decidedly, since the excess is excreted through this channel. There is no evidence that saturation of the tissues with vitamin C is essential to maximum health.

appears to be the amount utilized in the body per day in normal adult men.

Many surveys exist of the vitamin C status of samples of the populations of various countries. Unless a survey is recent, it should be regarded with some degree of caution because of changing food habits and new fortification practices. In surveys made in the United States,* including the recent National Nutrition Survey, borderline (or below) intakes of vitamin C were commonly found (ranging up to 10 to 30 percent of infants, children, and adults, especially in lower income groups). It is one of our most common examples of low vitamin intakes. Frank infantile scruvy is still seen in this country and Canada but in very limited numbers in recent years.

Various estimates have been made recently of the *actual daily intakes* of vitamin C in the United States. Friend states that in 1968, the average vitamin C *available* for consumption was 104 mg per day.[19] This does not take into account loss of vitamin C in food preparation, storage, or wastage, which can be appreciable, so one must conclude that large surpluses of the vitamin do not exist. Of real concern is the fact that average daily intakes of vitamin C have been steadily decreasing in the United States since the highest intake levels were reached in 1944–45 (about 125 mg).[20] Obviously from the nutritional status figures, many of our population take in far below these *average* intakes.

Very few normal American diets provide ascorbic acid in such limited amounts as would cause development of scurvy (though the intake may be less than optimal). In fact, since knowledge of the protective action of citrus fruits and other fresh fruits and vegetables has become widespread, actual epidemics of scurvy, as were seen centuries ago, have completely disappeared. Since rice is very low in vitamin C, persons eating extremely simple diets based on rice (such as the "macrobiotic"

diet) have been known to develop severe scurvy.

Requirement and Recommended Allowance

The absolute *minimum requirement* of vitamin C per day to prevent scurvy appears to be about 10 mg. To provide a margin of safety, the recommended allowance in Britain is 20 mg per day for adults, and the Canadian and Australian allowance for vitamin C is 30 mg[21] (see Appendix, Table 1B).

Although these levels of vitamin C intake will undoubtedly maintain adults in health and are practical in countries where fresh fruits and vegetables are not abundant, the Food and Nutrition Board of the United States[21] has set a higher recommended daily allowance at *60 mg per day* for adult males and *55 mg for females* in order to provide "a generous increment for individual variability and a surplus to compensate for potential losses in food." (This is 10 to 15 mg less than the 1963 recommendations.) The Food and Nutrition Board[21] also states, in introducing its bulletin, that the allowances "are not necessarily adequate to meet the additional requirement of persons depleted by disease, traumatic stress, or prior

Table 8–1. *Recommended Allowances for Vitamin C**

	Age	Allowance, mg/day
Males	1–12 years	40
	12–14 years	45
	14–18 years	55
	18 years and over	60
Females	1–12 years	40
	12–14 years	45
	14–18 years	50
	18 years and over	55
	Pregnant	60
	Lactating	60

*From the Food and Nutrition Board, 1968.[21]
See Appendix Table 1C for FAO recommendations.

*See references 10–13, Chapter 7, page 163.

dietary inadequacies," though recommended values for vitamin C still seem very generous. For values showing the slightly increased recommendation for pregnancy and lactation and for other details, see Table 8–1 and Table 1A of the Appendix. The recommended allowance for lactation (60 mg), based on newer evidence, is considerably less than the 100 mg figure recommended in 1963.

An undetermined amount of vitamin C activity is reaching the American public by a common and safe food additive, closely related to ascorbic acid, *erythorbic acid (scorbic acid)*, an antioxidant. This has about 5 percent of the activity of vitamin C.[22]

Distribution in Foods

For vitamin C we are dependent almost entirely on *fruits* and *vegetables*, and those that may be eaten fresh, uncooked, or previously frozen are the best sources.

Table 8–2. *Fruits and Vegetables as Sources of Vitamin C**

Food	Vitamin C (mg/100 gm, Edible Portion)
Fruits, fresh	
Strawberries	59
Oranges (or juice)	50
Frozen orange juice	45
Lemons (or juice)	46
Grapefruit (or juice)	38
Frozen orange-grapefruit juice	41
Cantaloupe	33
Honeydew melon	23
Berries (except strawberries and blueberries)	21
Pineapple, fresh	17
Avocados	14
Blueberries	14
Bananas	10
Cherries	10
Apricots	10
Peaches	8
Apples	
Grapes	
Pears	7
Plums	
Watermelon	

Milk contains small amounts of vitamin C but is an undependable source, especially if pasteurized. Much of the vitamin C in meats is destroyed in cooking; eggs, cereal grains, sugar, and fats, nuts, dried legumes, and dried fruits contain either very little or none at all.

Certain kinds of fruits and vegetables are unusually rich in vitamin C (see Table 8–2). Citrus fruits, strawberries, and cantaloupe lead the fruits in vitamin C content, with the exception

Table 8–2.   *Continued*

Food	Vitamin C (mg/100 gm, Edible Portion)
Vegetables	
Kale, leaves only	186
Turnip greens	139
Peppers, green	128
Broccoli	113
Brussels sprouts	102
Mustard greens	97
Collards	92
Cauliflower	78
Spinach	51
Cabbage	47
Rutabagas	43
Dandelion greens	35
Asparagus	33
Chard	32
Okra	31
Beet greens	30
Beans, lima, green	29
string, green	19
Peas, green	27
Radishes	26
Onions, young, green	25
mature	10
Tomatoes	23
juice, canned	16
Squash, summer	22
winter	13
Sweet potatoes	21
Potatoes	20
Lettuce, green	18
Parsnips	16
Corn, sweet	12
Cucumbers	11
Beets	10
Celery	9
Lettuce, head	6
Eggplant	5
Carrots	8

*Figures are from U. S. Department of Agriculture Handbook No. 8, *Composition of Foods—Raw, Processed, Prepared,* 1963. See Appendix for further details.

of two very rich sources rather uncommon in the United States except in "health food" stores. These are a West Indian cherry, the *acerola*, and a Peruvian jungle fruit called *camu-camu*.[23] (Rose hips are another concentrated, though variable, source of vitamin C, but they too are not widely available.) Green leafy vegetables, peppers, broccoli, and cauliflower have a high content of vitamin C and are very good sources of vitamin C, even after cooking. Raw cabbage, turnips, salad greens, and tomatoes (either fresh or canned) are also good sources. Potatoes contribute considerable amounts of ascorbic acid when eaten fresh and in large quantities, and they are still a principal source of dietary vitamin C in areas of the world where other sources are unavailable. Dehydrated potatoes are an undependable source, unless fortified with vitamin C (see Table 8–3). Most cooked and canned vegetables and fruits provide some vitamin C, but in smaller and more variable amounts than the corresponding fresh foods. Freezing, however, preserves most of the vitamin C activity.

Pure ascorbic acid is available in stores wherever vitamins are sold, in very inexpensive form—for as little as 0.5 cent or less per 100 mg (which is more than a day's supply).* This costs less than an equivalent amount in natural foods, but such foods (except for the "acerola" and "camu-camu" berries) also supply a variety of minerals and other vitamins and are to be preferred wherever possible. For this reason, we do not recommend the various high vitamin C, imitation fruit drinks on the market as routine sources of vitamin C for children or adults, except when no other source is available (which would be extremely rare).

It should be understood that there

---

*If bought in vitamin capsules which are sold by various pharmaceutical companies, the cost per unit may vary considerably. The natural active form of ascorbic acid is the L-isomer and this is equal in every way to the synthetic L-isomer, the usual form of commerce. Calcium and sodium salts of ascorbic acid are also readily available.

Table 8–3.   Retention of Vitamin C During Processing of Potatoes

State of Processing	Mean Total Vitamin C (fresh weight basis) mg per 100 gm
Raw potatoes	26.5
Fresh mashed	13.6
Reconstituted, dehydrated granules	6.7

*From Bring, S. V., and Raab, F. P.: J. Amer. Dietet. Assoc., 45:149, 1964.

is considerable variability in the vitamin C content of fruits and vegetables, and that the figures given in Table 8–2 represent only approximate mean values. The vitamin C content of plant foods varies greatly with different varieties of the same plant, with soil and climate, and especially according to the amount of exposure to sunlight and the degree of ripeness of the fruit. In general, the more mature a plant becomes, the less vitamin C it contains; the more sunlight a plant receives, the more vitamin C it contains. Different varieties of apples and oranges have been found to vary considerably in vitamin C content. Even allowing for variations, it can be seen that certain fruits and vegetables are much richer in this vitamin than others.

Losses in Processing

Further variations in the vitamin C content of table foods must be expected because of losses of this vitamin during *storage, processing* (canning or drying), and *cooking.* Vitamin C is very susceptible to destruction during cooking and processing, because it is so water-soluble, is easily oxidized, and is attacked by enzymes. Leafy vegetables (with large surface areas) lose more vitamin C on storage than do root vegetables or tubers. Refrigeration during storage reduces losses, and in markets, more of the vitamin is retained if vegetables are kept in crushed ice than if they are kept in a refrigerator.

In preparation for canning, quick freezing, or drying, a brief blanching with steam favors retention of vitamin C, because this process destroys the enzymes that hasten destruction of the vitamin in raw foods. There is least loss of vitamin C when foods are preserved by quick freezing as with frozen orange juice, an excellent practical source of vitamin C in countries where refrigerators are available. Most losses occur when foods are preserved by drying, especially if they are exposed to sunlight in the process. Commercially canned foods may compare favorably in vitamin C content with home-cooked products if the fruits or vegetables reach the cannery fresh from nearby fields and are heated quickly in vacuum-sealed cans. The vitamin C content of canned fruit juices will vary considerably, unless fortified with vitamin C or unless it is specially protected in canning.

Because vitamin C is water-soluble, considerable amounts of it may be lost in the liquid in which the food is canned, if this is discarded. In drying fruits, sulfuring before drying and rapid drying (away from sunlight) favor retention of the vitamin content, but dried fruits cannot be counted on as a source of much vitamin C.

In home cooking, there is a great deal of variation in the amount of vitamin C loss that takes place. However, if short boiling times and small amounts of water are used, and if the water is consumed, there is little loss. It has been reported that ascorbic acid in vegetables can be protected somewhat by boiling the cooking water for a minute before adding the food. This removes the oxygen dissolved in water, thus preventing oxidative destruction of some of the ascorbic acid.* For example, loss of

ascorbic acid from cabbage boiled 15 minutes starting in cold water is 25.5 percent compared with a 1.8 percent loss when cooked in water that has been boiled one minute.[24] The loss in vitamin C content in home cooking also depends on numerous factors, including the nature of the food, its reaction (acid or alkaline), the period and degree of heating, and especially the extent to which the food is exposed to water and to air in the cooking process. Retention of the vitamin is favored by cooking with peel left on or in large pieces and cooking with as much exclusion of air as possible (tightly covered vessel or pressure cooker). Increased losses of the vitamin result from contact with copper or iron in preparing or cooking the food, or from mashing the food and leaving it in a hot place or exposed to the air.

Practical Suggestions for Conserving Vitamin C in Foods in the Home

It is foolish to allow vitamin C, which is essential for health, to be lost before foods are served. Because this is the most easily destroyed of the vitamins, its conservation presents a special problem. Reasons for the following special *precautions* in handling fresh fruits and vegetables should be self-evident if one keeps in mind that vitamin C is water-soluble and easily destroyed by oxidation, and that heat, alkaline reaction, and above all, exposure to air hasten its destruction. These practical suggestions are also useful in preserving most water-soluble vitamins in foods in home cooking.

Buy fresh fruits and vegetables in small enough quantities so that they will be used promptly; keep them at low temperature (in refrigerator, if possible).

Prepare them (paring and cutting up) immediately before they are to be cooked or served raw; do not let them stand in water or exposed to air before cooking; serve promptly, *do not keep hot for long* (or reheat) before serving.

*Probably practical only where vitamin C is scarce and expensive and the value of one's time in the kitchen is not in question. The monetary value of the vitamin C gained by such a procedure (and which can easily be replaced by some other food or supplementary source) is less than the value of one moment's time in many countries. Of course, the flavor of the food may also be changed by these procedures, which also needs to be considered. (This points out again the necessity of nutrition education for all people who prepare food so that one can weigh these factors oneself.)

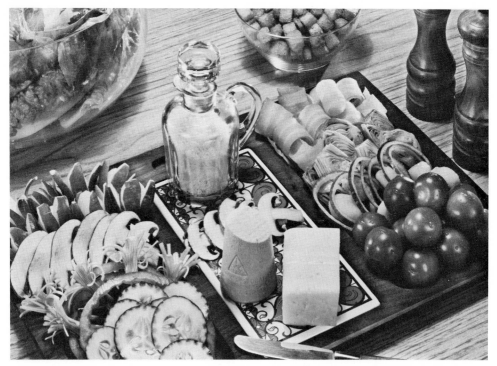

Figure 8–5. Fresh vegetables (including citrus fruits, not shown) are an excellent source of vitamin C. (Courtesy of Western Growers Association.)

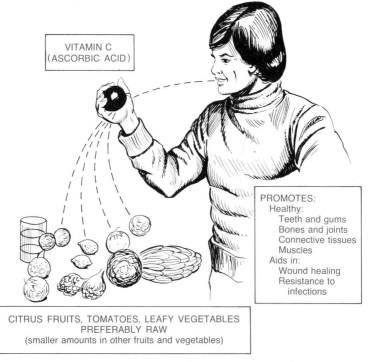

Figure 8–6.

Cook in as small a quantity of water and for as short a time as feasible; cook by steaming, or broiling (instead of boiling) and with "skins" left on when possible; keep cooking vessels tightly covered.

Never add soda in cooking vegetables and do not use copper cooking vessels if you want to preserve vitamin C (the presence of either alkali or copper hastens vitamin destruction).

Do not allow frozen foods to thaw out before cooking; keep them in refrigerator and start cooking in frozen state in limited amounts of boiling water.

Juices of fresh fruits are best prepared immediately before serving. However, acid juices (orange, grapefruit, tomato) may be left in a covered glass container in the refrigerator several days with little loss in vitamin C value; size of container should be chosen so liquid will about fill it, with minimum of air left in over liquid.

How to Get Allowance of Vitamin C in Diet

The best general rule to safeguard the diet with regard to vitamin C is to include each day one serving of either citrus fruit, tomato, or some other rich source of this vitamin. Other foods included in the normal diet, such as extra fruit and vegetables (both cooked and raw), usually supply sufficient vitamin C to make up the day's allowance. A six ounce glass of fresh or frozen orange juice supplies 80 to 100 mg of vitamin C, considerably more than the recommended daily allowance. Vitamin C is exceedingly well protected in citrus fruit products, because these products contain several constituents which inhibit its oxidation. Ascorbic acid oxidase, the enzyme which causes vitamin C oxidation, is not found in orange juice. Also, citrus fruits do not require cooking, and ordinary refrigerator temperatures prevent loss during short-term storage in the home.

There are many other ways to ensure adequate vitamin C intake (and variety is always to be recommended). This could be fresh strawberries, melon,

fresh tomato, or tomato juice, which supply 25 to 60 mg per 100 gm. Vegetables that are good sources of vitamin C may also be used as the main source, or in combination with a second good source (especially if citrus fruit is unavailable or not tolerated). Such vegetables are green peppers, broccoli, cauliflower, Brussels sprouts, and all dark green leafy vegetables. A serving of any of these provides 60 mg or more of vitamin C per 100 gm.

Table 8-2 lists a large variety of foods and their vitamin C content. Table 8-4 illustrates various fruit and vegetable combinations from this list which will furnish 55 mg or more of vitamin C. Combinations I and II represent a more expensive way to obtain vitamin C (i.e., fresh fruits, especially out of season), while combinations III and IV are examples of more economical sources of vitamin C, which are available throughout the year.

Table 8-4. Examples of Food Combinations That Furnish a Generous Day's Supply of Vitamin C

Food	Vitamin C (mg)
I	
Strawberries, ⅔ cup	60
Cooked summer squash, ½ cup	10
	70 mg
II	
Cantaloupe, ½ melon, 6 in. diam.	50
Asparagus, 4 stalks	18
	68 mg
III	
Tomato, 1 medium, fresh	35
Sweet potato, 1 medium, baked or boiled with skin	20
	55 mg
IV	
Grapefruit juice, ½ cup, canned	41
Lima beans, ½ cup cooked	14
Potato, 1 medium, baked or boiled with skin	16
	71 mg

Of interest are U.S. Department of Agriculture figures on food sources of vitamin C which the American public eats in a year*—a reflection of average food habits whether good or bad! The largest contributors were vegetables, which contributed almost 58 percent of our vitamin C (potatoes and sweet potatoes—20.3, dark green and deep yellow vegetables—8.2 and tomatoes and all other vegetables—29.1). Citrus fruits supplied 25.3 percent and all other fruits, including those fortified with synthetic vitamin C, 11.6 percent for a total of 36.9 percent. Thus, fruits and vegetables supply over 94 percent of our vitamin C intake in foods, which is a demonstration of the importance of this food group.

Similar figures on the percentage of vitamin C intake from synthetic sources are not readily available (but probably range between 20 to 30 percent of the total intake on a per capita basis). This varies considerably with each individual.

Bioflavonoids and Related Substances ("Vitamin P")

Various pigments and related compounds in citrus fruits and other plants are advertised widely in "health food" literature as sources of "vitamin P"—chiefly, certain *bioflavonoids, hesperidin,* and *rutin.* There is *no evidence* today that these compounds in otherwise nutritionally complete diets have activity similar to that of a vitamin, although they may serve as pharmaceuticals (they can protect against capillary fragility, for instance, under special experimental conditions in animals but this has not been demonstrated to take place in man). Nutritionists in this country and in most countries have not accepted "vitamin P" as either a separate entity or as a significant vitamin C-sparing factor.[25] The term "vitamin P," therefore, must be considered to be obsolete.

---

*1971 figures.

QUESTIONS AND PROBLEMS

1. From what materials was ascorbic acid first isolated as a pure substance? What type of chemical compound is it? Why was the name ascorbic acid given to it? Where does it occur in nature? In the human body? How stable is the substance when kept in dry, solid form? In water solution with alkaline reaction? In acid solution? What other conditions affect its stability, and why?

2. Why was scurvy a prevalent disease among crews on long sea voyages and early explorations? Why was it possible for Admiral Byrd to take men into the Antarctic for long periods without fear that any of them would succumb to scurvy? What foods or other substances were known to prevent or cure scurvy long before it was recognized that their efficacy in this respect was due to the presence in all of them of a definite compound that might be classed as a vitamin? Give the symptoms of acute scurvy and explain the widespread tissue damages in the light of one of the chief functions of vitamin C in the body—i.e., the formation and maintenance of intercellular and connective tissue substances.

3. Why do men and guinea pigs develop scurvy when the diet is lacking in vitamin C, while dogs, rats, and other animals do not? Do plants need vitamin C, and if so, how do they get it? Give three characteristic symptoms of subacute or latent scurvy in infants and three symptoms in adults that indicate the diet has furnished too little vitamin C. From consideration of the results of lack of this vitamin, what would you conclude are its main uses in the body?

4. What classes of foods contribute little or no vitamin C in the diet, at least in the condition in which they are eaten? What classes of foods furnish the major part of the vitamin C intake? Consult Table 8–2 and list the five fruits and five vegetables richest in vitamin C in the raw state. List the ten that have the next highest vitamin C content per 100 gm, either fruits or

vegetables, in order of their relative vitamin C content when raw. Rearrange these 20 fruits and vegetables in the order of the vitamin C contribution that is made by an *average serving* of each, fruits raw and vegetables with average allowance for loss of vitamin C in cooking, as given in Table 7 of the Appendix.

5. What is the recommended daily allowance of vitamin C for a normal woman? For a teen-age boy? For a pregnant woman? If 10 mg of vitamin C per day protects an adult against scurvy, what is the use of eating the recommended allowance? Is there any point in taking about twice the recommended allowance daily? Is a high level of vitamin C intake practical, or even possible, in some parts of the world? Name three countries in which the available foods and dietary customs make it probable that the average intake of vitamin C is low.

6. List five foods that provide vitamin C at low or moderate cost. Plan a day's diet, at low or moderate cost, that would furnish about 60 mg of vitamin C for an adult, following the dietary pattern given on page 15.

7. Plan a day's meals for yourself with some food that is a good source of vitamin C in each meal. Compute how many milligrams of vitamin C this diet would provide and compare with the standard allowance.

8. Give methods of conserving vitamin C in foods during storage and preparation for the table.

REFERENCES

1. Funk, C.: J. State Medicine, *20*:341, 1912 (as reprinted in Goldblith, S. A., and Joslyn, M. A.: *Milestones in Nutrition.* Westport, Avi Publishing Co. Inc., 1964, pp. 145–171); Holst, A., and Frölich, J.: Z. Hyg., *72*:1, 1912.

2. Hardin, A., and Zilva, S. S.: Biochem. J., *12*:408, 1918; Drummond, J. C.: Biochem. J., *13*:77, 1919.

3. Santos, F. O.: Proc. Soc. Exp. Biol. Med., *19*:2, 1921; McClendon, J. F.: J. Biol. Chem., *47*:411, 1921.

4. Drummond, J. C.: Biochem. J., *14*:660, 1920.

5. Szent-Györgyi, A., and Haworth, W. N.: Nature, *131*:24, 1933.

6. King, C. G., and Waugh, W. A.: Science, *75*:357, 1932; Waugh, W. A., and King, C. G.: J. Biol. Chem., *97*:325, 1932; and King, C. G.: Physiol. Rev., *16*:238, 1936.

7. Lind, J.: Treatise on Scurvy (first published in 1753). Reprinted, and edited by C. P. Stewart and Douglas Guthrie. Edinburgh University Press, 1953.

8. Editorial: Captain James Cook (1728–1779). J. Amer. Med. Assoc., *209*:1217, 1969.

9. Hodges, R. E., et al.: Amer. J. Clin. Nutr., *22*:535, 1969; *24*:432, 1971; Baker, E. M., et al.: Am. J. Clin. Nutr., *19*:371, 1966; *22*:549, 1969; *24*:444, 1971.

10. Chaudhuri, C. R., and Chatterjee, I. B.: Science, *164*:435, 1969; Chatterjee, I. B., et al.: Nature, *192*:163, 1961.

11. Holst, A., and Frölich, J.: J. Hyg., *7*:634, 1907.

12. Szent-Györgyi, A.: Biochem J., *22*:1387, 1928.

13. Levenson, S. M., et al.: Arch. Int. Med., *110*:693, 1962.

14. Menten, M. L., and King, C. G.: J. Nutr., *10*:141, 1935.

15. Pauling, L.: *Vitamin C and the Common Cold.* San Francisco, W. H. Freeman and Co., 1970; Pauling, L.: Proc. Nat. Acad. Sci., *67*:1643, 1970.

16. Margen, S.: J. Nutr. Educ., *2*:131, 1971; Hodges, R. E.: Amer. J. Clin. Nutr., *24*:383, 1971; Wilson, C. W. M.: Brit. Med. J., *1*:669, 1971; Diehl, H. S.: Amer. J. Public Health, *61*:649, 1971; Consumer Reports, *36*:113, 1971.

17. Mayer, J.: Postgrad. Med., *45*:268, 1969; Goldsmith, G. A.: J. Amer. Med. Assoc., *216*:337, 1971; Lamden, M. P.: New Eng. J. Med., *284*:336, 1971.

18. Brook, M., and Grimshaw, J. J.: Amer. J. Clin. Nutr., *21*:1254, 1968; Pelletier, O.: Amer. J. Clin. Nutr., *23*:520, 1970; *21*:1259, 1968.

19. Friend, B.: *National Food Situation.* U.S. Department of Agriculture, Economic Research Survey. Washington, D.C., Government Printing Office, Nov. 1969.

20. Parrish, J. B.: J. Nutr. Educ., *2*:140, 1971.

21. Food and Nutrition Board: *Recommended Dietary Allowances.* 7th Ed. Publication 1694, Washington, D.C., National Academy of Sciences, 1968.

22. Wang, M. M., Fisher, K. H., and Dodds, M. L.: J. Nutr., *77*:443, 1962.

23. Derse, P. H., and Elvehjem, C. A.: J. Amer. Med. Assoc., *156*:1501, 1954; Bradfield, R. B., and Roca, A.: J. Amer. Dietet. Assoc., *44*:28, 1964.

24. Roy, J. K., and Biswas, S. K.: Ind. J. Med. Res., *50*:259, 1962.

25. Lee, R. E.: J. Nutr., *72*:203, 1960; Brit. Med. J., *1*:235, 1969.

SUPPLEMENTARY READING

Reviews and History
(also see refs. 1–8)

Anonymous: How gold-rush-day doctors battled scurvy. Today's Health, Oct. 1965, p. 53.

Beeukwes, A. M.: The prevalence of scurvy among voyageurs to America, 1493–1600. J. Amer. Dietet. Assoc., *24*:300, 1948.

Burns, J. J., ed.: Vitamin C. Ann. New York Acad. Sci., *92*:1, 1961.

Crandon, J. H., Lund, C. C., and Dill, D. B.: Experimental human scurvy. New Eng. J. Med., *223*:353, 1940.

Dodds, M. L.: Vitamin C. In *Food*, Yearbook of Agriculture. Washington, D. C., Government Printing Office, 1959.

Harris, R. S., et al.: Ascorbic acid. In Sebrell, W. H., Jr., and Harris, R. S. (eds.): *The Vitamins*, Vol. 1, Ch. 2. New York, Academic Press, 1954.

Hess, A. F.: Recent advances in knowledge of scurvy and the antiscorbutic vitamin. J. Amer. Med. Assoc., *98*:1429, 1932.

King, C. G.: Early experiences with ascorbic acid—a retrospect. Nutr. Rev., *12*:1, 1954.

King, C. G.: Vitamin C, ascorbic acid. Physiol. Rev., *16*:238, 1936.

Lorenz, A. J.: The conquest of scurvy. J. Amer. Dietet. Assoc., *30*:665, 1954.

Shipley, P. G.: Our fathers and the "scorby." J. Amer. Dietet. Assoc., *5*:1, 1929.

Villiers, A.: That extraordinary sea genius, Captain James Cook. Nutr. Today, *4*:8, Autumn 1969.

Waife, S. O.: Lind, lemons, and limeys. J. Clin. Nutr., *1*:471, 1953.

Function and General

Ash, K. O.: Ascorbic acid: cofactor in rabbit olfactory preparations. Science, *165*:901, 1969.

Lockie, G. M.: Relative costs of different sources of vitamin C. Nutrition, *26*:8, 1972.

Pelletier, O.: Cigarette smoking and vitamin C. Nutr. Today, *5*:12, Autumn 1970.

Priest, R. E.: Formation of epithelial basement membrane is restricted by scurvy *in vitro* and is stimulated by vitamin C. Nature, *225*:744, 1970.

Richmond, V., and Stokstad, E. L. R.: Effect of ascorbic acid on guinea pig skin collagen synthesis: II. Neutral and acid soluble collagens, mucopolysaccharides, and amino acid composition. J. Dent. Res., *48*:83, 1969.

Schwartz, P. L.: Ascorbic acid in wound healing—a review. J. Amer. Dietet. Assoc., *56*:497, 1970.

Human Need and Status

Bailey, D. A., Carron, A. V., Teece, R. G., and Wehner, H.: Effect of vitamin C supplementation upon the physiological response to exercise in trained and untrained subjects. International J. Vitamin Res., *40*:435, 1970.

Baker, E. M.: Vitamin C requirements in stress. Amer. J. Clin. Nutr., *20*:583, 1967.

Gey, G. O., Cooper, K. H., and Bottenberg, R. A.: Effect of ascorbic acid on endurance performance and athletic injury. J. Amer. Med. Assoc., *211*:105, 1970.

Hodges, R. E.: What's new about scurvy? Amer. J. Clin. Nutr., *24*:383, 1971.

Hood, J., and Hodges, R. E.: Ocular lesions in scurvy. Amer. J. Clin. Nutr., *22*:559, 1969.

Kinsman, R. A., and Hood, J.: Some behavioral effects of ascorbic acid deficiency. Amer. J. Clin. Nutr., *24*:455, 1971.

Sherlock, P., and Rothschild, E. O.: Scurvy produced by a zen macrobiotic diet. J. Amer. Med. Assoc., *199*:794, 1967.

Srikantia, S. G., Mohanram, M., and Krishnaswamy, K.: Human requirements of ascorbic acid. Amer. J. Clin. Nutr., *23*:59, 1970.

Distribution and Stability

Eddy, T. P., Nicholson, A. L., and Wheeler, E. F.: Precooked frozen foods: The effects of heating on vitamin C. Nutrition, *22*:122, 1968.

Lopez, A., Krehl, W. A., and Good, E.: Influence of time and temperature on ascorbic acid stability. J. Amer. Dietet. Assoc., *50*:308, 1967.

Noel, G. L., and Robberstad, M. T.: Stability of vitamin C in canned apple juice and orange juice under refrigerated conditions. Food Technol., *17*:127, 1963.

Twomey, D. G., and Goodchild, J.: Variations in the vitamin C content of imported tomatoes. J. Sci. Food Agric., *21*:313, 1970.

Nutrition Reviews

Inadequacy of rose hips as a source of ascorbic acid. *23*:223, 1965.

Endothelial changes in scorbutic guinea pigs. *24*:179, 1966.

Ascorbic acid effect on blood lipids and lipoprotein lipase. *25*:183, 1967.

Ascorbic acid and the common cold. *25*:228, 1967.

Malabsorption, gastric surgery, and ascorbic acid. *25*:237, 1967.

Senile purpura, sublingual hemorrhages, and ascorbic acid. *25*:239, 1967.

Platelet function and capillary hemorrhage in scurvy. *25*:282, 1967.

Present knowledge of ascorbic acid (vitamin C) (by King, C. G.). *26*:33, 1968.

Vitamin C intakes in Great Britain. *27*:139, 1969.

Capillary hemorrhage in scorbutic guinea pigs. *27*:158, 1969.

nine

Fat-Soluble Vitamins
(A, D, E, and K)

The fat-soluble vitamins, as the term implies, are those four vitamins (A, D, E, and K) which are found in nature generally associated with fatty foods, such as butter, cream, vegetable oils, and the fats of meat and fish—substances usually containing only traces of B vitamins. These four vitamins are all soluble in fat and fat solvents, such as ether. As knowledge about the fat-soluble vitamins progressed, it was found that several forms of the vitamins were present in green leafy vegetables, not considered fatty foods, so the subject became somewhat complicated. As with the other vitamins, we can cover only some of the basic highlights in this chapter about these most interesting and important compounds, and we will attempt to unravel some of the complications.

Though the four fat-soluble vitamins have quite different chemical properties, they have a few general distinctive similarities:

1. They are more stable to heat than the B vitamins and are less likely to be lost in the cooking and processing of foods.

2. Fat-soluble vitamins are absorbed from the intestine along with fats and lipids in foods, so that anything that interferes with fat absorption results in lowered utilization of this class of vitamins.

3. Because these vitamins are not soluble in water, they are not excreted in the urine. Instead, they are *stored in the body*, chiefly in the liver, to a considerable extent. Hence deficiency symptoms may be slow in developing and low-grade shortages may be hard to detect.

4. Because fat-soluble vitamins can be stored in the body, toxicity can develop if too great an amount of vitamin A or D is ingested, for the excess cannot be excreted in the urine.

VITAMIN A

Vitamin A is probably the most important of all vitamins, if any single vitamin can be so distinguished from another. Its great importance is demonstrated dramatically in that, more than any other vitamin, deficiencies of vitamin A are still widespread throughout most developing countries of the world and involve millions of persons, especially children.

Discovery and Identification

Hippocrates, in ancient Greece, knew that the eating of liver was a treatment for night-blindness,[1] now known to be caused by a lack of vitamin A. Many other references to the disease, throughout the centuries (back to 1500 B.C.), are known. In 1904, Mori, of Japan, found that the night blindness-preventing substance was in fatty foods and suggested the use of cod-liver oil and chicken liver for its treatment in children.[1]

The presence of vitamin A in certain fats was first detected because of their effect in promoting growth. This discovery was made in 1913, independently by McCollum and Davis* and by Osborne and Mendel.[2] Rats, fed on purified foodstuffs with lard as the only fat, ceased to grow, developed soreness of eyes, and eventually died. With butterfat or ether extract of egg yolk in the diet, rats were protected from these ill effects. Further experiments showed that cod-liver oil was also very rich in this growth-promoting, health-protective factor, whereas most commercial fats and oils produced results more like those of lard. Eventually, in 1931, the structure of vitamin A was discovered by Karrer,[3] who received a Nobel prize for this and his work with riboflavin. (Vitamin A was the first vitamin to have its structure determined — see Appendix.) In 1937, it was isolated in crystalline form from fish-liver oils.[4] Shortly thereafter, it was synthesized, and today pure, inexpensive, synthetic forms of vitamin A are readily available and largely replace fish-liver oils as the primary source in food supplements.

Chemical Properties of Vitamin A

Vitamin A is almost *colorless, insoluble in water, soluble in fats* and fat solvents, and fairly *stable to heat,* but may be *destroyed by oxidation* (such as exposure to air at high temperatures) or by exposure to ultraviolet light. Fats and oils lose vitamin A content by oxidation as they become rancid. Substances that inhibit this oxidation (antioxidants) are often present in unrefined oils but are usually removed when oils are refined for food use. Hence, we depend mainly on storage in a cool, dark place (refrigerator) and on added antioxidants to protect fats and oils from vitamin A loss.

Several slightly different forms of this vitamin are found in nature. The two most common are *retinol* (formerly called just "vitamin A" or "vitamin A alcohol") and *dehydroretinol* (formerly vitamin A_2). The former is the traditional vitamin A commonly found in all the animal kingdom (but not in plants), while the latter occurs only in fresh-water fish and birds that feed on these fish. Since both forms of the vitamin have similar physiological effects, we need make little distinction between them. Both forms of the vitamin exist in nature in alcohol, aldehyde, and acid forms.† The term vitamin A properly

---

*McCollum later (J. Biol. Chem., 24:491, 1916) named his active material "fat-soluble A," which was the first use of a letter of the alphabet to designate any vitamin. This term was changed to vitamin A in 1920 at the suggestion of Drummond (Biochem. J., 19:660, 1920) and has been used ever since (see Chap. 6). McCollum did not observe the eye changes at first, but based his conclusions on the growth-promoting properties of the vitamin.

†Since 1969, new names have been adopted for the various vitamin A compounds. The natural aldehyde form (formerly called vitamin A aldehyde, retinal, or retinene) is now properly termed *retinaldehyde* and the corresponding acid form *retinoic acid.* Corresponding suffixes are used after the phrase "dehydroretin . . ." referring to dehydroretinol compounds. Several other active forms of the vitamin exist in nature or as synthetic isomers. In the body, vitamin A exists largely in the form of esters with fatty acids, known as "retinyl esters." The different forms of vitamin A are not necessarily interchangeable in protecting against a deficiency when fed to man or animals.

refers in a broad sense to the several compounds in the animal kingdom which have vitamin A activity when fed to animals, and the term is used in that sense here.

Provitamins A and Total Vitamin A Activity

Animals get their vitamin A either directly or indirectly from plant sources. (Plants are the only source in nature of the highly colored *provitamin A carotenoids*,* precursors of this vitamin. See next section.) Fish eat smaller fish or crustaceans which, in turn, have fed on marine plants that contain the provitamins A. Herbivorous animals eat green plants and convert these substances into the vitamin itself in their bodies. Carnivorous animals get the vitamin from feeding on plant-eating animals. The cow and the hen are useful to man by converting the provitamins A in plant foods into the vitamin A in milk fat, eggs, etc. Since some provitamin A activity in the diet escapes this conversion, *milk fat, egg yolk,* and other animal products contain a *mixture* of both vitamin A and its plant precursors (which we shall call *total vitamin A activity*). The relative amounts of each depend partly on the food of the animal and partly on its species, or even breed. For instance, milk from Holstein cows contains a higher proportion of vitamin A, and that from Guernsey cows carries less vitamin A and more of the provitamin A, which explains why Guernsey milk is more "golden" in color. Both milks have about the same amount of "total vitamin A activity," however.

Plants as Sources of Provitamin A Carotenoids

Vitamin A as such is not found in the plant kingdom. Instead, the pro-

vitamins A, which are converted to vitamin A in the body, are found in plants. They are bright *yellow* or *orange-yellow* pigments, which give the color to carrots, sweet potatoes, melons, squash, pumpkin, apricots, peaches, and yellow corn. They are also present in all green vegetables, although in these vegetables their color is masked by that of the green pigment, chlorophyll. The quantity of these vitamin A precursors roughly parallels that of chlorophyll, being found most richly in thin, green leaves.

Three of these provitamin A carotenoids are known as *carotenes*† (alpha-, beta-, and gamma-carotene), and a fourth is *cryptoxanthin*, the yellow pigment of corn. The structures of the carotenes were known several years before it was clear that they were associated with vitamin A.[5] Steenbock and Boutwell first showed that sources of carotene had vitamin A activity in the rat,[6] but this relationship was not fully understood until 1930.[7]

When the carotenes and cryptoxanthin are taken into the body, they are split in half, giving rise to vitamin A. The chief site of conversion of the provitamins to vitamin A in man is in the intestinal wall during absorption into the body and also in the liver. The site of conversion differs from one animal species to another. Although beta-carotene is theoretically capable of being split to give two molecules of vitamin A (twice as much as the other precursors), this is not done very efficiently in the human body. The amount absorbed and utilized depends on many factors—the amount of fat in the diet, the method of food preparation, the rate and completeness of digestion, the presence of vitamin E and the hormone thyroxine, and other factors. Then too, there are wide differences in species and in individuals as to how well they utilize carotenes. It

---

*1969 nomenclature (see J. Nutr., *101*:133, 1971).

†Carotene is deep red when in pure form and derives its name from carrots, from which it was first isolated and in which it exists at a level of about 0.01 percent.

is conservatively estimated that in man about one-sixth the carotene intake may be expected to be transformed into vitamin A.[8] This is on the basis that only about one-third of the carotene is absorbed and that only about one-half of this (or a total of only one-sixth) has vitamin A activity for man.

*Effects of Lack of Vitamin A
in Man and Animals*

Vitamin A is essential for growth, for vision, for maintenance of epithelial tissues in a healthy state, and for tooth development. Hence, a diet that contains insufficient amounts of total vitamin A activity to meet the needs of humans will in time cause *stunting of growth, lack of ability to see well in dim light* (night blindness) or more serious eye troubles, diseased conditions of the skin and membranes lining the *respiratory passages and the digestive and genitourinary tracts,* and abnormalities in the enamel-forming cells of the *teeth.*

The eye is one of the first organs to show effects of vitamin A deficiency because the vitamin is a *constituent of a pigment in the retina.* When light falls on the normal retina, this pigment—called visual purple (rhodopsin)—is bleached to another pigment known as visual yellow (retinaldehyde; see footnote, p. 188). As a result of this change, images are transmitted to the brain through the optic nerve. In the dark, the vitamin A-containing visual purple is rebuilt, but there is always some loss of degradation products, which necessitates new supplies of vitamin A brought by the blood (Fig. 9–1).*

If vitamin A is at a low level in the blood, normal vision will be restored slowly and *dark adaptation* of the eyes will be faulty. Dark adaptation is influenced by too many other factors to be an infallible index of the adequacy of vitamin A in the diet. But lack of vitamin A is one of the common causes of night blindness, and a good many cases do respond favorably to extra doses of this vitamin. If a person is suffering from vitamin A deficiency, night driving could prove to be hazardous, because vision would be impaired after exposure to the bright headlights of oncoming cars.

One of the chief functions of vitamin A is to maintain the health of *epithelial tissues*—namely the skin and membranes that line all passages which open to the

---

*A Nobel Prize in Medicine was awarded in 1967 to Dr. George Wald of Harvard University, who is primarily responsible for these studies on the role of vitamin A in vision.[9]

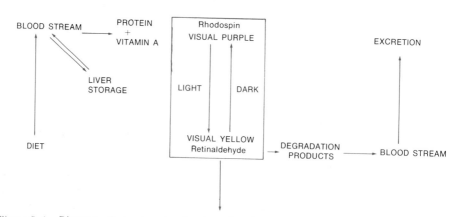

Figure 9–1. Diagram of visual cycle, showing why vitamin A from the blood stream is needed to rebuild the pigment, visual purple, in the eye after exposure to light. (From Gordon, E. S., and Sevringhaus, E. L.: *Vitamin Therapy in General Practice.* Chicago, Year Book Publishers, Inc., 1942.)

exterior of the body, as well as glands and their ducts. When deprived of an adequate supply of vitamin A, these tissues undergo changes that lead to a peculiar type of horny degeneration called *keratinization*. Damage to the mucous membranes lining the mouth, throat, nose, and respiratory passages is one of the earlier effects of vitamin A deficiency. In addition to general deterioration of the cells, these membranes lack their normal secretions, and there is loss of the little filaments called cilia, which by constant movement aid in keeping the membrane surface clean. As bacteria have easy access to these parts, susceptibility to infections, such as *sinus trouble, sore throat, and abscesses in ears, mouth, or salivary glands,* is a common manifestation of insufficient vitamin A in the diet. Similar damage to membranes lining the alimentary tract may allow bacteria to penetrate into the stomach or intestinal wall, whence they may be carried in the blood stream to other parts of the body. Deficient rats kept under special germ-free conditions live many months longer than similar rats under usual laboratory conditions.

The frequency of such infections (especially of the respiratory tract) in severe vitamin A deficiency has led to the use of concentrated preparations of this vitamin for their prevention and treatment, but obviously vitamin A is useful in such conditions only when they are due to a *deficiency* of vitamin A. Vitamin A shares with other vitamins in promoting health of tissues and is anti-infective only in the sense that it helps to keep healthy the lining membranes that are the first line of defense in preventing entrance of bacteria into the body. If there has been previous deficiency of this vitamin in the diet, extra doses of it are helpful in rebuilding stores of it in the liver and restoring damaged epithelial tissues to health.

A prolonged lack of vitamin A results in dry and scaly skin (follicular hyperkeratosis), with plugs of horny material

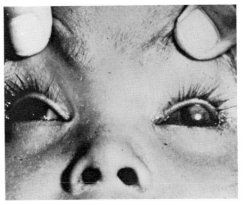

Figure 9–2. Eye changes (xerophthalmia) in a child from a developing country, being examined by a member of a survey team. It costs only 12 cents a year to fortify this child's powdered milk with adequate amounts of vitamin A. (From *NIH Record.*)

about the hair follicles, and in the eye disease known as *xerophthalmia* (see Figs. 9–2 and 9–3). In this disease, the secretion of tears is stopped, the eyes are sensitive to light, the lids become swollen and sticky with pus, and bacteria may invade the eye itself and cause ulcers of the cornea, which lead to blindness if the disease is not arrested. Xerophthalmia is a very common disease in *infants* or undernourished *children* in those parts of the world where the deficiency is prevalent, and it may be prevented by including in the diet a good source of vitamin A.

Vitamin A is also essential for proper formation and maintenance of tooth enamel and health of gums, and for health of the sex glands, uterus, and the membranes that line the bladder and urinary passages. Some investigators have found that nervous lesions develop in animals on vitamin A deficient diets. It is stated that the bony structure ceases to grow (owing to vitamin A deficiency) before growth of nervous tissue is inhibited, and that the resultant crowding of nerves in the bony cavities of the skull and spinal column is the cause of the nervous lesions. This vitamin is needed to ensure optimum *growth* (Fig. 9–4).

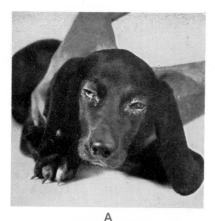

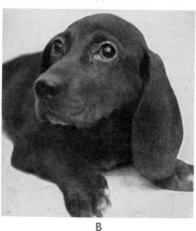

Figure 9–3. Xerophthalmia in a puppy due to feeding a vitamin A deficient diet. **A,** Note the swollen lids and sticky discharge from the eyes. **B,** Full recovery after administration of vitamin A. (Courtesy of Doctors Steenbock, Nelson, and Hart.)

Deficient animals show most, if not all, of the same symptoms that are described in man. *Reproductive* disorders (Figs. 9–5 and 9–6) are more readily observed in deficient animals with evidences of poor fertilization, abnormal embryonic growth, placental injury, and in severe deficiency, death of the fetus. Deficiencies have been obtained in all animal species studied — rat, fowl, pig, cow, sheep, dog, guinea pig, and others.

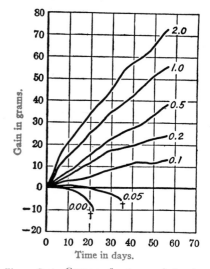

Figure 9–4. Curves of rat growth in pioneer nutrition studies show results due to differences in intake of vitamin A. Figures at end of each curve indicate amount of tomato (in grams) fed daily as the sole source of vitamin A. (Courtesy of Dr. H. C. Sherman, Dr. H. E. Munsell, and the *Journal of the American Chemical Society.*)

Vitamin A in the Body

ABSORPTION. Chemical and physical methods for detecting and measuring vitamin A in blood and tissues have enabled nutritionists to follow its course within the body. Most of the provitamin A carotenoids are split by a special enzyme in the intestinal wall, and these products, plus any dietary vitamin A itself, are absorbed along with fats* into the lymph to be emptied later into the blood. The presence of fat and bile favors their absorption. Any factor that lowers fat absorption may affect the absorption of fat-soluble vitamins unfavorably. In disorders such as jaundice and celiac disease, much of the vitamin A value of the diet may fail to be absorbed from the intestine. Bile

---

*Vitamin A is esterified in the mucosa of the intestine generally with palmitic acid (a fatty acid) to form retinylpalmitate, in which form it eventually reaches the liver.

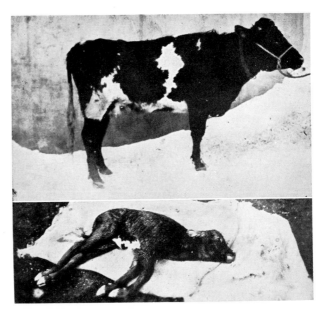

Figure 9–5. A disaster in reproduction caused by feeding a ration, now known to be deficient in vitamin A, made from wheat straw, wheat meal, and wheat gluten, with common salt. In this classic experiment, the cow was shaggy-coated, slow and sleepy in movement, and had a tendency to drag her hind feet. The calf was born prematurely and died. (From Research Bulletin 17, University of Wisconsin Agricultural Experiment Station, 1911.)

salts may be given to aid absorption in such cases, or preparations of *water-soluble vitamin A* may be given by mouth as a supplement. Water-soluble vitamin A is an *emulsion* of very finely divided droplets of vitamin A (usually in the form of the ester vitamin A palmitate in a gelatin matrix) in water, and in this state the vitamin is more rapidly absorbed by healthy persons, infants, or patients with faulty fat absorption than when it is given dissolved in oil.

Provitamin A and vitamin A in foods of animal origin are normally completely absorbed. Absorption of the provitamin A carotenoids from fibrous

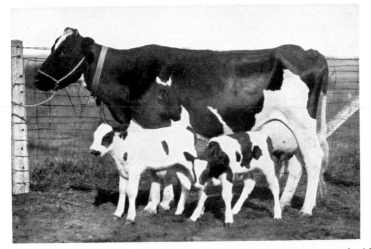

Figure 9–6. When the ration fed to cow shown in Figure 9–5 was supplemented with bone meal (2 percent), common salt (1 percent), and raw cod-liver oil (2 percent), its deficiencies were fully corrected. The cow was in excellent condition and produced twin calves weighing 124 pounds. (Courtesy of Doctors Hart and Steenbock.)

vegetable material is much less efficiently accomplished. Carotenes in green peas are better utilized than those in spinach, but both these vegetables, along with carrots, have much lower vitamin A activity, when taken as food, than equivalent quantities of the vitamin itself taken in cod-liver oil. Other experiments on the relative utilization of carotenes in vegetables showed that the carotenes in kale are 67 percent available, those in sweet potatoes 37 percent available, and those in carrots 35 to 40 percent available.[10] The degree to which provitamins in vegetable foods are available later as vitamin A in the body varies not only with the kind of food but also with different individuals and at various times.

The very high theoretical vitamin A activity of some green and yellow vegetables (as listed in tables) may be misleading; owing to incomplete absorption and conversion, they may be expected to yield only one-fourth to one-half as much vitamin A in the body as the listed amount.

The presence of significant amounts of *mineral oil* in the intestine interferes with the absorption of vitamin A, carotenes, and other fat-soluble vitamins, because they dissolve in this oil, which is nonabsorbable; thus they are excreted in the feces.[11] Therefore mineral oil should not be incorporated in foods (as in salad dressings) or taken too close to mealtimes.

STORAGE AND FUNCTION IN THE BODY. Both vitamin A (as retinyl palmitate) and any carotenoids not split in the intestinal wall are carried by the lymph system to the blood stream in man.* The *liver* takes up any excess of these substances from the blood and *stores reserves of this vitamin*. These can be released into the blood as retinol, attached to a specific protein† and carried to the

tissues later as needed. The level of vitamin A in the blood is thus kept fairly constant and would not be affected by a diet poor in vitamin A until the body reserves were about exhausted. Nearly 95 percent of these reserves are in the liver. How much vitamin A has been stored in the liver depends, of course, on whether the habitual diet has been rich or poor in vitamin A and its precursors. Liver reserves of vitamin A are usually lowest at birth and are built up with advancing years. In diseases of the liver—notably cirrhosis—these stores are markedly reduced.

Because reserve stores of vitamin A exist but are variable in amount in different individuals, it is natural that *symptoms due to a vitamin A deficiency should develop rather slowly* and that the time interval before deficiency symptoms appear differs according to the extent of the body stores available in time of need.

No vitamin A is excreted in the urine because it is not water-soluble, but considerable unabsorbed carotene is normally found *in the feces*. In disorders in which the stools are loose and frequent, or in which bile is lacking, most of the carotene and even some of the vitamin A intake may fail to be absorbed. During lactation, there is a considerable output of vitamin A in the milk secreted, so that the need for extra quantities of this vitamin is greater at this time than at others.

Interrelations in metabolism between vitamin A and other vitamins exist. Vitamin A and provitamin A can lose their potency by oxidation; both vitamin E and vitamin C are thought to spare vitamin A by acting as antioxidants—substances that enhance the preservation of vitamin A in its biologically active form.

The importance of vitamin A in maintaining the integrity of epithelial cells, in preventing eye disorders, in bone and teeth formation, and in growth and reproduction has been discussed. The classic studies on its role in vision were mentioned, but only

---

*Some animals, such as the rat, sheep, and pig, absorb no carotene at all.

†The human retinol-binding protein (RBP) in serum is a low molecular weight albumin rich in tryptophan and specific for this purpose.[12]

recently have clues been found to explain how vitamin A acts biochemically elsewhere in the body.

Vitamin A appears to be necessary for the formation of *mucopolysaccharides*, which are essential components of mucous membranes and without which epithelial membranes degenerate. Vitamin A appears to be essential for the release of a protein-splitting enzyme necessary for the formation of bone from cartilage, of ribonucleic acid (RNA), and of certain ovarian hormones (necessary for reproduction) in the rat.

Human Requirement and Standard Allowance

The total vitamin A activity (both for requirements and in food composition tables) is stated in *International Units* (IU) rather than in milligrams or in micrograms (for convenience, if not for ease in understanding).[8] One International Unit is defined as equal to 0.344 mcg of crystalline retinylacetate (which is equivalent to 0.300 mcg of retinol, or to 0.60 mcg of beta-carotene).* These standards are based on experiments which show that in rats only about 50 percent of the beta-carotene is converted to vitamin A. In man, however, beta-carotene is not as available as in the rat due to poorer absorption in the intestine and other factors. Only between 25 and 60 percent (an average of one-third is generally accepted) of the beta-carotene ingested is converted into vitamin A depending upon the type of food and other factors.[8, 13] Pure carotene and the carotene present in milk are completely absorbed, an exception to the rule. In other words,

the actual amount of vitamin A provided to humans by a standard allowance stated in terms of International Units varies according to whether the major part of the dietary intake is in the form of true vitamin A or the less efficient provitamin A.

Biologically, the most active isomers of the pure vitamin A compounds are all in the "trans" form. Various "cis" forms of the vitamin and provitamin do exist in foods in smaller amounts which are less active than the "trans" forms. This introduces additional complications, but is not of practical importance except in processed foods (see p. 199).

The average American diet is considered to contain roughly one-half of its total vitamin A activity in the active form and one-half as the provitamin, according to the Food and Nutrition Board.[8] The Board also states, "For practical purposes, within the United States, it is not considered to be necessary to further adjust the RDA of 5000 IU for variations in the proportions of preformed vitamin A and provitamin A in the diet."†

The 1968 recommended allowances of the U.S. Food and Nutrition Board are: 5000 IU (1.5 mg of retinol or equivalent) daily for all persons over 12 years of age, 1500 IU daily for infants, 4500 IU daily for boys and girls 10 to 12 years of age, 6000 IU daily dur-

---

*Attempts are now being made by international agencies to do away with the confusing International Units. However, until a fully accepted method is available for measuring total vitamin A activity by some useful weight unit (such as the proposed "retinol equivalents"), we shall continue to use the widely used IU here.

---

†This statement, however, apparently does not take into account some of the extreme variations in eating habits of the American public. Since only one-third of the carotene of many vegetable foods is available to the human body, the recommendation on the above basis for a complete vegetarian would be equal to 10,000 IU of provitamin A (carotene) per day, much higher than the Board probably intended. This is calculated from the assumption that the current RDA of 5000 IU is based on the activity of a half and half mixture of retinol and carotene—since one IU of retinol in man equals three IU of carotene (or 2500 IU plus 7500 IU). The RDA on this same basis for a person eating only animal vitamin A would be equivalent to 3330 IU (2500 IU plus 830 IU). We know of no evidence, though, that 5000 IU of provitamin A is insufficient, in spite of these calculations.

ing the fourth to ninth months of pregnancy, and 8000 IU during lactation. (See Appendix for more complete figures.) Allowances for infants and children are liberal in terms of minimum requirements in order to provide extra vitamin A for growth and to ensure adequate stores. Adults who depend heavily on vegetable sources that contain the provitamins would do well to take amounts more liberal than the recommended allowance (see footnote, right column, page 195).

Toxicity

Long-continued large doses of vitamin A have a *toxic* effect, and regular moderate intake (5000 to 10,000 IU per day) is better for building up stores in the liver. Toxic symptoms (hypervitaminosis A) may occur in children one to three years of age after they have received 75,000 IU or more of vitamin A daily for at least six months (or less, of the water-soluble forms). Such symptoms—which include excessive irritability, swellings over the long bones, and dry and itching skin—are relieved by discontinuing the dosages of supplementary vitamin A. In adults, the early symptoms of toxicity are headache, nausea, and diarrhea; a great excess of vitamin A may also lead to decalcification of bones with consequent bone fragility.

Livers of animals may concentrate so much vitamin A that they may be toxic when eaten in large amounts over long periods.[14] Early explorers in the Arctic, it is said, learned to avoid eating the liver of the polar bear because symptoms of toxicity were observed and were later found to be due to excessive vitamin A. Carotene, in contrast to vitamin A, is not toxic even when fed at high levels. In man, the only abnormal sign that might be seen when large amounts of carotene are eaten is a yellow skin (as is seen in some persons who consume high amounts of carrots or red palm oil, for example).

Extent of Vitamin A Deficiency

It is not difficult to get the recommended allowance of vitamin A in daily foods, if good foods are available and are wisely chosen. Although surveys show that it is not uncommon for the diet to fall slightly below the recommended allowance in the United States,[15] marked symptoms of vitamin A deficiency are not seen commonly. The allowances provide a large margin of safety above basic minimum requirements, so diets somewhat below the allowance figure are not necessarily deficient for body needs.

Generally, nutritionists do not become overly concerned unless intakes of vitamin A are less than two-thirds the recommended allowance. In any event, in the United States, it is clear from the references cited[15] that most of us are obtaining sufficient vitamin A in our diets. However, in the diets of teenage girls, pregnant women, and older persons, the level of vitamin A intake may often be too low to allow for a proper margin of safety. On the other hand, two studies of diets in several groups of infants indicated the vitamin A intake to be more than ample.[16]

Contrary to most other nutrients, the average amount of vitamin A available to each person per day in the United States has decreased from a level of 8700 IU in 1947–49 to the present level of 7800 IU.[17] These are *available units* and do not include amounts lost in food wastage or in food preparation or processing, but the figures nevertheless indicate a trend that ought to be reversed.

Vitamin A deficiency, unfortunately, is very widespread throughout the world, especially among children in countries where fat supplies are low and where there are few green vegetables in the diet. Night blindness, xerophthalmia, impaired vision, and blindness as a result of vitamin A deficiency are prevalent throughout Asia, the Middle East, India, Malaysia, and parts of Africa, South America, and

Latin America. It has been estimated that throughout the world (excluding Communist China) *about 80,000 children become blind each year from vitamin A deficiency,* and that about one-half of these die.*[18] For instance, in Indonesia, in 82 percent of the blind children below the age of ten, the cause was vitamin A deficiency.[19] Gopalan has stated that in South India, vitamin A deficiency accounts for 25 to 30 percent of all cases of clinical malnutrition and is often seen in association with protein deficiency.[20] Other dramatic examples are cited in the list of references. In older children and young adults, too low a supply of vitamin A predisposes the individual to tuberculosis, which is widespread in a number of countries.

It is difficult to determine when a person is deficient in vitamin A in the absence of the usual symptoms seen in more severe deficiency. Night blindness or dark adaptation tests are not always successful in diagnosing a deficiency. Most useful are measurements of serum vitamin A and carotene values in comparison with known standards. Serum levels of 10 to 19 mcg of vitamin A per 100 ml are considered low, as are 20 to 39 mcg or less of carotene.

Food Sources of Vitamin A

The most important animal sources of vitamin A are *liver, butterfat, and egg yolk.* Milk, cream, ice cream, and whole milk or most cheeses all carry vitamin A in smaller amounts. The vitamin A value of these foods varies widely according to the vitamin A value of the food of the animals that produced them. Livers from older animals and from animals fed on green fodder contain much larger stores of vitamin A. Butterfat in the milk of cows is usually yellower and of higher vitamin A value when the animals are grazing

in green pastures than when stall-fed in winter. However, improved feeds for dairy cattle, together with their ability to draw on stores of vitamin A in the liver, result in less seasonal variations in vitamin A content of milk and butter than were formerly common. The yellowness of egg yolks and butterfat is not an infallible guide to their vitamin A value, because they contain both the yellow provitamins A and the colorless vitamin A.

Margarine has been fortified by addition of carotene or vitamin A (also vitamin D) up to the level equal to a year-round average in butter (15,000 IU per lb, or 3300 IU per 100 gm). This makes it fully acceptable nutritionally as a less expensive substitute for butter.

Important plant sources of vitamin A value are the *green and yellow vegetables.* As the vitamin A value of plants is due entirely to yellow carotenoid pigments, either alone or found with chlorophyll, the depth of yellow or green color is a reliable index of their potential vitamin A value. Most thin green leaves (spinach, kale, turnip greens, etc.) have a vitamin A value from 5000 to 15,000 IU (average about 8000 IU) per 100 gm; bleached inner leaves of cabbage and lettuce, as well as bleached asparagus, are of low vitamin A value. Carrots may vary in vitamin A value from 2000 to 12,000 IU per 100 gm, and sweet potatoes also vary widely in vitamin A value (1500 to 7700 IU), according to the depth of their color. Average provitamin A values (in IU) of other green and yellow vegetables and yellow fruits are given in Table 9–1.

Grains (except for yellow corn), white flour, sugar, and the common colorless vegetable oils carry little or no vitamin A activity, while lean muscle meats, nuts, and many common fruits and vegetables provide only minor quantities. The body fat of animals is usually low in vitamin A, but that of fish may contain considerable amounts.

Combinations of *foods that provide the standard daily allowance of total vitamin A activity for an adult* are given in Table

---

*To say nothing of the grief and untold misery for parents, and lifetime disability for most of the survivors.

Table 9–1.   Total Vitamin A Activity of Typical Foods*

Food	IU Per 100 Grams, Raw	Size of Average Serving	IU Per Avg. Svg.
Liver, beef	43,900	2 slices, fried (74 gm)	40,050
Carrots, deep color	11,000	⅔ cup, diced, cooked (100 gm)	10,500
Apricots, dried	10,900	½ cup, cooked, with juice	4200
Sweet potatoes, deep color	8800	1 medium, baked (110 gm)	8910
Green leafy vegetables (4000–15,000), avg.	7870	½ cup, cooked (100 gm)	7870
Fruits, fresh:			
Apricots	2700	2–3 medium	2700
Nectarines	1650	2 medium	1650
Peaches, avg., yellow	1330	1 medium large	1330
Cherries	1000	15 large	1000
Watermelon	590	1/16 of 10 × 16 inch melon	2530
Others (trace to 400), avg.	135	Avg. serving (100 gm)	135
Squash, winter, boiled	3500	½ cup, boiled	3500
Cantaloupe, deep color	3400	½ melon (200 gm)	6800
Butter (2000–4000), year-round average	3300	1 avg. pat (10 gm)	330
Margarine, fortified	3300	1 avg. pat (10 gm)	330
Broccoli	2500	⅔ cup, cooked, or 1 large stalk	2500
Lettuce, green leaf	1900	2 lg. or 4–5 small leaves	950
Pumpkin	1600	½ cup, cooked	3840
Prunes, dried	1600	4 medium cooked, 2 tbsp juice	510
Cheese, cream	1540	1 oz avg. serving	460
Cheese, American Cheddar	1310	1 oz avg. serving	390
Eggs, whole	1180	1, avg. size (50 gm)	590
Tomatoes	900	1, medium size (150 gm)	1350
Asparagus, green	900	6 stalks, canned (100 gm)	900
Cream, thin, 20%	840	4 tbsp (60 gm)	500
Ice cream, plain, avg.	520	⅙ qt (100 gm)	520
Green vegetables, other than those listed above, avg.	500	Avg. serving (100 gm)	500
Yellow vegetables, other than listed above, avg.	330	Avg. serving (100 gm)	330
Milk, whole, fresh	140	1 pint	740
Other vegetables (10–90), avg.	50	Avg. serving (100 gm)	50

*Figures adapted from U.S. Department Agriculture Handbook No. 8: *Composition of Foods—Raw, Processed, Prepared,* 1963.

9–2. Each combination combines animal and plant sources, and furnishes somewhat more than 5000 IU of vitamin A.

There is danger that the diet will provide less than optimum amounts of total vitamin A activity unless green and yellow vegetables are used frequently, and in addition they are inexpensive sources of vitamin A for low-cost diets. This danger of inadequacy of the diet is illustrated by the list of foods in Table 9–3, which might seem to constitute the basis of a normal diet for one day, but which falls considerably short of the 5000 IU daily vitamin A allowance.

If one of the vegetables listed in Table 9–3 were of the green or yellow variety, the vitamin A value of this diet would be raised decidedly, usually up to the 5000 IU level or more, provided the vegetable chosen was strongly colored and an average-sized serving (100 gm) was eaten. Figure 9–7 shows sources of vitamin A in average American diets.

Table 9–2. *Food Combinations That Provide the Recommended Daily Allowance of Total Vitamin A Activity for an Adult**

Food	Amount
Whole milk	1 pint (480 gm)
Pumpkin pie	4-inch wedge (150 gm)
Vegetable-beef soup	1 cup
Margarine or butter	2 tablespoons
Broccoli	2/3 cup
Nectarines	2
Eggs	2
Apricots	2-4
Tomato juice	6 oz

*Each of these food combinations furnishes somewhat more than 5000 IU of total vitamin A activity.

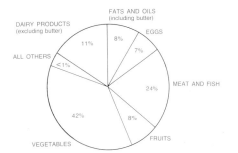

Figure 9–7. Percentages of vitamin A value contributed by various food groups in the average American diet. (From information supplied by U.S. Department of Agriculture, 1971.)

Effect of Cooking or Processing

Because vitamin A and its precursors (the carotenes) are *insoluble in water* and *stable to heat at ordinary cooking temperatures, most foods lose little of their total vitamin A activity, as measured chemically, in cooking or processing,* unless they are exposed to air. However, the biological value of the vitamin A activity of common processed vegetables may be reduced from 15 to 20 percent in green

Table 9–3. *A Food Combination Supplying an Inadequate Amount of Vitamin A Activity for Daily Adult Diet **

Food	Amount
Whole milk	1 pint
Butter or margarine	2 squares
Egg	1
Orange juice	4 oz
Apple	1 medium
Green beans	1/2 cup (3-4 oz)
Coleslaw (cabbage salad)	1/2 cup
Beets	1/2 cup

*This diet contains only about 3000 IU instead of 5000 IU of total vitamin A activity.

vegetables and as high as 30 to 35 percent in common yellow vegetables because of chemical changes in the carotene molecule (some *trans* forms are changed to other isomers).[21] Drying of eggs, vegetables, or fruits, with exposure to air, sunlight, or high temperatures, may cause serious loss of vitamin A value. Evaporation, pasteurization, or irradiation of milk has little or no effect on its vitamin A content. Vegetables should be stored at low temperatures to conserve their vitamin A value, and of course, quick freezing is an excellent means to this end. Animal fats should be kept in a cold dark place, and fish-liver oils should be protected from light by being put in a dark glass bottle.

By far the most potent sources of vitamin A today are the synthetic forms; they are also the most inexpensive. Vitamin A costs only 20 cents, or less, *per gram* of stabilized material (1 million IU), when purchased in large quantities. This is a 200-day supply for one person. The use of synthetic vitamin A and carotene to fortify certain foods accounts today for about 7 percent of all vitamin A intake in the United States. Many tons of synthetic forms of the vitamin are made each year. They are just as effective and safe as the natural forms, though of course they carry no other nutrients with them.

VITAMIN D

History and Identification

Rickets,* a bone disorder (also seen in calcium and phosphorus deficiency), has been known since 500 B.C. In industrial England rickets was very common in children in the crowded slums, and it became known as the "English disease." In 1824, cod liver oil, long used as a "folk medicine," was found to be important in the treatment of rickets (though it was not used universally for this purpose until nearly a century later). In 1889, in a unique nutrition education demonstration, rickets in young lion cubs in the London zoological gardens was dramatically treated with crushed bones and cod liver oil.

The importance of sunshine for good health of individuals was known by ancient civilizations and is probably one of the bases for sun-worship by primitive nations. In the 1890's it was found that sunshine was a specific cure for rickets[22]—though the exact reason for this was not known until the discovery of vitamin D in the 1920's (see below). Ever since, vitamin D has been popularly called "the sunshine vitamin," for good reason.

In 1918 Mellanby of London, in studies with puppies, provided the first experimental proof that rickets was a deficiency disease and he was able to cure it by feeding cod liver oil. McCollum and his co-workers[1, 23] found in 1922 that after destruction (by oxidation) of all the vitamin A in cod liver oil, it still retained its rickets-preventing potency. This proved the existence of a second fat-soluble vitamin, carried in liver oils and certain other fats, which he called the *calcium-depositing vitamin*

and, in 1925, *vitamin D.*† The first crystalline vitamin D was obtained in 1931,‡ and it was synthesized shortly thereafter. Soon it became evident that there are at least ten natural substances which exert vitamin D-like activity in varying degrees, but only two of these are of practical importance from the standpoint of their occurrence in foods —*ergocalciferol* (vitamin D₂) and *cholecalciferol* (vitamin D₃)—see formulas in the Appendix. Because they are closely related chemically and produce a like effect on the body, the term vitamin D is used collectively to indicate the *group* of substances that show this vitamin activity.

Ergocalciferol (D₂) and Cholecalciferol (D₃), and Their Precursors

Steenbock and Hess, in the 1920's, discovered independently that when certain foods are exposed to ultraviolet light, their ability to protect animals against rickets is increased. This meant that some foods must contain precursors of vitamin D—substances which are altered chemically by light of certain wave lengths (including sunlight) so that they become capable of functioning as vitamins in the body. We now know that the *provitamin D* in plants differs from the animal precursor and that each gives rise to a slightly different vitamin D when activated by light. In

---

*According to McCollum,[1] the word "rickets" is derived from the old English word "wrikken" (to bend or twist). In 1650 Glisson of Cambridge wrote a treatise about the disease and blamed it on bad home environment and hygiene.[1]

†The term "vitamin D" for the anti-rachitic vitamin was not suggested until 1924 by Sure (J. Biol. Chem., 58:693, 1924) and later by McCollum and co-workers (J. Biol. Chem., 64:161, 1925). This suggestion was quickly accepted, in spite of the fact that Funk and Dubin (J. Biol. Chem., 48:437, 1921, and Proc. Soc. Exp. Biol. Med., 19:15, 1921) had earlier used the term "vitamine D" to describe a new and different, water-soluble growth factor for the rat (and for yeast), a suggestion disregarded by others for some reason.

‡Crystals of vitamin D were first obtained by the Dutch chemists Reerink and van Wijk (Biochem. J., 25:1001, 1931).

plants, a substance known as *ergosterol**
is converted by light into ergocalciferol.
In animals, a derivative of *cholesterol*
(7-dehydrocholesterol) is the precursor
of cholecalciferol (as discovered by
Waddell in 1934). Birds respond much
better to cholecalciferol, but most animals can utilize either type of vitamin D.
Cholecalciferol occurs in fish-liver oils
and foods of animal origin, such as
eggs, butter, milk, and cream. It is
also available in low-cost, synthetic form
which is equal in activity to natural
forms of the vitamin.

The vitamin D group belong to the
class of organic substances known as
sterols — compounds with large molecules containing an alcohol group and
with the same solubilities as fats. They
are very stable compounds, resisting
destruction by heat and oxidation, as
well as by acids and alkalis. Obviously
they are sensitive to light, especially
that of shorter wave lengths (ultraviolet). They are the precursors in the
body of many important hormones.
Another common sterol in the body is
cholesterol.

Vitamin D is measured in terms of
International Units, as is vitamin A.
Crystalline cholecalciferol (D_3) was
adopted in 1949 as the standard reference material. *One International Unit
corresponds to the vitamin activity of
0.025 mcg* of this pure substance, and
400 units equals 10 mcg, a day's allowance, making this one of the most potent vitamins known. The U. S. Pharmacopeia (USP) unit, often used for
potency of medicinal preparations, is
the same as the International Unit (as
was also true for vitamin A).

*Formation of Vitamin D in the
Body by Sunlight*

The major precursor of the vitamin
(7-dehydrocholesterol) is present in

man and animals in the oily lubricating
material in the skin and on its surface.
Hence, it is not surprising that when
sunlight, in which there is light of short
wave lengths (ultraviolet light), falls
directly on the skin, some of the provitamins are converted into cholecalciferol, the major animal form of vitamin D.[22] The vitamin thus formed in
or on the skin is readily taken into the
local circulation and carried by the
blood to all parts of the body. Excess
formed over immediate body needs can
be stored in considerable amounts in
the liver and may be found also in the
fatty tissues, lungs, spleen, and brain.

Hess found that rickets could be prevented or cured by exposing children
(without clothing) to sunlight or the
rays of an *ultraviolet lamp,* since they thus
were enabled to manufacture vitamin D
in their own bodies. Today, however,
with the availability of foods enriched
with vitamin D and of other low-cost
food supplements, ultraviolet lamps or
sun lamps are not the most practical
way of obtaining this vitamin.

The lower animals also generate vitamin D in their bodies on exposure to
light. Steenbock kept chicks indoors on
a ration low in vitamin D, conditions
which led to stunted growth and leg
weakness. Exposure to sunlight for a
half hour daily served to protect the
chicks against the effects of vitamin D
deficiency in the diet (Fig. 9–8). The
discovery of cheap dietary sources of
vitamin D for farm animals (as substitutes for sunshine) was a major factor
in the ability to raise poultry, swine,
and cattle indoors and the year around,
resulting in the wide availability of
low-cost eggs, milk, and meat in developed countries. We could not raise cats
and dogs as pets in our homes without
this discovery of a "sunshine substitute."

Effects of Vitamin D Deficiency

The effects of a lack of vitamin D,
as seen most strikingly in children and

*The German chemist Adolph Windhaus re-
ceived the Nobel Prize in 1928 for his studies on
the vitamin activity of irradiated ergosterol. The
compound was named from ergot, a black fungus
which grows on the rye plant, from which ergosterol was first isolated in 1889.

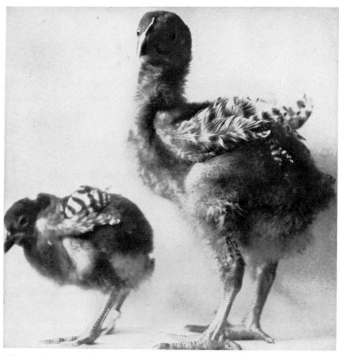

Figure 9–8. Effect of exposure to sunlight in stimulating growth. Both chicks received the same ration, which was poor in vitamin D, but the one on the right was exposed to sunlight one-half hour daily, thus permitting generation of the needed vitamin D in its body. (Courtesy of Dr. H. Steenbock, University of Wisconsin.)

young animals, are poor growth and lack of normal development of the bones. In the condition *rickets*, the metabolism of calcium and phosphorus is disturbed in such a way that the deposition in the bones of the inorganic salt calcium phosphate, which is responsible for bone rigidity, cannot proceed normally. Hence, this disease is characterized by weak bones, which readily develop curvatures when compelled to carry the weight of the body, and by overgrowth of the softer tissues (cartilage) at the ends of the bones. Rachitic deformities develop, such as *bowlegs, knock-knees, enlargement of* bones about the *joints,* and a *narrow, distorted chest* with beading of the ribs (Figs. 9–9 and 9–10). These deformities, not themselves causing death, may persist into adult life, at which time the shrunken chest may predispose to lung diseases, and a narrow pelvis may be one of the

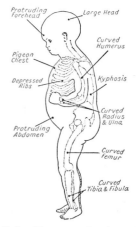

Figure 9–9. Diagram showing deformities that are symptoms of severe cases of rickets. (From Harris, L. J.: *Vitamins in Theory and Practice,* 4th Ed. London, Cambridge University Press, 1955.)

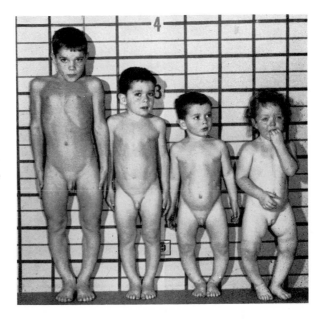

Figure 9–10. Hypophosphatemic vitamin D-refractory rickets of the simple type. Three brothers and a female first cousin. (From Fraser, D., and Salter, R. B.: *Pediatric Clinics of North America,* May, 1958.)

factors making childbearing difficult for such women. Milder cases of rickets, associated with less severe lack of vitamin D, may be detectable only by blood analyses (either the serum calcium or phosphate, or both, are below normal levels), by failure of bones to grow properly in length, and by x-ray pictures which show the characteristic failure of normal deposition of calcium phosphate in the ends of the bones. When healing takes place (usually as a result of giving vitamin D), new deposits of calcium phosphate are laid down in the cartilage along the line of demarcation between the head of the bone (*epiphysis*) and the main part or *shaft* of the long bone. This increase of mineral deposit near the ends of the bones is indicated by increased density in x-ray pictures (Fig. 9–11).

Though vitamin D deficiency is not common in adults, it does occur especially during pregnancy, lactation, old age, and in persons eating vitamin D–low diets who do not receive any sunshine (such as those who work at night, or heavily clothed persons).*[8] *Adult*

*Such as women of the Middle East and North Africa who are confined indoors by the custom of *purdah.*

rickets, or *osteomalacia* (a form of softening of the bone, see also p. 243), is caused by depletion of bone stores of calcium and phosphorus. This may be from either poor utilization of these mineral elements associated with vitamin D deficiency — or lack of sunshine — over very long periods (many years), from faulty absorption, from kidney defects, or possibly in old age from changes in activity of certain hormone-producing glands (especially the parathyroid and thyroid glands).

It should be obvious that rickets in any age may be caused also by *lack of either calcium or phosphorus,* since these are the building materials for the calcium phosphate upon which the rigidity and strength of bone depend. No amount of vitamin D will promote normal bone development unless the mineral elements necessary for building strong bones are provided in the diet in adequate quantities. Conversely, rickets may develop in persons on diets that supply plenty of calcium and phosphorus (e.g., in infants on milk diet) if *vitamin D is lacking.* The vitamin D may be supplied in food or an oil concentrate, it may be generated in the body by exposure to sunlight, or some may be

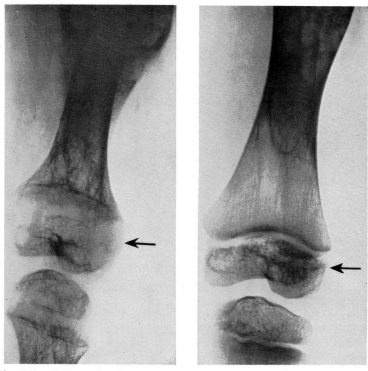

Figure 9–11. X-ray pictures of same joint in a 10-year-old Mexican boy, before and after treatment for rickets. **A,** Rarefication at ends of bones due to failure of normal deposition of calcium phosphate in rickets. **B,** One month later, showing increased density of bones and rapid healing of rachitic changes as the result of very large doses of vitamin D. (From McCune, in Wohl, M. S. (ed.): *Dietotherapy.* Philadelphia, W. B. Saunders Co., 1945.)

obtained from each source. A diet rich in one of the necessary mineral elements and poor in the other predisposes toward development of rickets. The best *protection* against this disease and the most favorable bone growth are secured when calcium and phosphorus are supplied in approximately equal amounts (as in milk) and when liberal quantities of vitamin D are available.

Vitamin D deficiency may also result in poor tooth development, muscular weakness, a protruding abdomen, listlessness, and an enlarged skull.

Vitamin D in the Body,
and Its Functions

Vitamin D, being fat-soluble, is absorbed from the intestine along with

fats. Bile aids in this process, and conditions unfavorable to fat absorption (lack of bile, disorders such as sprue and celiac disease, etc.) may result in poor utilization of vitamin D.

In common with other fat-soluble vitamins, vitamin D can be stored (in various chemical forms) in the body to an important extent. It can be passed from the mother's body to build up stores in the child before birth, or into breast milk on which the infant feeds, and in both these ways it may help to protect the infant against rickets. It is noticeable that the age at which rickets is most likely to develop (one to three years) coincides with a period of rapid growth (high need) and one in which there has been little chance to accumulate large body stores of vitamin D. The gradual accumulation of such stores with age doubtless accounts in large part for the infrequency of any evidences of vitamin D deficiency in adults.

The overall *functions* of vitamin D are to promote *growth* and proper *mineralization of the bones and teeth.* There is general agreement that the main result of its action is the *improvement of utilization of calcium and phosphorus* supplied in the food. Vitamin D increases the absorption of calcium, and secondarily also of phosphorus, from the intestinal tract. It is also involved with calcium mobilization from bones and with the preservation of phosphate by control of its excretion from the kidney (see Fig. 9–12). All these reactions help to keep the content of these two elements in the blood up to levels favorable to the deposition of calcium phosphate in the bones (the level of either or both of these elements in blood serum is depressed in rickets).

Some exciting discoveries have been made in recent years on the *metabolic and biochemical role* of vitamin D in the body. After vitamin D (cholecalciferol, D_3) is absorbed into the blood, it is carried to the liver by a specific vitamin D carrier protein (a globulin). Here it changes to an intermediary, more active metabolic form, newly discovered *25-hydroxycholecalciferol* (25-HCC) in which an OH group replaces an H atom on carbon number 25.* It is now known from studies

*Identified by DeLuca and co-workers of Wisconsin (Proc. Nat. Acad. Sci., *61*:1503, 1968; Amer. J. Clin. Nutr., *22*:412, 1969). DeLuca, now in charge of the laboratory of the late Dr. Steenbock, has also shown that ergocalciferol, D_2, is changed to a similar active metabolite in the liver—25-hydroxergocalciferol (25-HEC).

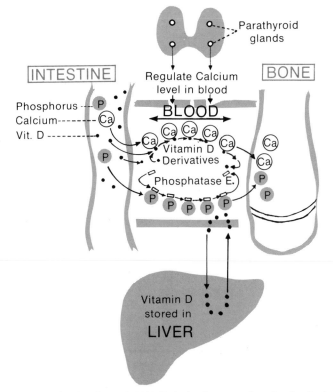

Figure 9–12. Diagram indicating how vitamin D derivatives may function in the body by increasing the absorption of calcium and phosphorus from the intestine, thus raising their level in the blood and promoting their deposition in bone. Reserves of vitamin D or their derivatives stored in the liver can be drawn on to keep up the level of this vitamin in blood and tissues during periods of low intake or extra need.

with chicks that this compound is transported in the blood by the same protein to the kidney where one more OH group is added, forming the compound *1,25-dihydroxycholecalciferol* (1,25-DHCC).[24] This appears to be the metabolically active form of vitamin D in the intestine and perhaps the bone. When ingested from food, it acts slightly more efficiently and rapidly than the parent compound.

The active compound (1,25-DHCC) has all the characteristics of a *hormone*, since it is a very active substance made in the body by one organ (the kidney) and transported in the blood to cells within target tissues. Vitamin D serves as a precursor, whether derived from the food or from the skin as a result of the action of light. (It is comparable, in a sense, to dietary essential amino acid precursors of several hormones, such as thyroxine.)

The new "hormone" (1,25-DHCC) appears to be the metabolically active form of the vitamin for increasing calcium absorption in the intestine and in serving other vitamin D dependent functions. For instance, a source of vitamin D is essential through this mechanism for the formation of a specific *ribonucleic acid*, necessary in turn for the formation of several important proteins including a *calcium-binding protein* in the cells of the intestine. This protein is essential for the absorption and transportation of calcium (along with the need for parathyroid hormone).

Vitamin D-active compounds appear, also, to be essential for the formation of at least two enzymes—*alkaline phosphatase* in intestinal lining (involved in calcium transport) and *adenosine triphosphatase*, which appears to be necessary for collagen formation in the bone (necessary for bone matrix). Vitamin D compounds also play a role, somehow, with other hormones, *in the regulation of amino acid levels* in the blood (by protecting against the loss of amino acids through the kidney) and of the *level of citric acid in tissues and bones.*

In some individuals, vitamin D from the food is not well absorbed, such as in "vitamin D-resistant rickets." The new metabolically active forms of vitamin D have been useful in the treatment of this and similar diseases in which there is a blockage of the conversion of natural vitamin D to the active forms.

Human Requirements

It is impossible to state the vitamin D requirements exactly. The amounts supplied by food can be estimated fairly well, but no one has been able to determine a way of knowing how much extra vitamin D is made in the body under the influence of sunlight.

Jeans and Stearns have made extensive studies of the effects of different levels of vitamin D intake on infants.[25] They have found that 135 IU daily prevents rickets, but that 300 to 400 IU daily results in more rapid growth (especially in length) and earlier eruption of teeth (if a supply of calcium and phosphorus is available, plentiful, and readily assimilable).

Less is known about the vitamin D requirements of older children than of infants. Jeans and Stearns showed that 300 to 400 IU daily in the form of cod liver oil favored calcium retention in children from 1 to 12 years of age. They state that in adolescence the need for this vitamin becomes "as universal and as great as in infancy." The Food and Nutrition Board (1968) recommends 400 IU of vitamin D daily from birth to 22 years of age, including breast-fed infants.[8]

The Board makes no recommendation for adults but states:[8] "The requirement of vitamin D in adult life is not known. The occurrence of deficiency states (though very rare) indicates that a small need exists, but it is considered that the amounts required are so small that under normal circumstances they are met by the vitamin D content of the usual mixed diet and by exposure to sunlight."

During pregnancy and lactation, supplemental vitamin D (400 IU daily) is recommended. A liberal supply at these periods is undoubtedly wise, because even though transmission to the fetus and milk is relatively low, the stores of vitamin D in the baby's body and the vitamin D content of milk are appreciably increased by vitamin D in the diet of the mother. In addition, optimum amounts of this vitamin promote the most efficient utilization by the mother of the calcium and phosphorus in her diet.

The amount of vitamin D that is made in the body through exposure to sunlight varies according to the *season*, the *locality* in which one lives, and one's *habits*. In the tropics bright sunlight is available the year round; nevertheless, rickets is still possible. In other parts of the world, sunlight is scarce during the winter months. Sunlight also is richer in ultraviolet rays in summer, and more of these rays get through to the "consumer" when the sun is directly overhead—between 10 A.M. and 2 P.M. On cloudy or foggy days and in cities troubled with "smog," almost all the ultraviolet rays are screened out before light penetrates to the people. Window glass and layers of clothing also effectively prevent ultraviolet rays from reaching the skin. Because only the ultraviolet rays (light of short wave length and high frequency) have the ability to bring about the chemical change by which vitamin D is formed, persons who live in cities can place little dependence on making this vitamin in their own bodies, especially in winter. Others who live and work outdoors in sunny regions manufacture a considerable amount of vitamin D with the aid of sunlight, and hence are less dependent on food for it. (See Fig. 9–13.)

Estimates of Vitamin D Intake and Nutritional Status

It is very difficult to estimate average vitamin D "intakes" of persons because of the difficulty of measuring that manufactured in the body by the effect of sunlight. Because of the widespread use of fortified milk and other foods, intakes of at least 400 IU daily must be the general rule in most persons. Filer[26] estimated, from studies with over 2000

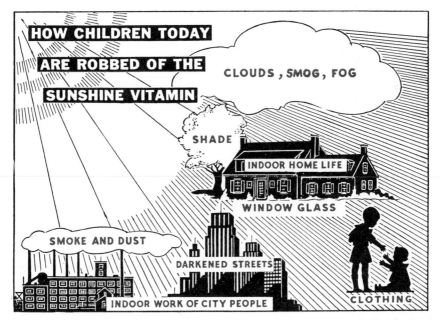

Figure 9–13. People in country districts and in the tropics can make vitamin D in their bodies through the agency of direct sunlight. This drawing shows some of the factors of modern life which screen out ultraviolet light and prevent people from exposure to sunlight, thus robbing them of the chance of making this vitamin in their bodies. (Courtesy of the Wisconsin Alumni Research Foundation.)

six-month-old infants, that they were receiving 390 IU from food alone (90 percent from enriched milk and 10 percent from egg). The Committee on Nutrition of the American Academy of Pediatrics pointed out that many older children may be receiving as much as 2000 to 3000 IU per day owing to the rather wide variety of fortified foods available.[27] This amount is considerably more than necessary.

Since the importance of vitamin D has been apreciated and the practice of giving vitamin D concentrates to young children has become widespread, severe cases of rickets are seldom seen in the United States, although mild rickets is still sometimes seen. The value of vitamin D administration is well illustrated by statistics of preschool children in Chicago, obtained from 1926 to 1932. Examination of the children before treatment showed 16 to 21 percent with definite evidence of rickets, but by 1935 the percentage had fallen to 7 percent with only 0.03 percent of cases of severe rickets. The incidence of severe rickets, on the basis of these 1935 figures, had been reduced to 3 cases per 10,000 children. The American Academy of Pediatrics made a survey in 1962 and found only 4 cases of rickets in every 10,000 pediatric admissions to hospitals.[28] Some of these may have been caused by mineral deficiencies or metabolic disorders, rather than by vitamin D lack. It is clear that rickets as a disease is well on the way to being eradicated in this country, but doubtless very many children do not achieve full growth and proper development of bones and teeth because of lack of optimum amounts of calcium, phosphorus, and/or vitamin D.

Public health nutritionists, nutrition educators, and all persons in countries who give nutrition advice to normal persons must always be alert to the possibility of indifference and forgetfulness concerning good nutrition habits. Vitamin D supplementation of infant diets is a case in point and has

become so routine that the importance of it might readily be forgotten. For instance, in Glasgow, Scotland, in 1963 there was an upswing in the incidence of rickets in infants.[29] Rickets in children has been recently observed in Canada (400 cases in only three pediatric hospitals in Montreal and Toronto in 1967 and 1968),[30] Greece (15 percent incidence in 330 infants), France (8 percent in aged persons in one hospital), Japan, South Africa, and Egypt, where it has been observed to a rather large extent in undernourished children in association with caloric deficiency. Fortification of milk and other foods with vitamin D has materially aided in preventing this problem in the United States and elsewhere.

Vitamin D in Foods

Nature's plan seems to have been that man should generate most of his supply of vitamin D by sunlight, for it is contained more sparsely in foods than is any other vitamin. In vegetable foods, it is present not at all or only in traces. It occurs with other fat-soluble vitamins in such foods of animal origin as egg yolk, butter fat, fatty fishes, and of course in liver, since this is the storage organ for it. The amounts found in these foods are small and vary widely according to the diet of the animal and the extent to which it has been exposed to sunlight. Because vitamin D is stable to heat and insoluble in water, there is little loss of it in the cooking or processing of foods.

Table 9–4 lists some typical food sources of vitamin D with the amount that may be counted on from an average serving, although the content in egg yolk and butter is higher if some rich source of vitamin D has been incorporated in the animals' feed, as is a common practice now. Eggs and dairy products furnish vitamin D in small quantities. Liver and fatty fish (sardines, salmon, mackerel) are good sources,

Table 9–4.   *Vitamin D Content of Typical Foods*

Food	Size of Serving	Avg. Vitamin D, IU
Fatty fish, canned:		
Herring	1 small fish (100 gm)	330
Salmon	100 gm	314
Tuna	5/8 cup solid (100 gm)	200–320
Eggs	1 medium-size egg	27
Butter	1 oz or 3 avg. pats (30 gm)	28
Liver, raw	2 lg. slices (100 gm)	15–45
Cream, light to heavy	1 oz or 2 tbsp	4–8
Milk, whole, fresh (enriched)	1 pint	200

but are infrequently used in U.S. diets. If the daily diet contains one egg, three tablespoons of butter, and a pint of un-enriched milk, one would get only about 65 IU of vitamin D from natural foods. Three ounces of salmon would provide about 300 IU. Most adults seem to get along at least fairly well on the small amounts furnished in foods, sup-plemented with the amounts they gen-erate under the influence of sunlight.

Human milk has only about 20 IU of vitamin D per liter, an insufficient amount to prevent rickets (even though calcium intake is adequate). Breast-fed infants require supplementation with vitamin D or exposure to ample sun-light.

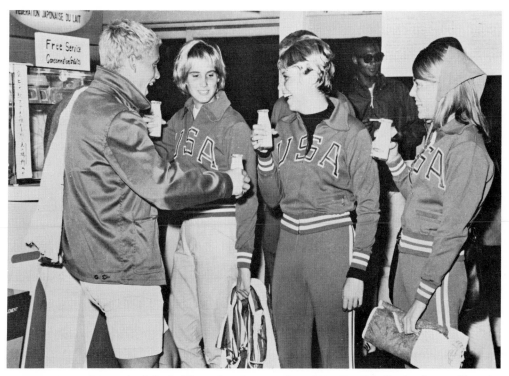

Figure 9–14.   A portrait of physical fitness based on sound nutrition. Don Schollander, former Olympic swimming champion, visits with members of the United States' women's swimming team at the Olympic games in Tokyo. (Courtesy of American Dairy Association.)

Enriched Foods and Other Rich
Sources of Vitamin D

Supplements of vitamin D for infants, usually in the presence of other vitamins and made from synthetic sources of vitamin D, are now readily available, replacing the older, more expensive, and less palatable fish-liver oil concentrates. Synthetic vitamin D can now be purchased in large wholesale lots for only 3 cents per million units (sufficient for seven years!), which is almost as cheap as sunshine itself and much more dependable. The cost of fortifying a quart of milk is therefore negligible (less than 1/100th of a cent). Vitamin D supplements vary greatly in concentration—often as little as one or two drops supply a full day's requirement. Other foods are quite widely fortified with vitamin D today, so much so that under certain situations there could be danger of getting too much vitamin D (see next section). About 85 percent of all fresh milk is fortified with 400 IU of vitamin D per quart, as is all evaporated milk.[27] Many breakfast foods are fortified (usually from 80 to 400 IU per serving) as are various margarines (125 to 250 IU per ounce) and milk flavorings (from 5 to 150 IU per glass of milk).

Recently, because of the dangers of overconsumption of vitamin D, the Committee of Nutrition of the American Academy of Pediatrics has become concerned about the widespread enrichment programs.[27, 31] Also, because of this, the Food and Drug Administration is considering making changes in its regulations by limiting the foods which may be enriched to milk products only. Obviously when vitamin D-enriched milk is used in the amount of one quart daily, no other source of the vitamin is required.

Toxicity

Enough is better than too much as far as vitamin D is concerned, and

mothers (especially mothers who believe in the practice of "overinsurance") should be warned of this fact in case they are giving high potency vitamin D preparations to their children. There is evidence that certain infants are especially sensitive to the toxic action of vitamin D and may be adversely affected by intakes as low as 3000 to 4000 IU per day (as shown by abnormally high calcium levels in the blood, loss of appetite, and retarded growth).[27, 31] With daily doses of 20,000 to 40,000 IU for infants, or 75,000 to 100,000 IU for adults, serious toxic symptoms may develop; these include vomiting, diarrhea, weakness, loss of weight, and kidney damage. The serum calcium is elevated to such a degree that deposits of calcium salts may be found in various organs.

Adults should be cautioned against the massive doses of this vitamin sometimes taken for arthritis and other diseased conditions over long periods. Even moderate overdosage with vitamin D is not good for the elderly. With water-soluble vitamins, overdosage is wasteful but not harmful because the excess is excreted in urine. With fat-soluble vitamins, the excess remains in the body in such quantities that, in the case of vitamin D and to a lesser extent with vitamin A, it may give rise to toxic conditions. Concentrated preparations of any of the fat-soluble vitamins should be used with caution and only under direction of a physician.

VITAMIN E

Vitamin E has recently become a household word. There is much interest in it because of newer knowledge showing its practical importance in human nutrition (but unfortunately much of the current enthusiasm for the vitamin is without experimental basis). Ever since its discovery it has been known as an important vitamin for laboratory and farm animals, so the current interest has some theoretical basis for support.

Discovery and Chemical Properties

In 1922, Evans and Bishop, of the University of California, discovered that a third unknown fat-soluble dietary factor (*factor X*) in lettuce and wheat germ was essential for successful *reproduction* in rats.[32] Several years later, Sure of the University of Arkansas suggested the term *vitamin E* for the factor, and this was widely accepted.[33] With use of the discovery of Olcott and Mattill that the vitamin was an alcohol and had *antioxidant properties,*[34] Evans* and his co-workers isolated crystalline vitamin E from wheat germ oil in 1936 and named it *tocopherol* (from Greek words meaning "to bear offspring").[35] The structures of the four natural forms of the tocopherols (alpha, beta, gamma, and delta) were soon determined, and synthesis was accomplished in the laboratory. (See formula of alpha-tocopherol in the Appendix. It is biologically the most active natural form.)

Four other closely related compounds with various degrees of vitamin E activity (from 1 to 50 percent) occur in food: the alpha-, beta-, gamma-, and delta-*tocotrienols*. Because foods contain significant amounts of almost all eight natural forms,[36] the milligrams of *alpha-tocopherol equivalent* has been recommended recently as a summation term for all vitamin E activity.† When this is done the nutrition student does not have to be concerned about the individual activity of the various forms (though the situation is still very complicated, especially since the antioxidant properties of the various compounds do not correspond well with other biological activities, and there are species differences).

The vitamin E compounds are light yellow, viscous oils, insoluble in water, stable to heat but readily destroyed by oxidation and ultraviolet light. They are not destroyed to any great extent by temperatures used in cooking, though some loss occurs in frozen foods and in processing. Because they are capable of taking up oxygen, vitamin E compounds function in the body to protect certain other compounds (such as vitamin A, carotenes, and unsaturated fatty acids) from oxidation by acting as an antioxidant. The tocopherols are the chief antioxidants in natural fats and oils and act to prevent fats from becoming rancid. They are often added to food to help stabilize other valuable nutrients. Vitamin E is available in over 40 forms with different degrees of activity but most commonly as the active alpha-tocopherol acetate. None of the forms are especially toxic, even when taken in relatively large amounts.

Effects of Vitamin E Deficiency

Studies by Horwitt and others have shown that man requires vitamin E for normal creatine excretion and for the prevention of blood disorders (including an anemia, and in a laboratory test, the rupturing of isolated red blood cells by oxidizing agents in the so-called "hemolysis" test).[8] There is no convincing evidence that vitamin E deficiency in man causes reduced athletic performance, heart disease, weakened sex drive, muscular dystrophy, sterility, or reduced longevity, as is often claimed.‡ Deficiencies of this vitamin

---

*Dr. Herbert Evans, who also was co-discoverer of the growth hormone, remained very active until his death in 1971. Dr. Katherine Bishop, a physician, still lives in Berkeley. Dr. Harold Olcott[34] and Dr. Gladys Emerson[35] are now on the University of California faculty at Davis and Los Angeles, respectively.

†See J. Nutr., *101*:133, 1971. This change should help eventually to eliminate the confusing "International Unit," a summation term used for many years in vitamin E measurements. Currently, nomenclature groups have tentatively recommended that the new International Unit of vitamin E be made equal to 0.60 mg of alpha-tocopheryl acetate, a much more stable chemical form than the free vitamin (J. Nutr., *101*:1278, 1971; Lipids, *6*:281, 1971). On this basis, 1 IU is equal to 0.55 mg of the natural alpha-tocopherol (or 1 mg equals about 1.8 IU). In other words, when using tables giving vitamin E values in IU, convert to milligrams of alpha-tocopherol equivalents by multiplying the IU value by 0.55 if this proposed conversion factor is used.

---

‡Nor would the reverse be true. In other words, extra amounts of vitamin E in a diet would not be expected to improve these conditions in man.

appear to be very rare, though the requirement is increased considerably by added polyunsaturated fatty acids (see p. 213).

In rats which have been deprived of vitamin E, the males become permanently sterile, and pregnant females are unable to carry their young to full term, because lack of this vitamin results in death and reabsorption of the embryos in the uterus. Fertility of female rats is not destroyed, however, and when given sufficient vitamin E later, they give birth to normal litters. Young rats (and other animals), after several months on diets deficient in vitamin E, *fail to grow normally* and also develop *weakness and degeneration of the skeletal muscles*, a condition known as *nutritional muscular dystrophy*, which may also be accompanied by paralysis. Lesions have also been found in heart muscle.

Deficiencies of this vitamin have been obtained in many species other than the rat. In the chick, brain lesions and muscular dystrophy occur. Liver damage and a number of other muscular symptoms have been seen in deficient mice, pigs, dogs, and other animals. It is a misnomer to call this the "reproduction vitamin," as is often done, because there are so many more specific symptoms of deficiency and because all vitamins are necessary for reproduction.

Relationship to Selenium

In 1957, a very interesting dietary relationship of vitamin E to a trace mineral was discovered when it became known that extremely low levels of *selenium* could replace the vitamin E need of animals under certain conditions.[37] The full significance of this discovery to human nutrition has not been worked out as yet, but there are large geographic areas in the United States, and in other countries, where farm animals (usually sheep or cattle) with "white muscle disease" are cured by injections or by feeding combinations of selenium and vitamin E (see Chap. 12).

Functions of Vitamin E

Vitamin E deficiency presents such a wide variety of symptoms in so many animals that one might assume that it would be a part of many enzyme systems. However, there is no known specific coenzyme form of the vitamin in tissues (in spite of claims to the contrary), nor does it seem to play a specific role in any enzymatic reaction. Symptoms of a deficiency may be prevented in experimental animals by other antioxidants or by much lower amounts of selenium. Several generations of animals have been reared without any vitamin E in the diet but with selenium and an antioxidant present. Therefore, the role of vitamin E in the body appears to be related entirely to its antioxidant role at the intracellular level. It is highly efficient in preventing cell membrane damage from naturally occurring *peroxides*, forms of toxic *free radicals* formed from fatty acids—substances that have been suggested as playing a role in the aging process.

Vitamin E protects both vitamin A and carotene from destruction by oxidation, especially in the alimentary tract. In this way, vitamin E spares the supply of vitamin A available to the body, which may be of importance if the intake of vitamin A is barely adequate for body needs.

Requirement for Vitamin E

The Food and Nutrition Board in 1968 (for the first time) set a recommended allowance for vitamin E.[8] The suggested daily allowances for college men and women, and older persons, are given in Table 9–5. Figures for other ages are given in Table 1 of the Appendix.

The requirement of vitamin E for man is known to vary with other ingredients in the diet, as it does for animals. For instance, the presence of large amounts of *linoleic acid* or other

Table 9–5. *Recommended Dietary Allowance for Vitamin E Activity* *

	Age	IU/DAY	Allowance ALPHA-TOCOPHEROL† EQUIVALENTS/DAY (MG)
Males	14–18 years old	25	14
	18 years and over	30	16.5
Females	14 years and over	25	14
	Pregnant	30	16.5
	Lactating	30	16.5

*From Food and Nutrition Board, 1968[8] (except last column).
†Calculated on basis of second footnote, page 211.

polyunsaturated fatty acids in the diet markedly increases the requirement. This has significance in today's dietary pattern in which large amounts of vegetable oils are widely used. Also, the presence of rancid fats, oxidizing substances, and selenium would be expected to modify the requirement for vitamin E. The recommended level is very generous and should cover all contingencies. Adults eating low amounts of polyunsaturated fatty acids need only 10 IU alpha-tocopherol equivalents per day, according to the Food and Nutrition Board.

Nutritional Status

Naturally occurring vitamin E deficiencies in adult man in the United States are extremely unusual. In the classic experiments with men volunteers in Illinois by Horwitt and associates,[38] a deficient diet was fed about three years before any symptoms became evident. However, low blood or tissue levels of vitamin E, indicative of too low an intake and/or destruction by excessive polyunsaturated fatty acids, have been observed in infants and adults in this country.[8, 39] This should not be too surprising in light of the losses of vitamin E in food processing and because of high polyunsaturated fat intakes. Estimates of vitamin E intake in the United States appear to average about 10 to 20 IU, less than the current recommended allowance. In Britain, recent studies[40] show the vita-

min E content of the majority of diets to be less than 10 IU per day (similar to intakes in Japan and India).

Obviously, many persons are consuming less than recommended amounts of vitamin E, but our state of knowledge is such that one cannot say such persons will develop a deficiency. The allowance may be set too high this first time. In the absence of enough knowledge it would be prudent, nevertheless, to consume diets with enough vitamin E sources to supply the recommended level. However, there is no reason to consume more than this under normal circumstances, as has been explained.

Vitamin E deficiencies in man have also been seen in other parts of the world. Leonard found 15 percent of a group of 490 Uganda African subjects to be deficient in vitamin E as measured by the *hemolysis test*.[41] Others have reported an anemia from vitamin E deficiencies associated with kwashiorkor (protein deficiency) in infants in Egypt.[42]

Vitamin E in Foods

In a typical American diet, about 66 percent of the intake of vitamin E comes from salad oils, shortening, margarines, and other fats and oils. (Normally, then, persons eating extra polyunsaturated fats will also consume extra vitamin E.) The rest of the vitamin E in our diet comes mainly from whole grains, liver, beans, and fruits and vegetables.[36, 43]

Only recently has it been possible to

measure with reasonable accuracy the various forms of vitamin E in foods[36] (see Table 9–6 for representative values). However, there is not sufficient knowledge as yet to know the vitamin E activity in many of these various forms, so one must be very cautious in interpreting such values. Because of the lack of general availability of figures for vitamin E in food, however, Table 9–7 gives the alpha-tocopherol content of representative foods based on recent methods. Use of these figures in calculating one's intake will give a conservative value (somewhat lower, in most cases, than the total vitamin E activity), since other, lower potency forms of the vitamin are disregarded. In general, most seeds and oils from these seeds are the best sources of vitamin E. Some vegetables are also good sources, especially green leafy vegetables. Wheat germ oil is one of the richest natural sources. Synthetic forms of vitamin E are the least expensive sources, although we recommend that vitamin E be consumed in a regular diet in so far as possible, in order to get all the other essential nutrients also.

The vitamin E activity of foods may be considerably reduced in processing, storage, and packaging.[36, 43] For instance, as much as 80 percent or more may be lost in converting whole wheat to white bread. Freezing of vegetables is also known to cause some destruction of vitamin E — a finding rather unique among the vitamins.

VITAMIN K

The fourth, but not the least, of the fat-soluble vitamins was discovered in studies with the chick in 1935 by Dam* of Copenhagen, and a few months later independently by Almquist and Stokstad of the University of California.[44] Because the vitamin is essential for the proper coagulation of blood, Dam proposed that it be called the *Koagulation vitamin* (the Danish and German spelling of the word), from which the term *vitamin K* was derived.† Vitamin K was isolated in pure form in 1939, and shortly thereafter it was synthesized and its chemical structure determined. Deficiencies are rare in man, except in infants or persons re-

---

*Dam, still living in Copenhagen, received the Nobel Prize for this in 1943 with Dr. Doisey of St. Louis (who first determined the structure of vitamin K_2).

†Vitamins I and J, now obsolete terms for other vitamins, were proposed also in 1935, so that the use of the latter K was in alphabetical order.

The terms vitamin L (for "lactation"), vitamin M (now folacin), vitamin N, vitamin P (for the bioflavonoids), and vitamins R, S, T, U, and V have since appeared in the literature but are all obsolete.

Table 9–6.   *Several Common Forms of Vitamin E in Representative Oils**

	Alpha-tocopherol	Alpha-tocotrienol	Beta-tocopherol	Gamma-tocopherol	Delta-tocopherol
Relative biological potency (estimated)	100	20–30	35	1	1
Food Sources:		mg/100 gm			
Corn oil	11	5	5	60	2
Cottonseed oil	39	–	–	39	–
Palm oil	26	14	–	32	7
Peanut oil	13	–	–	21	2
Safflower oil	39	–	–	17	24
Soybean oil	10	–	–	59	26
Wheat germ oil	133	3	71	26	27

*Adapted from Slover.[36]

Table 9–7. Alpha-tocopherol Content of Representative Foods*

Food	mg/100 gm	Food	mg/100 gm
Seeds		*Vegetables and fruits*	
Almond	27.0	Asparagus, fresh	1.8
Barley	0.5	Carrots, fresh	0.5
Corn	0.6	Beans, dry	0.1 to 0.7
Oat	0.5	Mango, ripe	1.0
Rice, white	0.1	Potatoes	0.1
Rice, whole	0.3	Green leafy (most)	1 to 10
Wheat	1.4	Corn, fresh	0.1
Peanuts	10.0	Most fruits, fresh	0.1 to 1.0
Peas	0.5		
		Other foods	
Oils		Potato chips	2.1
Coconut	0.5	Sugar cookie	2.0 to 5.0
Cod liver	29.0	Eggs	1.0
Corn	11.0	Liver	2.0
Cottonseed	39.0	Cod fish	0.2 to 1.2
Olive	5.0	Beef	1.0
Palm	26.0	Lobster	1.7
Peanut	13.0	Butter	2.0
Rapeseed	18.4	Lard	1.2
Safflower	39.0	Margarine	10.0
Soybean	10.0	Shortening (vegetable)	10.0
Sunflower	49.0	Milk (cow's)	0.1
Walnut	56.0	Yeast	0
Wheat germ	133.0	Infant cereals	0.1 to 1.0
		Wheat flour	0.2
		Wheat germ	13.0
		Bread	0.2

*Most values adapted from Slover[36] and Dicks.[43] (Values are for alpha-tocopherol only.)

ceiving antagonists (see p. 130) or with clinical problems related to absorption. Considerable use, however, is made of synthetic substances which act as *antagonists* of vitamin K (such as dicoumarol, an anticoagulant) to prevent clotting of the blood in patients with certain circulatory disorders. The antagonists are also, interestingly enough, used as very potent rat killers (such as warfarin) which destroy the rat by preventing its blood from clotting.

Properties and Distribution

Vitamins K_1 and K_2* are two forms of chemicals known as *quinones* (see formula of vitamin K_1 in Appendix) which exist naturally in plants (especially green leaves) and in foods which have undergone bacterial fermentation. Several synthetic forms, such as menaquinone (formerly menadione) and its various water-soluble derivatives, are converted to vitamin K_2 in the body, and thus have similar vitamin K activity when fed to animals (but unlike the natural forms, are toxic when given in large amounts). All forms of the vitamin are yellow and are quite stable to heat, air, and moisture, but not to light. Cooking destroys very little of the vitamin because it is not water soluble.

Food sources of vitamin K include all the green leafy vegetables, egg yolk, soybean oil, and liver.[45] Lettuce, spinach, kale, cauliflower, and cabbage are

*Most recent nomenclature rules (J. Nutr., *101*:133, 1971) use the chemical name *phytylmenaquinone* (formerly phylloquinone) for vitamin K_1 and *multiprenylmenaquinones* for the several vitamins K_2 (all derivatives of menaquinone). Vitamin K_1 is the natural form generally found in plant foods, whereas the several vitamins K_2 appear to be the active forms present in bacteria and the animal body.

excellent sources; the inner leaves of cabbage have about one-fourth as much as the outer leaves. Very little vitamin K is present in most cereals, fruits, carrots, peas, meats, or highly refined foods.

Effects of Deficiency

The first studies with vitamin K were made with chicks. When vitamin K is absent, they develop delayed blood clotting, causing hemorrhages under the skin, serious internal bleeding, and if not corrected, death. Deficiencies have also been produced in cattle, pigs, rats, dogs, man, and all other species studied. Often a drug, such as a sulfa drug or an antibiotic, is added to the diet of the experimental animal in order to reduce biosynthesis of the vitamin by intestinal organisms. Also, experimentally, the animals sometimes are raised in a "germ-free" environment; hence, they have no intestinal flora and no vitamin K deficiency.

Vitamin K deficiency formerly was quite common in commercial poultry flocks in this country because of the widespread use of sulfa drugs and antibiotics for the prevention of disease and for growth promotion. In spite of the many natural foodstuffs that poultry rations contained, they were surprisingly quite low in vitamin K, especially when dried alfalfa was not included. Today, synthetic forms of vitamin K or alfalfa are widely used in such diets for supplementary purposes and suc-

cessfully prevent signs of deficiency. The lesson of this for human nutrition is quite obvious.

Role in the Body

The primary function of vitamin K in the body is the formation in the liver of a protein called *prothrombin*, which is necessary for the clotting, or coagulation, of blood. Several other substances, or "factors,"* needed for blood clotting also depend on vitamin K.

Prothrombin is converted to its active form—*thrombin*—which in turn is necessary for the formation of fibrin, a protein which is the basis for a blood clot, as is illustrated by the simplified diagram at the bottom of the page.

Without vitamin K, or when an antagonist is given, prothrombin (and several related substances) cannot be formed, and the blood will not clot. The exact biochemical mechanism for the formation of prothrombin in the liver, and the role of vitamin K, is being studied now. Various mechanisms for its clotting action have been proposed involving a role in important cellular enzymes at the ribosome level, but a biochemical role is still unknown. Vitamin K appears not to be useful to the body other than its role in clotting.

---

*Known as Factors VII (proconvertin), IX (Christmas factor), and X (Stuart factor), all proteins apparently. Prothrombin is also known as Factor II.

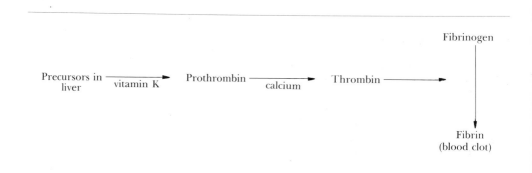

*Requirement and Nutritional
Status*

No allowance for vitamin K has been set as yet by the Food and Nutrition Board because of the "lack of reliable information concerning human intakes of vitamin K" and for other reasons.[8] Apparently, bacteria in the intestine provide considerable vitamin K for most persons. The Board states that "deficiency is likely to occur in premature or anoxic infants and in those born to mothers receiving anticoagulants." A large, corrective oral dose of 1 to 2 mg used for the infant in such cases is probably considerably higher than the minimum requirement.[46] Giving the vitamin to the infant appears to be superior to supplying extra amounts of it to the mother before childbirth.

Deficiencies have been seen in babies receiving drugs for diarrhea or intestinal infections. A normal infant's requirement must be about 15 mcg per day, the amount present in 1 liter of human milk. The adult minimum requirement must be around 30 mcg per day, since this amount was necessary to restore clotting in a group of vitamin K-depleted adults.[47] (This makes this vitamin among the most potent of all the vitamins.) On the basis of the requirement of the rat, humans would need about 50 mcg per day as a minimum.

Vitamin K deficiency, as evidenced by internal hemorrhages, has occurred in man under situations in which absorption of the vitamin is hindered or prevented, as in any condition in which bile flow is disturbed, such as obstructive jaundice, or after injuries or surgical operations (as with the other fat-soluble vitamins). Under such conditions, extra doses of vitamin K given with bile salts have proved effective in raising the level of prothrombin in the blood, thus restoring the normal clotting ability of the blood, even though there may be sufficient vitamin K in the diet otherwise. Unless these abnormal conditions exist, vitamin K deficiency would seldom be seen in man. There appears to be no reason for a normal individual eating a varied diet of traditional foods to feel that his diet does not contain

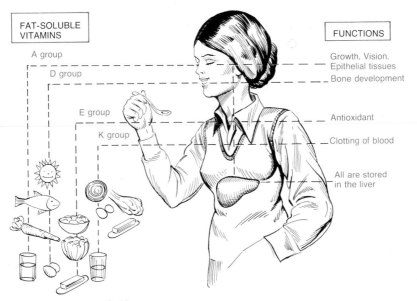

Figure 9–15. Fat-soluble vitamins and their functions.

an adequate supply of this vitamin. Vitamin K has proved ineffective in hemophilia—an inherited condition causing abnormal hemorrhaging in man.

Toxicity

Synthetic menaquinone and its various derivatives (vitamin K_3) have produced certain toxic symptoms in rats and jaundice in human infants when given in relatively low amounts (over 5 mg).[8, 46] Consequently, the Food and Drug Administration of the United States requested in 1963 the removal of all menaquinone (even 1 mg levels) from all food supplements, including prenatal vitamin capsules. The natural forms of vitamins K_1 and K_2 may still be used for this purpose, because they have not exhibited signs of toxicity even when given in large amounts.

QUESTIONS AND PROBLEMS

1. Tell in a general way how fat-soluble vitamins differ from water-soluble ones in each of the following respects: solubilities, types of food in which they are carried, losses in cooking and processing of foods, conditions necessary for good absorption from intestine, path or paths of excretion, and ability to be stored in the body.

2. Name four fat-soluble vitamins and give for each one its chief use (or uses) in the body and the effects of moderate and severe lack of it in the diet. How does its function in nutrition account for the type of symptoms that result from an insufficient supply?

3. What is meant by provitamins or vitamin precursors? Name the precursors of vitamin A, and tell in what classes of foods they are found. How and to what extent are they made into vitamin A in the body? What foods contain both the provitamins A and vitamin A? Which contain only provitamins A? What determines whether the vitamin A value of eggs, milk, and butter is high or low? Is the depth of color of egg yolk and milk fat a reliable index of their vitamin A value? Why? Does the depth of color of green and yellow vegetables indicate their relative vitamin A value, and why?

4. List ten vegetables and three fruits of high vitamin A value. List the five foods of animal origin that are the richest sources of vitamin A (consult Table 9–1 and tables in the Appendix for vitamin A values of individual foods).

5. Plan a diet that will furnish 2500 IU of vitamin A (total activity). Modify this diet so that it provides 5000 IU of vitamin A. Substitute foods or add some rich sources of vitamin A, so that the diet as modified supplies 10,000 IU (or more) of vitamin A. Is it difficult to get as much as 5000 IU (recommended daily allowance for adults) in the diet? What will happen if the diet supplies 2500 IU one day and 10,000 IU the next day? Of what advantage is it to have an intake of vitamin A considerably in excess of the minimum requirement?

6. What are the earliest symptoms of vitamin A deficiency? What course would you recommend for getting rid of such symptoms?

7. What are the precursors of vitamin D and where are they found? By what means are they transformed into vitamin D? Under what circumstances can this vitamin be made in the body? Under what conditions will persons make little of this vitamin in their bodies and so be dependent almost entirely on food sources for their supply of vitamin D? What foods carry small and variable amounts of vitamin D? How may the natural low content of vitamin D in foods be increased? What foods have been reinforced as to their vitamin D content?

8. At what periods of life is the need for vitamins A and D relatively high, and why? What rich source (or sources) of these vitamins is usually given at these periods to insure a plentiful supply of vitamins A and D? Why does a

baby that is breast fed derive more benefit if supplementary vitamins A and D are given to it directly than if they are given to its mother?

9. How can rickets be prevented? How can it be cured? Discuss why rickets is no longer a common disease.

10. What are the chief symptoms of deficiency of vitamin E; of vitamin K? Why are such deficiencies seldom seen in man? What are the chief functions of vitamins E and K in the body?

11. Which fat-soluble vitamins may be toxic if taken over long periods in large doses?

12. Describe some important research now underway with any of the fat-soluble vitamins.

REFERENCES

1. McCollum, E. V.: *A History of Nutrition.* Boston, Houghton Mifflin Co., 1957.
2. McCollum, E. V., and Davis, M.: J. Biol. Chem., *15*:167, 1913; *19*:245, 1914; *23*:181, 1915; Osborne, T. B., and Mendel, L. B.: J. Biol. Chem., *15*:311, 1913; *16*:423, 1913–1914.
3. Karrer, P., et al.: Helv. Chim. Acta, *14*:1036, 1431, 1931; Chem. Rev., *14*:17, 1934.
4. Holmes, H. N., and Corbet, R. E.: J. Amer. Chem. Soc., *59*:2042, 1937.
5. Karrer, P., et al.: Helv. Chim. Acta, *12*:1142, 1929.
6. Steenbock, H., and Boutwell, P. W.: J. Biol. Chem., *41*:81, 1920; *42*:131, 1920.
7. Moore, T.: Biochem. J., *24*:692, 1930.
8. Food and Nutrition Board: *Recommended Dietary Allowances.* 7th Ed., Publ. 1694, Washington, D.C., National Academy of Sciences, 1968.
9. Wald, G., et al.: Vitam. Horm., *1*:195, 1943; *18*:417, 1960; Fed. Proc., *12*:607, 1953; Nature, *219*:800, 1968; Science, *162*:230, 1968.
10. Callison, E. C., et al.: J. Nutr., *37*:139, 1949.
11. Rountree, J. I.: J. Nutr., *3*:345, 1931; Dutcher, R. A., et al.: J. Nutr., *8*:269, 1934; Smith, M. C., and Spector, H.: Ariz. Agric. Expt. Sta. Tech. Bull., *84*:375, 1940; Becker, G. L.: Amer. J. Dig. Dis., *19*:344, 1952.
12. Peterson, P. A.: J. Biol. Chem., *246*:34, 1971; *246*:44, 1971.
13. Report of a joint FAO/WHO Expert Group: *Requirement of Vitamin A, Thiamine, Riboflavin, and Niacin.* FAO Nutr. Meet. Rep. Ser. No. 41, Rome, 1967; Rao, C. N., and Rao, B. S. N.: Amer. J. Clin. Nutr., *23*:105, 1970.
14. Seawright, A. A., and English, P. B.: Nature, *206*:1171, 1965; Herbst, E. J.: Science, *100*:338, 1944.
15. Morgan, A. F.: J. Home Econ., *52*:631, 1960; Kelsay, J. L.: J. Nutr., *99* (No. 1, Part II, Suppl. 1): 119, 1969; Davis, T. R. A., Gershoff, S. N., and Gamble, D. F.: J. Nutr. Educ., *1* (Fall, Suppl. 1): 39, 1969; Schaefer, A. E.: J. Amer. Dietet. Assoc., *54*:371, 1969; Nutr. Today, *4*:2, 1969.
16. Guthrie, H. A.: J. Amer. Dietet. Assoc., *43*:120, 1963; Filer, L. J., Jr., and Martinez, G. A.: Clin. Pediat., *3*:633, 1964.
17. Friend, B.: *National Food Situation.* Washington, D.C., Government Printing Office, November, 1970.
18. McClaren, D. S.: Medical World News, Jan. 26, 1968.
19. Roels, O. A., et al.: Amer. J. Clin. Nutr., *12*:380, 1963.
20. Gopalan, C., et al.: Amer. J. Clin. Nutr., *8*:833, 1960.
21. Sweeney, J. P., and Marsh, A. C.: J. Amer. Dietet. Assoc., *59*:238, 1971; Heierli, C.: Internat. J. Vit. Res., *40*:515, 1970.
22. See reviews by Chick, H.: Lancet, Aug. 13 and 20, p. 325 and 377, 1932; Powers, G. V., et al.: J. Amer. Med. Assoc., *78*:159, 1922; Stein, H. B., and Lewis, R. C.: Amer. J. Dis. Child., *41*:62, 1931.
23. McCollum, E. V., et al.: J. Biol. Chem., *53*:293, 1922.
24. DeLuca, H. F., et al.: Biochem., *10*:2799, 1971; *10*:2935, 1971; Proc. Nat. Acad. Sci., *68*:803, 1971; Lawson, D. E. M., et al.: Nature, *230*:228, 1971.
25. Jeans, P. C., and Stearns, G.: J. Pediat., *13*:730, 1938; J. Amer. Med. Assoc., *11*:703, 1938; Jeans, P. C.: J. Amer. Med. Assoc., *143*:177, 1950.
26. Filer, L. J., Jr., and Martinez, G. A.: Clin. Pediat., *3*:633, 1964.
27. American Academy of Pediatrics, Committee on Nutrition: Pediatrics, *31*:512, 1963.
28. American Academy of Pediatrics, Committee on Nutrition: Pediatrics, *29*:646, 1962.
29. Arneil, G. C., and Crosbie, J. C.: Lancet, 2:423, 1963.
30. Report of Canadian Council on Nutrition: Canadian Nutr. Notes, *24*:85, 1968.
31. American Academy of Pediatrics, Committee on Nutrition: Pediatrics, *40*:1050, 1967.
32. Evans, H. M., and Bishop, K. S.: Science, *56*:650, 1922.
33. Sure, B.: J. Biol. Chem., *58*:693, 1924; *62*:371, 1924; *63*:211, 1925.
34. Olcott, H. S., and Matill, H. A.: J. Biol. Chem., *93*:59, 1931; Olcott, H. S.: J. Biol. Chem., *110*:695, 1935.
35. Evans, H. M., Emerson, O. H., and Emerson, G. A.: J. Biol. Chem., *113*:319, 1936.
36. Slover, H. T.: Lipids, *6*:291, 1971.
37. Schwarz, K., and Foltz, C. M.: J. Amer. Chem. Soc., *79*:3292, 1957.

38. Horwitt, M. K.: Amer. J. Clin. Nutr., *8*:451, 1960; J. Amer. Dietet. Assoc., *38*:231, 1961; Fed. Proc., *24*:68, 1964.
39. Hassan, H., et al.: Amer. J. Clin. Nutr., *19*: 147, 1966; Ritchie, et al.: New Eng. J. Med., *279*:1185, 1968; Oski, F. A., and Barness, L. A.: J. Pediatrics, *70*:211, 1967; Harris, P. L.: Proc. Soc. Exp. Biol. Med., *107*:381, 1961.
40. Smith, C. L., et al.: Brit. J. Nutr., *26*:89, 1971.
41. Leonard, P. J.: Trans. Roy. Soc. Trop. Med. Hyg., *58*:517, 1964.
42. Sandstead, H. H., et al.: Amer. J. Clin. Nutr., *17*:27, 1965.
43. Booth, V. H., and Bradford, M. P.: Brit. J. Nutr., *17*:575, 1963; Bunnel, R. H., et al.: Amer. J. Clin. Nutr., *17*:1, 1965; Dicks, M. W.: *Vitamin E Content of Foods and Feeds for Human and Animal Consumption.* Bulletin 435, Agric. Expt. Stat., Univ. Wyoming, 1965; Dicks-Bushnell, M. W., and Davis, K. C.: Amer. J. Clin. Nutr., *20*:262, 1967.
44. Dam, H.: Nature, *135*:652, 1935; Biochem. J., *29*:1273, 1935; Almquist, H. J., and Stokstad, E. L. R.: Nature, *136*:31, 1935; J. Biol. Chem., *111*:105, 1935.
45. H. J. Heinz Co.: *Nutritional Data.* 6th Ed. Pittsburgh, 1965, p. 29.
46. American Academy of Pediatrics, Committee on Nutrition: Pediatrics, *28*:501, 1961.
47. Frick, P. G., et al.: J. Appl. Physiol., *23*: 387, 1967.

SUPPLEMENTARY READING

General (Vitamins A, D, E, and K)
(also see references at end of Chap. 6)

Bauernfeind, J. C., Rubin, S. H., Surmatis, J. D., and Ofner, A.: Carotenoids and fat-soluble vitamins: Contribution to food, feed and pharmaceuticals. Internat. J. Vit. Res., *40*:391, 1970.
DeLuca, H. F., and Suttie, J. W. (eds.): *The Fat-Soluble Vitamins.* Madison, University of Wisconsin Press, 1970.
Morton, R. A.: The history of vitamin research. Internat. J. Vit. Res., *38*:5, 1968.
Ostwald, R., and Briggs, G. M.: Toxicity of the vitamins. In Food Protection Committee, Food and Nutrition Board: *Toxicants Occurring Naturally in Foods.* Washington, D.C., National Academy of Sciences Publ. No. 1354, 1966.

Nutrition Reviews

Early experiences with fish oils—a retrospect (by Bills, C. E.). *13*:65, 1955.
Lipids and fat soluble vitamins in cellular metabolism. *24*:272, 1966.

Vitamin A
(also see refs. 1–21)

General, History, and Reviews

McLaren, D. S.: Present knowledge of the role of vitamin A in health and disease. Trans. Roy. Soc. Trop. Med. Hyg., *60*:436, 1966.
Morton, R. A. (chairman): Symposium: Vitamin A. Proc. Nutr. Soc., *24*:127, 1965.
Olson, J. A.: The metabolism of vitamin A. Pharm. Rev., *19*:559, 1967.
Rodriguez, M. S., and Irwin, M. I.: A conspectus of research on vitamin A requirements of man. J. Nutr., *102*:909, 1972.
Roels, O. A.: Vitamin A physiology. J. Amer. Med. Assoc., *214*:1097, 1970.
Wolf, G. (chairman): International symposium on the metabolic function of vitamin A. Amer. J. Clin. Nutr., *22*:897, 1969.

Other References

Bieri, J. G., McDaniel, E. G., and Rogers, W. E., Jr.: Survival of germfree rats without vitamin A. Science, *163*:574, 1969.
Chopra, J. G., and Kevany, J.: Hypovitaminosis A in the Americas. Amer. J. Clin. Nutr., *23*:231, 1970.
Cleland, J., and Southcott, R. V.: Hypervitaminosis A in the Antarctic in the Australasian Antarctic expedition of 1911–1914: A possible explanation of the illnesses of Mertz and Mawson. Med. J. Australia, *1*: 1337, 1969.
DeLuca, L., Kleinman, H. K., Little, E. P., and Wolf, G.: RNA metabolism in rat intestinal mucosa of normal and vitamin A-deficient rats. Arch. Biochem. Biophys., *145*:332, 1971.
Ehrlich, H. P., and Tarver, H.: Effects of beta-carotene, vitamin A, and glucocorticoids on collagen synthesis in wounds. Proc. Soc. Exp. Biol. Med., *137*:936, 1971.
Figueira, F., et al.: Absorption of vitamin A by infants receiving fat-free or fat-containing dried skim milk formulas. Amer. J. Clin. Nutr., *22*:588, 1969.
Gal, I., Parkinson, C., and Craft, I.: Effects of oral contraceptives on human plasma vitamin-A levels. Brit. Med. J., *2*:436, 1971.
Ganguly, J., et al.: Studies on the metabolism of vitamin A: The effect of vitamin A status on the content of some steroids in the ovaries of pregnant rats. Biochem. J., *123*: 669, 1971.
Greaves, J. P., and Tan, J.: Vitamin A and carotene in British and American diets. Brit. J. Nutr., *20*:819, 1966.
Hellström, V.: Calculation of the total vitamin A value of human diets. Internat. J. Vit. Res., *38*:131, 1968.

High, E. G.: Some aspects of nutritional vitamin A levels in preschool children of Beaufort County, South Carolina. Amer. J. Clin. Nutr., 22:1129, 1969.

Hoppner, K., et al.: Vitamin A reserves of Canadians. Canad. Med. Assoc. J., 101:736, 1969.

Kothari, L. K., Lai, K. B., Srivastava, D. K., and Sharma, R.: Correlation between plasma levels of vitamin A and proteins in children. Amer. J. Clin. Nutr., 24:510, 1971.

McLaren, D. S.: To eat to see. Nutr. Today, 3:2, January, 1968.

Muenter, M. D., Perry, H. O., and Ludwig, J.: Chronic vitamin A intoxication in adults. Amer. J. Med., 50:129, 1971.

Murray, T. K., and Erdody, P.: The utilization of vitamin A and of β-carotene by rats of increasing age. Nutr. Rep. Intl., 3:129, 1971.

Patwardhan, V. N.: Hypovitaminosis A and epidemiology of xerophthalmia. Amer. J. Clin. Nutr., 22:1106, 1969.

Paul, A. A.: The calculation of nicotinic acid equivalents and retinol equivalents in the British diet. Nutr. J. Dietet., Food Catering, Child Nutr., 23:131, 1969.

Raica, N., Jr., et al.: Vitamin A concentration in human tissues collected from 5 areas in the United States. Amer. J. Clin. Nutr., 25:291, 1972.

Swaminathan, M. C., Susheela, T. P., and Thimmayamma, B. V. S.: Field prophylactic trial with a single annual massive dose of vitamin A. Amer. J. Clin. Nutr., 23:119, 1970.

Underwood, B. A., Siegel, H., Weisell, R. C., and Dolinski, M.: Liver stores of vitamin A in a normal population dying suddenly or rapidly from unnatural causes in New York City. Amer. J. Clin. Nutr., 23:1037, 1970.

Witschi, J. C., Houser, H. B., and Littell, A. S.: Preformed vitamin A, carotene, and total vitamin A activity in usual adult diets. J. Amer. Dietet. Assoc., 57:13, 1970.

Zile, M., and DeLuca, H. F.: Vitamin A and ribonucleic acid synthesis in rat intestine. Arch. Biochem. Biophys., 140:210, 1970.

Nutrition Reviews

Transport of vitamin A in the lymphatic system. 24:16, 1966.

Present knowledge of vitamin A (by Roels, O. A.). 24:129, 1966.

Vitamin A transport in man. 25:199, 1967.

Vitamin A deficiency and mitochondrial lipids in rat liver. 27:144, 1969.

Protein synthesis in intestinal mucosa of rats deficient in vitamin A. 27:320, 1969.

On the physiopathology of vitamin A deficiency (by Hayes, K. C.). 29:3, 1971.

Vitamin A and the synthesis of a lipid containing mannose in rat liver. 29:67, 1971.

Effect of calcitonin on bone resorption induced by excess vitamins A and D. 29:150, 1971.

Effect of processing on the carotenoid provitamins. 30:95, 1972.

Vitamin D
(also see refs. 1, 8, 22–31)

General, History, and Reviews

Avioli, L. V.: Absorption and metabolism of vitamin D_3 in man. Amer. J. Clin. Nutr., 22: 437, 1969.

DeLuca, H. F.: Mechanism of action and metabolic fate of vitamin D. Vit. Horm., 25: 316, 1967.

Lawson, D. E. M.: Vitamin D: New findings on its metabolism and its role in calcium nutrition. Proc. Nutr. Soc., 30:47, 1971.

Norman, A. W.: The mode of action of vitamin D. Biol. Rev., 43:97, 1968.

Somogyi, J. C., and Kodicek, E. (eds.): Nutritional aspects of the development of bone and connective tissue. Biblio. Nutr. Dietet., 13:1, 1969.

Other References

Arneil, G. C.: The return of infantile rickets to Britain. World Review Nutr. and Dietet., 10:239, 1969.

Blunt, J. W., DeLuca, H. F., and Schnoes, H. K.: 25-Hydroxycholecalciferol. A biologically active metabolite of vitamin D_3. Biochem., 7:3317, 1968.

Dale, A. E., and Lowenberg, M. E.: Consumption of vitamin D in fortified and natural foods and in vitamin preparations. J. Pediat., 70:952, 1967.

Drescher, D., and DeLuca, H. F.: Possible precursor of vitamin D stimulated calcium binding protein in rats. Biochem., 10:2308, 1971.

Ebel, J. G., Taylor, A. N., and Wasserman, R. H.: Vitamin D-induced calcium-binding protein of intestinal mucosa. Amer. J. Clin. Nutr., 22:431, 1969.

Fraser, D. R., and Kodicek E.: Unique biosynthesis by kidney of a biologically active vitamin D metabolite. Nature, 228:764, 1970.

Holick, M. F., DeLuca, H. F., and Avioli, L. V.: Isolation and identification of 25-hydroxycholecalciferol from human plasma. Arch. Intern. Med., 129:56, 1972.

Inman, R. E., Ingersoll, R. B., and Levy, E. A.: Vitamin D metabolism: The role of kidney tissue. Science, 172:1232, 1971.

Kligman, A. M.: Early destructive effect of sunlight on human skin. J. Amer. Med. Assoc., 210:2377, 1969.

Neer, R. M., et al.: Stimulation by artificial lighting of calcium absorption in elderly human subjects. Nature, 229:255, 1971.

Ney, R. L., Kelly, G., and Bartter, F. C.: Actions of vitamin D independent of the parathyroid glands. Endocrinology, 82:760, 1968.

Norman, A. W., et al.: Basic studies on the mechanism of action of vitamin D. Amer. J. Clin. Nutr., *22*:396, 1969.

Norman, A. W., Mircheff, A. K., Adams, T. H., and Spielvogel, A.: Studies on the mechanism of action of calciferol. III. Vitamin D-mediated increase of intestinal brush border alkaline phosphatase activity. Biochim. Biophys. Acta, *215*:348, 1970.

Ponchon, G., and DeLuca, H. F.: The role of the liver in the metabolism of vitamin D. J. Clin. Invest., *48*:1273, 1969.

Scriver, C. R.: Vitamin D dependency. Pediatrics, *45*:361, 1970.

Seelig, M. S.: Are American children still getting an excess of vitamin D? Clin. Pediat., *9*: 380, 1970.

Seelig, M. S.: Vitamin D and cardiovascular, renal, and brain damage in infancy and childhood. Ann. N.Y. Acad. Sci., *147*:537, 1969.

Silvers, D. N., and Cohen, H. J.: Cutaneous effects of sun exposure. J. Amer. Med. Assoc., *211*:1377, 1970.

Stearns, G.: Early studies of vitamin D requirement during growth. Amer. J. Pub. Health, *58*:2027, 1968.

Watney, P. J. M., Chance, G. W., Scott, P., and Thompson, J. M.: Maternal factors in neonatal hypocalcaemia: A study in three ethnic groups. Brit. Med. J., *2*:432, 1971.

Wergedal, J. E., and Bylink, D. J.: Factors affecting bone enzymatic activity in vitamin D-deficient rats. Amer. J. Physiol., *220*:406, 1971.

Nutrition Reviews

Vitamin D and protein synthesis. *24*:18, 1966.

Safe levels of vitamin D intake for infants. *24*:230, 1966.

Nutrition and metabolic bone disease in the elderly. *25*:71, 1967.

Mode of action of vitamin D. *25*:180, 1967.

Vitamin D₃-biologically active metabolites. *25*: 207, 1967.

Present knowledge of vitamin D (by Forbes, G. B.). *25*:225, 1967.

An hypothesis for the action of vitamin D on bone. *26*:183, 1968.

Parathyroid hormone and hyperaminoaciduria of human vitamin D deficiency. *26*:200, 1968.

Rickets in Greece. *27*:51, 1969.

Vitamin D therapy of hypoparathyroidism. *27*:71, 1969.

Vitamin D sulfate. *28*:73, 1970.

Dibutyryl cyclic AMP, vitamin D, and calcium absorption. *28*:265, 1970.

Vitamin D stimulation of calcium-dependent adenosine triphosphatase. *28*:269, 1970.

Intestinal calcium transport mediated by vitamin D. *29*:41, 1971.

Metabolism of vitamin D. *29*:165, 1971.

Vitamin D: A new look at an old vitamin (by DeLuca, H. F.). *29*:179, 1971.

1,25-dihydroxycholecalciferol, a biologically active metabolite of vitamin D₃ *30*:14, 1972.

Vitamin E
(also see refs. 1, 8, 32–43)

General, History, and Reviews

Ames, S. R.: Isomers of alpha-tocopheryl acetate and their biological activity. Lipids, *6*:281, 1971.

Binder, H. J., et al.: Tocopherol deficiency in man. New Eng. J. Med., *273*:1289, 1965.

Darby, W. J.: Tocopherol-responsive anemias in man. Vit. Horm., *26*:685, 1968.

Draper, H. H., and Csallany, A. S.: Metabolism and function of vitamin E. Fed. Proc., *28*: 1690, 1969.

Fitch, C. D.: Experimental anemia in primates due to vitamin E deficiency. Vit. Horm., *26*:501, 1968.

Green, J., and Bunyan, J.: Vitamin E and the biological antioxidant theory. Nutr. Abs. Rev., *39*:321, 1969.

Herting, D. C.: Perspective on vitamin E. Amer. J. Clin. Nutr., *19*:210, 1966.

Horwitt, M. K.: Vitamin E in human nutrition—an interpretative review. Borden's Rev. of Nutr. Res., *22*:1, 1961.

Olson, R. E., et al.: Symposium: Interrelationships among vitamin E, coenzyme Q, and selenium. Fed. Proc., *24*:55, 1965.

Other References

Anonymous: Vitamin E as a biological antioxidant. Dairy Council Digest, *42*:19, 1971.

Binder, H., and Spiro, H. M.: Tocopherol deficiency in man. Amer. J. Clin. Nutr., *20*: 594, 1967.

Blackburn, H.: A critical review of Shute, W. E.: *Vitamin E for Ailing and Healthy Hearts.* New York, Pyramid House, 1969. In New Eng. J. Med., *283*:214, 1970.

Bunnell, R. H.: Modern procedures for the analysis of tocopherols. Lipids, *6*:245, 1971.

Chadd, M. A., and Fraser, A. J.: Vitamin E deficiency in premature infants. Internat. J. Vit. Res., *40*:604, 1970.

Gross, S., and Guilford, M. V.: Vitamin E-lipid relationships in premature infants. J. Nutr., *100*:1099, 1970.

Herting, D. C., and Drury, E. E.: Vitamin E content of milk, milk products, and simulated milks: Relevance to infant nutrition. Amer. J. Clin. Nutr., *22*:147, 1969.

Hoppner, K., Phillips, W. E. J., Murrary, T. K., and Campbell, J. S.: Data on serum tocopherol levels in a selected group of Canadians. Canad. J. Physiol. Pharmacol., *48*:321, 1970.

Kelleher, J., and Losowsky, M. S.: The absorption of α-tocopherol in man. Brit. J. Nutr., *24*:1033, 1970.

Leonard, P. J., and Losowsky, M. S.: Effect of alpha-tocopherol administration on red cell survival in vitamin E-deficient human subjects. Amer. J. Clin. Nutr., *24*:388, 1971.

McCay, P. B., et al.: A function for α-tocopherol: Stabilization of the microsomal membrane from radical attack during TPNH-dependent oxidations. Lipids, *6*:297, 1971.

Melhorn, D. K., Gross, S., Lake, G. A., and Leu, J. A.: The hydrogen peroxide fragility test and serum tocopherol level in anemias of various etiologies. Blood, *37*:438, 1971.

Sharman, I. M., Down, M. G., and Sen, R. N.: The effects of vitamin E and training on physiological function and athletic performance in adolescent swimmers. Brit. J. Nutr., *26*:265, 1971.

Tulloch, J. A., and Sood, N. K.: Vitamin E deficiency in Uganda. Amer. J. Clin. Nutr., *20*:884, 1967.

Whitaker, J. A., Fort, E. G., Vimokesant, S., and Dinning, J. S.: Hematologic response to vitamin E in the anemia associated with protein-calorie malnutrition. Amer. J. Clin. Nutr., *20*:783, 1967.

Witting, L. A.: Recommended dietary allowance for vitamin E. Amer. J. Clin. Nutr., *25*:257, 1972.

Nutrition Reviews

Vitamin E status of adults on a vegetable oil diet. *24*:41, 1966.

Vitamin E and amino acid transport. *24*:203, 1966.

Present knowledge of vitamin E (by Roels, O. A.). *25*:33, 1967.

Peroxidized fatty acid absorption and vitamin E. *26*:315, 1968.

Compounds with vitamin E activity. *27*:92, 1969.

Methionine, vitamin E, and selenium toxicity. *29*:48, 1971.

Vitamin E and heme synthesis in the rat. *29*:100, 1971.

Pitfalls in calculating the vitamin E content of diets. *30*:55, 1972.

Vitamin K

(also see refs. 1, 8, and 44–47)

General Reviews

Barnes, R. H., and Fiala, G.: Effects of the prevention of coprophagy in the rat. VI. Vitamin K. J. Nutr., *68*:603, 1959.

Dam, H.: Historical survey and introduction. Vit. Horm., *24*:295, 1966.

Kornberg, A., Daft, F. S., and Sebrell, W. H.: Mechanism of production of vitamin K deficiency in rats by sulfonamides. J. Biol. Chem., *155*:193, 1944.

Matschiner, J. T.: Occurrence and biopotency of various forms of vitamin K. Chap. 25 in DeLuca, H. J., and Suttie, J. W. (eds.): *The Fat-Soluble Vitamins.* Madison, University of Wisconsin Press, 1970 (also see Chaps. 26–30 of this book).

Other References

Bell, R. G., and Matschiner, J. T.: Warfarin and the inhibition of vitamin K activity by an oxide metabolite. Nature, *237*:32, 1972.

Filer, L. J., Jr., et al.: Vitamin K supplementation for infants receiving milk substitute infant formulas and for those with fat malabsorption. Pediatrics, *48*:483, 1971.

Garrison, W.: Vitamin K, savior of bleeding babies. Today's Health, Sept. 1969, p. 42.

Goldman, H. I., and Amadio, P.: Vitamin K deficiency after the newborn period. Pediatrics, *44*:745, 1969.

Hill, R. B., et al.: Vitamin K and biosynthesis of protein and prothrombin. J. Biol. Chem., *243*:3930, 1968.

Matschiner, J. T., and Doisy, E. A., Jr.: Vitamin K content of ground beef. J. Nutr., *90*:331, 1967.

Matschiner, J. T., Hsia, S. L., and Doisy, E. A., Jr.: Effect of indigestible oils on vitamin K deficiency in the rat. J. Nutr., *91*:299, 1967.

Nammacher, M. A., Willemin, M., Hartmann, J. R., and Gaston, L. W.: Vitamin K deficiency in infants beyond the neonatal period. J. Pediat., *76*:549, 1970 (as seen in J. Amer. Dietet. Assoc., *57*:263, 1970).

Owen, G. M., et al.: Use of vitamin K_1 in pregnancy. Amer. J. Obstet. Gynecol., *99*:368, 1967.

Sutherland, J. M., Glueck, H. I., and Gleser, G.: Hemorrhagic disease of the newborn. Amer. J. Dis. Child., *113*:524, 1967.

Suttie, J. W.: Control of clotting factor biosynthesis by vitamin K. Fed. Proc., *28*:1696, 1969.

Udall, J. A.: Human sources and absorption of vitamin K in relation to anticoagulation stability. J. Amer. Med. Assoc., *194*:127, 1965.

Nutrition Reviews

The antagonistic effect of vitamin A on vitamin K in the germfree rat. *24*:125, 1966.

Vitamin K deficiency in adults. *26*:165, 1968.

Response of human beings to vitamin K_1. *27*:287, 1969.

ten

Water and Electrolytes (Sodium, Potassium, and Chlorine)

The body is composed of *chemical elements* in many different combinations. The chemical elements are thus the basic building stones of the human body.

Oxygen constitutes over half the body weight, while oxygen and hydrogen together make up three-fourths the body weight (Fig. 10–1). The prominence of these two elements is largely accounted for by the fact that about half the body consists of water. Four nonmetallic elements—oxygen, carbon, hydrogen, and nitrogen—make up 96 percent of the body weight. The other elements present in the body are commonly referred to as the mineral elements, as inorganic salts or, sometimes, as ash because they are the portion left after the organic or combustible matter is burned.

It should be clearly understood, however, that while a certain amount of the minerals may exist in foods or tissues as inorganic salts, a considerable amount of them is found in combination in organic compounds. The bulk of body calcium and phosphorus is concentrated in the mineral salts found in bones and teeth but the portion—

1 percent of calcium and 20 percent of phosphorus—present in the soft tissues and fluids plays a vital role in the structure and metabolism of all cells, for example. Most metallic elements needed in trace amounts appear to function as a part of enzymes or hormones required to bring about specific chemical reactions in the tissues. The body fluids consist mainly of water in which inorganic salts, protein, and some organic compounds are dissolved.

WATER

Water, a simple compound of two atoms of hydrogen with one of oxygen, has unique features that make it absolutely necessary for life. It has special solvent properties that alter the configuration of substances dissolved in it and thus change their behavior in cellular systems. In spite of its small molecular size, water is liquid at body temperatures (carbon dioxide, a much heavier molecule, is a gas, by way of comparison). For these reasons water is an ideal medium for transporting dissolved nutrients and wastes throughout

224

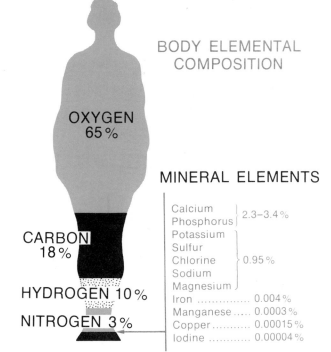

Figure 10-1. The nonmetallic elements oxygen, carbon, hydrogen, and nitrogen together make up 96 percent of the body weight, leaving only 4 percent for all the various mineral elements. Calcium and phosphorus are the mineral elements present in largest amounts, but these amounts vary considerably depending on the reserves of these two elements stored in the bones. Iron, manganese, copper, zinc, cobalt, and iodine are present in minute quantities, though vitally important. Many other elements are present in the body in trace amounts, but most of these are considered to be nonessential.

BODY ELEMENTAL COMPOSITION

OXYGEN 65%

MINERAL ELEMENTS

Calcium	
Phosphorus	2.3–3.4%
Potassium	
Sulfur	
Chlorine	0.95%
Sodium	
Magnesium	
Iron	0.004%
Manganese	0.0003%
Copper	0.00015%
Iodine	0.00004%

CARBON 18%

HYDROGEN 10%

NITROGEN 3%

the body. A relatively large amount of heat is needed to vaporize it. It takes about 600 kcal (2500 kJ) to evaporate 1 kg of water, which makes sweating a very effective means of dissipating body heat. Water also participates in some chemical reactions in the body. The splitting of starch into sugar by addition of water is one such instance.

Water is second only to oxygen in importance to the body. One may live for weeks without food but only for a few days without water. One can lose all reserve carbohydrate (glycogen) and fat, and about half the body protein without real danger, but a loss of 10 percent of total body water is serious, while a loss of 20 to 22 percent is fatal. With a depletion of up to 10 percent of water, one can perform some physical work, although efficiency is decreased and exhaustion takes place earlier. With greater depletion of body water, weakness precludes physical efforts.

The fact that the water content of the body must be replenished from with-out to make up for continuous loss of this substance is a matter of common knowledge. Water is excreted from the body by the kidneys in the urine, by the lungs as water vapor in the expired air, and by the skin as sensible or insensible perspiration (Fig. 10-2). Lesser amounts are regularly lost in the stools. The relative amounts which are excreted through these different channels vary somewhat, as discussed in Chapter 14. Ordinarily more water is excreted in the urine than by other channels, but in hot weather a larger amount is evaporated as perspiration in the effort to regulate the body temperature (see p. 335), and a smaller volume of more concentrated urine is secreted. The amount lost through all channels averages 2 to 2½ liters per day.

Water Replacements

This loss must be made up by the water furnished from three different sources:

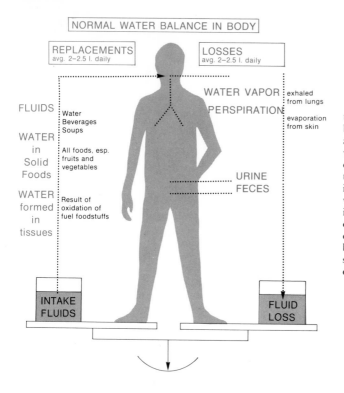

NORMAL WATER BALANCE IN BODY

REPLACEMENTS
avg. 2–2.5 l. daily

LOSSES
avg. 2–2.5 l. daily

FLUIDS
Water
Beverages
Soups

WATER
in
Solid
Foods
All foods, esp.
fruits and
vegetables

WATER
formed
in
tissues
Result of
oxidation of
fuel foodstuffs

WATER VAPOR : exhaled
                           from lungs
PERSPIRATION
                           evaporation
                           from skin

URINE
FECES

INTAKE
FLUIDS

FLUID
LOSS

Figure 10–2. Normally the intake and output of water from the body are approximately in balance. If much water is drunk, the volume of urine excreted increases. If water intake is low or the amount lost in perspiration is high (with exercise or in hot weather), the urine will be reduced in volume. With fever, vomiting or diarrhea, there is excessive loss of water. Any excessive loss should be made up by taking more fluids so that body stores of water are not depleted.

(1) by the fluids taken (water, beverages, soup, etc.);

(2) by the water contained in solid foods; and

(3) by the water produced in the body as a result of the metabolic processes.

Solid *foods* contain a good deal of water—ranging from about 5 percent in very dry foods such as crackers to over 90 percent in juicy fruits and vegetables such as tomatoes, eggplant, cauliflower, lettuce, strawberries, and watermelon. Even such a solid food as bread contains water to the extent of about 31 to 36 percent of its weight.

Also many people do not realize that we form water in our own tissues as a product of the oxidative processes which are necessary to sustain life (see chapter on metabolic processes). Water is always one of the products formed when fuel foods are burned in the tissues to get energy, and this so-called *metabolic water* may amount to 300 to 400 ml per day.

However, in addition to the water obtained from these two sources, we

need to take in *fluids* to replenish the water content of the body, and the amount taken in this form should usually be about 5 to 6 glasses daily. If a good deal of milk, tea, coffee, or soup is taken, one may not need to drink as large an amount of water, but within reasonable limits, an excess of water intake over the actual need is a good thing. There is no objection to drinking water with meals. Large quantities of an iced beverage, however, may cause some mild, temporary gastric distress. Hard water is not injurious, and may even supply significant amounts of needed minerals if large quantities are drunk, but mineral waters should be taken only on advice of a physician.

BODY FLUID COMPARTMENTS

At birth, the human body is about 77 percent water. Water content falls to about 63 percent in infants during the first year of life, 59 percent in children and 45 to 65 percent in healthy

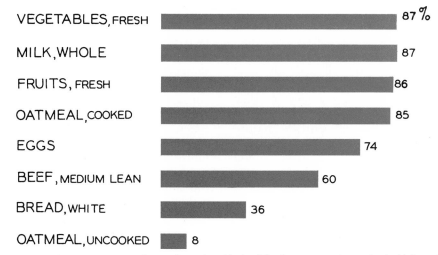

Figure 10–3.   Average content of water in various kinds of foods, on a percentage basis. (Adapted from Cooper, Barber, Mitchell, et al.: *Nutrition in Health and Disease*, 14th Ed. Philadelphia, Lippincott, 1963.)

young adults. Men have more water and less fat in their bodies than do women, on the average, and both show a steady decline in total body water with advancing age. Men over 60 have about 50 to 54 percent of body weight as water, and women, 42 to 49 percent.[1]

The body water is not a continuous mass but is divided roughly into two main compartments, the *intracellular fluid* (ICF) and *extracellular* fluid (ECF). About 60 percent of the total body water is found within the cells (the intracellular fluid); the other 40 percent is in various compartments outside the cells (the extracellular fluid). Less than one-fifth of the extracellular fluid is found in the circulatory system; blood plasma constitutes a bit less than 5 percent of body weight in healthy adults, or about 3 to 3.5 liters of fluid. Some of the extracellular fluid is in hollow organs and joints and some is in bone, but by far the largest amount surrounds and bathes the cells. The water inside each cell is also subdivided into yet smaller compartments which are discontinuous, rather like a sponge.[2]

The composition of the fluids within and outside of the cells is quite different. The extracellular fluid contains a large amount of sodium and chlorine and is equivalent to a 0.9 percent solution of common salt (sodium chloride). Small amounts of potassium, calcium, magnesium, phosphorus and sulfur are also present. This composition is about the same as is thought to have been present in the pre-Cambrian sea from which man's remote ancestors emerged to walk on land, a similarity that has fostered the idea that the extracellular fluid is a small pond that a man has brought with him to land.[3] Although this view is not fully supportable in the light of modern knowledge, the composition of this fluid compartment does indicate a marine ancestry.[4] Besides these inorganic salts, extracellular fluid contains dissolved carbon dioxide, protein, a small amount of organic acids, and, of course, other organic compounds.

The intracellular fluid is high in potassium and phosphorus. It contains more magnesium, sulfur, and protein than does the extracellular fluid but less carbon dioxide and much less sodium.

It is surprising that the concentration of a substance as freely moving as water is different in these separate compartments. One factor involved is the nature of the membranes that surround the cells. These membranes are semipermeable; they are freely permeable to water and small molecules like the mineral salts diffuse through them, but other substances with larger molecules (like proteins) are held back. The membranes within the cells and the nature of the adjacent water layer also play regulatory roles that are only beginning to be understood.[2]

The salt content of the fluids also affects movements of water into or out of the tissues. The salts present in body fluids belong to the class of substances known as *electrolytes*.* When in water, the molecules of electrolytes separate into two or more electrically charged particles called *ions*, while nonelectrolytes (such as glucose and urea) do not. The chief electrolytes in body fluids are the positively charged ions (cations), sodium and potassium, plus small amounts of calcium and magnesium, and the negatively charged ion (anion) chloride; there are smaller amounts of the anions, sulfate, carbonate and phosphate. The ionization of sodium chloride may be represented simply as follows:

$$NaCl \leftrightarrows Na^+ + Cl^-$$

Because *osmotic† pressure* is directly pro-

portional to the number of particles in a solution, substances that ionize (separate into two or more particles) have much greater osmotic pressure than do those that do not ionize.

Conditions in a living system are never constant; some products are being formed and others degraded at all times. These products have different electrical charges, and some may ionize and others not. Adjustments are constantly taking place so that within the limits of a dynamic system. fluids within a compartment are balanced with respect to positive and negative ions. The compartments contain different ions and different total amounts of electrolytes but in spite of these differences in salt content, the osmotic pressure of the compartments is very nearly the same.

Movement of substances between blood and extracellular fluids and between these fluids and tissue cells, is due to the influence of osmotic pressure, which in turn is due chiefly to the content of mineral salts.

Both sodium and potassium will diffuse through cell membranes. It is thought that the content of sodium inside the cell is kept low by an active energy-requiring process of pumping the sodium out.[5] The sodium-pump, by moving a small number of sodium ions, shifts a large volume of water because of the requirement to achieve equal osmotic pressure. Differences in protein content of the compartments also participate in osmotic regulation of fluid. The fact that plasma contains more protein than does the ECF outside the blood vessels enables fluid to remain in the circulatory system under the force of pressure needed to circulate the blood, and to recollect there from the tissues. Thus, fluid moves continuously in and out of cells, carrying in nutrients, oxygen and other chemical compounds and carrying out wastes and other soluble substances formed by the cells.

There are many other instances in which the exchange of water across

---

*When an electric current is passed through an aqueous solution of certain compounds, some elements collect at the positive pole and others at the negative side. This indicates that the elemental particles bear electric charges. Substances that behave in this way are called electrolytes.

†When a permeable membrane is interposed between two salt solutions of different concentrations, the salt and the water both diffuse from their area of higher concentration to the lower one until equilibrium is attained. If the membrane is semipermeable, the water will move from its area of higher concentration (the dilute solution) more rapidly than will the salt; that is, osmosis will occur. The amount of excess pressure which must be imposed on the solution to prevent the passage of the water through the membrane is called the osmotic pressure of the solution.

body membranes is important and is influenced at least in part by the relative amounts of salts on the two sides of the membrane. These instances include absorption and reabsorption of water across the membrane lining the intestine; passage of water (with dissolved nutrients) from the blood stream into the tissues and from the tissues (laden with waste products or intermediate metabolic products) to the blood stream; and the excretion of water into urinary tubules and its partial reabsorption back into the blood stream. All these processes permit the use of water over and over by the body for various purposes.

Loss of body water is always accompanied by some loss of the soluble mineral salts, but under certain circumstances the two may not be commensurate. Suppose a sailor is cut off from his water supply. His water losses continue and the loss is mainly from the extracellular compartment. The ECF then becomes a more concentrated salt solution, which change triggers the sensation of thirst and initiates some hormonal changes that direct the kidney to conserve water and make more concentrated urine. If the water loss is not then replaced, the ECF becomes still more concentrated and osmosis drives water out of the intracellular compartment until the ECF is diluted to the same concentration as the ICF. The cells are then dehydrated, and ultimately death will ensue. Present-day seawater is a much more concentrated salt solution than is ECF, so it is apparent that drinking sea water can only worsen the man's condition.

Excessive sweating at high air temperatures causes loss of water and sodium chloride (salt) from the body. If all the water is replaced and not the salt, the ECF becomes more dilute than normal and water will move from the ECF to the more concentrated ICF. The cells will be overhydrated and cramps (formerly called *stoker's disease*, after the coal stokers in steamships) may de-

velop because of salt depletion. However, if only enough water is drunk to bring the ECF back to normal osmotic concentration, without taking any salt, the total ECF volume will have shrunk but the state of cellular hydration will be unchanged. When the ECF volume falls, much of the body's protection against water and salt deprivation is gone; and if the loss of ECF is severe, the blood pressure will also fall, to the point of faintness.

Sometimes salt is retained excessively, under hormonal influences or due to kidney or liver disease. Then, water is also retained to dilute it and the ECF volume increases. The tissues may then become edematous because of the large amount of water surrounding the cells.

Normal Functioning of Muscles and Nerves

We are not usually conscious of the part salts play in the exchange of body fluids unless conditions become abnormal; the same is true of the role of salts in maintaining *normal irritability of the nervous tissues and contractility of muscular tissues.* Neither muscles nor nerves function properly unless they are bathed in tissue fluids which contain certain amounts of mineral salts. Calcium ions seem to have a stimulating effect, which tends to counterbalance the more or less relaxing or depressing effects of ions of magnesium, sodium, and potassium. Reduced or imbalanced concentrations of these ions can result in paralysis or convulsive movement. Ordinarily, the content of the different salts in the blood and tissue fluids is regulated (chiefly by hormones) to a nice balance and a constant level so that the muscles and nerves function normally. The rhythmic alternate contractions and relaxations of the heart muscle constitute an example of this regulation and are dependent on the maintenance of a normal concentration of all the necessary mineral salts in the blood.

ACID-BASE BALANCE

The cells function best in a slightly alkaline medium, and will be unable to function if the pH* within the cells or in fluids surrounding the cells differs too widely from the optimum. Hence, there are elaborate mechanisms for keeping the blood and tissue fluids within a narrow pH range (7.35 to 7.45). Proteins act as buffer substances capable of uniting with either acids or bases in such a way as to prevent their affecting blood neutrality (Chapter 5). Mineral elements also participate in regulating body neutrality, in that some of them are acidic and others are basic, and these can be paired to form neutral salts.

---

*Acids are compounds of electronegative substances (anions) plus ionizable hydrogen (H^+); bases are compounds of electropositive substances (cations) plus ionizable hydroxyl groups (OH^-). Acidity is, then, the concentration of H-ions in solution. In the physiologic range the concentration of H-ions is much less than one; so for convenience in expressing values the pH unit was devised. pH is the negative logarithm of the H-ion concentration. pH 7.0 is neutral; values below 7 are in the acid range and above 7, the alkaline range.

Table 10–1. The Chief Acid- and Base-Forming Components of the Diet

Acid-Forming	Base-Forming
Elements	
Phosphorus	Sodium
Sulfur	Potassium
Chlorine	Calcium
	Magnesium
Foods	
Meat	Most fruits
Eggs	Vegetables
Cereal products	Milk
Bread	Nuts
Corn	
Cranberries,* plums	

*These are acidic due to their content of one organic acid, benzoic acid, that yields an acidic end-product in metabolism. Most other organic acids are converted to carbon dioxide and water.

The principal mineral elements may be classified as to their acidic or basic properties (Table 10–1). When sulfur and phosphorus are taken in proteins or other organic compounds, these elements are oxidized to sulfuric and phosphoric acid residues in metabolism. Carbon is oxidized to carbon dioxide whenever organic compounds are burned for energy, and this in turn reacts with water to form carbonic acid (H_2CO_3). These three acidic substances are constantly being formed in tissue metabolism and must be neutralized by basic substances to form salts. Chlorine, another acid-forming element, is taken into the body almost entirely in the form of neutral salts, chiefly common salt or sodium chloride.

Many basic elements are present in foods in organic combinations, the organic part of which can be oxidized, leaving the basic element free to combine with acids and form salts. For instance, many of the basic elements in fruits are present as salts of organic acids, such as citric and malic acids (e.g., potassium malate in apples). Most of the calcium in milk exists as a salt of the protein casein (calcium caseinate). The carbon chains of protein, organic acids, or other organic matter is oxidized in metabolism to yield carbon dioxide and water, leaving the basic elements free to combine with acids taken in food or formed in metabolism. Thus, it is easier to maintain body neutrality if the acid-forming and base-forming elements in the diet approximately balance each other.

Foods may be classified as acid-forming or base-forming, that is, whether they will furnish a preponderance of acid-forming or base-forming elements after the organic part of the food is oxidized in the tissues. The acid-forming foods usually are high in protein which contains sulfur and phosphorus; most fruits and vegetables are base-forming because they contain a preponderance of basic elements, either as inorganic salts or as salts of organic acids that can be burned in the body.

The maintenance of pH in the blood and tissues, however, is too important a matter to be left solely to chance selection of diet. In fact, there are several mechanisms for coping with excess acid or base. Because acids are constantly formed in metabolism, usually the problem is to dispose of excess acid products.

Proteins and carbonates act as buffer* substances in the blood which means that considerable amounts of either acid or alkali can be taken up by them in such a way that the pH remains constant. A large amount of carbon dioxide is removed normally in expired air. When CO_2 production is excessive and the carbonic acid content of blood rises the respiratory center responds, increasing breathing rate so that more CO_2 is ventilated. The kidney disposes of the remainder of excess acid by excreting the phosphate, sulfate, and chloride ions as salts, chiefly of sodium and potassium. If the supply of base is limited, ammonium and hydrogen ions formed by the kidney are substituted for sodium.† The urine then becomes more acid.

Excess base is rarely a problem, because the kidney very effectively removes any extra sodium or potassium by forming a more alkaline urine. This condition may occur with loss of chloride due to severe vomiting or with overdosage of alkalizing agents.

SODIUM

The importance of salt as an item of commerce dates back to ancient times. It was used as a flavoring agent and preservative, and in the making of glass. Sodium (Na), from the word "soda" (or *natrium* in Latin) was first isolated by Davy (see page 238) in 1807. It is a very active soft, white, silvery metal which burns on exposure to air. Although it had long been believed by many to be a dietary essential, final proof was not obtained until after 1905 in experiments with animals. Ordinary table salt (NaCl) and baking soda ($NaHCO_3$) are common and familiar forms of the element.

We have seen that sodium is a key element in regulation of body water and acid-base balance. Because the body has such effective means of conserving sodium when it is scarce and of ridding the body of any excess via the urine, it is quite difficult to establish a minimum daily requirement for this nutrient or to set upper limits of tolerance. The average daily American intake is 10 to 15 gm of salt, or about 5 gm of sodium. (Salt is approximately 40 percent sodium and 60 percent chlorine.) There is no evidence as to the desirability of this intake. Where habitual sodium intake is much higher, in Japan, for instance,[6] there is an increased incidence of high blood pressure. In a strain of rats that is prone to develop the condition, a high sodium intake has been proved to induce high blood pressure.[7] This suggests that sodium should be treated cautiously, and certainly there is no demonstrated benefit from high intake of sodium in healthy people.

The minimum requirement for sodium can be related to the amount of so-

---

*Buffers are mixtures that have the ability to resist change in H-ion concentration. Usually they are mixtures of weak acids (such as carbonic acid) with their salts of strong bases (such as sodium or potassium). Phosphates behave similarly to carbonate in buffer systems. Proteins can react with acid (by means of their NH_2 groups) or with alkaline substances (by means of their COOH groups) in such a way that hydrogen or hydroxyl are bound and not free to form ions.

†In the kidney, H^+ is substituted for Na^+ by the following reaction:

$$H_2CO_3 + Na_2HPO_4 \longrightarrow NaH_2PO_4 + NaHCO_3$$

Still more base may be conserved by substitution of ammonium ion as symbolized by the following reactions:

$$2\ NH_3 \text{ (from amino acids)} + 2\ H_2CO_3 + Na_2HPO_4 \rightarrow (NH_4)_2HPO_4 + 2\ NaHCO_3$$

In both cases the H-ion comes from a shift of carbonic acid to bicarbonate.

dium lost from the body when none is fed. Under this condition, all available mechanisms are operating maximally to conserve sodium and excretion falls to less than 200 mg per day. There is no question of this being a safe level of intake, by virtue of the fact that it represents output by an individual who is already depleted and it provides no safety margin against changing day-to-day needs. A safe lower intake level is thought to be about 2.5 gm per day under temperate conditions. Continued sodium depletion leads to shifts in body fluid compartments previously described; there is muscle cramping, loss of appetite, mental apathy, convulsions, and, ultimately, coma and death.

If sweating loss is high there may be need for additional salt in the diet, but the usual daily intake, 10 to 15 gm of salt, is more than sufficient to cover the loss that occurs with most physical work or moderate heat exposure. Sweat contains up to 1 gm of sodium per liter, so the usual sodium intake (5 gm per day) allows for at least 4 liters of sweat after all other sodium needs are met. For persons who do moderate to heavy work in a hot climate *and* under hot conditions, *salt* intake should be increased by about 7 gm per day.[8] This is best accomplished by salting food heavily or by adding salt to the drinking water that is taken to replace the water lost as sweat. Sweat is hypotonic, that is, it contains a lower concentration of salt than the physiological saline level (0.9 percent), so the fluid drunk for replacement must also be less concentrated than the extracellular fluid. A good solution should have 2 gm of salt per liter (two scant teaspoons of salt per gallon).

Most of the sodium in the diet is added to foods as salt. Not only do we appreciate the taste of salt, but it is probably the oldest of all chemical preservatives. With the increased use of prepared and "convenience" foods, less option is open to the individual in setting his own salt intake and there is less salt added to foods in the home. This change in food pattern can reduce

the effectiveness of iodization of salt (a public health measure; see Chapter 12) unless both household and commercial salt are fortified with iodine. Other sources of added sodium are monosodium glutamate (MSG), soy sauce, and baking powder. Cheese, milk, and shellfish are good sources of sodium, and meat, fish, poultry, and eggs make significant contributions. Cereals, fruits, and vegetables are low in this nutrient unless it is added in processing. Water supplies are quite variable in sodium content but may add significantly to the daily total intake. See Table 10-2 for some more detailed values of the sodium content of foods.

POTASSIUM

Potassium (K) was named in 1807 by Davy, its discoverer, from the word "potash" (Latin *kalium*), the alkaline ash of vegetable substances. Potassium is widely used as a fertilizer for plants and is one of the more abundant elements.

It was not until 1938 that McCollum (using the rat) obtained proof that potassium is an essential nutrient, although this had been suggested earlier.

Potassium is a nearly constant component of lean body tissue, so much so that one method of estimating the amount of lean tissue in a living person is by measuring the amount of potassium present. (This is done by counting the amount of radioactive potassium which is naturally present in a constant ratio to ordinary potassium.) The need for potassium is increased when there is growth or deposition of lean tissue, and potassium is lost whenever muscle is broken down due to starvation, protein deficiency, or injury. Deficiency of potassium results in muscular weakness or paralysis; the intestinal muscle is also affected so that normal movement ceases and the abdomen becomes distended with gas. Finally the heart muscle stops. The ordinary diet usually contains enough potassium if energy and protein intake are adequate, be-

Table 10–2. Sodium and Potassium Content of Some Representative Foods*

Food, 100 gm	Sodium, mg	Potassium, mg
Apple	1	110
Banana	1	370
Bread, salted	527	273
Bread, unsalted†	28	120
Broccoli, cooked	10	267
Butter, salted	987	23
Butter, unsalted	<10	<10
Carrot, raw	47	341
Cheese, Cheddar	700	82
Chicken, broiled	66	274
Corn, canned with salt	236	97
Corn, diet pack	2	97
Egg, poached	271	128
Hamburger, cooked	47	450
Liver, calf, fried	118	453
Milk, whole	50	144
Orange	1	200
Pickle, dill	1428	200
Popcorn, plain	3	660
Popcorn, with oil and salt	1940	512
Potato, French fried	6	853
Potato, French fried with salt	236	853
Potato chips, salted	up to 1000	1130
Rice, parboiled, cooked	358	43
Spinach	50	324
Wheat, puffed, without salt	4	340
Wheat, puffed, with salt and sugar	161	99

*From Watt, B. K., and Merrill, A. L.: *Composition of Foods: Raw, Processed, Prepared.* Washington, D.C., U.S.D.A. Handbook No. 8, 1963, except where noted. Where unspecified, values refer to foods cooked without salt.
†From *Diet Manual.* Nashville, Vanderbilt University Press, 1961.

cause potassium is widely distributed in foods of both plant and animal origin. Deficiency results from a combination of poor diet and excessive loss of potassium due to severe diarrhea, in most cases. For this reason, potassium de-

ficiency is often present in children suffering from kwashiorkor.

Persons given an experimental diet low in potassium excrete about 1.5 gm per day. Most of this is lost in the urine, but there is a substantial amount in feces and a little in sweat. A reasonable lower level of intake is thought to be 2.5 gm per day. The usual American diet has about 0.8 to 1.5 gm of potassium per 1000 kcal, little if any above this suggested lower limit.

The same animal model that provides evidence of an adverse effect of sodium on blood pressure (see above) shows that blood pressure may be lowered to a more normal level if potassium is increased along with the increased level of sodium in the rat diet The best response in these rats resulted from a simultaneous increase of potassium and a reduction of sodium. It is prudent to maintain a closer ratio of sodium to potassium in the diet than is present in the typical American diet. A more desirable 1:1 ratio can be achieved by either lowering salt intake or increasing the intake of potassium, or perhaps both.

Meats and other lean muscle tissue are good dietary sources of potassium. Milk is also a good source but not cheese, as much of the potassium is lost in whey. Many fruits are outstanding sources of potassium, especially dried dates, bananas, cantaloupe, apricots, and citrus fruits. Tomato juice and the dark green leafy vegetables are also high in this nutrient. Other vegetables, many fruits and all cereals make smaller contributions of potassium. See Table 10–2 for more details.

CHLORINE

Chlorine, a common water purifier and bleach, is also an essential element for all higher animals and man. Discovered in 1774 by Scheele and named by Davy in 1810, chlorine (Cl) is a very toxic yellow-green gas in its elemental form. In nature it always exists combined. A common form is salt (NaCl— sodium chloride).

We tend to forget that chlorine is an essential nutrient because it comes into the diet so automatically along with sodium in the salt we add to foods. Chlorine has a special function in forming the hydrochloric acid (HC1) present in gastric juice. This acid is necessary for proper absorption of one of the vitamins (B-12) and iron, and it suppresses growth of microorganisms that enter the stomach with food and drink. Chloride ion is also involved in the acid-base economy of the body as noted above. Loss of chloride generally parallels that of sodium, and a separate deficiency occurs only when there is loss of chloride due to vomiting. Persons whose sodium intake is severely restricted (owing to diseases of the heart, kidney, or liver) may need an alternative source of chloride; a number of chloride-containing salt substitutes are available for this purpose.

QUESTIONS AND PROBLEMS

1. Which elements are most abundant in the body? What substances are classed as mineral or ash? Why? How much mineral is found in the body?

2. How much water is present in the body? How does water content change with age? Into what compartments is water divided? Is water necessary for building and maintaining tissues? Why? Name and discuss three ways in which water acts as a regulator of body processes.

3. By what routes is water lost from the body? What conditions determine the relative amounts of water lost through the skin and in the urine? What conditions make for excessive loss of water from the body? What is the normal loss of water from the body daily (approximate)? How much heat is required to evaporate 1 kg of water? How much additional water would be needed to compensate for the amount lost as sweat due to playing tennis for one hour indoors? (Use the data on energy cost of activities given in Chapter 2.)

4. Keep a record of your total intake of water for one day—that is, the amount taken as water, soup, tea, coffee, and milk. How does your intake compare with the amount that most persons should take either in beverages or as drinking water? What is meant by "metabolic water"?

5. What is an electrolyte? Which ions are most abundant in the extracellular fluid? The intracellular fluid? How are these differences maintained? What is meant by osmotic pressure? How does it relate to the exchange of substances between fluid compartments?

6. What changes occur in the body when water intake is insufficient? Why must salt and water be replaced when sweating is heavy? What is a good way to take extra salt when it is needed?

7. What foods are high in sodium content? Which are low? How much sodium should be taken daily? What percentage of salt is sodium? What other element is found in common salt? What function does it have in the body?

8. What foods are high in potassium content? Which are low? How does potassium deficiency occur? What are the symptoms? How much potassium should be taken daily?

9. What is meant by acid-base balance? How is it regulated? Which elements and foods are acidic? Which basic?

REFERENCES

1. Korenchevsky, V.: *Physiological and Pathological Ageing.* New York, Hafner Publishing Co., 1961.
2. Robinson, J. R.: Water, the indispensable nutrient. Nutrition Today, 5:16, Spring 1970.
3. Bunge, G.: *Lehrbuch der Physiologischen und Pathologischen Chemie.* Leipzig, 1889.
4. Elkinton, J. R.: The relationship of water and salt. Proc. Nutr. Society (Great Britain), *16*:113, 1957.
5. Schmidt-Nielsen, B.: Symposium: Comparative aspects of transport of hypertonic, isotonic and hypotonic solutions by epithelial membranes. Introduction. Fed. Proc., *30*:3, 1971.
6. Dahl, L. K.: Possible role of chronic excess salt consumption in pathogenesis of es-

sential hypertension. Amer. J. Cardiol., 8:571, 1961.

7. Meneely, G. R., and Ball, C. O. T.: Experimental epidemiology of chronic sodium chloride toxicity and the protective effect of potassium chloride. Amer. J. Med., 25: 713, 1958; Dahl, L. K., Heine, M., and Tassinari, L.: Effects of chronic excess salt ingestion. Evidence that genetic factors play an important role in susceptibility to experimental hypertension. J. Exper. Med., 115:1173, 1962.

8. Lee, D. H. K.: Terrestrial animals in dry heat: Man in the desert. In Code, C. F. (ed.): *Handbook of Physiology*, Section 4, Chap. 35. Baltimore, Williams and Wilkins for Amer. Physiol. Society, 1964.

SUPPLEMENTARY READING

Adolph, E. F.: Regulation of water intake in relation to body water content. In Code, C. F. (ed.): *Handbook of Physiology*, Section 6, Vol. I, Chap. 12. Baltimore, Williams and Wilkins for Amer. Physiol Society, 1967.

Alleyne, G. A. O.: Studies on total body potassium in malnourished infants. Factors affecting potassium repletion. Brit. J. Nutr., 24:205, 1970.

Anderson, J. W., Herman, R. H., and Newcomer, K. L.: Improvement in glucose tolerance of fasting obese subjects given oral potassium. Amer. J. Clin. Nutr., 22:1589, 1969.

Baker, E. M., Plough, I. C., and Allen, T. H.: Water requirements of men as related to salt intake. Amer. J. Clin. Nutr., 12:394, 1963.

Bell, T. A., Etchells, J. L., Kelling, R. E., and Hontz, L. H.: Low-sodium pickle products for modified diets. J. Amer. Dietet. Assoc., 60:213, 1972.

Birge, S. J., Jr., Gilbert, H. R., and Avioli, L. V.: Intestinal calcium transport: The role of sodium. Science, 176:168, 1972.

Crawford, R., and Crawford, M. D.: Prevalence and pathological changes of ischemic heart disease in a hard and in a soft water area. Lancet, 1:229, 1967.

Dahl, L. K.: Salt intake and salt need. New Eng. J. Med., 258:1152, 1958; Salt and hypertension. Amer. J. Clin. Nutr., 25:232, 1972.

Daly, C., and Dill, D. B.: Salt economy in humid heat. Amer. J. Physiol., 118:285, 1937.

Denton, D. A.: Salt appetite. In Code, C. F. (ed.): *Handbook of Physiology*, Section 6, Vol. I, Chap. 31, Baltimore, Williams and Wilkins for Amer. Physiol. Society, 1967.

Dluhy, R. G., Underwood, R. H., and Williams, G. H.: Influence of dietary potassium on plasma renin activity in normal man. J. Appl. Physiol. 28:299, 1970.

Fitzsimons, J. T.: Thirst. Physiol. Rev., 52:468, 1972.

Flynn, M. A., Hanna, F. M., and Lutz, R. N.: Estimation of body water compartments of preschool children. Amer. J. Clin. Nutr., 20:1125, 1967.

Food and Nutrition Board, NAS/NRC: Minimal allowances of water and food for fallout shelter survival, 1962.

Gamble, J. L.: The water requirements of castaways. Proc. Amer. Philos. Soc., 88:151, 1944.

Grande, F., et al.: Water exchange in men on a restricted water intake and a low calorie carbohydrate diet accompanied by physical work. J. Appl. Physiol., 12:202, 1958.

Gros, G., Weller, J. M., and Hoobler, S. W.: Relationship of sodium and potassium intake to blood pressure. Amer. J. Clin. Nutr., 24:605, 1971.

Holmes, J. H.: Thirst and fluid intake as clinical problems. In Code, C. F. (ed.): *Handbook of Physiology*, Section 6, Vol. I, Chap. 11. Baltimore, Williams and Wilkins for Amer. Physiol. Soc., 1967.

Malhotra, M. S.: Salt and water requirement of acclimatized people working outdoors in severe heat. Indian J. Med. Res., 48:212, 1960.

Osnes, J., and Hermansen, L.: Acid-base balance after maximal exercise of short duration. J. Appl. Physiol., 32:59, 1972.

Pitts, G. C., Johnson, R. E., and Consolazio, C. F.: Work in the heat as affected by intake of water, salt and glucose. Amer. J. Physiol., 142:253, 1944.

Prior, I. A. M., et al.: Sodium intake and blood pressure in two Polynesian populations. New Eng. J. Med., 279:515, 1968.

Rubini, M. E.: Mariposa, salt and thirsting. Amer. J. Clin. Nutr., 23:861, 1970.

Schmidt-Nielsen, K.: *Desert Animals: Physiological Problems of Heat and Water*. Oxford, Oxford University Press, 1964.

Schroeder, H. A.: Relationship between mortality from cardiovascular disease and treated water supplies. J. Amer. Med. Assoc., 172:1902, 1960.

Share, L., and Claybaugh, J. R.: Regulation of body fluids. Ann. Rev. Physiol., 34:235, 1972.

Stevenson, J. A. F.: Central mechanisms controlling water intake. In Code, C. F. (ed.): *Handbook of Physiology*, Section 6, Vol. I, Chap. 13. Washington, Amer. Physiol. Soc., 1967.

Walker, J. S., et al.: Water intake of normal children. Science, 140:890, 1963.

Nutrition Reviews

Body water in kwashiorkor. 24:75, 1966.

Food and water intake regulation of rats with Walker tumors. 24:111, 1966.

Arterial enzymatic activity on a high salt diet. *24*:159, 1966.

Renal control of acidosis. *24*:340, 1966.

Regulation of salt intake in rats. *25*:91, 1967.

Lateral hypothalamic function in sodium chloride appetite regulation. *25*:187, 1967.

Tissue electrolytes in dehydrated children. *25*: 205, 1967.

Thirst in rats resulting from hypovolemia and hyperosmolarity. *25*:246, 1967.

Hormonal influences and salt restriction. *25*:311, 1967.

Dehydration with high protein tube feeding. *26*: 271, 1968.

Sodium intake and blood pressure. *27*:280, 1969.

Salt in infant foods. *29*:280, 1971.

eleven

Calcium, Phosphorus, and Magnesium

In the last chapter we discussed the body's need for water and the electrolytes (sodium, potassium, and chlorine). These three elements plus *calcium*, *phosphorus*, and *magnesium* make up the six important *macro inorganic minerals* essential in our diets (also called the *macrominerals*).* They are present in the body in relatively large amounts and are required in the diet in considerably larger quantities than the "trace elements" (Chapter 12).† Inorganic forms of the six macrominerals take care of all dietary needs (organic forms are not required or of any added benefit).

CALCIUM AND PHOSPHORUS

Because calcium and phosphorus are so closely associated in the formation and upkeep of the *bones and teeth*, these two elements are conveniently considered together.

Discovery of Dietary Requirement

The knowledge of the antirachitic properties and other health benefits of milk, ground dry bones, and other calcium- and phosphorus-rich sources goes back to ancient times, in both the Asian and Middle Eastern cultures.

Calcium was among the first substances known to be essential in the diet. A Frenchman, Chossat, showed experimentally as long ago as 1842 that calcium salts were required by the pigeon. Many other experiments, before 1920, proved the need by all animals for both calcium[1] and phosphorus.[2] Well-controlled experiments with man were not made until more recent years.

---

*There is as yet no standard nutritional nomenclature to distinguish macrominerals from trace elements. We use the word "mineral" here in deference to common usage, though whether some of the essential elements are "minerals" or gases is a moot point. In common usage we generally speak of our "mineral needs" rather than our "element needs," and of "minerals" in foods or diets rather than "elements."

The element sulfur is also need by the body, but is utilized in the organic rather than inorganic form (see Chap. 5).

†All six macrominerals are required by the human diet in amounts over 100 mg per day. This serves as a convenient dividing line between macrominerals and trace elements.

Calcium (Ca) was discovered in 1808 by Sir Humphry Davy, the English chemist.* It exists in nature only in the combined form, often with phosphorus, in such common substances as chalk, limestone, granite, egg shell, sea shells, "hard" water, and bone (all of which can serve as a source of calcium in the diet). Calcium makes up about 1.5 to 2.2 percent of the human body, more than any other mineral.

Phosphorus (P), a nonmetallic element, was first identified in urine in 1669 by a German alchemist, Brand. It created much interest, since this element, in the unnatural free form, glows in the dark, is very toxic, breaks into fire spontaneously, and is used in making matches and smoke screens. Fortunately, it exists in nature only in the combined forms (usually with calcium) in such sources as bone and rock phosphates. It is widely used in detergents and in fertilizers. Phosphorus is present in the body at a level of about 1 percent. It is one of the most important nutrients known, taking part in almost every reaction in the body.

Absorption and Retention in Body

Calcium and phosphorus in digested food material (either taken as salts in food or liberated from organic combinations to free soluble forms) are absorbed through the intestinal wall and carried by the blood in the more soluble forms to all parts of the body.

Absorption of calcium and phosphorus from the intestinal tract varies with different individuals and under different conditions, but it is not as

*Sir Humphry Davy (1778–1829) not only named and identified calcium but also potassium, sodium, chlorine, and boron. He is also recognized as the discoverer of free magnesium and barium. Of interest is the fact that in his home town of Penzance, Cornwall, a statue in the center square honors him in tribute not to his work with these highly important elements but for his invention of the miner's safety lamp, of greater importance to this mining community.

complete as for some other nutrients. In the first place, any calcium or phosphorus that is in organic combination must be set free in soluble form before it can be absorbed; and second, various substances or conditions in the intestinal tract may contribute to the formation of insoluble (and hence unabsorbable) compounds of one or the other of these two elements. On a mixed diet under ordinary conditions, about 70 percent of the phosphorus intake is thought to be absorbed but only 20 to 40 percent of the calcium intake is absorbed. Under special conditions or with individual foods the relative absorption may be either higher or lower. Some of the factors which either favor or hinder the absorption of calcium or phosphorus from the intestinal contents are listed briefly in Table 11–1.

The fact that *oxalic acid* in certain foods (e.g., rhubarb, cocoa, and spinach) forms an insoluble salt with calcium (calcium oxalate), and that *phytic acid* in the outer coats of cereals can tie up much of the calcium and phosphorus in insoluble compounds, is not considered of major practical importance, provided the supply of these elements in the diet is liberal enough that sufficient absorbable calcium and phosphorus remain to meet body needs.

Excessive amounts of fatty acids in the intestine can also tie up calcium by forming insoluble "soaps," but this, too, appears to have little practical significance when persons are eating normal diets (see Chapter 18). The amount of *vitamin D* available in the body, however, does play an important role in both the *absorption* and *utilization* of calcium and phosphorus, especially calcium.

Possibly even more potent factors influencing the relative amounts of calcium and phosphorus that are *absorbed* and *retained in the body,* are the body's *need* for these elements, especially calcium, and the *level of intake* to which the body has become adapted. If a person regularly takes in large amounts of calcium, his body adjusts

Table 11–1. *Absorption of Calcium and Phosphorus from the Intestinal Tract*

Factors Favoring Absorption	*Factors Hindering Absorption*
Acid reaction in upper intestinal tract	Alkaline reaction in lower intestinal tract.
Normal digestive activity and normal motility of intestinal tract.	Large amounts of fiber in diet.
	Laxatives or any circumstances that induce diarrhea or hypermotility of the intestine.
Calcium and phosphorus in diet in about equal amounts.	Large excess of either element in comparison with the other (Ca:P ratio unbalanced).
The fat-soluble vitamin D.	With excess calcium present, insoluble Ca salts may be formed with phytin (complex P compound in cereals), oxalic acid (in certain leafy vegetables), and unabsorbed fatty acids.
Need for higher amounts of these mineral elements by the body.	Excess of iron, magnesium, or aluminum forms insoluble phosphates.

by absorbing less calcium. On the other hand, people may adjust to a lower level of calcium intake by more efficient absorption and decreased excretion of this element, thus conserving sufficient calcium for upkeep of body tissues, but in the case of calcium the readjustment process may take many weeks, or months. Again, the amount absorbed is largely dependent on *body need*. In an infant or young child (or during healing of bone fractures), absorption of calcium is relatively more efficient, so that a larger percentage of the intake is available for the building or strengthening of bone tissues. The same is true in pregnancy or in an adult after a fairly long period on a low-calcium intake, in which body stores of this element are likely to be depleted. If higher calcium intake is provided, a relatively larger amount of calcium is absorbed and retained in the body than if the previous diet had furnished calcium in liberal quantities. Thus, the relative amounts of calcium and phosphorus retained in the body vary, depending on the age of the person, his previous dietary habits, and the level of the current supply.

Distribution in Body

Ninety-nine percent of the calcium and about 80 percent of the phosphorus in the body are in the bones and teeth. The remaining 1 percent of calcium is present mostly in the blood and extracellular tissues, with very small amounts in the soft tissues and organs. On the other hand, the 20 percent of phosphorus content of the body not involved in bones is present mostly in the soft tissues, with some phosphorus in every cell and vitally involved in cell functions.

Calcium is a relatively inert element, while phosphorus is itself highly reactive and imparts this property to substances with which it is combined. Phosphorus is present in or combines readily with proteins, lipids, or carbohydrates. Chemically inert substances such as glucose and fats become highly reactive in tissue metabolism and more readily transported in body fluids by combination with phosphate (PO_4^{---}) radicals. In the blood, from one-third to one-half of the calcium is in the serum as inorganic salts (chiefly phosphates or bicarbonates) that ionize, while the remainder is combined with protein, does not ionize, and must be split off by enzymes before use in metabolism. From one-half to two-thirds the phosphorus in blood is contained within the red cells.

Functions in Body

Although the amounts of calcium and phosphorus in the blood are small by comparison with those contained in the bony structure, each element has a vital role to play. ***Calcium*** in blood plasma is one of the essential factors for blood clotting, markedly affects muscle tone and irritability, and is required for normal nerve transmission. The proper balance between calcium ions on the one hand and sodium, potassium, and magnesium ions on the other is necessary for normal rhythmic contraction and relaxation of the heart muscles. Regulation of blood calcium to a normal level is an important function of the parathyroid glands and of the hormone *calcitonin* which regulates the release of calcium from bone. When the blood level of calcium is low, calcitonin is stimulated to promote withdrawal of some calcium from the stores in the bones. A high blood calcium level appears to inhibit the action of the parathyroids and to promote excretion of calcium. There is a dynamic equilibrium between the calcium in the skeletal structure and in the blood. Calcium also activates several enzymes important in metabolism.

Phosphorus performs an important role in combining with calcium in the formation and strengthening of bone tissues. Inorganic phosphates in the blood act as buffer substances that assist in maintaining blood neutrality and the acid-base balance of the blood (p. 230). Phosphorus (as phosphate radicals) is an essential constituent of nucleic acids and nucleoproteins in cell nuclei and cytoplasm, which play a key role in reproduction, transmission of hereditary traits, cell division, and protein synthesis within the cells. Phosphates are also a component of phospholipids, which promote the emulsification and transport of fats and fatty acids, as well as permeability of cell membranes. Also, phosphates are indispensable to the oxidation of carbohydrates by which much of the energy for body processes is obtained, links with glycogen and glucose to activate them for oxidation, and is a part of several enzymes or coenzymes that are essential to this oxidation. Adenosine mono-, di-, and triphosphates are among the most vital of all body substances, for regulation of hormone activity and in providing quick release of energy in muscular contraction.

Metabolism and Excretion

The turnover of mineral elements in metabolism is much slower than that of carbohydrates, fats, and proteins. It has been estimated that there is a daily exchange of about one-third of 1 percent of the body protein, as against one-eighth of 1 percent of the phosphorus and one-twentieth of 1 percent of the calcium. The metabolism of bones and teeth is especially slow. Formerly the calcium phosphate stored in these tissues was thought of chiefly as inert material which, although it to some extent constituted *reserve stores* of these minerals, was drawn on only in cases of great need. The stores of these two elements in the bones, especially that in the ends of bones (epiphyses), has now been shown to be much more readily available for use in the body than formerly thought; in fact, it is continuously in dynamic equilibrium with these elements as carried in blood and interstitial fluids.

Bones and teeth have a very interesting structure. Bones are about 70 percent mineral matter and 30 percent organic material (protein, nucleoprotein, and the substances in bone marrow). The mineral part is comprised of tiny crystals of complex calcium salts, mainly phosphates (but also small amounts of carbonates, magnesium, and fluorine). These are arranged in honeycomb fashion around the soft matrix and bathed in intracellular fluid (with blood vessels within the marrow)—an arrangement which favors exchange of mineral elements and nutrients between the tissues and body fluids. The same type of structure occurs in the teeth, except that the mineral crystals in the enamel and

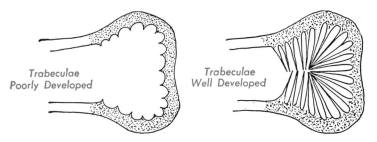

Figure 11–1. Diagrammatic representations of bone trabeculae showing poor or good development according to whether the food calcium intake is low or liberal. (From Sherman, H. C.: *Chemistry of Food and Nutrition.* New York, Macmillan Co., 1952.)

dentine are larger and more densely packed, which makes for relatively slower metabolism in teeth. Once the teeth are laid down and calcified, their composition is difficult to alter by changes in diet.

The most labile supply of calcium and phosphorus in bones is found in the *trabeculae*—columns of crystalline calcium compounds that grow from the inner surface of the cavity at the bone's end and project toward the center in such a way as to act as braces in strengthening the end of the bone. Within the cavity, blood vessels and interstitial fluid come into intimate contact with the mineral material in the trabeculae, so that it may be readily taken up by the blood stream to meet minor fluctuations in blood calcium. The more abundant the supply of calcium in the food, the greater is the development of bone trabeculae, while on a low-calcium diet over a consider-able period these structures may be practically absent (Fig. 11–1).

The levels of calcium and phosphates in the blood are controlled by the action of calcitonin and other hormones, and represent a balance between the amounts of the elements absorbed, the demand of the various tissues, the amounts contributed from bone and by discarded cells, and the amounts excreted (see Fig. 11–2). Any excess quantities of these two elements are excreted in part as soluble salts in the *urine* and in part by secretion across the intestinal membrane into the *fecal material*. The feces thus contain some calcium and phosphorus that remained unabsorbed from the food, along with some that has been metabolized and excreted into the intestine. The relative amounts that leave the body by the urinary or intestinal route vary with numerous conditions. It has been estimated that about 175 mg per day of

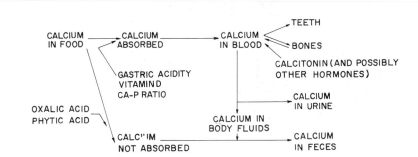

Figure 11–2. Absorption and utilization of calcium. (From McHenry, E. W.: *Basic Nutrition.* Philadelphia, Lippincott, 1963.)

calcium is lost in the urine in adults and about 125 mg in the feces, for a total of at least 300 mg.[3]

Minor amounts of calcium may be lost in perspiration (at least 20 mg per day), but they need be taken into account only in cases of excessive sweating due to physical activity at high environmental temperatures.

The amount of phosphorus excreted per day would be expected to be about in this same relative amount, but more studies are needed.

Effects of Dietary Deficiencies of Calcium and Phosphorus

In *children or young animals*, who need calcium and phosphorus in relatively large amounts for building bones and teeth, an insufficient supply of either element or both produces effects that are readily seen or otherwise demonstrated. The effects of such deficiencies during the growth period may be manifested in one or more of the following ways:

1. By stunting of growth.
2. By poor quality of bones and teeth.
3. By malformation of bones (rickets).

When calcium lack has not been too severe, no effect may be noted in the size of the body, but the bones may be either delicate and brittle, or remain soft and pliable because too little mineral salts are deposited in them. The skeleton of the smaller rat in Figure 11–3 shows both stunting in size of bones and their poor quality as exemplified in brittleness and certain deformities. The child suffering from rickets shown in Figure 11–4 evidences the bone deformities peculiar to that disease—narrow chest, enlargement of bones at their ends (seen at knees), and bow-legs resulting from inability of soft bones to bear the body weight. This disease can be caused by lack of either calcium, phosphorus, or vitamin D, or combinations of all three nutrients. The bone deformities of rickets may persist in later life, the narrow pelvic cavity being a complicating factor in pregnancy.

The *teeth* are largely formed during the latter part of fetal life and during infancy. Any lack of calcium or phosphorus during this period is likely to result in malformed teeth and jaws, or in poor quality teeth that are more subject to decay in later life. Many instances of poor quality teeth or of teeth crowded too closely in a narrow jaw may be attributable to the mother's insufficient supply of calcium, phos-

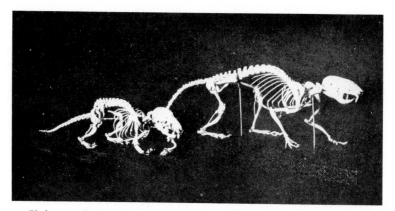

Figure 11–3. Skeletons of twin albino rats, showing influence of calcium content of the diet on the growth and character of the bones. **Right,** This rat, fed a diet adequate in calcium, attained full growth and had strong bones. **Left,** This rat received a diet deficient in calcium. Its growth was stunted, and its bones were soft, fragile, and more or less deformed. (Courtesy of Sherman and MacLeod and the *Journal of Biological Chemistry*.)

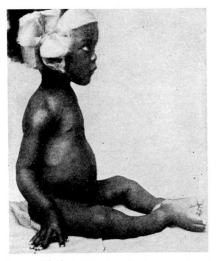

Figure 11–4. Rachitic child—note bowlegs with enlargement of bones about joints, deformity of chest, and enlargement of abdomen. (From Morse: *Clinical Pediatrics.*)

phorus, or other dietary essentials during pregnancy or to the child receiving an insufficient supply of these dietary essentials during its first years of life. It is difficult, by good diet in later life, to undo the effects of such deficiencies during the formative periods. Figure 11–5 shows the effects on the facial bones and teeth resulting from severe and prolonged deficiency of calcium and phosphorus in the diet, contrasted with those children whose diets have supplied these elements liberally.

In parts of the world where food supplies and living conditions are poor, conditions that indicate calcium or phosphorus deficiency may be found frequently, both in children and in adults. When milk and meats are scarce or unavailable, a large proportion of the diet must come from vegetable sources, especially cereal grains. Such diets are usually low in calcium, as well as deficient in the quantity and biological value of the proteins supplied. Populations do adapt to low-calcium diets, their children grow, and bone disease is not common among them. However, the children in such countries are often as much as three years behind in growth rate, as compared with well nourished children, and the shorter stature attained by many of the adults suggests strongly that the low level of calcium intake (probably accompanied by other dietary lacks) may have prevented them from developing the full height of which they were genetically capable. Children of such parents, when given a more nutritionally adequate diet, respond with increased growth rate and are considerably taller by adulthood than the stature of their parents.

A lifetime of a low-calcium intake may be a contributing factor to a state of gradual demineralization of bony tissues known as *osteoporosis*. This disorder is characterized by porosity, thinness, and fragility of the bones. Apparently in the continuous remodeling of bone, calcium has been withdrawn for body use or mandatory excretion over a long period and the calcium has not been adequately replaced. Recent work has established the fairly common occurrence of this disorder among older people both in this country and elsewhere. Women are more liable to develop osteoporosis than men, perhaps because their diets are apt to be lower in calcium content than those of men. A recent radiographic survey of 100 aged women disclosed symptoms of osteoporosis in 26 percent, with hip fractures in 15 percent. Some cases may respond to an increased calcium intake by showing calcium storage (positive balance), but it seems probable that, in addition to calcium insufficiency, a lack of sex hormones or of protein may be causative factors.

A disease with somewhat similar symptoms, *nutritional osteomalacia*, occurs fairly commonly in parts of the world but is largely due to lack of vitamin D (rather than calcium and/or phosphorus—but these also may be lacking).

Phosphorus deficiency sometimes occurs in cattle grazing on soil that has been depleted of phosphates (by crops, leach-

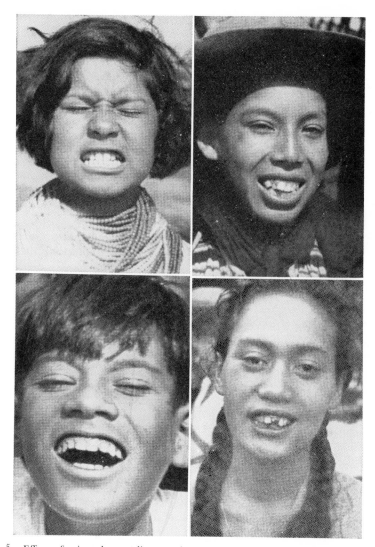

Figure 11–5. Effect of mineral-poor diets on the teeth and facial bone structure. **Top,** Two Seminole Indian children in Florida. **Bottom,** Two Polynesian children. Note the broad faces, well developed jaws, wide dental arches, and splendid teeth in the two children at left, both of whose families used native diets. Families of the two children at right had adopted modern diets through contact with white civilization. Note the narrowing of the face and jaws (especially lower jaw), crowding of teeth due to narrow dental arch, and dental caries that resulted from diets rich in highly milled cereals and sweet foods. (From W. A. Price: *Nutrition and Physical Degeneration.* New York, P. B. Hoeber, 1939.)

ing, etc.), for the grass grown on such soil is of low phosphorus content. Such a deficiency is evidenced by decrease or distortion of the appetite (desire to eat bones, wood, etc.), emaciation, weakness, and eventually death. Phosphorus deficiency seldom, if ever, develops in normal humans because of its wide distribution in food. Deficiencies are seen in man in certain clinical conditions, in persons receiving antacids over long periods, and in certain stress situations such as bone fractures. Such persons may show weakness, bone pain, demineralization of bone, and loss of calcium.

Calcium and phosphorus are continuously being lost from the body through excretion in the urine and feces (to a small extent through the skin), and smaller amounts are required for the interchange between bone tissues and interstitial fluids. The *minimum requirement* in the case of adults is the amount needed to balance these losses.

Attempts to fix a minimum requirement were at first based on balance experiments similar to those described for nitrogen balance (pp. 83–84), but in the case of calcium this method proved to have many drawbacks. While it is possible to obtain some mean value or rather narrow range within which the majority of subjects attain balance, there are many cases in which inexplicable variations occur. Even after two or three weeks on a basal diet of known calcium content, when the calcium intake is lowered in attempting to find the minimum requirement, some subjects maintain equilibrium on the lowered intake, while others are in either negative or positive balance. Knowing as we do that absorption of calcium is influenced by body need and that previous patterns of excretion are carried over into the later periods because of slow adaptations to changed levels of intake, this would have to be expected. For instance, a person whose calcium intake was liberal, when placed on the lower level of intake has less efficient absorption of calcium and carries over his pattern of high excretion, drawing on his already built-up stores of body calcium (called the *labile calcium pool*) to make up the difference. Hence, he responds to the lowered level by showing a negative balance, although the stores of calcium in his body were excellent.

With such obvious drawbacks in the balance method, investigators have been unable to give an exact figure for the minimum calcium requirement of adults. Estimates of the minimum requirement range from about 400 to 650 mg per day for an adult of average weight with ideal absorption and other ideal conditions.

Several well-known earlier studies[4] have claimed that men can adapt, with time, to lower calcium intakes and to maintain calcium balance on intakes as low as 200 to 400 mg daily. Although it is true that a higher proportion of calcium is utilized on a low intake than when it is liberally supplied, most of the national groups cited as in equilibrium on such low calcium intakes either live in tropical or semitropical areas (where abundant sunlight favors calcium utilization by forming vitamin D in the body) or may have hitherto unrecognized sources of calcium in the diet, such as white clay quite commonly consumed by some cultures (a practice known as *pica*); the lime-steeped corn used for making tortillas in Mexico; or the "stone powder," which is essentially calcium carbonate, added to rice during its milling in Formosa. In a review of the extensive literature on calcium balance experiments, Ohlson states, "Few adults eating diets characteristic of our society are in equilibrium on intakes of less than 500 mg (0.5 gm) per day."[5] It is known that calcium requirements are influenced by levels of protein intake—the greater the protein intake, the greater the calcium loss.

The Food and Nutrition Board in 1968 kept its *recommended allowance for calcium* at 800 mg per day for adults.[3] This allowance provides a factor of safety above the bare maintenance requirement and covers individual differences of need and of the ability to utilize calcium from the diet. Despite the usually lesser weight and lighter skeletal structure of women, the same amount is recommended for women as for men in order to cover menstrual losses and to provide a reserve store in the body to meet needs of pregnancy and lactation. Table 11–2 gives the recommended dietary allowances for growing children and adults of all ages

Table 11–2. *Recommended Dietary Allowances per Day for Calcium and Phosphorus**

	Age	Calcium, mg	Phosphorus, mg
Males	10–12 years	1200	1200
	12–18 years	1400	1400
	18 years or over	800	800
Females	10–12 years	1200	1200
	12–18 years	1300	1300
	18 years or over	800	800
	Pregnant		
	12–18 years	1700	1700
	18 or over	1200	1200
	Lactating		
	12–18	1800	1800
	18 or over	1300	1300

*Food and Nutrition Board (Canada) 1968.[3]

for both calcium and phosphorus (see more details in Appendix, Table 1). The recommended allowances of calcium vary from country to country (see Appendix, Table 1B), ranging from as low as 400 mg a day up to 1000 mg. These differences are to be expected until more research is done on the subject. At this time, we would advise a student to use that figure for himself recommended by the highest nutrition authority in his own country (in the United States it is the Food and Nutrition Board) because of different dietary and environmental conditions in each country.

An FAO/WHO Expert Committee has proposed intakes of calcium between 400 and 500 mg per day as "suggested practical allowances" for adults, especially for countries where calcium-rich foods such as dairy products are either not plentiful or unavailable.[6]

It appears obvious that a large proportion of the population can adjust to levels of calcium intake of 0.5 to 0.6 gm per day without any disadvantageous symptoms, and if their reserves of calcium in skeletal tissue are less than optimum, it is difficult to detect or measure any such depletion. In fact, 10 to 40 percent of the mineral material in bones may be withdrawn for body use before a decrease in bone density can

be detected by x-ray pictures. It is evident that the recommended allowance of the United States has a considerable factor of safety for most adults.

For the first time, in 1968, the Food and Nutrition Board[3] gave specific *recommended dietary allowances for phosphorus*. Without other evidence available, the allowances for phosphorus were made the same as for calcium (except for infants). See Table 11–2 and Table 1 of the Appendix. The allowance for a normal adult is 800 mg a day. About twice as much calcium as phosphorus is present in bones and teeth, but because of the much higher amounts of phosphorus in soft body tissues and in our food supply, it is estimated that the requirement is similar to that for calcium. These figures should be considered only as preliminary, since much more research needs to be done in this area before more specific recommendations can be made.

Allowances During Childhood, Pregnancy, and Lactation

Adults need calcium and phosphorus only for maintenance of a body already built, but children need also a "growth quota." Extra amounts of these ele-

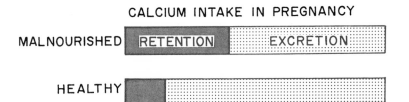

Figure 11–6.   Some women enter into pregnancy with too low reserves of those nutrients that can be stored in the body because of previous inadequate diets. Calcium is one of the nutrients most likely to be furnished in less than optimum amounts in American diets. This diagram shows that, when given a relatively rich supply of calcium during pregnancy, the previously malnourished woman retained a good percentage of it, thereby building up her body reserves of this element. The woman whose diet before pregnancy had been adequate and whose stores of calcium were therefore higher had less need to store it and hence retained a smaller percentage of the calcium furnished by the diet than the other woman. (Adapted from Macy and Williams: *Hidden Hunger.* Jacques Cattell Press, Lancaster, Pa., 1945.)

ments are required not only for the *growth* of bones but also for their *strengthening* by further deposits of calcium phosphate. The bones of a newborn infant are more flexible and of lower mineral content than those of an adult, a provision of nature which makes birth easier. As the child grows, the relative proportion of calcium phosphate in the bones must be increased, so that they will become stronger and more rigid, in order to bear the weight of the body, and to be less easily broken. The teeth are formed and partially calcified in the latter months of fetal life, and their calcification is practically completed by the time the child is two to three years old. For children from two to six years of age, the calcium and the phosphorus allowances are the same as for adults (800 mg), and from ages six to ten the allowances are 1000 mg (1 gm). Per unit of weight, growing children may need two to four times as much calcium as does an adult.

Children will continue to grow on diets that supply less than desirable amounts of calcium or phosphorus, but the bones and teeth will not be of as good quality, or growth may not be so rapid as with a more liberal allowance of these elements. If the quantity of either element is too limited, growth may be stunted. During the rapid growth in the period of preadolescence and puberty (10 to 18 years), a higher intake is recommended (1200 to 1400 mg; see Table 11–2). At levels of 1 to 1.5 gm daily of each of these elements in the diet, children have shown "maximum retention"—that is, as much calcium and phosphorus is provided as the body can store.[7] Higher levels would normally be excreted by the body.

Women in the latter half of pregnancy and those who are nursing their babies have considerably higher calcium and phosphorus needs than do normal adults, since the mineral needs of the growing fetus or infant must be met through the mother's body. For mothers, as well as for growing children, there should also be a *plentiful supply of vitamin D,* a vitamin that helps assure good absorption and assimilation of the mineral elements provided in the diet. A liberal intake of calcium is especially important during lactation, in order to provide for the secretion of calcium-rich milk without undue drain on the reserve stores of calcium in the mother's own body (Fig. 11–6). Specific allowances for children of different ages and for pregnant and lactating women are found in Chapters 19 and 20, devoted to diet for these conditions, and also are found in Table 1 of the Appendix.

Foods as Sources of Calcium and Phosphorus

In planning a diet that will furnish enough calcium and phosphorus (or

Table 11–3. Foods Richest in Calcium and Phosphorus

Calcium (in milligrams)			Phosphorus (in milligrams)		
FOOD	PER AVG. SVG.	PER 100 GM	FOOD	PER AVG. SVG.	PER 100 GM
Sesame seeds, whole, ¼ cup	348	1160			
Milk, 8 oz glass, ½ pint	285	118	Liver, fried, 2 sl., 75 gm	311	358
Salmon, red, canned					
with bones, ⅖ cup	259	259			
Cheese, Am. Cheddar, 1 oz	225	750	Milk, 8 oz glass, ½ pint	227	93
*Leafy vegetables, avg.			Cod steak or sole, 100 gm	220	220
½ cup cooked	140	167	Lamb, leg, roast, 2 sl., 100 gm	208	208
Ice cream, plain, avg. ¾ cup	123	123	Beef, rib roast, 1 sl., 100 gm	186	186
†Molasses, med., 2 tbsp	116	290	hamburger, ¼ lb, 85 gm	165	194
Artichokes	102	51	Baked beans, canned, ½ c.	120	92
Broccoli, ⅔ cup	88	88	Cheese, Am. Cheddar, 1 oz	140	478
Baked beans, canned with			Peanut butter, 2 scant tbsp	118	393
molasses, ½ cup	82	56	Shredded wheat, 1 biscuit	102	360
tomato sauce, ½ cup	70	49	Whole wheat cereal, ½ c., ck.	113	83
Cream, light, 7 tbsp	74	97	Oatmeal, ⅔–¾ c. cooked	105	57
Orange, 1 medium	62	40	Cottage cheese, 2 rd. tbsp	108	189
‡Cottage cheese, 2 rd. tbsp	52	96	Egg, 1 large	101	210
String beans, ⅔ c., ck.	50	50	Ice cream, plain, avg., ¾ c.	99	99
Parsnips, ½ c. cooked	44	57	Cream, light, 7 tbsp	77	77
Lima beans, ½ c. cooked	38	47	Broccoli, ⅔ cup	76	76
Salad greens, raw, avg.			Nuts, mixed, 1–12 nuts, ½ oz	67	446
2 lg. or 4-5 sm. leaves	34	68	Parsnips, ½ c., cooked	62	80
Sesame seeds, hulled, ¼ cup	33	110			
Egg, 1 large	26	54	Lima beans, ½ c., ck.	97	121
Figs, dried, 1 large	25	125	Peas, canned, ½ cup	62	77
canned, 3, with juice	13	13	Corn, canned, ½ cup	43	52
Bread, whole wheat, 1 slice	23	96	Cauliflower, ¾ cup, ck.	42	72
white, 1 slice (4%			Leafy vegetables, ½ c. ck., avg.	45	45
milk solids)	19	79	Bread, whole wheat, 1 slice	60	263
Peanut butter, 2 scant tbsp	22	74	white, 1 slice		
Peas, canned, ½ c.	20	25	(4% milk solids)	21	92
Apricots, dried, ck.,			Apricots, dried, ck., 3 halves	34	34
4 halves	20	22	Figs, dried, 1 large	33	111
Orange juice, 6 oz	20	25	canned, 3, w/juice	21	35
Dates, 3-4 pitted, 1 oz	22	72	Prunes, 4-5 medium, ck.	27	40
Prunes, 4-5 medium, ck.	17	25	Dates, 3-4 pitted, 1 oz	18	60
Grapefruit, ½ medium	16	16	Orange, 1 small	37	37
Cereal, whole-grain, avg.			String beans, ⅔ c., ck.	19	23
⅔–¾ c., cooked	8-15	9	Grapefruit, ½ medium	16	16

*Including dandelion, mustard, turnip greens, collards, and kale, but excluding spinach, beet greens, and chard, in which calcium is in a poorly utilizable form.

†The calcium in molasses is due to addition of lime to neutralize acid in refining sugar; it is in lowest concentration in light molasses and highest in the blackstrap variety.

‡Calcium content of cottage cheese varies according to whether it is made from sour milk or by addition of rennin to sweet milk.

other mineral elements) to meet body needs, one must take into account three main factors:

1. How much of the mineral element is present in different foods.

2. What foods furnish it in an easily utilizable form.

3. Which of the foods are rich enough in it or can be eaten in sufficient quantity to contribute substantially to the daily quota.

In Table 11–3, the first column of figures under each mineral element gives the amount furnished in an *aver-*

age serving of each food in the condition in which it is eaten (cooked or raw). The second column shows the number of milligrams present in 100 gm of the food substance. Thus, Cheddar cheese ranks highest in calcium (750 mg) on a 100 gm basis, but an average serving, or 1 oz portion, would contribute only 225 mg, which is slightly less than the amount furnished by an 8 oz glass of milk. As a source of calcium, it would pay us to eat more liberal portions of cheeses (e.g., Cheddar or American). On a weight basis, milk (which is 87 percent water) is not so high in calcium and phosphorus as dried beans or dried figs, but it is at or near the top of the list for both elements in amount furnished in an average serving. Two other good sources of these minerals do not contribute as much as one might expect in the diet, because dried fruits ordinarily are eaten in small quantities and dried beans increase in water content on cooking. One process used to change regular farina into a quick-cooking product adds nearly 0.5 gm each of calcium and phosphorus per 100 gm of dry product (which is a good demonstration of why nutrient labeling of food products is important).

CALCIUM. To generalize, we may group foods according to their contributions of calcium in the ordinary diet as follows:

Excellent sources — hard cheeses, milk, most dark green leafy vegetables, and soft fish bones.

Good sources — softer cheeses, ice cream, broccoli, baked beans, dried legumes, and dried figs.

Fair sources — cottage cheese, light cream, oranges, dates, salad greens, nuts, lima beans, parsnips, and eggs.

Poor sources — most other fruits and vegetables, grains, and meats.

Eggs and nuts (which are high in phosphorus) are of only moderate calcium content, while meat, poultry, and fish are calcium-poor. Most fruits and vegetables, bread, and breakfast cereals contain relatively minor quantities, but if eaten in considerable quantities, may add appreciably to the calcium intake.

About 75 percent of all the calcium in the American food supply comes from dairy products (other than butter). The rest is about equally distributed between meat, eggs, vegetables, beans, and cereals. Enrichment of foods with calcium is not as yet widely done in this country.

PHOSPHORUS. Phosphorus is associated chiefly with protein-rich foods and cereal products. It is found in many foods that contribute little calcium, as well as along with calcium in milk and its products. Rich sources of phosphorus in the diet are meats (especially organs), fish, and poultry, eggs, cheeses and milk, nuts, legumes, and all foods made from grains (especially whole grains). Fruits (especially dried ones) and vegetables contribute lesser amounts of phosphorus to the diet. In general, edible roots, stems, and flowerets of plants contain similar amounts of both calcium and phosphorus, but plants concentrate calcium in the green leaves and phosphorus in the seeds (grains). The darker green leaves have higher calcium content than light green ones (e.g., the inner leaves of head lettuce).

It is seen that phosphorus is carried in foods more liberally than is calcium, and many foods that provide little calcium (such as meats) are excellent sources of phosphorus. Since its distribution follows that of protein, a diet that supplies adequate amounts of protein is usually adequate for phosphorus.

In the American food supply, over 60 percent of the phosphorus comes from dairy products and meat, poultry, and fish. Flour and cereal products contribute 12 percent of the supply. The rest comes largely from eggs, potatoes, vegetables, and beans. Sugar and fats provide only trace amounts of calcium and phosphorus.

*How to Get the Recommended
Allowance of Calcium in the Diet*

Of the various nutrients required, calcium is one of those most likely to be provided by the diet in less than recommended or optimal quantities. However, it is not difficult to obtain the recommended allowance of 800 mg daily if one includes 2 cups (1 pint) of milk (or its calcium equivalent in milk products other than butter). In Table 11–4, four groups of foods are given, each of which furnishes the recommended calcium allowance for a day, with the amount of milk decreasing in each group from left to right (from 1½ pints, which furnishes more than the day's allowance, to none). It should be noted that, with lesser amounts of milk (or none in group 4), cheese or ice cream, as well as green leafy vegetables and broccoli, are depended on as major sources of calcium.

Other foods in an average diet (some of which are classed as fair, moderate, or even poor sources of calcium) may together contribute significant amounts toward the day's total intake. Two servings each of fruit and vegetables (other than green leafy ones or broccoli) might contribute somewhere in the neighborhood of 100 to 150 mg cal-cium, while four to six slices of bread or a serving of cereal might contribute 75 to 150 mg, especially if whole grain cereals or bread made with added milk solids are used. The typical American dietary pattern of bread and butter, meat and potatoes, other vegetable, salad or fruit, and dessert can be expected to supply about 300 mg of calcium daily. Two cups of milk in the daily diet would bring the total intake up to the recommended allowance, yet less than one-fifth the women in a dietary survey had this amount of milk in their diet, even when that in cream soups, white sauce, puddings, and ice cream was taken into account.[8]

It is also important to consider which foods carry calcium in forms that are readily absorbed from the intestine and hence available for use in the body. The calcium in milk is highly utilized by man, and its availability is not altered by pasteurization. Broccoli, cauliflower, and kale rank almost with milk in availability of their calcium content, while that in carrots, lettuce, string beans, and almonds has been shown to be only slightly less well assimilated. Leafy vegetables with fairly well utilized calcium include kale, cabbage, collards, turnip greens, and probably also mustard and dandelion greens. Spinach,

*Table 11–4. Foods That Furnish the Adult Recommended Calcium Allowance
(800 mg daily)*

(1)	Calcium, mg	(2)	Calcium, mg	(3)	Calcium, mg	(4)	Calcium, mg
Milk, 1½ pts	855	Milk, 1 pint	570	Milk, ½ pint	285	Cheese, Am.	
		Cottage cheese, 2 rd. tbsp	52	Cheese, Am. Cheddar, 1 oz	225	Cheddar, 1½ oz	337
		Bread, w. w., 4 slices	92	Bread, w. w., 5 slices	95	Ice cream, plain, ⅙ qt	123
		Orange, 1 med.	62	Orange juice, 8 oz	24	Bread, w. w., 4 slices	92
		Green beans, ¾ c., ck.	45	Broccoli, ⅔ c.	88	Turnip greens, ½ c., ck.	138
			821	Carrots, diced, ⅔ c.	33	Beans, baked, with molasses, ½ c.	82
				Cream, light, 4 tbsp	61	Egg, 1 med.	27
					811	Hamburger, lean, 85 gm	10
							809

chard, and beet greens have much of their calcium in insoluble combination with oxalic acid, and hence in a form unavailable to the body, but this is no menace if there is plenty of absorbable calcium in the diet, and these greens are valuable sources of iron and vitamin A.

The inclusion of at least a pint of milk daily in the diet of adults is urged as the chief means for obtaining the calcium quota, as well as for the high quality proteins and vitamins that milk provides. For those who do not drink milk it should be incorporated in cooked foods wherever possible, and the more common use of cheese would also be advantageous. Hard cheeses have much higher calcium content than soft cheeses with higher water content; cottage cheese has only about one-seventh as much calcium as a hard cheese like Cheddar (American), but ½ cup of it can take the place of a scant half cup of milk in calcium value. The wider use of green leafy vegetables (including salad greens) would help to reinforce the diet in calcium, as well as in other minerals and vitamins.

How adequate are freely chosen diets in the United States as to the amount of calcium they supply? The answer to this depends upon which index, or standard, is used and which age and sex group. Then, too, a survey of an *average* population does not mean too much, since adequate calcium intakes are so dependent upon the consumption of milk or milk products by individuals, which varies widely. Whenever milk intake is low, calcium intakes are very likely to be low unless other calcium sources are substituted. Fifteen to 25 percent of the American population consume very little, or no, milk, which is directly indicative of the extent of inadequate calcium intakes.

Within a family, fathers and adolescent boys are most likely to eat food that meets the recommended allowances of calcium, while mothers, pregnant and lactating women, and adolescent girls are least likely to do so. Statistics in the United States[9-13] show that girls from age 11 up, on the average, consume less than 75 percent of the recommended allowances of calcium. After age 35 this drops to 66 percent or less.[11] Since this is an *average* figure, it means that there is no question that calcium intakes are too low in many individual females. Males tend to consume more calcium than females at all age periods, no doubt due to their greater total intake of food.

Overall, it appears that at least 10 percent of the American population is consuming less than one-half of the recommended allowance of calcium,[12-13] an inadequate amount. Anywhere from 15 to 40 percent of men in the population may eat less than two-thirds of the recommended amount of calcium; 50 percent of adolescent girls and 75 percent of women 38 to 80 years of age fall into this category of calcium intake.

Records of growth of children, and osteoporosis (soft bones) in older individuals, are as useful an indicator of calcium (and phosphorus) deficiencies as any available. The recent Ten State Survey in the United States[14] showed averages of from 10 to 50 percent of low income children (six years old or less) in different states with "one or more standard deviations below Iowa growth standards." In a recent study in Tennessee on 300 preschool children from poor black families, half of the children were found to be below the twenty-fifth percentile (of "normal" values) for height.[15] These differences are probably largely due to calcium deficiency (though this remains to be proved). The existence of osteoporosis in older females is known to be very high, but exact figures are not available.

Suggestions have been made for reinforcing the calcium content of some staple foods. The most commonly used of these is the addition of nonfat milk solids to bread in amounts of either 2, 4, or 6 percent. The 6 percent level brings the calcium content nearly up to that of bread made with whole wheat. However, the addition of milk solids is

not mandatory, and because of inadequate nutritional labeling of our bread
supply (i.e., calcium level per slice or
per pound), the consumer has much
difficulty in knowing the calcium content of any bread. Even whole-wheat
bread does not contribute considerable
amounts of calcium.

If calcium is taken in pills (by doctor's advice), it should be in the form of
some soluble salt, such as calcium lac-
tate. Unless there is some excellent
reason (e.g., an allergy to milk or intolerance to appreciable amounts of
lactose), it is far better to revise the diet
so as to include more calcium-rich
foods, which furnish, along with calcium, other minerals, vitamins, and
amino acids essential for body welfare.

Phosphorus deficiency is very uncommon in the United States (except
in some clinical situations and through
long-term use of antacids[16]) because of
its widespread distribution in food supplies. However, persons consuming
typical vegetarian-type diets (especially
those low in milk products) might easily
be deficient in this element (as well as
other nutrients). It is well known that
farm animals fed diets composed only
of grains, legumes, and green leafy
feeds must have supplementary phosphorus (as well as calcium) in order to
have adequate growth and bone structure.

MAGNESIUM

Magnesium (Mg) is a silvery-white
metal related closely to calcium and zinc.
Much has been learned in nutrition the
past few years about this very vital
mineral.

Magnesium is the eighth most plentiful element in the earth's crust (2.1
percent) and the third most abundant
and lightest structural metal. We see it
all about us in a modern world as magnesium alloys (usually containing over
75 percent of this mineral) in air planes,
parts of cars (up to 90 pounds in a

Volkswagen), ladders, portable tools,
luggage, vacuum cleaners, and as the
silver-like material which provides the
light in flares, flash bulbs, and fireworks.
It is said that more magnesium is in
orbit than any other mineral, since it is
the major component of space ships.
It is also the major mineral in asbestos,
talcum powder, and dolomite limestone
(a fertilizer).

More important to nutritionists, magnesium has dozens of essential biological functions in the plant and animal
body. As the central component of
chlorophyll, the well-known green pigment of all higher plants, it is absolutely essential in plants for making
glucose and oxygen from sunlight
(energy source), water, and carbon
dioxide (photosynthesis) without which
life itself could not exist. Magnesium
is a major mineral component of seawater (0.13 percent) from which life
and chlorophyll originally evolved. It
is estimated that each cubic mile of
seawater, a good industrial source,
contains 6 million tons of magnesium,
so it appears that we will have enough
in the future to take care of our needs!

Discovery and Identification as a Nutrient

We are all familiar with "milk of magnesia" (magnesium hydroxide) and
Epsom salts* (magnesium sulfate).
Salts of magnesium have been known
through the ages for their healing properties. A Roman, whose name is unknown to us, claimed many centries
ago that "magnesia alba" (white magnesium salts from the district of Magnesia in Greece, from which the element was eventually named) cured
many ailments. The Scottish chemist
Joseph Black, working with this sub-

*Named after Epsom, a village south of Lon-
don, found in 1618 to have a water supply with
wound-healing properties and with a laxative
effect. "Epsom salts" were the substance formed
after evaporation of the water.

stance (now known to be magnesium carbonate), discovered in 1755 that magnesium was an element. It was first isolated in 1808 by Sir Humphry Davy, the same person who first isolated many other elements (see p. 238).

Though magnesium was found to be present in the human body in the 1850's, it was not until 1926 that Leroy, in France, could first prove that magnesium is an essential nutrient for the animal body (he used the mouse).[17] Later, McCollum and co-workers[18] described the wide range of deficiency signs in rats and dogs, including *magnesium tetany*, a form of convulsions in which the nerves and muscles are affected. Indications that magnesium was required by man were published shortly thereafter (1933–1944).[19] More complete proof of man's need for the element has since been shown by a number of workers.[3, 20] At this time, it is a very active field of research.

Absorption and Distribution in the Body

Magnesium salts (like those of calcium) are usually rather insoluble, so that their absorption is relatively low and occurs in the small intestine. About a third of ingested magnesium is normally absorbed. The use of high levels of salts such as magnesium sulfate as laxatives depends on the fact that they draw much water into the gut by osmosis because they are so poorly absorbed. In active transport across the intestinal membrane, magnesium salts seem to use the same route as calcium salts, so that a high intake of either interferes with the absorption of the other. Unlike calcium, there is little excretion of magnesium through the intestine, except that which is unabsorbed from the food. When extra amounts of magnesium are given after long-continued magnesium-poor diets, a considerable amount is retained and stored in the bones, so the body seems to have re-

serve stores of magnesium as well as of calcium.*

The human body contains about 20 to 28 gm of magnesium, over half of which is found in the complex salts that make up bone. The remainder is chiefly found in the cells of soft tissues (especially the liver and skeletal muscles) where it is second only to potassium in abundance. Small amounts of magnesium are present in the body fluids and take part in the transfer by osmosis of water into and out of the cells, and they also take part in the regulation of the acid-base balance of the body. Mostly, magnesium circulates in body fluids in ionic form, but about 35 percent of serum magnesium is bound to protein.

Role in the Body and Deficiency Signs

The role of magnesium in animal metabolism is mainly as an activator of various enzymes, especially those which bring about the linking of phosphate groups to glucose in the formation and breakdown of glycogen and release of energy. It is essential for the transfer of "high-energy phosphate groups" (as in adenosine triphosphate, ATP). It is essential for maintenance of DNA and RNA structure. Magnesium is necessary also for regulation of temperature of the body, contractions of nerves and muscles, and synthesis of protein. The rate of its excretion in the urine seems to be influenced by aldosterone, one of the hormones of the adrenal cortex.

Symptoms of deficiency in animals are first, failure to grow, followed by pallor, weakness, low serum magne-

---

*Strontium is a nonessential mineral, of the same chemical family as calcium and magnesium, which is also deposited in bone tissue if it is introduced into the body. Normal foods carry only minute amounts of it (not enough to do harm), but much discussion has been raised as to its presence in the atmosphere (strontium-90, radioactive) as an aftermath of an atomic explosion, and toxic effects it might produce if absorbed into foods and then deposited in the bones.

sium, excessive irritability of nerves and muscles, irregular heart beats, heart and kidney damage, and convulsions or seizures (tetany), especially when the animal is suddenly disturbed. Death can result in a few weeks' time in small animals fed magnesium-deficient diets.

In man, similar nervous and muscular excitability is seen in magnesium deficiency. Behavioral disturbances, delirium, and depression are seen, as well as weakness, tremors, vertigo, and tetany (spasms, convulsions, or other forms—similar to that seen clinically in calcium deficiency).

Allowances and Nutritional Status

The magnesium requirement depends upon body size and composition of the diet. High calcium in the diet, for instance, is known to compete with the absorption of magnesium. Protein, phosphorus, and vitamin D levels also influence the requirement. Requirements are higher in pregnancy and lactation.

Because of new knowledge on requirements, the Food and Nutrition Board has recently added magnesium to its list of dietary allowances. These are summarized in Table 11–5 and are given in detail in Table 1 of the Appendix. The allowances are roughly 50 percent higher than minimal require-

*Table 11–5. Recommended Dietary Allowances of Adult for Magnesium**

	Age	Magnesium, mg/day
Males	12–14 years	350
	14–22 years	400
	22 years or over	350
Females	12–22 years	350
	22 years or over	300
	Pregnant	450
	Lactating	450

*From Food and Nutrition Board (Canada), 1968.[3]

ments (which range between 200 and 300 mg per day for adults) to allow for individual differences, normal stresses, and variations in diet composition.

Deficiency symptoms are slow to develop in humans because of reserve stores in the body; they have been observed chiefly in alcoholics (because of excessive urinary secretion induced by alcohol consumption). Magnesium deficiency also occurs in infants with kwashiorkor. Low serum magnesium levels have been seen in diabetes, in malabsorption conditions, in certain surgical patients with restricted diets, and in patients receiving high levels of diuretics over long periods. The normal kidney is able to conserve magnesium in borderline intakes, thus preventing more deficiencies from occurring. Acute kidney failure is accompanied by the reverse picture—namely high serum magnesium and depression of the central nervous system, as seen in uremic coma.

Magnesium deficiencies do not occur in normal persons eating a variety of the traditional wholesome foods. Only when one is eating a very limited diet of white rice or a mixed diet consisting only of limited amounts of highly processed foods (such as a "tea and white toast" diet) would magnesium deficiency be possible, and then only in conjunction with deficiencies of many other nutrients. Magnesium deficiency is known to occur in persons who have malfunctioning kidneys or who are alcoholics. Persons eating little or no foods over long periods (as in extreme fasting) are known to become depleted in magnesium.[21]

Food Sources

Distribution of magnesium in foods tends to follow that of protein and phosphorus. Whole grains, nuts, beans, and green leafy vegetables are good sources. Animal products including meat and milk are only poor to fair sources. Processing of foods can result in high

Table 11–6. Examples of Magnesium Distribution in Common Foods*

Food	Magnesium in Edible Portion, mg/100 gm	Food	Magnesium in Edible Portion, mg/100 gm
Apples, raw, unpared	8	Lettuce	11
Bananas, raw	33	Liver, beef	13
Beans, white, canned, baked	37	Macaroni, cooked	20
Beans, snap, frozen	21	Milk, whole	13
Beef cuts	18	Oatmeal, cooked	21
Beef, hamburger, broiled	25	Orange juice, frozen	10
Beet greens, raw	106	Peaches, raw	10
Bread, white	22	Peanuts, roasted	173
Bread, whole wheat	78	Peas	35
Cabbage, raw	13	Potatoes, unpeeled	34
Carrots, raw	23	Rice, brown, cooked	29
Chard, Swiss, raw	65	Rice, white, cooked	8
Cheese, cheddar	45	Soybeans	265
Chicken, white meat, stewed	19	Spinach, raw	88
Chocolate, sweet	107	Sweet potatoes	31
Cocoa, dry powder	420	Tomatoes, raw	14
Coffee, instant, dry powder	456	Turnip greens, raw	58
Corn flakes	16	Walnuts, black	190
Eggs, whole	11	Wheat bran (breakfast cereal)	420
Flour, whole wheat	133	Wheat germ	336
Flour, all-purpose	25	Yeast, brewer's	231

*Watt, B. K., and Merrill, A. L.: *Composition of Foods: Raw, Processed, Prepared.* Washington, D.C., U.S.D.A. Agric. Handbook No. 8, 1963. See this source for more detailed figures.

losses. Thus, there is little left in rice and white flour (about 20 percent of that in the whole grain) and none, of course, in sugar, alcohol, or fats and oils. Boiling of vegetables can cause losses if the water is discarded. Table 11–6 gives figures for magnesium distribution in some common foods.

An average American diet contains about 340 mg per day—about the recommended allowance. In such a diet, most of the magnesium comes from milk (23 percent), vegetables—including potatoes (20 percent), cereal products and flour (18 percent), meat and eggs (13 percent), coffee and cocoa (9 percent), fruit (6 percent), and dry beans, nuts, and legumes (11 percent)*.

QUESTIONS AND PROBLEMS

1. In what special tissue or tissues is most of the calcium and phosphorus

*National Food Situation, United States Department of Agriculture, November 1971.

in the body found? What function do they serve in this tissue? In what other tissues do these mineral elements occur, and what are their special roles in these tissues?

2. Can the body build up reserve stores of calcium and phosphorus, provided the diet supplies more than enough to meet current body needs? Where are these elements stored? What are the bone trabeculae and what is the advantage of having them well developed?

3. Why do growing children store more calcium and phosphorus than adults? In addition to the rate of growth what other factors influence the relative amount of the calcium intake that is retained in the body? What special advantages are there in a liberal intake of both calcium and phosphorus for young children? Why are the needs for these two elements higher in pregnant women and nursing mothers than in other adults?

4. Describe the relationship of the

hormone calcitonin to calcium nutritional needs.

5. Give the minimum requirement and recommended allowance for calcium and phosphorus in normal adults. Explain why the minimum requirement for calcium varies rather widely in different individuals. Why is the recommended allowance for calcium set as high as it is? If it varies with body size and amount of bony tissue, why is the allowance for women the same as for men? Explain how the body may adapt to varying levels of calcium intake.

6. Compare the average extent to which calcium in the food is utilized with the degree of utilization of proteins, fats, and carbohydrates in foods. Why does the absorption of mineral elements tend to be less complete? Name three factors that have a favorable influence and three that have an unfavorable influence on absorption of calcium from the intestinal contents. What vitamin exerts an important influence on the utilization of calcium and phosphorus?

7. Name the two classes of foods that are the richest sources of calcium; of phosphorus. Name five specific foods that are comparatively rich in calcium and five rich in phosphorus. Which foods are used in large enough quantities in the average diet to contribute largely in making up the calcium quota for the day? Which classes of food contribute phosphorus liberally but carry little calcium? Why is the average diet less likely to be high in calcium than in phosphorus?

8. Keep an individual record of all foods eaten in a certain day, with the quantities of each consumed. Using either Table 11–3 or the table in the Appendix which gives nutritive values of average servings or common measures of foods, calculate the quantity of calcium furnished by this day's diet (either in milligrams or grams). How does the total compare with the standard allowance for calcium? If it is lower than the standard, how could it best be reinforced as to its calcium content?

9. What symptoms may develop in growing children as the result of a deficient supply of calcium or phosphorus in the diet? Why do adults seldom show recognizable signs of such deficiency? What signs of deficiency may appear in adults after long-continued diets that furnish too little calcium for body needs? At what periods in life is the character of the teeth most affected by any deficiency in these mineral elements?

10. What is the function of magnesium in the body? Is a deficiency likely to occur in your own diet? Why? What common foods contain little or no magnesium, based on your own knowledge of foods?

REFERENCES

1. Osborne, T. B., and Mendel, L. B.: J. Biol. Chem., *34*:131, 1918.
2. McCollum, E. V.: Amer. J. Physiol., *25*:120, 1909; Hart, E. B., McCollum, E. V., and Fuller, J. G.: Univ. Wisc. Agric. Exp. Stat. Res. Bull. No. 1, 1909; Plimmer, R. H. A.: Biochem. J., 7:34, 1913; Forbes, E. B., and Keith, M. H: Ohio Agric. Exp. Stat. Tech. Series Bull. No. 5, 1914.
3. Food and Nutrition Board: *Recommended Dietary Allowances.* 7th Edition, Publication 1694. Washington, D.C., National Academy of Sciences, 1968.
4. Hegsted, D. M., Moscoso, J., and Collazos, C.: J. Nutr., *46*:181, 1952; Nicolaysen, R., et al.: Physiol. Rev., *33*:424, 1953.
5. Ohlsen, M. A.: J. Amer. Diet. Assoc., *31*:333, 1955.
6. FAO Nutrition Meetings Report: *Calcium Requirements.* Series No. 30, Rome, 1962.
7. Sherman, H. C., and Hawley, E.: J. Biol. Chem., *53*:375, 1922; Daniels, A. L., et al.: J. Nutr., *10*:373, 1935; Stearns, G., and Jeans, P. C.: Proc. Soc. Exp. Biol. Med., *32*:428, 1934; and Stearns, G.: J. Amer. Med. Assoc., *142*:478, 1950.
8. Swanson, P. P., et al.: Fed. Proc., *21*:308, 1962.
9. Morgan, A. F. (ed.): *Nutritional Status, U.S.A.* Calif. Agric. Exper. Stat. Bull. 769, 1959.
10. Ohlson, M. A., and Stearns, G.: Fed. Proc., *18*:1075, 1959.
11. U.S.D.A. Consumer and Food Economics Res. Div.: *Food Intake and Nutritive Value of Diets of Men, Women, and Children in the United States, Spring 1965* (A Preliminary Report). Washington, D.C., Agric. Res. Serv., Publ. No. ARS 62–18, 1969.
12. Davis, R. A., Gershoff, S. N., and Gamble, D. F.: J. Nutr. Educ., *1*(No. 2, Suppl. 1): 41, 1969.

13. Kelsay, J. L.: J. Nutr., *99*(No. 1, Suppl. 1, Pt. II):123, 1969.
14. Center for Disease Control: *Ten-State Nutrition Survey in the United States, 1968–1970* (Preliminary Report). Washington, D.C., U.S. Department of Health, Education, and Welfare, 1971.
15. Zee, P., Walters, T., and Mitchell, C.: J. Amer. Med. Assoc., *213*:739, 1970.
16. Lotz, M. E., Zisman, E., and Bartter, F. C.: New Eng. J. Med., *278*:409, 1968.
17. Leroy, J.: Compt. rend. Soc. Biol., *94*:431, 1926.
18. Kruse, H. D., Orent, E. R., and McCollum, E. V.: J. Biol. Chem., *96*:519, 1932; *100*: 603, 1933; Orent, E. R., Kruse, H. D., and McCollum, E. V.: Amer. J. Physiol., *101*: 454, 1932; J. Biol. Chem., *106*:573, 1934.
19. Hirschfelder, A. D.: J. Clin. Invest., *12*:982, 1933; J. Amer. Med. Assoc., *102*:1138, 1934; Daniels, A. L., and Everson, G. J.: J. Nutr., *11*:327, 1936; Miller, J. F.: Amer. J. Dis. Child., *67*:117, 1944.
20. Flink, E. B.: J. Amer. Med. Assoc., *160*: 1406, 1956; Suter, C., and Klingman, W. O.: Neurology, *5*:691, 1955; Vallee, B. L., Wacker, W. E. C., and Ulmer, D. D.: New Eng. J. Med., *262*:155, 1960; Durlach, J.: Lancet, *1*:282, 1961; Montgomery, R. D.: Lancet, *2*:264, 1960; Leverton, R. M., et al.: J. Nutr., *74*:33, 1961.
21. Drenick, E. J., Hunt, I. F., and Swendseid, M. E.: J. Clin. Endocrin. Metab., *29*:1341, 1969.

SUPPLEMENTARY READING
General, History, and Reviews

Anonymous: Nutritional implications of osteoporosis. Dairy Council Digest, *41*:25, 1970.
Clark, I.: Metabolic interrelations of calcium, magnesium, and phosphate. Amer. J. Physiol., *217*:871, 1969.
Donaldson, C. L., et al.: Effect of prolonged bed rest on bone mineral. Metabolism, *19*: 1071, 1970.
Fox, H. M., et al.: Diets of preschool children in the North Central region: Calcium, phosphorus, and iron. J. Amer. Dietet. Assoc., *59*:233, 1971.
Garn, S. M.: Nutrition Society Symposium: Nutrition and bone loss. Fed. Proc., *26*:1716, 1967.
Gitelman, H. J., and Welt, L. G.: Magnesium deficiency. Ann. Rev. Med., *20*:233, 1969.
Hankin, J. H., Margen, S., and Goldsmith, N. F.: Contribution of hard water to calcium and magnesium intakes of adults. J. Amer. Dietet. Assoc., *56*:212, 1970.
Leitch, I., and Aitken, F. C.: The estimation of calcium requirement: A re-examination. Nutr. Abs. Rev., *29*:393, 1959.
McCollum, E. V.: Early speculations on the significance of phosphorus in nutrition. J. Amer. Dietet. Assoc., *27*:650, 1951.
Murphy, E. W., Page, L., and Watt, B. K.: Major mineral elements in Type A school lunches. J. Amer. Dietet. Assoc., *57*:239, 1970.
Ohlson, M. A.: The calcium controversy. J. Amer. Dietet. Assoc., *31*:333, 1955.
Pechet, M. M., Bobadilla, E., Carroll, E. L., and Hesse, R. H.: Regulation of bone resorption and formation. Amer. J. Med., *47*: 696, 1967.
Roy, C. C., and O'Brien, D.: Calcium and phosphorus: Current concepts of metabolism. Clin. Pediat., *6*:19, 1967.
Sherman, H. C.: *Calcium and Phosphorus in Foods and Nutrition.* New York, Columbia University Press, 1947.
Shohl, A. T.: Mineral metabolism in relation to acid-base equilibrium. Physiol. Rev., *3*:509, 1923.
Stewart, C. P., and Percival, G. H.: Calcium metabolism. Physiol. Rev., *8*:283, 1928.
Zook, E. G., and Lehmann, J.: Mineral composition of fruits. II. Nitrogen, calcium, magnesium, phosphorus, potassium, aluminum, boron, copper, iron, manganese, and sodium. J. Amer. Dietet. Assoc., *52*: 225, 1968.

Calcium

American Medical Association Council on Food and Nutrition: Symposium on human calcium requirements. J. Amer. Med. Assoc., *185*:588, 1963.
Avioli, L. V.: Intestinal absorption of calcium. Arch. Intern. Med., *129*:345, 1972.
Begum, A., and Pereira, S. M.: Calcium balance studies on children accustomed to low calcium intakes. Brit. J. Nutr., *23*:905, 1969.
Bhattacharyya, A. K., et al.: Dietary calcium and fat. Effects on serum lipids and fecal excretion of cholesterol and its degradation products in man. Amer. J. Clin. Nutr., *22*:1161, 1969.
Bierenbaum, M. L., Fleishman, A. I., and Raichelson, R. I.: Long term human studies on the lipid effects of oral calcium. Lipids, *7*:202, 1972.
Bronner, F. (ed.): Symposium: Calcium absorption. Amer. J. Clin. Nutr., *22*:375, 1969.
Bullamore, J. R., Wilkinson, R., Gallagher, J. C., and Nordin, B. E. C.: Effect of age on calcium absorption. Lancet, *2*:535, 1970.
Cohn, S. H., Dombrowski, C. S., Hauser, W., and Atkins, H. L.: High calcium diet and the parameters of calcium metabolism in osteoporosis. Amer. J. Clin. Nutr., *21*: 1246, 1968.
Epstein, F. H.: Calcium and the kidney. Amer. J. Med., *45*:700, 1968.
Haymovits, A., and Rosen, J. F.: Calcitonin: Its nature and role in man. Pediatrics, *45*: 133, 1970.
Hirsch, P. F., and Munson, P. L.: Thyrocalcitonin. Physiol. Rev., *49*:548, 1969.
Katz, S. H., and Foulks, E. F.: Mineral metabolism and behavior: Abnormalities of cal-

cium homeostasis. Amer. J. Phys. Anthrop., *32*:299, 1970.

Lutwak, L.: Tracer studies of intestinal calcium absorption in man. Amer. J. Clin. Nutr., *22*:771, 1969.

Neer, R. M., et al.: Stimulation by artificial lighting of calcium absorption in elderly human subjects. Nature, *229*:255, 1971.

Nicolaysen, R., et al.: Physiology of calcium metabolism. Physiol. Rev., *33*:424, 1953.

Nordin, B. E. C.: Clinical significance and pathogenesis of osteoporosis. Brit. Med. J., *1*: 571, 1971.

Pilac, L. M., Abdon, I. C., and Mandap, E. P.: Oxalic acid content and its relation to the calcium present in sone Philippine plant foods. Phil. J. Nutr., *24*:21, 1971.

Rasmussen, H., and Pechet, M. M.: Calcitonin. Sci. American, *223*:42, 1970.

Rubin, R. P.: The role of calcium in the release of neurotransmitter substances and hormones. Pharmacol. Rev., *22*:389, 1970.

Shenolikar, I. S.: Absorption of dietary calcium in pregnancy. Amer. J. Clin. Nutr., *23*: 63, 1970.

Walker, A. R. P.: The human requirement of calcium: Should low intakes be supplemented? Amer. J. Clin. Nutr., *25*:518, 1972.

Phosphorus

Boelens, P. A., Norwood, W., Kjellstrand, C., and Brown, D. M.: Hypophosphatemia with muscle weakness due to antacids and hemodialysis. Amer. J. Dis. Child., *120*: 350, 1970.

Coburn, J. W., and Massry, S. G.: Changes in serum and urinary calcium during phosphate depletion (in dogs): Studies on mechanisms. J. Clin. Invest., *49*:1073, 1970.

Patton, M. B., et al.: The relation of calcium-to-phosphorus ratio to the utilization of these minerals by 18 young college women. J. Nutr., *50*:373, 1953.

Reiss, E., and Canterbury, J. M.: The role of phosphate in the secretion of parathyroid hormone in man. J. Clin. Invest., *49*:2146, 1970.

Schofield, F. A., et al.: Utilization of calcium, phosphorus, riboflavin and nitrogen on restricted and supplemented diets. J. Nutr., *59*:561, 1956.

Spencer, H., Menczel, J., Lewin, I., and Samachson, J.: Effect of high phosphorus intake on calcium and phosphorus metabolism in man. J. Nutr., *86*:125, 1965.

Summers, J. D., Slinger, S. J., and Cisneros, G.: Some factors affecting the biological availability of phosphorus in wheat by-products. Cereal Chem., *44*:318, 1967.

Magnesium

Anonymous: Magnesium in human nutrition. Dairy Council Digest, *42*:7, 1971.

El Shahawy, M.: Role of magnesium in myocardial function. New Eng. J. Med., *286*: 217, 1972.

Flink, E. B., and Jones, J. E. (eds.): The pathogenesis and clinical significance of magnesium deficiency. Ann. N.Y. Acad. Sci., *162*:707, 1969.

Hathaway, M. L.: *Magnesium in Human Nutrition.* Washington, D.C., U.S.D.A. Home Econ. Res. Rep. No. 19, 1962.

Krehl, W. A.: Magnesium. Nutrition Today, *2*: 16, September 1967.

Paddle, B. M., and Haugaard, N.: Role of magnesium in effects of epinephrine on heart contraction and metabolism. Amer. J. Physiol., *221*:1178, 1971.

Rook, J. A. F., and Storry, J. E.: Magnesium in the nutrition of farm animals. Nutr. Abst. Rev., *32*:1055, 1962.

Schroeder, H. A., Nason, A. P., and Tipton, I. H.: Essential metals in man, magnesium. J. Chron. Dis., *21*:815, 1969.

Seelig, M. S.: The requirement of magnesium by the normal adult. Summary and analysis of published data. Amer. J. Clin. Nutr., *14*:342, 1964.

Shils, M. E.: Experimental production of magnesium deficiency in man. Ann. N.Y. Acad. Sci., *162*:847, 1969.

Wacker, W. E. C., and Parisi, A. F.: Magnesium metabolism. New Eng. J. Med., *278*:658, 712, 772, 1968.

Wacker, W. E. C., and Vallee, B. L.: The magnesium deficiency tetany syndrome in man. Borden's Rev. Nutr. Res., *22*:51, 1961.

Nutrition Reviews

Human renal calculus formation and magnesium. *24*:43, 1966.

Magnesium deficiency and cell transplant. *25*: 151, 1967.

Calcium and serum cholesterol. *25*:298, 1967.

Hypermagnesemia. *26*:12, 1968.

Present knowledge of calcium, phosphorus, and magnesium (by Hegsted, D. M.). *26*:65, 1968.

Phosphates and dental caries. *26*:81, 1968.

Relation of the crystallinity of bone to its metabolic capability. *26*:118, 1968.

Magnesium and thiamine deficiency. *26*:347, 1968.

Renal defect in magnesium deficiency. *28*:72, 1970.

A physiological function for thyrocalcitonin. *28*: 99, 1970.

Calcium and magnesium absorption in the germ-free rat. *28*:101, 1970.

Parathyroid mediation of magnesium-calcium interrelationships. *28*:129, 1970.

Magnesium deficiency and the parathyroid. *28*: 167, 1970.

Dietary calcium and lead toxicity. *29*:145, 1971.

Effect of bed rest on bone mineral loss. *30*:11, 1972.

Maternal magnesium deprivation. *30*:97, 1972.

twelve

Trace Elements (Iron, Iodine, Copper, Manganese, Zinc, Fluorine, and Others)

TRACE ELEMENTS, GENERAL

The *essential trace elements* can be defined simply as those elements necessary in the diet of man or animals in trace* amounts—less than 100 mg per day in man (an arbitrary dividing line of more use to students and teachers than to the animal body). Among the trace elements the range of requirements runs from milligram quantities for iron, zinc, and manganese down to microgram quantities for some of the newly discovered *micronutrient elements* such as selenium, chromium, and vanadium. A combined total of only about 25 to 30 gm of all trace elements (about 1 ounce) exists in the human body (compare with over 1000 gm of calcium alone).

The trace element field is one of the most active and interesting areas of nutrition today, with important discoveries constantly being made. Since the last edition of this textbook, four new essential trace elements have been identified—vanadium, nickel, silicon, and tin—and others, not identified yet, are believed to be essential.

There is no convenient single way to classify trace elements in nutrition, because they vary so much in function, distribution, level of need, and chemical properties. To call them the "minor elements" is very misleading. Table 12–1 lists the 13 essential trace elements in about the order of discovery of their nutritional importance: the order we will use in this chapter to study them. Understandably, this happens also to be roughly their order of decreasing quantitative needs, with some exceptions—especially iodine, which is needed in less than milligram amounts.

---

*The word "trace" was given to these elements by early nutritionists before modern methods of analysis of food and tissues were available. The levels present were just barely discernible in a qualitative way only and, therefore, said to be present in "trace amounts."

Table 12–1.   *Trace Elements, Essential and Nonessential*

Trace Elements Essential for Higher Animal Species	*Examples of Trace Elements Present in Food for Which No Essential Role is Known in Higher Animals*	
1. Iron	*Element known to have a biological role in plants or lower organisms:*	
2. Iodine		
3. Copper	Boron	
4. Manganese		
5. Zinc		
6. Fluorine	*No biological role yet known:*	
7. Cobalt*	Aluminum	Lead
8. Molybdenum†	Arsenic	Lithium
9. Selenium†	Barium	Mercury
10. Chromium	Bismuth	Rubidium
11. Nickel†	Bromine	Silver
12. Tin†	Cadmium	Strontium
13. Vanadium†	Germanium	Titanium
14. Silicon†	Gold	Zirconium

Total: 14 essential
trace elements

*Needed by man only in the organic form, as vitamin B-12.
†The need by man has not yet been proved, though this can be assumed from their role in animals (see text).

Table 12–1 also lists other trace elements known to be present in plants and in the animal body for which no biological function is known at this time in higher animals.

Because the field is so relatively new, in this chapter we will discuss each trace element known to be essential by any higher animal species, even though its role in human nutrition is not yet proved. From past experience, it would be most unlikely for man not to require a trace element which has a vital function in another higher mammal.[1] We can assume the delay in proof is simply one of (fortunately) not being able to experiment in man as one can in animals. These distinctions will be pointed out as each element is studied.

Role in Plant Nutrition—"Organic" vs. Inorganic Foods

Because we hear so much today about "organic" foods (short for "organically grown foods"),* it is important to look briefly at the role of trace elements in the nutrition of plants used as food sources. Of the essential trace elements listed in Table 12–1, only iron, copper, manganese, zinc, molybdenum, and boron (and rarely, silicon and selenium) are essential for the growth of plants. From these elements in inorganic form, plus inorganic nitrogen, sulfur, calcium, phosphorus, potassium, magnesium, water, carbon dioxide, and sunlight (energy), the plant is able to grow

*Sellers of "organic" foods state that food labeled "organic" is produced with the use of humus and organic fertilizers, and without the use of chemical pesticides, herbicides, hormones, antibiotics, or food additives. There is no easy way to corroborate most of these claims, and except for the possibility that certain trace elements might be present in higher levels, there is no basis for claiming significant nutritional superiority of such foods (see text). "Organic" foods are not likely to be any less free of contamination with filth, mold or bacterial growth, natural toxins, or heavy metals (such as mercury or lead) than the same natural foods sold at regular food stores at much lower prices.

normally and make within its own tissues all the carbohydrates, fiber, protein, fat, vitamins, pigments and flavors which make up plant foods as we know them.

None of the substances known to be required in the soil for plant growth are needed in the organic form—in fact, organic sources of the elements must first be broken down to inorganic forms before they can be absorbed by the plant root tips. (Certain organic plant hormones in soil can be exceptions.) This explains why the term "organically grown foods" is a misnomer. Especially, the term "organic food" is very misleading, because all foods of plant origin are basically organic in the chemical sense.

The confusion that many people seem to have about these terms comes from the fact that plants, fortunately, have the ability to absorb from the soil into their tissues, trace elements which they do not need, but which can later serve as sources of these trace elements for animals that eat such plants. Examples of such elements carried along from the soil are iodine, fluorine, cobalt, selenium (needed by some plants), chromium, and the macrominerals sodium and chlorine. The level of these trace elements in plant tissues (and to a small extent the level of certain other minerals, protein, and vitamins) can be influenced to some extent by the level of these trace elements in the soil. In some cases, such as the levels in food of iodine, copper, zinc, chromium, and selenium, the extent of influence of soil elements can be considerable. Climate, temperature, and other environmental conditions can also affect plant composition.

Thus, theoretically, plant foods raised on soils with "natural" or organic fertilizers containing many trace elements (such as compost and farm manures) could be nutritionally superior in terms of their content of certain trace elements to plant foods raised on trace element-deficient soil. But this possibility is true only if such foods make up a major part of a person's diet over a long period of time, and if other sources of these trace elements are not available. This is very unlikely to be the case, practically speaking. In terms of your own nutritional needs, keep in mind that those few trace minerals affected by the soil (such as iodine and chromium):

1. Are generally present in adequate amounts in a mixed diet consisting of a variety of foodstuffs and iodized salt;

2. Are not usually in short supply in farm soils (and if they are, they can be added as inorganic fertilizers); and

3. Can be added to foods by other means such as enrichment programs (though this is not done now except for iron and iodine).

This is not meant to depreciate the value of compost, farm manures, and other organic fertilizers (since they are very useful for plant growth, though not at all necessary), but is given as a reminder that, nutritionally speaking, "organically grown" foods have no special magic. Furthermore, the amount of organic fertilizer available is greatly insufficient to take care of fertilizer (phosphorus, nitrogen, and potassium) needs in the United States or anywhere in the world.

Distribution in Foods and Effect of Processing

As explained in the last section, the composition of many trace elements in plants (especially the micronutrients) depends to some extent on the soil on which it is raised. For that reason we will not attempt to provide tables of distribution in plant foods of most of the trace elements discussed in the following sections. Such information would be quite meaningless. However, as a general rule, since plant cells require certain trace elements for their growth and activity and will not grow without them, the natural plant foods, such as grains, beans, fruits, and vegetables (when eaten as a mixture) are reasonably good sources of all these elements, and most always are good sources of the other trace elements not required by plants. Also, animal foods (such as eggs, milk, meat, and fish) are more likely to contain fairly uniform amounts of all essential trace elements because the animal will not grow if they are absent from the diet. This is one of the major reasons nutritionists recommend some animal foods as part of a normal diet.

The processing of foods, if severe and if anything is discarded, can be just as detrimental to trace minerals as to the vitamins. Boiling or blanching of foods (and discarding the water) or removal of the endosperm of grains are examples of processes which can remove trace elements. Few trace elements are present in sugar, starch, gelatin, fats and oils, or in foods made from these products, such as soft drinks, desserts, or hard candies.

Absorption and Utilization

Except for cobalt, all the trace elements are absorbed (or can be) in the inorganic form before being utilized by the animal body. Minerals present in organic forms in the food, in general, must be split off to the free inorganic form before absorption (the iron in meat is an exception). It is also a general rule that trace elements in food may not be readily available to the body and, in such cases, are only partially absorbed. Because such small amounts of trace elements are present in the gut, their availability to the body can be greatly affected by the level of other minerals as well as the presence of various organic compounds such as

oxalates, phytates,* or other organic *chelating*† compounds (natural or synthetic compounds which can chelate, or "tie up" an element, thus preventing its absorption). Specific exceptions and examples will be discussed individually.

Function in the Body

The trace elements have no common biological role other than that they function in the body at the cellular level, often as constituents of enzymes or as enzyme activators. Their function is not unlike that of vitamins in some ways, except that they can be absorbed by the body in the inorganic form. Most function as constituents in the body of important organic compounds such as iron in *hemoglobin*, and iodine in the hormone *thyroxine*.

The specific role of each element, where known, will be discussed individually. The function of some of the newly discovered essential elements is unknown.

Nutritional Status and Deficiencies of Trace Elements

Iron deficiency (anemia, etc.) is probably the most common deficiency of all nutrients in the United States, and as such illustrates the importance of the trace minerals. The only other trace elements known to be of any nutritional importance in the United States are iodine (deficiency results in goiter) and fluorine (needed to prevent tooth decay), since many areas of the country have soils and water supplies low in these elements. Deficiencies of the other trace elements are either very rare (such as copper, zinc, or chromium) or are unrecognized in man because of lack of sufficient scientific studies.

---

*The phytates are especially abundant in whole wheat but also in other grains.
†From the Greek, meaning claw of a crab.

From what we know about the widespread distribution of trace elements in foods, and the effect of processing, we can assume that any person eating a varied diet of traditional foods, including animal products, will receive sufficient (if not abundant) amounts of the other trace elements. The risk that deficiencies of trace elements would ever occur in man in the United States (except for iron, fluorine, and iodine) is very slight.[1]

IRON

Iron and its alloys such as steel are very familiar substances to everyone. Iron is the major element of the total earth (35 percent, greater than oxygen at 30 percent and silicon at 15 percent), making up the major part of the earth's interior.

Since iron (Fe, its chemical symbol from the Latin *ferrum*) is easy to obtain, its discovery is lost in the history of man, many thousands of years ago. The early Greeks were aware of the health-giving properties of iron. It has been one of the favorite health tonics ever since and a major ingredient in old-time patent medicines (whether based on good reason or not). Iron was found to be a specific treatment for anemia in man as early as the seventeenth century in England.[2] Reasons for its beneficial properties began to become clear in the 1700's when it was discovered to be a component of the body and, later, the blood.[3] It was soon found that about 3 to 5 gm of iron is present in the human body, most of which is in the blood as an essential component of the red protein *hemoglobin* of the red blood cells (of this color because of the iron content).

Experimental evidence of the *essential nature of iron* in nutrition was provided by the French chemist, Boussingault, in 1867.[3, 4] Later, further proof was obtained by many others in Europe and the United States. It became clear, gradually, that inorganic iron could be as effective as organic forms as a dietary source, thus opening the door to the field of inorganic trace elements in nutrition. Tables on the iron composition of common foods were published late in the nineteenth century.

It is paradoxical that although the need for iron was discovered long ago and although it is the most common and cheapest of all metals, more deficiencies of iron (mainly in the form of anemia) exist in the United States and most other developed countries than of any other nutrient. The extent of deficiency lies somewhere between 10 and 25 percent of the total population. Refining and processing of our food supply and the great decrease in use of cast iron cooking equipment in food manufacturing and in our homes have been major reasons for this. Deficiencies of iron in underdeveloped countries are also very common. As a result, iron is now one of the most pressing (and popular) topics among nutritionists. Many basic and applied studies are now in progress around the world on how to improve the iron nutriture of man. Increased food enrichment with iron is one partial solution to the problem. (See Chap. 17.)

Absorption and Availability

The body guards its iron stores very carefully and reuses any which is broken down in the body over and over again. Only the small amounts of iron lost in the urine, sweat, hair, sloughed off skin, and nails, and by menstruation need to be replaced—normally only about 1 or 1.5 mg a day.

Because considerable iron is needed when large amounts of blood are lost (as in bleeding from wounds), the body has a unique built-in control mechanism which allows the intestine to absorb more iron when the need is greatest and to inhibit absorption, in part, when there is an excess.[5, 6] Normally, only about one tenth of the iron in the diet is absorbed. This means, for practical purposes, that about 10 times the amount of iron must generally be eaten than the 1 or 1.5 mg a day which the body actually uses in its tissues. The rest is excreted in the feces unabsorbed.

The situation is further complicated by the fact that not all dietary forms of iron are equally *available* to the body; that is, their chemical state also affects the amount absorbed over and above the body's normal control mechanism. Many factors are known to affect the availability and absorption of iron, such as the form of iron in food, conditions in the gut, composition of the food, iron status and needs of the body (as in pregnancy), age, sex, hormonal factors, and presence of infections and parasites (hookworm infection, for example, is known to greatly increase iron requirements).

Both inorganic and some organic forms of iron can be utilized by the body. Hemoglobin iron from red meats (veal, beef, lamb) may be absorbed directly into the mucosal cells before the iron is released. Even elemental iron, when added to the diet in fine enough particles and when ionized in the gut, is available to the body. This explains why cast iron cooking ware can supply iron to food (as could rust or common nails, if ground up fine enough). Iron is more readily absorbed in the less oxidized form—as ferrous rather than ferric iron. Ferrous sulfate, a fully available chemical form, is generally used as a standard in absorption studies, and is usually absorbed at nearly the maximum rate of 20 to 40 percent (not more because of the control mechanisms). Ferric citrate is also a highly available iron source, being converted to the ferrous form before absorption. Factors favorable for absorption are normal acidity of the gastric juice secreted in the stomach, the presence of reducing substances (such as ascorbic acid) that can change ferric

iron to the more readily absorbable ferrous form, and a well balanced diet in which a fair proportion of the iron is provided in meat or eggs and not too high amounts in fibrous vegetable foods in which the iron is not very available. Green leafy vegetables, then, such as spinach, formerly famous for its iron content, are relatively poor sources of iron (only 2 to 5 percent of its iron is absorbed). Phytin, found especially in grains, militates against absorption by forming insoluble compounds with iron, as with calcium. This accounts for the poor absorption of iron from whole wheat (also about 2 to 5 percent), which explains the high incidence of anemia in countries whose population depends on whole wheat as its major carbohydrate source. The iron in rice, corn, and beans (except for soybeans) is likewise poorly absorbed. When these plant foods are eaten with meat, their iron availability is approximately doubled. Because there are wide individual differences in the efficiency of iron absorption and the number of variables affecting absorption of food iron are so numerous, it is difficult to equate the true body requirement with the amount needed in the diet to meet this requirement.

In the small intestine, the epithelial cell lining the intestinal wall (the *mucosal* cell) is the key to the *mechanism of iron absorption* (see Fig. 12–1). This cell takes in iron by regulatory procedures not fully understood (possibly hormonal regulation). It appears that a protein called *gastroferrin*,[7] present in normal gastric juice, is involved in the regulation of the absorption of iron by the mucosal cell.

Once iron is inside the mucosal cell, it can be either transferred (and later released) to the tissues with the aid of a protein known as *transferrin*,[2, 8] or it can be stored in the mucosal cell or other body cells in the form of a unique protein called *ferritin*. Ferritin, a golden brown protein discovered in 1937, is a major form in which iron is stored in

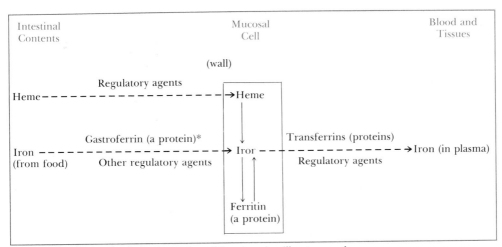

*The role of gastroferrin in absorption of free iron is still not proved.

Figure 12–1. Absorption of iron from the intestine (simplified).

the body, representing about 10 to 20 percent of all the iron stores. It contains about 20 percent of iron in its molecule (whereas hemoglobin has only 0.34 percent). No other biological substance has this great capacity to store a heavy metal. The ferritin in the mucosal cell is no longer believed to assist directly in the absorption of iron but is no doubt important in the regulation of body stores.

Iron in the blood serum circulates not only bound to transferrin and to certain other proteins but also to the citrate molecule, as ferric citrate.

Distribution and Role in the Body

Iron is distributed throughout the body, being a component of essential metabolic enzymes in every cell. The adult human body contains a total of about 4 to 5 gm of iron. Most of this, about 65 to 70 percent, is present in the blood as *hemoglobin* in the red blood cells. Hemoglobin is a red compound consisting of two parts: *globin*, a protein tightly connected to a nonprotein substance called *heme*, containing iron in the ferrous state. Each molecule of hemoglobin can carry four molecules

of oxygen and is essential for oxygen transfer in the blood. A total of about 800 to 900 gm (2 pounds) of hemoglobin is present in an adult man. Normally it is present in blood at a level of from about 11 to 14 percent (except in anemic persons in whom the amount is lower—down to as low as 5 to 8 percent in rare instances). Hemoglobin contains about 0.33 percent of iron.

The next largest concentration of iron is that stored in combination with proteins (such as ferritin and *hemosiderin*) in the liver, spleen, and bone marrow, which normally constitutes about 25 to 30 percent of that in the whole body.

The minor quantities of iron (about 5 percent) found in other tissues are nevertheless vitally important as is evidenced by the localities in which they exist:

1. In the chromatin network in cell nuclei.

2. In *cytochrome* (an iron-containing pigment) in protoplasm of cells, and in numerous enzymes that help catalyze oxidation-reduction processes in body tissues.

3. In *myoglobin* in muscles, which is closely related in chemistry and function to blood hemoglobin but is fixed

266

in muscle tissue (and which constitutes about 3 percent of the total body iron).

In all these sites, the iron-containing compounds are involved in the vital life processes of cells and tissues (Fig. 12–2).

Iron owes its usefulness in the body to its special ability to be reversibly oxygenated— that is, to take on oxygen and later give this oxygen up to other substances. By means of this property, the iron-containing hemoglobin in red blood cells can take on extra oxygen when blood circulates through the lungs, can then carry oxygen to the tissues, and there can pass it on to the tissue cells for oxidative processes necessary to their life. Venous blood, which owes its bluish color to the presence of reduced hemoglobin, takes on excess carbon dioxide (a waste product of tissues) and is returned to the lungs, where it loses carbon dioxide and takes on another load of oxygen, becoming bright red again when *oxyhemoglobin* is formed. When insufficient iron is available to the body, less hemoglobin is formed (anemia), and these oxygen-carrying mechanisms are reduced, giving rise to many physiological problems (see later section).

The iron-containing pigments and enzymes in the tissues serve to bring about transfers of oxygen within cells in much the same manner. The cytochromes and *cytochrome oxidases* (enzymes which contain iron) have been estimated to be responsible for about 90 percent of the energy transfers associated with the oxidative phases of tissue respiration. *Catalase*, another example of an iron-containing enzyme (in the form of heme, also present in hemoglobin), is present in relatively high concentrations in red blood cells and in other tissue cells. The level of catalase in cells is reduced in an iron deficiency.

Among the billions of red blood cells (about 4½ to 5 million per cubic centimeter of blood), there are continual casualties and calls for replacements; the lifetime of such cells has been determined by use of isotopes to be about four months. They are formed in the bone marrow and destroyed chiefly in the spleen. Not only is iron needed for their formation, but also protein (for the protein part of hemoglobin), and other materials for the *stroma*—the body of the cell in which hemoglobin is embedded. When these cells disintegrate, the main nonprotein portion of hemoglobin is split into an iron-containing substance (*hematin*) and a pigment (*bilirubin*). Almost all the iron and much of the bilirubin are saved to be used over again in new red corpuscles.

Only traces of iron are excreted in the urine, and the excreted iron lost to the body in the feces amounts ordinarily to less than 1 mg daily. More than half this loss is from cells sloughed off from the intestinal mucosa and the minimal intestinal blood losses. In girls and women between puberty and menopause, there is an extra loss of iron during menstruation which needs to be taken into account.

The body has a store of readily available iron, a "labile pool of iron,"[9] made up of recently absorbed iron plus that recently released by the breaking down of red blood cells. This iron is used by preference for hemoglobin in building new red cells. Older stores of iron (as in the liver) may be somewhat less readily available, and the fixed iron in tissue cells is not drawn upon even in times of great need for this element.

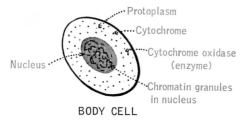

BODY CELL

Figure 12–2. Small amounts of iron are found in every tissue cell—in chromatin granules in the cell nucleus and in the protoplasm as the pigment, cytochrome, and the enzyme, cytochrome oxidase. These iron-containing substances are largely responsible for the uptake of oxygen by the cells and in the use of oxygen in their life processes.

Iron Deficiency Symptoms: Anemia

The most common sign of iron deficiency in man is *iron deficiency anemia,* in which the level of hemoglobin in the red cells is reduced, and the red cells themselves are smaller.* Some other symptoms of iron deficiency, though, are now known to occur even in the absence of anemia—such as faulty digestion, measurable changes in levels of various enzymes containing iron, cellular damage, and low iron stores.

Because the body uses iron so economically and has opportunity to build up considerable reserve stores of it over long periods, any deficiency due to an iron-poor diet or to poor absorption of the iron in the food is likely to develop only after a long period or under conditions in which the need for iron is unusually high—as in the infant (see Chap. 20), the growing child, in pregnancy, and after severe loss of blood by hemorrhage. Diarrhea over long periods, hemorrhoids, peptic ulcers, malignancies, subnormal acidity of the gastric juice (fairly common in older persons), and excessive loss of blood during menstrual periods are clinical situations in man which can appreciably increase iron needs and the severity of symptoms.

Iron deficiency anemia, like anemias from other causes, reduces the oxygen-carrying capacity of the blood, resulting, if severe, in such symptoms as paleness of the skin, weakness, shortness of breath, lack of appetite, and a general slowing-up of vital functions of the body. Severe iron deficiency over long periods is known to cause death, as would be expected.

Iron deficiency anemia may be precipitated in young girls whose diets are on the borderline of adequacy for iron when the onset of menstruation results in increased losses of iron from the body. More common with very young women than outright anemia is the low stores of body iron with which they come into the period of possible pregnancy. Pregnancy is a period during which iron deficiency anemias may

---

*Called technically a *microcytic hypochromic* anemia (small cells and reduced color).

be precipitated because of the increased need for iron both for blood in the unborn child and for building up a store of iron in the placenta and in the infant's liver. The child may be born with a good store of iron in its own liver, but this may be at the cost of depletion of the mother's store. Repeated pregnancies are especially costly to iron stores in the mother's body.

Anemias Due to Blood Losses

Anemias may also be brought about by excessive loss of blood. Average menstrual losses amount to 0.6 mg iron per day, but are highly variable with different individuals. It is estimated that in about 20 percent of women these losses exceed 1 mg per day[10], and in some they may be considerably higher. Excessive menstrual bleeding may constitute a continual drain on body iron stores, which may be hard to replace unless the diet is high in available iron and iron absorption is relatively efficient.

Unusually high iron needs may be precipitated by hemorrhages (either sudden loss of much blood or long-continued pathologic bleeding such as with ulcers) or by the donation of blood for transfusions. Such losses may occur in either sex. The body tends to replace a major loss of iron (for hemoglobin building) at a rate far in excess of that supplied in the diet and for this it mobilizes stored iron, especially the more labile types. The need for extra iron under these circumstances is far in excess of the amounts supplied by normal absorption of dietary iron from the intestine. This in turn promotes more efficient absorption of food iron. A diet which provides a plentiful supply of all substances needed for rebuilding blood (especially protein and including some rich sources of iron, such as liver, meats, and eggs) often is adequate, provided there are normal reserves of iron in the body.[11] If the previous diet has been too low in iron to provide such reserve stores, or if the current diet is low in iron, extra iron supplements would be needed to promote rapid blood regeneration.

Requirement and Recommended Allowances

It is difficult to fix any exact figure as to the minimal requirements for iron, because of the many variables concerned which we have mentioned previously. Chiefly because of the very limited absorption and availability of iron, the recommended intake has to be much higher (about 10 times) than the actual tissue requirements.

Taking all these variables into consideration, the United States Food and Nutrition Board recommends (1968) a 10 mg per day allowance for men and postmenopausal women and an 18 mg per day allowance for other women.[1] In discussion of the scientific bases for its recommended allowances, this Board states:[1] "Recommended dietary intake is predicated on the basis of 10 percent absorption of food iron. This seems optimal in permitting individual adjustment of absorption between 2 and 20 percent and in permitting the creation of iron stores."

The United States Food and Nutrition Board feels that its recommendations are reasonable and that a larger margin of safety may make for better health. The recommended iron allowances of the Food and Nutrition Board for both sexes and different periods of life are given in Table 12–2 and, in more detail, in Table 1 of the Appendix.

Any period in which growth takes place calls for an additional allowance of iron; such periods include pregnancy, lactation, and childhood from infancy through adolescence. With infants, requirements for iron to support rapid growth are relatively high per unit of body weight, but because of small weight, not high quantitatively (see Chap. 20). The iron requirements for small growing children are relatively

high, as is the requirement for older boys and girls during the growth spurt that occurs in the teen-age period (12 to 18 years). The U.S. recommended allowance of 18 mg per day during the ages of 12 to 18 is designed to permit optimum storage of iron against possible drains on iron reserves, especially in young women because of menstruation, pregnancy, and lactation. Recommendations of iron intake differ in different countries, as would be expected, and it is hoped that international standards will soon be published.[12] This standardization among countries is difficult because of the influence of so many factors on the iron requirement, including levels of intake of animal foods (which have iron of high availability).

Most other countries currently advise iron intakes of about 7 to 10 mg a day for men and 12 mg or higher for women of child-bearing age (see Appendix, Table 1B). The FAO/WHO recommendations for women of child-bearing age, in countries where intakes of animal foods are less than 10 percent, is set at 28 mg per day.[12]

Iron Content of Foods

Figures for the amount of iron in some typical foods, both in milligrams

Table 12–2. *Recommended Daily Iron Allowances**

	Age in Years	Iron (in mg)
Children	½–3	15
	3–10	10
Males	10–12	10
	12–18	18
	18 on	10
Females	10–55	18
	55 on	10
	Pregnant	18
	Lactating	18

*From Food and Nutrition Board, 1968.[1] See Appendix Table 1C for FAO recommendations.

Table 12–3.   *Typical Foods as Sources of Iron**

Food	Size of Serving	Iron, in Milligrams	
		PER AVG. SERVING	PER 100 GRAMS OF FOOD
Liver:			
Lamb, broiled	2 slices (75 gm)	13.4	17.9
Beef, fried	2 slices (75 gm)	6.6	8.8
Chicken, cooked	¼ cup (50 gm)	4.3	8.8
Meats (lean or med. fat):			
Beef, round, cooked	1 lg. hamburger (85 gm)	3.0	3.5
rib roast, cooked	3 slices (100 gm)	2.6	2.6
Pork, chop, cooked	1 med. lg. chop (80 gm)	2.5	3.1
Lamb, shoulder chop	1 chop, cooked (90 gm)	1.6	1.8
Baked beans, canned with			
pork and molasses	½ cup (130 gm)	3.0	2.3
pork and tomato	½ cup (130 gm)	2.3	1.8
Fruits, dried (uncooked)			
Apricots	4 halves, (30 gm)	1.7	5.5
Prunes	4–5 medium, (30 gm)	1.2	3.9
Figs	2 small (30 gm)	0.9	3.0
Raisins	2 tbsp (20 gm)	0.6	3.5
Legumes:			
Soy beans, dry	½ cup scant, cooked (30 gm dry)	2.5	8.4
Peanut butter	2 tbsp scant (30 gm)	0.6	2.0
Lima beans, fresh	½ cup, cooked (80 gm)	2.0	2.5
Peas, fresh, green	½ cup, cooked (80 gm)	1.4	1.8
Molasses, med.	1 tbsp (20 gm)	1.2	6.0
Eggs, whole	1 med. (50 gm)	1.2	2.3
Leafy vegetables:			
Spinach	½ cup, cooked (90 gm)	2.0	2.2
Beet greens	½ cup, cooked (100 gm)	1.9	1.9
Chard	½ cup, cooked (100 gm)	1.8	1.8
Kale (leaves only)	½ cup, cooked (55 gm)	0.9	1.6
Turnip greens	½ cup, cooked (75 gm)	0.8	1.1
Vegetables:			
Potatoes, sweet	1 med., baked (110 gm)	1.0	0.9
white	1 med., baked (100 gm)	0.7	0.7
Broccoli	⅔ cup (100 gm)	0.8	0.8
Brussels sprouts	5–6 med. (70 gm)	0.8	1.1
Cauliflower	¾ cup, cooked (100 gm)	0.7	0.7
Carrots	⅔ cup, diced, cooked (100 gm)	0.6	0.6
String beans	¾ cup, cooked (100 gm)	0.6	0.6
Beets	2, 2-in. diam. (100 gm)	0.5	0.5
Bread:			
White, enriched	1 slice	0.6	2.5
Whole-wheat	1 slice	0.5	2.3
White, unenriched	1 slice	0.2	0.7
Cereals, whole grain (oats, corn, wheat, rice):	See label on package—range from 0.2 to 0.7 mg unenriched, up to 10 mg enriched, per serving.		
Fresh fruits and fruit vegetables	100 gm serving, mostly	0.3–0.6	
Milk, whole, fluid, cow's	½ pint, or 8 oz glass (244 gm)	0.10	0.04
Human	½ pint, or 8 oz (244 gm)	0.24	0.1

*Most of these data from *Composition of Foods*, Agriculture Handbook No. 8, U.S. Department of Agriculture, 1963. (See also Table 2 of the Appendix.)

per 100 gm and in an average serving, are given in Table 12-3 (see also Table 2 of the Appendix for other foods). In many instances, the distribution of iron follows that of other mineral elements, as it is relatively high in foods of low moisture content and low in fresh fruits and vegetables, which contain large amounts of water and fiber. Milk, which is one of the best sources of many other nutrients, is poor in iron, while organ meats, such as liver and the blood-forming organs (spleen and bone marrow, seldom consumed in this country), are unusually rich in iron. Good sources of iron are eggs, lean meats, legumes, nuts, dried fruits, whole grains or enriched cereal foods, and all green, leafy vegetables. Such foods as dark molasses, raisins, and nuts (often featured as rich sources of iron) are used infrequently or in small servings, so that they do not constitute sources of this element as important as some staple foods of lower iron content (such as whole grain or enriched breads and cereals).

The addition of iron salts to bread, breakfast cereals, flour and other cereal products in conjunction with the enrichment program, has been a considerable help in raising the available iron content of the American diet. Approximately 30 percent of our total iron intake comes from enrichment sources (see Chap. 17). Unfortunately, not all states of the United States have enrichment regulations. Unenriched highly milled cereals or bread, sugar, and fats are either very low or lacking in iron.

The amount of iron in a food can be quite variable, and too much trust should not be put in food composition tables as far as iron content of foods is concerned. The iron content of processed and manufactured foods is extremely variable unless iron is added. The use of iron cooking utensils in food manufacture, as used to be the case with molasses, is a factor, as are iron cooking utensils used in the home.[13]

Some water supplies are high in iron, but this is not a dependable source. The student should learn to read food labels and, if in doubt about the iron content of a manufactured food, he should write to the manufacturer.

However, the extent of the body's *need* for iron still remains the *primary* factor that controls the relative amount of the iron content of all types of food in the diet that will be absorbed; this makes differences in degree of utilization of iron from different types of food of less importance. If the margin between the total amounts needed and those furnished by the food intake is small, the relative utilization from all types of food will be "stepped up." If only small amounts of iron are needed for body maintenance, less will be absorbed and much of the food iron will remain unabsorbed to be discarded in the feces—that is, the degree of availability will be lower for all types of food. Minor differences will remain as to the relative availability of iron in different foods, but the determining factor of body need will affect the ultimate utilization of all types of food—for example, iron from leafy vegetables may be only about 5 percent absorbed when small amounts of iron are needed for maintenance in an adult, but at times of great body need (rapid growth or restoring depleted body reserves) the amount of iron utilized from these sources may be increased to 20 percent (or even more).

How To Get Recommended Allowance of Iron in the Diet

In Table 12-4 are listed two groups of common foods, in average servings, that furnish respectively 10 mg iron (daily allowance for a man and for a 3 to 10 year old child), and 18 mg (daily allowance for younger women and for boys 12 to 18 years of age). It is apparent that if two or three servings of some relatively iron-rich foods are in-

Table 12–4. *Groups of Foods That
Furnish Iron at Levels of 10 and 18 mg*

(1)	Iron mg	(2)	Iron mg
Hamburger, 1 avg. (85 gm)	3.0	Liver, beef, broiled, 2 sl. (75 gm)	13.4
Beet greens, ½ c. cooked	1.9	Beans, snap, ¾ c., canned	1.5
Bread, whole-wheat, 3 slices	1.5	Milk, 1 pint	0.2
Egg, 1 med. lg.	1.2	Dried apricots or prunes, ½ c., cooked	2.1
Potato, 1 med.	0.7		
Beets, 2 small	0.5		
Banana, 1 med.	0.7	Bread, white, 2 slices	1.2
Orange, 1 med.	0.6		
Milk, 1 pint	0.2		18.4
	10.3		

cluded, other normal items of the diet that provide minor amounts of iron will make up the desired total. On days when liver is used, the total iron intake will probably be higher than the standard allowance, but the excess can be stored to make up for a day when a slightly less than normal amount is taken. Liver can be ground up and mixed with hamburger to make a very palatable mixture rich in iron.

Because it is important, both for body welfare and for good utilization of iron, that the diet be adequate in all nutritive essentials, the groups of foods listed under (1) of Table 12–4 represent a well balanced diet. If one follows the recommendation to include in the daily diet one pint of milk, one serving of meat, one egg, three or four slices of whole wheat or enriched bread, one serving of potato, two servings of other vegetables (using colored and leafy vegetables fairly often), and two servings of fruit (one citrus or tomato), these foods alone provide 9 to 12 mg of iron daily. To bring the daily iron intake up to 18 mg requires either more liberal use of meats (liver or other organ meat eaten once a week is good insurance), increased amounts of eggs, green leafy vegetables, legumes, nuts, or enriched bread and cereals, or the use of

a special iron supplement (especially for persons with reduced caloric intakes). The Food and Nutrition Board states:[1] "The borderline state of iron balance is indicated by the greatly reduced or absent iron stores in two thirds of menstruating women[14] and in the majority of pregnant women. It is impractical to supply these needs with ordinary food, and iron supplementation is required. For these groups, it is desirable to increase the iron content of the diet through fortification." The proposal in 1972 to increase the level for iron in enriched flour in the United States to 40 mg per pound (88 mg per kg)—about 2½ times the present level—will be followed with interest in this connection.

Iron Intakes and Nutrition Status

Failure of the iron content of the diet to be adequate for actual body needs, as evidenced by the occurrence of nutritional anemia, is found frequently in the United States. The amount of iron in a normal American diet averages about 6 mg for every 1000 kcal.[1,15] This means that women who are restricting themselves to 1500 to 2000 calories per day are apt to receive too little iron. As mentioned previously, iron deficiency anemia is the most common overt nutritional deficiency in the United States[16] (with an incidence of over 15 percent) and in many developing countries. The most vulnerable age groups are infants and young children, young pregnant teenagers, women of child-bearing age, and older persons on reduced food intakes. Iron deficiency affects rich and poor alike.

When cost limits the amount of meat and eggs used, greater dependence for iron is placed on legumes and cereals, so that the use of whole-grain or enriched cereal products may mean the margin of safety in low-cost diets.

Toxicity of Iron

As with all trace elements, the toxic level of iron is easily reached by taking in sources outside of a normal food supply. The safe range with most of the trace elements is within about 10 to 50 times the requirement.

Iron toxicity is known, for example, in certain members of the Bantu tribe in South Africa who have used iron utensils in cooking and the brewing of alcoholic beverages. In the United States, toxicity from the normal iron in foods is unknown except in a rare genetic disease in which iron accumulates.*

Some people find they have very limited tolerance for single doses of highly ionizable forms of iron (such as ferrous sulfate) if eaten in a supplement in amounts much over 250 mg a day, a nontoxic dose. Such a level each day, over long periods of time, could cause accumulation of excessive iron stores in the body.[17]

IODINE

Discovery as a Nutrient

Goiter, a condition caused by an enlarged thyroid gland in the neck, was known in China as early as 3000 B.C. and was treated effectively by feeding seaweed or burnt sponge. In 1820 Coindet,[18] a physician in Switzerland, provided evidence that the then newly discovered iodine† (isolated from seaweed by Courtois in 1811) was the curative agent in seaweed and burnt sponge.[3] Though the idea was not universally accepted then, in retrospect it is clear that iodine was one of the first nutrients,

if not the first, to be recognized as essential for man or animals. Vitamins and amino acids were unknown at the time.

Distribution and Role in the Body

Iodine is absorbed in the inorganic form (as iodide ions) in the upper part of the intestine. It is freely available; even organic forms are well utilized after being released in the intestine. It may also be absorbed through the skin, if applied. Estimates of the total amount in the body range from 15 to 30 mg (about the size of a matchhead), and of this small amount about three-fifths is concentrated in the thyroid gland (the rest is mostly in the circulating blood). Iodine serves but one purpose in the body—namely, to form an integral part of the thyroid hormones *thyroxine* (discovered by the American, Kendall, in 1915) and *triiodothyronine* (a more active but less abundant form discovered in 1952).‡ These hormones are manufactured in the thyroid gland from its stored iodine (which must be obtained originally from sources outside the body, of course) and the amino acid tyrosine, and they are released in small amounts into the blood. When carried to the tissues, these hormones are quantitatively the most important single factor in determining the *rate* of *basal metabolism*. The thyroid hormones also have other vital roles in health and reproduction which, from a nutritional viewpoint, are likewise essential roles of dietary iodine (see Chap. 15). (Without iodine in the thyroxine molecule, the compound is completely ineffective.) Control of the level of the thyroid hormones in the blood

---

*Hemochromatosis.

†Iodine (I_2) is related chemically to the halogens chlorine, bromine, and fluorine. Its name is derived from the Greek word *iodes*, meaning violet color, from the color of the fumes of iodine (which also have a distinctive odor).

‡Thyroxine is formed by the union of two tyrosine molecules and the substitution of four iodine atoms for four hydrogens. Triiodothyronine is exactly the same except that it carries three, instead of four, iodine atoms in the molecule. Kendall later received the Nobel Prize for his work on this and other hormones.

is effected by release or suppression of a stimulating hormone from the pituitary gland.

Iodine is supplied to the body by intake of foods or water, in which it is contained in minute amounts. Dietary iodine is absorbed from the alimentary tract, after which approximately 30 percent is removed by the thyroid gland (where most of it is stored as the complex protein *thyroglobulin*), and the remainder is excreted in the urine (with minor amounts in the feces).

Iodine Deficiency: Goiter

Simple (or endemic) goiter is an enlargement of the thyroid gland in the neck due to an insufficiency of iodine supply. The gland enlarges in an attempt to compensate for the shortage of iodine, which is an essential ingredient for making its hormones (see Fig. 12–3). This disorder was prevalent for centuries before its cause was recognized. Although others had suspected iodine,[3] attention to the thyroid gland and its

relation to iodine was received by the accidental discovery in Germany by Baumann in 1895 that the thyroid gland was especially rich in iodine. This eventually led to final proof that iodine was essential for goiter prevention, for thyroxine formation, and as an essential nutrient for man and animals. Research began in earnest then on finding the mechanism of action of iodine and on correlating the iodine content of water and soil with the incidence of goiter in certain areas.

French, American, and Swiss chemists, in whose countries there was a high incidence of simple goiter, (especially in isolated mountain valleys) found that in these valleys, both water and soil are low in iodine. The inhabitants subsisted almost entirely on products grown in the locality. Iodine (added to salt) became a popular treatment for goiter in these areas both for man and animals.

Two sets of events around 1918 directed the attention of the public and of scientists to the distribution of simple goiter in different parts of the United States (Fig. 12–4). One was the pub-

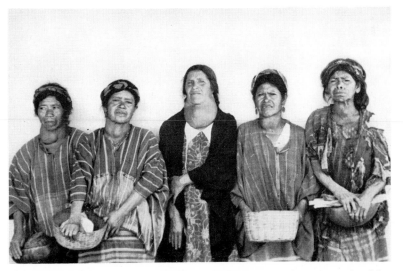

Figure 12–3. A group of women from a goitrous region in Guatemala, an example of the prevalence of simple goiter in many isolated sections of the world today. (Courtesy of Dr. N. S. Scrimshaw and the Institute of Nutrition of Central America and Panama.)

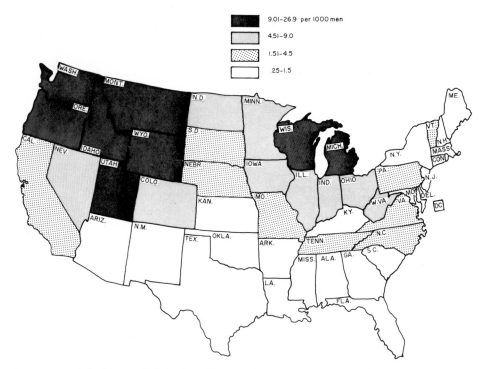

Figure 12–4. A "goiter map" of the then 48 states, showing (in black) the regions where goiter among draftees in 1917–18 was most prevalent. It also occurred fairly commonly in the cross-barred states, but was almost totally absent in the states in white. The use of preventive measures (iodine in drinking water and iodized salt) has greatly reduced the incidence of simple goiter, even in the states where it was most prevalent. However, in recent years the incidence in some of these states, plus several states in the South (Texas and Louisiana), has increased somewhat (see text). (From Love and Davenport: *Geographic Distribution of Simple Goiter Among Drafted Men,* 1917–18. U.S. Department of Public Health.)

lication of figures on the incidence of goiter among men drafted during World War I, which showed that this disorder was most prevalent in the basin of the Great Lakes and in the Pacific Northwest in the United States and Canada. In areas adjacent to the ocean (where both soil and foods grown on it were relatively iodine-rich, and sea foods were commonly eaten) goiter proved to be almost nonexistent. The second disclosure was that farm animals in goitrous regions showed the same evidences of iodine deficiency as humans, and their tendency to produce stillborn or weak and sickly young was a source of financial loss and concern to farmers. In 1918, Hart and Steenbock published results of a study of the "hairless pig malady," a condition in which apparently normal sows gave birth to stillborn young that were nearly hairless and had thick, goitrous necks.[20] This condition was found to be the result of iodine deficiency, and the addition of iodide to the feed enabled the sows to produce normal young. The condition is similar to *endemic cretinism* in severely handicapped and dwarfed children born with underdeveloped thyroids due to a deficiency of iodine in their mothers during the first three months of pregnancy or before conception.

This report and other evidence stimulated Marine and Kimball[21] to see whether beneficial results might follow administration of small doses of iodide given to school children in Akron, Ohio, where mild goiter was common among adolescent girls (females are more subject to goiter than males, and it is most likely to make its appearance at such periods as adolescence and pregnancy). Small doses of potassium iodide were given during two 10-day periods each year to about 800 girls, while about 1800 untreated girls of the same age group served as controls. No goiter developed in the treated group, while 26 percent of the control group developed enlarged thyroids in the same time period. Similar treatment with iodides, undertaken among the school children in three cantons of Switzerland, produced a tremendous decrease in the incidence of adolescent goiter. These studies and others established without question the practicability of prevention of simple goiter by administration of small quantities of some iodine compound (Fig. 12–5). It was finally decided that iodized salt (refined salt to which sodium or potassium iodide has been added in amounts up to 0.01 percent) offered the best

preventive, because salt is a low-cost food which is commonly used by all people. The use of iodized salt (or some other carrier) is now recommended in all localities where simple goiter is endemic, and iodization of salt is required by law in Switzerland, Canada, Colombia, Guatemala, and other countries. In the United States, the iodization of salt is not legally mandatory but is very common, and educational campaigns have wisely encouraged its widespread use. Under a 1972 Food and Drug Administration regulation, iodized table salt must be labeled, "This salt supplies iodide, a necessary nutrient." Uniodized salt will be labeled, "This salt does not supply iodide, a necessary nutrient."

Because the cause and means of prevention of endemic goiter have thus been well known since 1920 and much progress toward its eradication has been made in certain countries, it is perhaps surprising that goiter is still one of the most prevalent nutritional deficiency diseases in the world. Many millions of persons (200 million has been esti-

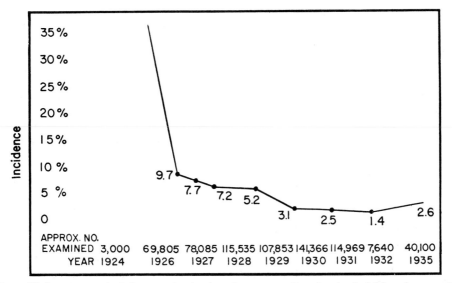

Figure 12–5. The marked decrease in simple goiter among Detroit school children between 1924 and 1935, due to the use of iodized salt. (From Kimball, O. P.: *Journal of American Medical Association*, 1937.)

mated) are affected today. Occurrences in the United States, though not common, are increasing rather than decreasing (see next section). Much remains to be done in clearing up the last of it even in more advanced countries, and it is still rife in many developing countries and out-of-the-way places, such as isolated valleys of Austria, northern India, South and Central America, and Yugoslavia. There remains much work yet to be done by educational, medical, and public health agencies before its final eradication is accomplished.

It should be stressed that once a goiter has developed in adult life, taking supplementary iodine will not decrease the size of an enlarged thyroid gland. Persons on low-salt or salt-free diets, may need some other source of supplementary iodine (prescribed by physician) especially in the case of pregnant women. Iodized oil, by injection, can serve this purpose in endemic areas.[22]

Mention should be made of the fact that enlarged thyroid glands (goiter) can also be caused by the eating of large proportions of foods such as turnips, cabbage, and rutabaga over long periods of time. Such foods contain natural *goitrogens* (anti-thyroid compounds) which inhibit the formation of thyroid hormones. The normal use of these foods, as in this country, is in no way harmful. Certain drugs such as thiouracil and several sulfa drugs also have a goitrogenic effect, and there are known inherited defects which can cause goiter.

Iodine Needs and Sources

It is evident that iodides are present in the body and in foods in amounts small enough to be counted as "traces," and naturally the requirement (to replace losses in the urine) is very small.

Recommended allowances for iodine have been set (for the first time) in the United States at about two times the minimal amount essential to maintain a normal balance in order to ensure a margin of safety. The recommendation for young men (age 18 to 35) is 140 mcg (0.14 mg) per day; it is 100 mcg for young women (age 18 to 35).[1] The needs are raised during pregnancy and lactation (see Appendix, Table 1, for the details of needs of other age groups). Iodine intakes at this level have no harmful effects and serve to build up a reserve store of this element in the thyroid gland for use in emergencies. Possibly the smallness of the quantities of iodine required may best be appreciated from the statement that the standard allowance of iron for an adult woman for two days (36 mg) would weigh about the same as a whole year's allowance (36.5 mg) of iodine. It is truly a "trace" element.

For intakes of iodine to replace losses, man is dependent on the amounts present in foods, soil, and water. Iodine in drinking and cooking water varies widely in different regions; in some areas (near the sea) it is high enough to meet the daily requirement. The iodine content of foods also varies widely, depending chiefly on the iodine content of the soil or that of animal feeds (to which iodide salts are routinely added in most countries). Because these amounts, stated in *parts per billion* of fresh material, are so small and variable, it seems wiser to confine oneself to general statements as to the relative value of different foods as sources of this element.[2] To put iodine values in food composition tables would be most misleading for reasons explained previously. In general, marine fish, shellfish, dried seaweed (in countries where it is used), and cod-liver oil are relatively rich in iodine; butter, milk, cheese, and eggs may be good sources when animals have been fed on iodine-rich rations; vegetables grown in soils of at least moderate iodine content are fairly good sources; cereal grains, legumes, and fresh fruits (even from nongoitrous regions) are of low iodine content.

Highly refined foods are generally very low or devoid of iodine, unless it has been added in some way.

Persons living in nongoitrous areas are practically certain to get enough iodine to meet their requirement on any well balanced diet (one not too high in cereals and highly refined foods) plus that in drinking water. Those living in goitrous regions may supplement their diet with seafoods and vegetables or other foods shipped in from regions where there is more iodine in the soil. However, by using iodized salt, persons in almost any area may be assured of getting their quota of this element without considering the small and variable amounts provided by the diet.

Nutritional Status

As mentioned, iodine deficiency is rampant throughout many areas of the world in spite of the extremely low amounts needed and the low cost (less than a few cents a year). In the United States, lessons learned in the past are easily forgotten and nutrition education programs are only beginning to be truly effective. The recent National Nutrition Survey[16] uncovered significant numbers of American children with goiter due to iodine deficiency — incidences of as high as up to 5 percent in some low-income areas.

It would appear logical to require *universal* enrichment of salt with a stable form of iodine (0.5 to 1 part per 10,000) in goitrous areas of the United States, along with new education programs and better labeling of food products. Regulations also should be required for mandatory use of iodized salt in food manufacturing. At the present time less than half of the salt used by the food industry is iodized.

Iodine Toxicity

As with the other trace elements, there is not too great a spread between iodine requirements and detrimental levels. In man, high levels (25 to 50 times the recommended levels over long periods of time) are known to depress the thyroid in acting as a goitrogen. Treating oneself with compounds of iodide or concentrates of iodine in dried seaweed over long periods is a hazardous procedure.

COPPER

The discovery of copper (Cu) goes back to prehistoric times (8000 B.C., during the Late Stone Age).* Its unexpected essential role as a nutrient for mammals was not discovered, however, until 1928, when Hart and associates[23] found that iron alone was not sufficient to prevent anemia in rats fed a milk diet. They found that a cure could be effected by adding to the food the ash of either lettuce or liver. They noticed the ash had a pale blue color. Suspecting that this color might be due to copper, they fed this element with iron to a deficient rat, and in just a few days' time there was a marked improvement in hemoglobin formation and growth. They were as surprised that copper was effective as we would be today to find a similar effect with, say, such common elements as aluminum, silver, or lead (although copper had been known to be essential for certain marine invertebrates).

Shortly thereafter, in 1931, Josephs[24] provided evidence that copper was more effective than iron alone in overcoming the anemia of milk-fed infants. Though not accepted at first, there is now convincing evidence that copper deficiency can exist in special situations in milk-fed infants.[25] Such deficiencies in in-

---

*The later Bronze Age (3000 to 1000 B.C.) takes its name from the use during this period of bronze — an alloy of copper and tin. The word "copper" is derived from the Latin *cuprum*, a corruption of cyprium, named after the island of Cyprus (which was a source of much copper about 3000 B.C.).

fants are most generally complicated with chronic diarrhea or metabolic diseases, while deficiencies in adult man are unknown either naturally or experimentally. However, because the copper content of refined foods is not a certain entity, because of the recognition of copper deficiency in infants, and because of the current very high interest in this trace element in human nutrition, it is important to have an understanding of its role in the body and distribution in food.

Distribution in Body and Function

A usual day's intake of copper for an adult is about 2 to 5 mg, most of which is in food as the organic form. About 30 percent of this is absorbed in the upper small intestine or stomach (as the inorganic ion, after digestion). A total of 75 to 150 mg of copper is present in the entire human adult body, most of it bound to various essential proteins. Most of the body copper is in blood and muscle, though the brain, heart, liver, eye, hair, and kidney have higher concentrations, suggestive of important functions in these tissues.[2]

In the blood serum most of the copper is present in the protein *ceruloplasmin* (also known as *ferroxidase I*), which is essential for iron utilization.[26, 27] Excess copper is excreted normally through the bile.

Copper is present in several important enzymes,* thus playing a role in many essential reactions in the body, including the synthesis of hemoglobin (or release of iron for this purpose), the metabolism of glucose and release of energy, the formation of phospholipids in the nerve wall, and the formation of connective tissue.

In copper deficiency in animals a variety of symptoms are known to occur besides anemia, including skeletal defects, gray or depigmented hair (see Fig. 12–6), faulty wool or hair structure, degeneration of the nervous system, cardiovascular lesions, and reproductive disorders.[1, 2] Many useful pioneer studies have been made with copper-deficient swine, especially at the University of Utah by Cartwright and Wintrobe. In deficient infants, low copper levels in the blood ("hypocupremia") and other tissues are observed, as well as other blood and bone disorders.

Requirement, Food Sources, and Nutritional Status

The Food and Nutrition Board (U.S.) states that "a copper intake of 2 mg per

---

*Copper is present in such enzymes as tyrosinase, monoamine oxidase (essential in elastin formation), and cytochrome-C oxidase. It is also a constituent of the protein erythrocuprein (probably an enzyme) in the red blood cell.

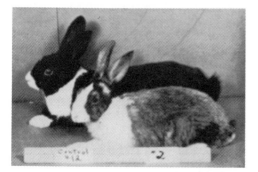

Figure 12–6. The rabbit in the back received sufficient copper in his diet. The rabbit in the foreground, after six weeks on a copper-deficient diet, displayed smaller size and depigmentation. (From Hunt, C. E., and Carlton, W. W.: J. Nutr., 87:385, 1965.)

day appears to maintain balance in adults and ordinary diets provide 2 to 5 mg per day," and that preadolescent girls maintain adequate balance with 1.3 mg per day.[1] The Board recommends an intake of 0.08 mg per kg of body weight for infants and children (equal to 0.8 mg for a 10-kg, or 22-pound child). If we compare this amount of copper needed daily (about 2 mg) with the amount in one copper cent which weighs over 3 gm (3000 mg), we see that one cent contains sufficient copper to supply the needs of one person for over 1500 days, or over four years. Obviously, if the time ever comes when we need to enrich our foods with copper, it will not be expensive. Deficiencies of copper are known in farm animals grazing on copper-deficient soils, so copper is routinely added to most commercial farm rations.

Copper occurs along with other mineral elements in most natural foods (richest sources are organ meats, crustaceans, shellfish, nuts, dried legumes, and cocoa). Cow's milk is a very poor source of this element (as are many foods). Human milk contains an adequate amount. The amount of copper in the diet depends both on the choice of foods and the locality in which they are produced.[28, 29] Copper may be added to foods in processing, as in the pasteurization of milk by passing it over copper rollers, or from cooking in copper utensils. Copper levels may be reduced, on the other hand, by the refinement of food. It would be extremely difficult, though, if not impossible, to get too little copper in one's diet when eating a variety of foodstuffs. Natural drinking water often supplies the entire requirement, for example.

Toxicity

There is more tolerance for higher levels of food copper than there is of many of the other trace elements. Since copper cooking utensils are rarely used now, there is little danger of toxic intake.[17] Mention should be made of *Wilson's disease*,[30] a rather rare chronic metabolic disease in man in which the body has great difficulty in disposing of excess copper; the copper is stored in the liver and other tissues (such as the eyes), finally resulting in toxic concentrations. The level of serum ceruloplasmin is usually very low in this disease. Copper-low diets of "normal foods" have been developed which are used as part of the clinical management of the disease.

MANGANESE

Manganese (Mn) is easily confused with *magnesium* (Mg) (see Chap. 11) because the names are similar, and both are essential nutrients. However, most of the similarity stops there. This gray metal is the twelfth most abundant element on the earth's crust and a necessary component of steel as well as plants and animals.

Inorganic manganese has been known to be essential for all higher animals ever since the original discovery in several laboratories (Hart, McCollum, and their associates) in 1931 that it was essential for rats.[31] Later it was shown to be essential for poultry (deficiency resulted in a tendon and bone disorder), swine, guinea pigs, cattle, and other animals.[2]

Though no experimental manganese deficiency has been studied in man, it is undoubtedly an essential nutrient. The requirement is so low in comparison with the abundant amounts in our environment and in most foods that a deficiency has never been known (and would be quite unlikely).

Manganese has many essential functions in each cell of the body.[2, 27] The highest concentrations in the body are in the pituitary gland, lactating mammary glands, liver, pancreas, kidney, intestinal wall, and bone.

Manganese is an important catalyst and is a cofactor or component of many enzymes in the body.* On the basis of its relationship to these enzymes, it is needed for synthesis of complex carbohydrates (mucopolysaccharides) in cells, for utilization of glucose, for lipid synthesis and metabolism, cholesterol synthesis, normal pancreas development, muscle contraction, prevention of skeletal defects, prevention of sterility, and other vital functions. Few elements have as many metabolic functions (though the mechanisms are still quite unknown).

Manganese deficiency has either occurred spontaneously (in fowl fed natural grain and legume diets) or been induced in several species of animals on manganese-low diets, with symptoms too numerous to itemize.[3] In general, manganese deficiency is associated with failure to grow, interference with sexual processes, and inability to produce normal young.[32] In rabbits, there are deformations of bone. In fowls, a manganese-deficient ration proved to be the chief cause of a disorder called "slipped tendon," resulting in deformed legs, which was a source of economic loss to poultry producers. The addition of small amounts of this element to the ration prevented development of this disease (55 mg per kg of diet is needed by fowl, a relatively high level compared with the normal need of mammals). Adult male humans appear to be in manganese balance with 6 to 8 mg of this element per day, and adult females 3 to 5 mg (the amount in usual diets).[29, 33] About 30 to 50 percent is absorbed.

Manganese is widely distributed in foods of plant and animal origin,[29, 33] though it is lost along with other trace elements in food refining. It is relatively nontoxic. There is no recommended daily allowance for it, since a human deficiency has not yet been obtained.

ZINC

Interest in zinc as an essential trace element has been renewed since the 1960's when evidence for its need by man was shown,[2, 34] and since the discovery that both animals and man can become deficient under so-called "natural" conditions, when eating foods of plant origin.[2]

Zinc alloys have been known for centuries (it is a constituent, with copper, of brass) and since the 1700's as a silver-blue mineral.† We see zinc around us commonly as the coating of "galvanized" iron and inside flashlight batteries. About 2 gm is present in an adult human body—about a 200-day supply for nutritional needs.

Its need in the diet of mammals was first proved by Wisconsin nutritionists working with rats in the 1930's.[35] Zinc is now known to be very important in the diet of all animal species studied, including rat, cattle, sheep, dog, pig, mouse, and poultry (see Fig. 12–7).

Distribution in Body and Role

Concentrations of zinc in the human body are highest in the liver, bones, epidermal tissues, prostate gland, testes, sperm cells, hair, nails, eye, and blood, and there is rapid metabolism of it in the pancreas, kidneys, and pituitary

---

*Manganese is present in such enzymes as *pyruvate carboxylase*, and *superoxide dismutase* (which also contains copper), and is a cofactor in the metabolism of liver arginase, phosphoglucomutase, polymerase (in mucopolysaccharide formation), galactotransferase, acetyl-CoA carboxylase, and others.

---

†The name "zinc" comes from the common name of its ore "zincium" found originally in Poland.

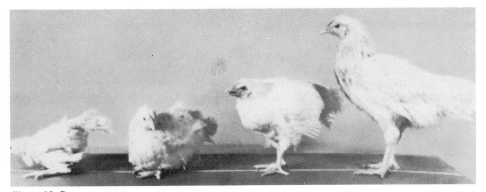

Figure 12–7. These four chickens are all 10 weeks old. From left to right, they were fed increasing amounts of zinc. Note the retarded growth, poor feathering, and difficulty in standing up in the deficient animals. (Courtesy of the American Zinc Institute.)

gland. In the blood, 75 percent of the zinc is in the red cells.

In animals, a diet low in zinc, especially one high in calcium or *phytates* (as in whole grains and beans), predisposes to zinc deficiency, symptoms of which may be retarded growth, loss of appetite, skin disorders, many reproduction problems,[36] and abnormal bone metabolism.[2] In zinc-deficient pigs, an increase of zinc intake prevents or cures a disease characterized by roughening of the skin and hair loss, called *parakeratosis*, which formerly caused economic losses. Zinc is now added routinely to commercial poultry and swine diets.

Zinc is a constituent of the hormone *insulin*, secreted by the pancreas and concerned in carbohydrate metabolism. Two hormones, which are secreted by the anterior pituitary (follicle-stimulating and luteinizing hormones) and play a role in the female reproductive cycle, have their action enhanced by the presence of zinc.

In enzyme systems, zinc plays an important role as an active component of the enzyme *carbonic anhydrase*, which functions in maintaining equilibrium between carbon dioxide and carbonic acid ($CO_2 + H_2O \rightleftharpoons H_2CO_3$) in tissues and catalyzes the reaction by which hydrogen may be split off from car-

bonic acid. This reaction not only is important in the transport of carbon dioxide by the blood but also may be involved (by the liberation of hydrogen ions) in the secretion of high concentrations of hydrochloric acid into the gastric juice. Zinc also activates enzymes which function in digestion of proteins by hydrolyzing specific peptide linkages. It is a constituent or activator of a number of other enzymes.[2] It plays an essential role in the formation of RNA and DNA in the synthesis of protein in the cell.

In man, zinc is essential for normal growth of the genital organs, prevention of anemia, general growth of all tissues (and prevention of "dwarfism," or greatly reduced stature), and wound healing.[27, 34] Zinc deficiencies are rarely seen in the United States but have been seen in the Middle East (in studies made by Dr. Prasad, then of Vanderbilt University in Nashville, and coworkers).

Requirement and Food Sources

The average American diet supplies about 10 to 15 mg of zinc per day, about half of which is absorbed. This is sufficient to prevent deficiencies, although diets limited only to vegetable sources of protein may be low or inadequate.[1,2] There is no "recommended allowance," but about 6 mg has been suggested as a tentative requirement for children.[1]

Zinc occurs widely in plant and animal tissues. It is present, therefore, in all natural foods, but it is low in fruits, vegetables, and refined foods (see Table 12–5).[29 (a, b, and d), 37] Oysters are an unusually rich source of the element. Fortunately zinc is not a particularly toxic element, though poisoning is known to occur (presumably from zinc) from drinking acid fruit drink stored in galvanized containers.

Low levels of serum zinc have been found in persons with alcoholic liver diseases or tuberculosis and in women who are pregnant or taking contraceptives, indicative of borderline intakes. It is most likely that other evidences of zinc deficiencies in man will be found as the quality and number of analytical studies improve.

FLUORINE

Fluorine (F),* now accepted as an essential nutrient for man, is still a most lively topic. One can get very strong reactions from it both in the chemical laboratory or by pointing out the advantages of the fluoridation of public water supplies to those who are opposed to the practice.

Fluorine is a very reactive gas, closely related to the other halogen gases—chlorine, iodine, and bromine. It has been known to be widely distributed, in combined forms, in natural ores such as fluorspar. It is also present in rock phosphate (a fertilizer which con-

*The name is derived from the Latin word *fluere*, meaning to flow—a property of fluorspar, one of its ores, when it is heated. This ore also "fluoresces" (from which the name of the common "fluorescent" lamp comes). Fluorine was first isolated in 1886 by the Frenchman Moissan.

*Table 12–5.   Approximate Zinc Content of Representative Foods**

	mg/100 gm		mg/100 gm
Whole grains	1.5–5	Potatoes	0.3
Germ	10–20	Cereal flakes	0.1–0.2
Bran	7–13		
Bread, whole wheat	2	Bread, white	0.7
Dry legumes	2–5	Vegetables	0.2–0.8
Nuts	2–4	Fruits	0.1–0.3
Muscle meats, fish, fowl	1.5–5	Milk	0.1–0.6
Eggs	1.5		

*Schlettwein-Gsell, D., and Mommsen-Straub, S.: Internat. J. Vit. Res., *40*:659, 1970.[37]

tains 3 to 4 percent of fluorine), in soil, water, teeth, and bones, and in small amounts in almost all natural animal and plant foods in varying amounts (in its ion form, fluoride). Like many others of the trace elements, too large amounts of it have toxic effects.

Discovery in Water Supplies

Interest in the element was at first concerned with the harmful effects of abnormally high concentrations of fluorine in drinking water in certain areas of the world, since consumption of such waters was shown to be the cause of mottled enamel of teeth (chalky spots which later stain dark brown), which appears in the teeth of children and persists into adult life.[38] In the United States, this tooth disorder was endemic in certain areas in Arizona, Colorado, the Texas Panhandle, and elsewhere. Although disfiguring, this mottling of teeth seemed to do no harm, and later studies indicated that children living in these areas had teeth which were *more resistant to decay* (dental caries) than the teeth of children in areas where drinking water was of lower fluorine content.[2, 3, 39]

Attention, which had previously been focused on possible ways of reducing the fluorine concentration in drinking water, now turned to the possible effect of raising the fluorine level in water supplies where it was low to a point where it might provide protection against dental caries without being harmful. If the fluorine concentration was over about 2 parts per million (2 mg per liter of water), mottling of the enamel of teeth was evident; if it was about 1 part per million, no harmful effects were observed and the incidence of dental decay in children's teeth was markedly reduced by 50 percent or more.

Regulation of the fluorine content of water by addition, or removal, of fluorides in localities where there is a deficiency, or excess, to a range of 0.7 to 1.2 parts per million (allowing for seasonal temperature changes) for prevention of tooth decay is now a fully scientifically accepted, safe, economical, and efficient public health measure for supplying this element.[1, 40] Artificially fluoridated water is now available to over 40 percent of the United States population and to millions in other parts of the world. About nine million additional American citizens and many elsewhere have naturally fluoridated water at about the recommended level (0.7 to 1.2 parts per million). (See Chap. 22 for further discussion of the dental aspects of fluoridation.)

Role in the Body

There is no known metabolic role in the body for fluorine, although it is known to activate certain enzymes and to inhibit others. All that can be said with certainty is that fluorine is necessary for maximal resistance to dental caries as a structural component of normal teeth.* For this reason, the Food and Nutrition Board, and rightly so, considers fluorine to be an "essential nutrient".[1] This reasoning appears

sound on the basis of recent work of Schwarz. He demonstrated growth retardation in rats kept under special fluorine-low conditions, thus confirming its essential need.†

There is much discussion today concerning the possibility that dietary fluorine may also be important for maintenance of strong bone structure in humans and in the prevention, with other minerals, of osteoporosis, or demineralization of the bones (see calcium).[41] As yet, no proved relationship exists.[1, 2]

Fluorine is readily absorbed from the intestine and is distributed widely in the body with highest concentration in the teeth and bones (where concentrations up to 0.5 percent are possible on a dry basis). The urine is the main route of excretion (about 80 percent of ingested fluorine is excreted in children and up to 98 percent in adults).

Distribution in Food and Requirement

Very few foods contain more than 1 to 2 parts per million of fluorine (unless such foods are raised in a high fluorine environment) and most contain less.[2, 42] Seafood, such as fish eaten with bones, and tea (about 0.2 to 0.3 mg per cup) are among the highest sources. Bone meal, sometimes used as a mineral supplement, is very rich in fluorine (normally 300 to 600 parts per million). A normal day's diet in the United States contains about 0.3 to 0.6 mg of fluorine (as fluorides), not including the amount in drinking water. Including drinking water, a normal intake would be 1 to 2.5 mg per day.

No specific values for food are given here, because the composition of fluorine in plant foods or animal products is dependent largely upon the level in

---

*The form of fluorine in teeth and bones is chiefly *fluorapatile* ($CaF_2 \cdot 3\ Ca_3(PO_4)_2$).

†Schwarz, K. S., and Milne, D. B.: Bioinorganic Chem., *1*:331, 1972.

the environment (such as soil, water, and air) or the amount in the feed.[42] Fluorine is not an essential element for plants, so it is not always present in important amounts in foods from such plants.

The most reliable sources of fluorine, therefore, are fluoridated water (at a level of 0.7 to 1.2 parts per million), or fluoridated salt (or other staple food) used in some countries as a means of providing fluorine to children. Sea salt is not a reliable source. Breast milk is very low though adequate. Fluorine tablets and fluorine toothpastes are available which can serve as a reliable, though expensive, source of this element.

Toxicity

Fluorine has a small safety range — as small as about any element. However, the range is "wide enough for safe accommodation of normal fluctuations in the fluoride content of foods without risk of inducing the first identifiable indication of an excess — slight mottling of the enamel."[1] Several million Americans live in communities with water levels of natural fluorine from 1.2 to 4 parts per million (higher than recommended amounts)[1] without any handicap other than slight mottling of the teeth (though public health authorities are working to reduce these concentrations where possible). Their general health is otherwise satisfactory.

When animals or humans are exposed to levels of fluorine higher than about 6 to 10 parts per million over long periods of time, or when there is environmental contamination, it can result in toxicity (*fluorosis*), manifested by deformed teeth and bones and other toxic symptoms.[2, 43] That fluorine in drinking water, when present at about 1 part per million, is not harmful to man or animals regardless of the amount of water consumed, has been fully demonstrated.

COBALT

Cobalt (Co)* is the seventh trace element to be recognized as a dietary essential. In 1935, it was discovered that soils and plants of various areas of Australia, Canada, New York, Florida, and elsewhere where farm animals grazed were very low in cobalt. Sick sheep and cattle grown in these areas responded to additions of cobalt. Without the cobalt they developed progressive anemia, muscular atrophy, listlessness, extreme emaciation, and eventually death (sometimes called wasting disease). About 2 mg of cobalt added per kilogram of feed is all that was needed to overcome the deficiency.[2]

In 1948, the important discovery was made that cobalt was an essential structural part of the vitamin B-12 molecule, present at a level of 4 percent by weight (see Chap. 7). Studies since then have shown that the major role of cobalt in the body (if not the only role) is to serve as part of vitamin B-12. When vitamin B-12 was injected into deficient cows and sheep, all symptoms were overcome, whereas injection of equivalent amounts of cobalt had no effect. In other words, cobalt had been effective in much larger levels fed or injected (excessive amounts were returned to the gut) because these made it possible for rumen microorganisms to synthesize vitamin B-12. Without cobalt there was no synthesis.

Obviously then, a dietary source of inorganic cobalt is essential for vitamin B-12 production in the gut only by those animals (such as sheep, cattle, goats, deer, horses, guinea pigs, and

---

*The name cobalt is thought to have been derived in the 1500's from the German word *Kobold*, meaning goblin or mischievous spirit, from the difficulty found in working with cobalt ores. It was first isolated in 1742 by the Swedish chemist Brandt (though salts of cobalt had been used for centuries for the blue color in decorative glass and pottery).

rabbits) that normally live on plant substances alone and that are not otherwise given a vitamin B-12 source. To some extent, humans also have this ability to synthesize vitamin B-12 from cobalt by microorganisms. This probably explains why true vegetarians can live many years without vitamin B-12 itself in the diet. Synthesis in the gut is not a sure thing in man at all, so we generally regard man's need of cobalt in terms of the intact vitamin B-12 molecule and not in terms of inorganic cobalt itself.

Physiologically speaking, since no animal can manufacture vitamin B-12 in its tissues (but only in the intestine), the specific need in the body for cobalt is only in the organic form—as vitamin B-12. Inorganic cobalt in the diet, then, serves only indirectly, but this can be very important, nutritionally, for many animals if not for man.

There is no evidence that humans must ever be concerned about their intake of inorganic cobalt. In other words, a cobalt deficiency has never been described for man and would be difficult if not impossible to obtain. A normal day's intake of 150 to 600 mcg of inorganic cobalt[44] is far greater than any possible requirement. Cobalt ions are distributed throughout the body, especially in the liver and heart, and they do not accumulate with age.

Cobalt is present in almost all foods in varying amounts,[2, 44] but since analytical techniques are still uncertain and since we really do not have to worry about it (there appears to be no shortage, and our concern, actually, in human nutrition is about vitamin B-12 and not cobalt), to present figures would serve no purpose. Undue amounts of cobalt in the diet of man and animal species other than ruminants cause stimulation of bone marrow, with excessive production of red corpuscles (polycythemia) and higher than normal hemoglobin. Toxic reactions from unusually large levels in food (in this case, beer) have been known.[45]

MOLYBDENUM

With the discovery in 1953 that *molybdenum* (Mo)* is a component of the essential enzyme *xanthine dehydrogenase*[46] (and later other enzymes), a new era of essential microelement research was ushered in which still continues.

Needs for this element are minute, and human deficiencies are not known. Certain animals (rats, poultry, and sheep) rendered deficient by artificially low levels of molybdenum intake (and often with use of the antagonistic action of other trace elements such as copper or tungsten) produce weak and malformed young.[2, 47]

Molybdenum is widely distributed in foods in very small amounts. About the only foods known to contain as much as 0.6 part per million are legumes, cereals, organ meats, and yeast.[48] Inorganic forms of molybdenum in the diet are well utilized by the body, and the main route of excretion is the urine.

A normal day's intake is about 0.1 to 0.4 mg, which must be slightly greater than the human requirement (which is still an unknown entity). A deficiency is unlikely to occur under normal conditions.[2] Schroeder and co-workers[48] present evidence that marginal or deficient intakes of molybdenum are a possibility if one were to choose by accident the wrong mixture of low value foods, emphasizing again the importance of choosing diets containing a variety of traditional foodstuffs. The Food and Nutrition Board has not yet set a recommended allowance.

SELENIUM

Since the last edition of this book, hundreds of research papers have been

---

*From the Greek word *molybdos* for lead. Molybdenum was first obtained in pure form in the late 1700's. It is a hard silver-white material used widely in alloys. It is essential for the growth of all higher plants.

published on the subject of selenium in experimental nutrition. Yet, since 1957, when Schwarz and coworkers discovered that selenium had a vital role in animals,[49] too few years have elapsed for its role in human nutrition to be fully evaluated. Selenium is in all probability required by the human organism, just as it is for all experimental animals studied (rat, poultry, sheep, cattle, pig, rabbit, horse, mouse, and others). However, final experimental proof of its need for man has not yet been obtained. There is no evidence to indicate that it is not an essential trace element for man, and the probability that it is essential has been pointed out by the Food and Nutrition Board,[1] by Sandstead and coworkers,[27] and others. It certainly appears to be as important a nutrient for man as better-known trace elements such as zinc, copper, and manganese.

The rapidly evolving story of selenium in nutrition is most fascinating, and only a few highlights can be given here (for further reading, see the references at end of this chapter and current publications).

Discovery and Toxicity

The element selenium (Se) was discovered and named by the Swedish chemist Berzelius in 1817.*[50] It is closely related chemically to sulfur but is much less abundant. Animal scientists first became interested in selenium when it was determined in the 1930's[2] that soils and certain plants in parts of western North America and in other parts of the world contained levels of this element which were toxic to farm animals. Grazing animals in such *se-*

leniferous areas (areas with toxic levels of selenium) developed symptoms of "alkali disease" or "blind staggers" characterized by stiffness and lameness, loss of hair, deformed hoofs, blindness, paralysis, and eventually death. Toxic symptoms are also known in man not unlike the animal symptoms, but including an increased incidence of dental caries.

It was with considerable surprise, then, that an element as toxic, or more so, as mercury and lead (as we know them today) would be found to be nutritionally essential. In the early 1950's Dr. Schwarz and coworkers produced *dietary liver necrosis* (death of liver tissue due to a deficiency), *poor growth*, and *death* in rats[2, 49] fed special diets containing torula yeast (which is very low in selenium and vitamin E). Schwarz found that an unidentified water-soluble substance in brewer's yeast and kidney appeared to be needed which greatly reduced or eliminated the vitamin E need of the rat. Less than 0.5 part per million of selenium, when it was identified as the missing component, was found to be as effective as 50 parts per million of vitamin E, which it replaced (see Fig. 12–8). Later work has shown that selenium has specific functions in addition to its vitamin E sparing effect (in fact, it now would appear that much of the need for vitamin E is to spare the selenium requirement).

Deficiency Signs in Animals and Function

Besides poor growth and liver necrosis in rats, a wide variety of deficiency signs were found in animals deficient in both selenium and vitamin E. Extensive *striated muscular degeneration*, known widely as "white muscle disease," or "nutritional muscular dystrophy," occurs in young sheep, cattle, horses, and rabbits under farm conditions. This occurs in many areas of the United States (mainly west of the Rocky Mountains and east of the Mississippi River—

---

*Named for the Greek word *selene*, or moon, since selenium was closely associated with the element tellurium, named for the earth. Selenium is important in making photoelectric cells, exposure meters, rectifiers, photocopying machines, and in the ceramics industry. Also it is often used to produce red glass, so it has many industrial uses.

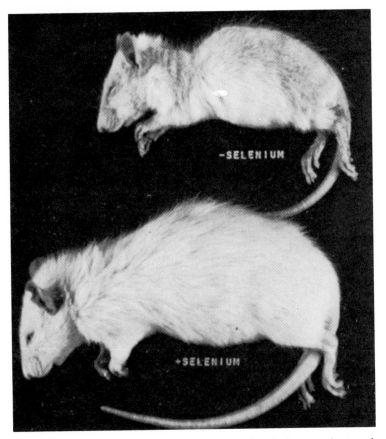

Figure 12–8. Selenium-deficient rat (above) compared with selenium-supplemented rat (below). (From Hurt, H. D., Cary, E. E., and Visek, W. J.: J. Nutr., *101*:761, 1971.

see Fig. 12–9) and other parts of the world where soils are deficient in this element. As many as 20 to 30 percent of all lambs in some flocks may be affected, for example. Deficient chicks develop large greenish-blue spots under the skin due to leakage of the blood from capillaries and soon die. Deficient mice develop damaged hearts. Pigs deficient in selenium and vitamin E develop diseased livers and die suddenly. Selenium, in the absence of much higher amounts of vitamin E (the requirement of which is greatly reduced by selenium) is essential for reproduction in all animals studied. Selenium additions are widely made to livestock in deficient areas by injection or by the addition of selenium-rich foods to the diet.

Selenium, though closely related to vitamin E in its function, is now known to have a specific essential role of its own in nutrition even when vitamin E is present in the diet.[2, 51] Why selenium is needed is not known as yet, but it appears to function (combined in organic form in the body) as a powerful cellular antioxidant protecting cellular membranes. No doubt it has other catalytic functions. The amounts of selenium needed by animals in the diet are exceedingly small, in the range of only 0.05 to 0.5 part per million. (This is only about 50 to 500 mcg per kilogram of diet, making it more active than

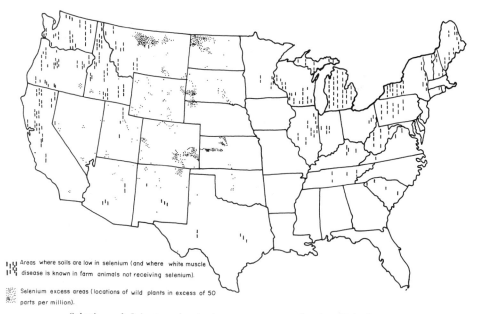

Areas where soils are low in selenium (and where white muscle disease is known in farm animals not receiving selenium).

Selenium excess areas (locations of wild plants in excess of 50 parts per million).

Figure 12–9. Selenium deficient and selenium excess areas in the United States (approximate). (Adapted from U.S. government figures. See Muth and Allaway: J. Amer. Vet. Med. Assoc., *142*:1379, 1963; and Kubota, et al.: J. Agric. Food Chem., *15*:448, 1967.)

many of the vitamins.) Toxic levels in animal diets start at about 5 to 10 parts per million, which is not much of a margin of safety.

Selenium in Food and Nutritional Status of Man

Selenium, probably bound to protein, occurs naturally in all seafood, meat, and those grains raised on selenium-containing soils. Fruits and vegetables are very low in it. Levels in most plants depend quite entirely on the level of selenium in the soil.[2, 50, 52] Variations of over 100-fold are known to occur (so general tables of the selenium content of food are quite useless). The few wild plants* which accumulate the element in selenium-rich soils contain toxic levels (up to 0.1 to 1 percent of selenium) for any grazing animals which might consume them.

———————————
*Gray's vetch and woody aster.

Considerable losses of selenium can occur in processing, refinement of foods, and cooking.

A person eating a mixed diet of foods of different origins would most likely be getting about 50 to 100 mcg of selenium per day. This amount appears to be more than the amount needed. No recommended daily allowance has been set. People eating very poor diets in selenium-deficient areas may well be low in this element, but this is only a supposition based on animal studies.

Several studies have shown that selenium is low in the diet or in the blood of severely malnourished children in developing countries,[2, 27, 50, 53] but additional studies are needed to establish specifically the essential nature of this element in man.

Besides the toxic symptoms previously mentioned, selenium has produced tumors in certain strains of rats fed 2 to 3 parts per million over long periods of time (about 10 times, or more, the requirement). Other studies have indicated that selenium can protect against tumors in other situations in the rat. Obviously food and drug administrators are being very careful in permitting selenium additions to any feed or food.

CHROMIUM

Very few persons would have guessed before 1959 that chromium, the mineral most of us know as that which makes the shiny "chrome"-plated bumpers and strips on automobiles, is essential in the diet of mammals, including man.

Chromium (Cr), originally discovered in 1797,* has been known for many years to be present in food and animal tissues. In 1959, Schwarz and Mertz,[54] then of the U.S. National Institutes of Health, made the important discovery that very small amounts of chromium (only when in the stable trivalent state, as Cr^{3+}) were necessary in the diet for normal metabolism of blood glucose in the rat. Over 47 different elements were tested by Schwarz and Mertz before the specificity of chromium was announced as the *glucose tolerance factor* (GTF), as it was called.

Sufficient evidence now exists, both direct and indirect, to include chromium among the essential trace elements for man. It has a variety of functions, including (1) the stimulation of enzymes involved in glucose and energy metabolism, (2) the stimulation of the synthesis of fatty acids and cholesterol in the liver, (3) an involvement in insulin metabolism, and (4) a role as a part of several other enzymes including one of the protein-digesting enzymes in the intestine.[54] In rats, mice, and monkeys,

a deficiency results in decreased growth and increased mortality, as well as decreased rate of glucose removal from the blood. Inorganic chromium is thought by Mertz to be a precursor of a still-unknown organic compound in the body (the "glucose tolerance factor"[54]).

Poorly nourished children in several parts of the Middle East (Turkey and Lebanon, where chromium levels of some soils and water supplies appear to be low) show signs of poor glucose utilization correctable in some instances by the addition to the diet of small amounts of chromium (250 mcg).[55] This was explained on the basis of the role of chromium in insulin metabolism. Similar effects have been seen in a few diabetic adults who apparently were deficient in chromium. Recent indications that chromium may play a role in the prevention of atherosclerosis in man and cholesterol metabolism in animals are interesting but require confirmation.

The human body contains a total of only a small amount of chromium—less than 6 mg,[27] with a decline with age. A typical daily intake in the United States usually ranges between 50 and 120 mcg. Only a small amount of that ingested is absorbed (1 to 5 percent). The biologically active form is quite nontoxic and is rapidly excreted.

Good *food sources* of chromium are fats such as corn oil (in which it exists as an impurity) and meats. Fruits, vegetables, sea food, and drinking water are generally poor sources. The amount of chromium in plant foods depends to a large extent on the amount in the soil, although tables of chromium content of representative foods are available[57] (but not to be trusted). Processing and refinement reduce the chromium content of foods considerably. For instance, white sugar contains very little, and white flour has much less than whole wheat. Of significance in considering food sources of chromium are the early studies of Mertz and Schwartz, who produced a chromium deficiency in rats

---

*Discovered by the French chemist Vauquelin (who also isolated the first amino acid) and named from the Greek word *chroma* for color. Most salts of chromium are brightly colored and are used widely as pigments. The red color of the ruby and the green color of the emerald are due to salts of chromium. It is an important component of stainless steel (with 10 to 18 percent chromium).

by feeding commercial stock diets of crude feedstuffs.

Good food sources of chromium are about the same as other trace minerals—foods of animal origin and a mixed diet of the traditional wholesome natural foods. The human requirement is not known but is probably in the range of 20 to 50 mcg per day, an amount present in the diet of almost all Americans (with the exception of persons eating largely of highly refined foods).

NICKEL

Nickel (Ni)* is included among the essential trace elements largely on the basis of reports of its presence in a serum protein in rabbits and man (called *nickeloplasmin*)[58] and of its apparent requirement by chickens.

Deficient chickens were said by Nielsen (1970) of the United States Department of Agriculture[2, 59] to have slightly enlarged hocks, thickened legs, bright orange leg color (instead of pale yellow-brown), a dermatitis, and a "less friable liver." Nickel at a level of 3 to 5 mg per kilogram of diet corrected these minor abnormalities. (This study requires confirmation.) Nickel is also known to activate several enzyme systems, although whether this is a specific function is not known. It is present in high levels in ribonucleic acids for reasons that are not yet clear.[2]

Nickel is widely distributed in foods, especially plant foods. The deficiency in chickens was produced after careful removal of all extra sources of nickel (although corn was one of the ingredients of the diet). A deficiency in man has never been seen and would be unlikely to occur except under unusual conditions. A normal diet could supply about 0.3 to 0.6 mg per day, and any require-

ment for the element must be less than this.

Nickel has not yet been proved to be needed by plants but is required by several microorganisms. Nickel is only moderately toxic for animals.

TIN

Tin (Sn)† is included among the essential elements on the basis of the discovery in 1970 by Schwarz and coworkers of its important growth-promoting effect in deficient rats.[60] By using rats under highly isolated conditions free of contamination with tin, a reduced growth rate was produced within two weeks after the start of the experiment. Supplements of tin at levels of about 1 mg per kg of diet increased growth in several different experiments by as much as 30 to 60 percent in only four weeks' time.

No studies showing a requirement for tin by man have been made as yet, but the above results with rats provide good evidence for its need. Tin is widely distributed in foods of animal and plant origin, and a deficiency in man or animals under normal conditions would not be expected to occur.

Tin is not very toxic, and if acid fruit juices or similar products dissolve appreciable amounts of tin from a tin-plated can it is not well-absorbed by man (though the iron might be).[61] High levels of tin—from 43 to 114 parts per million—have been found in canned pineapple and citrus juices,[29b] although such amounts do not appear to be toxic. Generally, such cans containing acid juices are now lacquered. A normal tin intake is probably in the range of 1.5 to 5 mg a day, depending on the amount of canned food eaten.[2] The requirement for man is not known but would

---

*Discovered originally in 1751 by Cronstedt and named nickel for "Old Nick," a demon. It is the same nickel that our five-cent piece is named after, and the element has wide use in industry.

†From the Latin word for tin, *stannum.* Tin has been known since the Bronze Age (since bronze is an alloy of tin and copper). Its most common use is in the "tin can," in which a thin inner coat of tin lines the steel can.

be expected to be slightly less than 1 mg a day on the basis of the rat studies.

VANADIUM

The thirteenth trace element needed by higher animals was shown to be *vanadium* (V)* in 1970 and 1971, although its essential nature has been suspected for many years. It has long been known to be present throughout the plant and animal kingdoms and to be required by several lower organisms.

Its need by higher animals was amply demonstrated in the laboratory of Dr.

Schwarz[62] of the Veterans Administration Hospital in Long Beach, California (the same Dr. Schwarz who with his coworkers had previously discovered the need for selenium, chromium, and tin; see Fig. 12–10). The growth of rats raised on special deficient diets in "ultraclean" conditions was increased over 40 percent in a 21 to 28 day period by the addition of 0.25 to 0.5 mg of vanadium (as sodium orthovanadate) per kilogram of diet. No specific deficiency signs were observed other than poor growth. Vanadium is known to be a catalyst in several biological systems and to be present in higher than normal concentrations in teeth.[2]

Earlier preliminary studies in 1970 by U.S.D.A workers, Hopkins and Mohr, with chickens (showing reduced growth of feathers) and with rats, by Purdue University workers, had indicated that vanadium was an essential trace element.[63]

---

*Vanadium was identified in 1831 by Sefström, of Sweden, who named it after the Norse goddess of beauty, Vanadis (from the beautiful color of its compounds). Earlier studies on it had been made by Del Rio in Mexico. It was not obtained in pure form until 1927. It has many industrial uses, especially in vanadium steel.

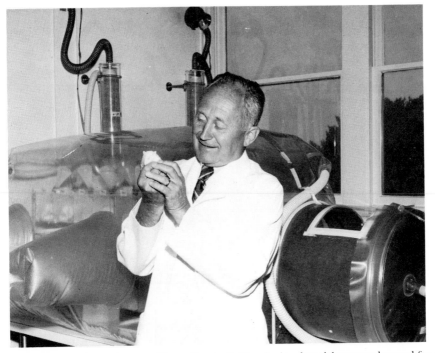

Figure 12–10. Dr. Klaus Schwarz, of Long Beach, California, in whose laboratory the need for selenium, chromium, tin, and vanadium was demonstrated.

No figure can be given for the vanadium requirement of man, but it would be about in the range of only 0.1 to 0.3 mg per day. Normal diets contain about 10 times this amount, so deficiencies would be very rare under usual conditions. The amount of vanadium in our foods and in the environment appears to be considerably lower than the toxic level.[2]

SILICON

The most recent essential trace element shown to be essential for the animal (chick and rat) is silicon (Si). This element (from the Latin word *silex*, meaning flint) is the most abundant mineral element in the earth. Its most common form is silicon dioxide (SiO_2), or sand from which glass is made. It was originally discovered as an element by Berzelius in 1823.

Edith Carlisle, nutritionist at the University of California (Los Angeles), reported in 1972 that silicon is needed in microgram amounts for normal growth and bone development in the chick.* Silicon has long been known to be required by certain lower forms of life and, apparently, by some plants, but its need by animals was unexpected and constitutes a major nutrition discovery.

Silicon is widely distributed in foods. Because of this, deficiencies in man (assuming that it is needed) would be virtually impossible on the basis of present knowledge of its distribution.

NONESSENTIAL TRACE ELEMENTS (FOR HIGHER ANIMALS)

Many other trace elements (at least 50) are known to be present in plants and animals. Any of these could con-

---

*Carlisle, E.: Fed. Proc., *31*:700, 1972 (abstract). Confirmed in rat studies by Schwarz, Nature, in press.

ceivably be shown to be essential in the diet at some time in the future (see Schwarz[60b]), although this is only conjecture at this point. There are small pieces of evidence (such as a requirement by plants or lower organisms, or a catalytic role demonstrated in isolated systems) for a possible future role in nutrition for some, such as *boron* (known to be required by certain plants), and the element *cadmium* (found associated with zinc in at least one natural protein).[2] These elements are relatively nontoxic in small amounts. They are widely distributed in nature in most plant and animal foods in minute amounts, as are *aluminum, arsenic, barium, bromine, germanium, niobium, rubidium, silver, strontium, titanium,* and *zirconium.*[2] In spite of their widespread occurrence, there is no evidence as yet that any of these elements plays any biological role in higher animals, and they must be considered as nonessential elements at this time. Likewise, such elements as gold, antimony, cesium, lead, lithium, and mercury are widely distributed in nature but this does not prove, or even indicate, any biological function. (However, it is well to remember that tin, nickel, selenium, chromium, silicon, and vanadium were listed with these nonessential elements just a few years ago.)

Toxicity of Micronutrients at Higher Levels of Intake

It is both interesting and important to call attention to the fact that, although small amounts are required for body welfare, all of these micronutrients are toxic when too large amounts of them are taken into the body. Sometimes the margin between optimal intake and toxic amounts is not very wide. Too large doses of iodine may overstimulate the thyroid gland, or too small an intake results in enlargement of this gland in simple goiter. With fluorine, about twice the amount which provides protection against dental caries will cause mottling of teeth. All the metallic elements are stored in the liver, so that the amount in the body may accumulate to toxic levels.

Especially of interest today are *mercury*, *lead*, and *cadmium* because of their presence in toxic amounts in certain segments of the environment.[2] Mercury, though naturally occurring in small amounts, has increased in concentration because of industrial wastes. It has been found to be close to toxic levels in some samples of sea foods. Toxic levels have been known to be reached in isolated instances in Japan and the United States. The highest permissible level in American foods is 0.5 part per million.

Lead has been found in high concentrations in plants and soils near highways due to discharges of lead from automobile engines. Lead toxicity is a well-known syndrome in children who have chewed on window sills, toys, or other surfaces painted with lead-containing paints. Another source of lead toxicity is lead glazes on dishes. (Acid fruit juices should not be kept more than a few hours in any suspected dishes or pitchers; in fact, dishes suspected of having lead glazes should be discarded.)

One cannot avoid eating traces of toxic elements no matter how carefully one attempts to do so, but it does not help to ignore the possibilities and sources of toxicity. We recommend keeping in close touch with (and taking an active interest in) government agencies whose job it is to control levels of toxins in our food and environment.

Pica

Pica (pronounced "pie-ca") is the name for an unnatural craving, most commonly seen in women and young children, to eat laundry starch, clay, ashes, dirt, ice, or similar material. It probably is due, in part, to a natural craving for trace minerals, especially iron. Pica is commonly seen in times of stress such as pregnancy or lactation. It is sometimes a source of toxic elements such as lead and should be avoided as much as possible. Its cessation can only come about with nutrition education and good eating habits.

QUESTIONS AND PROBLEMS

1. In what special tissue is most of the iron in the body found, and in what special substance in this tissue? What function does it fulfill in this tissue, and what chemical property enables it to carry out this function? How do the smaller amounts of iron located in tissue cells help in oxidation-reduction processes vital to the life of cells?

2. What is the Recommended Dietary Allowance for iron daily for a grown man? A woman? At what periods of life is the need for this element increased, and why? Why is iron sometimes referred to as "the one-way element"? Explain how iron is conserved by the body and how a liberal supply of it in the diet can build up reserve stores that serve to protect the body in times of extra need.

3. What are the symptoms of iron deficiency anemia, and under what conditions may it be caused? Does the existence of anemia necessarily mean that the diet furnished less than normal amounts of iron? Explain reasons for your answer. What other nutritional factors besides iron are important in prevention of anemia?

4. Can the body utilize either inorganic or organic iron equally well? In what form or forms is iron most readily absorbed from the intestine? Mention three factors that favor and three that are unfavorable for iron absorption. To what extent may the degree of availability and absorption of iron be influenced by the relative need of the body for iron?

5. Why is iodine essential in small

amounts for body welfare? In what tissue is this element concentrated, and what is its function there? Can iodine be stored in the body and, if so, where? What is a ductless gland? A hormone? The names of the two iodine-containing hormones of the thyroid gland? The influence of these hormones on body metabolism (tissue oxidations)?

6. Simple goiter is a deficiency disease caused by lack of what element? In what regions is it most prevalent, and why? At what periods of life is it most likely to develop, and why? What public health measure has been used successfully in preventing simple goiter?

7. Name five foods that are relatively rich in iron. Three that are relatively rich in iodine. What kinds of food are poor in iron? In iodine?

8. Is copper an essential element? For what special purpose is it necessary? Why does a rat become anemic if kept a long time on a diet consisting only of milk? Why can such an anemia not be cured by giving either iron alone or copper alone? If a baby developed nutritional anemia, would it be of assistance in curing the anemia to give some copper along with some form of iron? Explain why most people are sure of getting enough copper in their food to meet their requirement for this element.

9. Is some form of cobalt essential for humans? For what animals is it essential? What are the symptoms of cobalt deficiency and how may it be caused? In what vitamin is cobalt found, and why is anemia a prominent symptom in cobalt deficiency in ruminants such as sheep or cattle?

10. Record all the foods you ate on a typical day, with quantities of each, and calculate the amount of iron furnished by this day's diet. Use either Table 12-3 for iron content of foods or tables in the Appendix for nutritive values of foods in average servings. Does the amount of iron in this day's diet come up to the recommended allowance? If not, what changes could be made to furnish more iron?

11. Is fluorine an essential nutrient? In what body tissues is it concentrated? What is the effect of too high an intake of this element, and at what level of fluorine in drinking water do such effects occur? What level of fluorine in water supplies is safe and yet provides protection against tooth decay? Why has fluoridation of public water supplies met opposition in some communities, and is such opposition warranted?

12. Name four trace elements, other than those mentioned in the preceding questions, that are accepted as essential nutrients for man. On what types of evidence is their acceptance as essential based? Can you name two enzymes which contain and presumably are activated by some of these elements? How many of the micronutrients listed in this chapter are beneficial and essential in small quantities but toxic at higher levels of intake? Why may it be unsafe to take tablets or capsules as vitamin-mineral supplements if the kinds and amounts of minerals they contain are not specified in exact terms? Why is it usually unnecessary to take such supplements, if one eats a normal mixed diet?

REFERENCES

1. Food and Nutrition Board: *Recommended Dietary Allowances.* 7th Ed., Publ. No. 1694. Washington, D.C., National Academy of Sciences, 1968.
2. Underwood, E. J.: *Trace Elements in Human and Animal Nutrition.* 3rd Ed. New York, Academic Press, 1971.
3. McCollum, E. V.: *A History of Nutrition.* Boston, Houghton Mifflin Co., 1957.
4. Boussingault, J. B.: Compt. Rend., *64*:1353, 1867.
5. McCance, R. A., and Widdowson, E. M.: Lancet, 2:680, 1937.
6. Hahn, P. F., Whipple, G. H., et al.: J. Exper. Med., *70*:443, 1939; Hahn, P. F., et al.: Amer. J. Physiol., *143*:191, 1945; Moore, C. V., Dubach, R., Minnich, V., and Roberts, H. K.: J. Clin. Invest., *23*:755, 1944.
7. Multani, J. S., Cepurneek, C. P., Davis, P. S., and Saltman, P.: Biochem., *9*:3970, 1970.
8. Holmberg, C. G., and Laurell, C. B.: Acta Chem. Scand., *1*:944, 1947; Bates, G. W.,

and Wernicke, J.: J. Biol. Chem., *246*: 3679, 1971.

9. Greenberg, G. R., and Wintrobe, M. M.: J. Biol. Chem., *165*:340, 1946.

10. Beaton, G. H., et al.: Amer. J. Clin. Nutr., *23*:275, 1970.

11. Leverton, R. M., et al.: J. Amer. Dietet. Assoc., *20*:747, 1944; *24*:480, 1948.

12. FAO/WHO: *Requirements of Ascorbic Acid, Vitamin B₁₂, Folate, and Iron.* WHO Technical Report Series No. 452. Geneva, WHO, 1970.

13. White, H. S.: J. Home Econ., *60*:724, 1968.

14. Pritchard, J. A., and Mason, R. A.: J. Amer. Med. Assoc., *190*:879, 1964.

15. Monsen, E. R., Kuhn, I. N., and Finch, C. A.: Amer. J. Clin. Nutr., *20*:842, 1967.

16. Davis, T. R. A., Gershoff, S. N., and Gamble, D. F.: J. Nutr. Educ., *1*(No. 2, Suppl. 1):40 1969; U.S. Department of Health, Education and Welfare: Ten-State Nutrition Survey in the United States, 1968–1970 – Preliminary Report to the Congress, April 1971; Kelsay, J. L.: J. Nutr., *99*(No. 1, Suppl. 1, Part II):123, 1969; Schaefer, A. E., and Johnson, O. C.: Nutr. Today, *4*:2, 1969.

17. Roe, D. A.: N.Y. State J. Med., *66*:1233, 1966; MacDonald, R. A.: Amer. J. Clin. Nutr., *23*:592, 1970.

18. Coindet, J. R.: Ann. de chim. et de phys., *15*:49, 1820.

19. Baumann, E.: Zeit. Physiol. Chem., *21*:319, 1895.

20. Hart, E. B., and Steenbock, H.: J. Biol. Chem., *33*:313, 1918.

21. Marine, D., and Kimball, O. P.: Arch. Int. Med., *25*:661, 1920; J. Amer. Med. Assoc., *77*:1068, 1921.

22. Buttfield, I. H., et al.: Lancet, *2*:767, 1965; Kevany, J., and associates: Amer. J. Pub. Health, *60*:919, 1970; Amer. J. Clin. Nutr., *22*:1597, 1969.

23. Hart, E. B., Steenbock, H., Waddell, J., and Elvehjem, C. A.: J. Biol. Chem., *77*:797, 1928.

24. Josephs, H. W.: Bull. Johns Hopkins Hosp., *49*:246, 1931 (also see Lewis, M. S.: J. Amer. Med. Assoc., *96*:1135, 1931: Usher, S. J., MacDermott, P. N., and Lozinski, E.: Amer. J. Dis. Child., *18*:642, 1935).

25. Sturgeon, P., and Brubaker, C.: Amer. J. Dis. Child., *92*:254, 1956; Cordano, A., Baertl, J. M., and Graham, G. G.: Pediatrics, *34*:324, 1964; Cordano, A., Placko, R. P., and Graham, G. G.: Blood, *28*:280, 1966; Cordano, A., and Graham, G. G.: Pediatrics, *38*:596, 1966; Graham, G. G., and Cordano, A.: Johns Hopkins Med. J., *124*:139, 1969; Holtzman, N. A., et al.: Johns Hopkins Med. J., *126*:34, 1970; Al-Rashid, R. A., and Spangler, J.: New Eng. J. Med., *285*:841, 1971.

26. Holmberg, C. G., and Laurell, C. B.: Acta Chem. Scand., *2*:550, 1948; Frieden, E.:

Nutr. Rev., *28*:87, 1970; Osaki, S., Johnson, D. A., and Frieden, E.: J. Biol. Chem., *246*:3018, 1971.

27. Sandstead, H. H., Burk, R. F., Booth, G. H., Jr., and Darby, W. J.: *Current concepts on trace minerals, clinical considerations.* Med. Clin. N. Amer., *54*:1509, 1970.

28. Lawler, M. R., and Jelenc, M. A.: J. Amer. Dietet. Assoc., *57*:420, 1970; Hook, L., and Brandt, I. K.: J. Amer. Dietet. Assoc., *49*:202, 1966.

29. Murthy, G. K., and Rhea, U. S.: J. Dairy Sci., *54*:1001, 1971 (milk and infant foods); Meranger, J. C.: Bull. Env. Cont. Tox., *5*:271, 1970 (fruit juices and carbonated beverages); Zook, E. G., and Lehmann, J.: J. Amer. Diet. Assoc., *52*:225, 1968 (fruits); Gormican, A.: J. Amer. Dietet. Assoc., *56*: 397, 1970.

30. Wilkins, R. H., and Brody, I. A.: Arch. Neurol., *25*:179, 1971 (which reprints the original paper by Wilson, S. A. K.: Brain, *34*:295, 1912).

31. Kemmerer, A. R., Elvehjem, C. A., and Hart, E. B.: J. Biol. Chem., *92*:623, 1931; Orent, E. R., and McCollum, E. V.: J. Biol. Chem, *92*:651, 1931 (also see McCarrison, R.: Indian J. Med. Res., *14*:641, 1927).

32. Hurley, L. S., and associates: J. Nutr., *74*: 274, 1961; J. Nutr., *79*:23, 1963; Plumlee, M. P., et al.: J. Animal Sci., *15*:352, 1956; Rojas, M. A., Dyer, I. A., and Cassatt, W. A.: J. Animal Sci., *24*:664, 1965; Shrader, R. E., and Everson, G. J.: J. Nutr., *94*:269, 1968.

33. Schroeder, H. A., Balassa, J. J., and Tipton, I. H.: J. Chron. Dis., *19*:545, 1966; Schlettwein-Gsell, D., and Mommsen-Straub, S.: Int. J. Vit. Nutr. Res., *41*:268, 1971.

34. Prasad, A. S., et al.: J. Lab. Clin. Med., *61*: 537, 1963; Prasad, A. S., et al.: Amer. J. Clin. Nutr., *12*:437, 1963; Sandstead, H. H., et al.: Amer. J. Clin. Nutr., *20*: 422, 1967; Prasad, A. S.: Amer. J. Clin. Nutr., *20*:648, 1967; Carter, J. P., et al.: Amer. J. Clin. Nutr., *22*:59, 1969.

35. Todd, W. R., Elvehjem, C. A., and Hart, E. B.: Amer. J. Physiol., *107*:146, 1934; Stirn, F. E., Elvehjem, C. A., and Hart, E. B.: J. Biol. Chem., *109*:347, 1935.

36. Millar, M. J., Fischer, M. I., Elcoate, P. V., and Mawson, C. A.: Canad. J. Biochem. Physiol., *36*:557, 1958; Hurley, L. S., and Swenerton, H.: Proc. Soc. Expt. Biol. Med., *123*:692, 1966; Swenerton, H., and Hurley, L. S.: J. Nutr., *95*:8, 1968; Agpar, J.: Amer. J. Physiol., *215*:160, 1968; J. Nutr., *100*:470, 1970.

37. Schlettwein-Gsell, D., and Mommsen-Straub, S.: Int. J. Vit. Res., *40*:659, 1970; Tusl, J.: J.A.O.A.C., *53*:1190, 1970. (Also see p. 434 of Prasad, A. S.: *Zinc Metabolism*, book listed under zinc supplementary reading.)

38. Smith, M. C., Lantz, E. M., and Smith, H. V.:

Univ. Ariz. Agric. Expt. Stat. Tech. Bull. 32, 1931; Churchill, H. W.: Ind. Eng. Chem., *23*:996, 1931.

39. Dean, H. T., et al.: Pub. Health Rep., *56*: 761, 1941.

40. McClure, F. J.: *Water Fluoridation.* Washington, D.C., Superintendent of Documents, 1970; McClure, F. J.: *Fluoride Drinking Waters.* Public Health Service Publication 825, Washington, D.C., Superintendent of Documents, 1962; various authors of papers published in J. Amer. Dent. Assoc., *80*:697–786, 1970; National Academy of Sciences–National Research Council Publication 294: *The Problem of Providing Optimum Fluoride Intake for Prevention of Dental Caries,* Washington, 1953; British Ministry of Health: *Report on the Five Year Fluoridation Studies in the United Kingdom,* July 3, 1962; Roy. Soc. Health J., *82*:173, 1962. (Also see suggested reading lists and Chap. 22 for other references on fluoridation.)

41. Bernstein, D. S., et al.: J. Amer. Med. Assoc., *198*:499, 1966; Cohn, S. H., Dombrowski, C. S., Hauser, W., and Atkins, H. L.: Amer. J. Clin. Nutr., *24*:20, 1971; Editorial: Brit. Med. J., *3*:660, 1970; Faccini, J. M.: Calc. Tiss. Res., *3*:1, 1969; Hegsted, D. M.: J. Amer. Dietet. Assoc., *50*:105, 1967; Iskrant, A. P.: Amer. J. Pub. Health, *58*:3, 1968.

42. Waldbott, G. L.: Amer. J. Clin. Nutr., *12*: 455, 1963; Sengupta, S. R., and Pal, B.: Ind. J. Nutr. Diet., *8*:66, 1971 (gives content of Indian foods); McClure, F. J.: *Fluorine in Foods: Survey of Recent Data.* Washington, D.C., Superintendent of Documents, 1949.

43. Roholm, K.: *Fluorine Intoxication, A Clinical Hygienic Study,* London, H. K. Lewis and Co. Ltd., 1937; Committee on Animal Nutrition: *The Fluorosis Problem in Livestock Production,* Washington, D.C., National Academy of Sciences–National Research Council, 1955.

44. Schlettwein-Gsell, D., and Mommsen-Straub, S.: Int. J. Vit. Res., *40*:673, 1970; Schroeder, H. A., Nason, A. P., and Tipton, I. H.: J. Chron. Dis., *20*:869, 1967.

45. Kesteloot, H., et al.: Circulation, *37*:854, 1968; Sullivan, J., Parker, M., and Carson, S. B.: J. Lab. Clin. Med., *71*:893, 1968.

46. Richert, D. A., and Westerfeld, W. W.: J. Biol. Chem., *203*:915, 1953; deRenzo, E. C., et al.: J. Amer. Chem. Soc., *75*:753, 1953.

47. Higgins, E. S., Richert, D. A., and Westerfeld, W. W.: J. Nutr., *59*:536, 1956; Reid, B. L., Kurnich, A. A., Svacha, R. L., and Couch, J. R.: Proc. Soc. Expt. Biol. Med., *93*:245, 1956; Leach, R. M., Jr., and Norris, L. C.: Poultry Sci., *36*:1136, 1957; Ellis, W. C., and Pfander, W. H.: J. Animal Sci., *19*: 1260, 1960.

48. Schroeder, H. A., Balassa, J. J., and Tipton, I. H.: J. Chronic Dis., *23*:481, 1970; Westerfeld, W. W., and Richert, D. A.: J. Nutr., *51*:85, 1953.

49. Schwarz, K., and Foltz, C. M.: J. Amer. Chem. Soc., *79*:3292, 1957; Schwarz, K., Bieri, J. G., Briggs, G. M., and Scott, M. L.: Proc. Soc. Expt. Biol. Med., *95*:621, 1957; Patterson, E. L., Milstrey, R., and Stokstad, E. L. R.: Proc. Soc. Expt. Biol. Med., *95*: 617, 1957.

50. Schroeder, H. A., Frost, D. V., and Balassa, J. J.: J. Chron. Dis., *23*:227, 1970.

51. Bull, R. C., and Oldfield, J. E.: J. Nutr., *91*: 237, 1967; McCoy, K. E. M., and Weswig, P. H.: J. Nutr., *98*:383, 1969; Thompson, J. N., and Scott, M. L.: J. Nutr., *97*:335, 1969; *100*:797, 1970; Hurt, H. D., Cary, E. E., and Visek, W. J.: J. Nutr., *101*:761, 1971.

52. deMondragon, M. C., and Jaffe, W. G.: Arch. Lat. Amer. Nutr., *21*:185, 1971; Morris, V. C., and Levander, O. A.: J. Nutr., *100*:1383, 1970.

53. Schwarz, K.: Lancet, *1*:1335, 1965; Majaj, A. S., and Hopkins, L. L., Jr.: Lancet, *2*:593, 1966; Burk, R. F., Pearson, W. N., Wood, R. P., and Viteri, F.: Amer. J. Clin. Nutr., *20*:723, 1967; Levine, R. J., and Olson, R. E.: Proc. Soc. Expt. Biol. Med., *134*:1030, 1970.

54. Schwarz, K., and Mertz, W.: Arch. Biochem. Biophys., *85*:292, 1959; Fed. Proc., *20*: 111, 1961; Mertz, W.: Fed. Proc., *26*:186, 1967; Physiol. Rev., *49*:163, 1969.

55. Hopkins, L. L., Jr., Ransome-Kuti, O., and Majaj, A. S.: Amer. J. Clin. Nutr., *21*:203, 1968; Gürson, C. T., and Saner, G.: Amer. J. Clin. Nutr., *24*:1313, 1971.

56. Schroeder, H. A., Nason, A. P., and Tipton, I. H.: J. Chronic Dis., *23*:123, 1970; Schroeder, H. A.: J. Nutr., *97*:237, 1969; Staub, H. W., Reussner, G., and Thiessen, R., Jr.: Science, *166*:746, 1969.

57. Schlettwein-Gsell, D., and Mommsen-Straub, S.: Int. J. Vit. Res., *41*:116, 1971.

58. Nomoto, S., McNeely, M. D., and Sunderman, F. W., Jr.: Biochem., *10*:1647, 1971.

59. Nielsen, F. H.: Fed. Proc., *29*:696, 1970 (abst.); Nielsen, F. H., in *Newer Trace Elements in Nutrition* (edited by Mertz, W., and Cornatzer, W. E.). New York, Marcel Dekker Inc., 1971.

60. Schwarz, K., Milne, D. B., and Vinyard, E.: Biochem. Biophys. Res. Comm., *40*:22, 1970; Schwarz, K., in *Newer Trace Elements in Nutrition* (edited by Mertz, W., and Cornatzer, W. E.), New York, Marcel Dekker Inc., 1971.

61. Calloway, D. H., and McMullen, J. J.: Amer. J. Clin. Nutr., *18*:1, 1966.

62. Schwarz, K., and Milne, D. B.: Science, *174*: 426, 1971.

63. Hopkins, L. L., Jr., and Mohr, H. E., in *Newer Trace Elements in Nutrition* (edited by Mertz, W., and Cornatzer, W. E.), New York, Marcel Dekker Inc., 1971; Fed. Proc., *30*: 462, 1971; Strasia, C. A., and Smith, W. H.: J. Anim. Sci., *31*:1027, 1970 (abst.).

SUPPLEMENTARY READING

Trace Elements — General

General, History, and Reviews

Bowen, H. J. M.: *Trace Elements in Biochemistry.* New York, Academic Press, 1966.

Hoekstra, W. G. (chmn.): Nutrition Society Symposium: Trace elements in the metabolism of connective tissue. Fed. Proc., *30*: 983, 1971.

Kay, H. D.: Micro-nutrient elements — a recapitulation. J. Food Technol., *2*:99, 1967.

Mertz, W., and Cornatzer, W. E. (eds.): *Newer Trace Elements in Nutrition.* New York, Marcel Dekker, Inc., 1971.

Sandstead, H. H., Burk, R. F., Booth, G. H., Jr., and Darby, W. J.: Current concepts on trace minerals — clinical considerations. Med. Clin. N. Amer., *54*:1509, 1970.

Sauchelli, V.: *Trace Elements in Agriculture.* New York, Van Nostrand Reinhold Co., 1969.

Underwood, E. J.: *Trace Elements in Human and Animal Nutrition.* 3rd Ed. New York, Academic Press, 1971.

Effect of Soil on Plant Composition

Anonymous: Soil fertility is important in nutrient content of foods. United Fresh Fruit Veg. Assoc. Supply Letter, p. 7, March 1967.

Barmes, D. E., Adkins, B. L., and Schamschula, R. G.: Etiology of caries in Papua, New Guinea: Associations in soil, food and water. Bull. World Health Org., *43*:769, 1970.

Crooke, W. M., and Knight, A. H.: Crop composition in relation to soil pH and root cation–exchange capacity. J. Sci. Food Agric., *22*: 235, 1971.

Hopkins, H. T., Stevenson, E. H., and Harris, P. L.: Soil factors and food composition. Amer. J. Clin. Nutr., *18*:390, 1966.

McClendon, J. F., and Gershon-Cohen, J.: Reduction of dental caries and goiter by crops fertilized with fluorine and iodine. Agric. Food Chem., *33*:72, 1955.

Price, N. O., and Moschler, W. W.: Residual lime effect in soils on certain mineral elements in barley, fescue, and oats. J. Agric. Food Chem., *18*:5, 1970.

Warren, H. V.: Medical geology and geography. Science, *148*:534, 1965.

Other References

Asling, C. W., and Hurley, L. S.: The influence of trace elements on the skeleton. Clin. Orthop., *27*:213, 1963.

Cohen, N. L., and Briggs, G. M.: Trace minerals in nutrition. Amer. J. Nurs., *68*:807, 1968.

Engel, R. W., Price, N. O., and Miller, R. F.: Copper, manganese, cobalt, and molybdenum balance in pre-adolescent girls. J. Nutr., *92*:197, 1967.

Gormican, A.: Inorganic elements in foods used in hospital menus. J. Amer. Dietet. Assoc., *56*:397, 1970.

Hammer, D. I., et al.: Hair trace metal levels and environmental exposure. Amer. J. Epidemiol., *93*:84, 1971.

Murphy, E. W., Page, L., and Watt, B. K.: Trace minerals in Type A school lunches. J. Amer. Dietet. Assoc., *58*:115, 1971.

Neri, L. C., Hewitt, D., and Mandel, J. S.: Risk of sudden death in soft water areas. Amer. J. Epidemiol., *94*:101, 1971.

Prasad, A. S., Oberleas, D., and Rajasekaran, G.: Essential micronutrient elements: Biochemistry and changes in liver disorders. Amer. J. Clin. Nutr., *23*:581, 1970.

Price, N. O., Bunce, G. E., and Engel, R. W.: Copper, manganese, and zinc balance in preadolescent girls. Amer. J. Clin. Nutr., *23*:258, 1970.

Ratcliff, J. D.: Do traces of metal decide our fate? Today's Health, *44*:34, 1966.

Schroeder, H. A.: Losses of vitamins and trace minerals resulting from processing and preservation of foods. Amer. J. Clin. Nutr., *24*:562, 1971; A sensible look at air pollution by metals. Arch Environ. Health, *21*: 798, 1970.

Schroeder, H. A., and Mitchener, M.: Scandium, chromium (VI), gallium, yttrium, rhodium, palladium, indium in mice: Effects on growth and life span. J. Nutr., *101*:1431, 1971.

Schroeder, H. A., Mitchener, M., and Nason, A. P.: Zirconium, niobium, antimony, vanadium and lead in rats: Life term studies. J. Nutr., *100*:59, 1970.

Schroeder, H. A., and Nason, A. P.: Trace-element analysis in clinical chemistry. Clin. Chem., *17*:461, 1971.

White, H. S., and Gynne, T. N.: Utilization of inorganic elements by young women eating iron fortified foods. J. Amer. Dietet. Assoc., *59*:27, 1971.

Zook, E. G., and Lehmann, J.: Total diet study: Content of ten minerals — aluminum, calcium, phosphorus, sodium, potassium, boron, copper, iron, manganese, and magnesium. J.A.O.A.C., *48*:850, 1965.

Nutrition Reviews

Inhalation and absorption of metals. *25*:159, 1967.

Present knowledge of iron and copper (by Peden, J. C., Jr.). *25*:321, 1967.

Interaction between copper and molybdenum. *26*:338, 1968.

Calcium-fluoride interactions in kittens. *27*:295, 1969.

Copper, molybdenum, sulfate: The nature of their interactions. *28*:82, 1970.

Ceruloplasmin, a link between copper and iron metabolism (by Frieden, E.). *28*:87, 1970.

Nutritional trace element research. *29*:90, 1971.

Metals as constituents of enzymes. *29*:97, 1971.

Iron
(also see references 1–17)

General, History, and Reviews

Blix, G. (ed.): *Symposia of the Swedish Nutrition Foundation VI. Occurrence, Causes and Prevention of Nutritional Anaemia.* Uppsala, Almqvist & Wiksells, 1968.

Bothwell, T. H., and Finch, C. A.: *Iron Metabolism.* Boston, Little, Brown & Co., 1962.

Elwood, P. C.: Utilization of food iron—an epidemiologist's view. Nutr. Dieta, *8*: 210, 1966.

Fairbanks, V. F., Fahey, J. L., and Beutler, E.: *Clinical Disorders of Iron Metabolism.* New York, Grune & Stratton, Inc., 1971.

Laurell, C.-B.: Plasma iron and the transport of iron in the organism. Pharmacol. Rev., *4*:371, 1952.

Ministry of Health: *Reports on Public Health and Medical Subjects No. 117. Iron in Flour.* London, Her Majesty's Stationery Office, 1968.

Moore, C. V.: The importance of nutritional factors in the pathogenesis of iron-deficiency anemia. Amer. J. Clin. Nutr., *3*:3, 1955.

Pla, G. W., and Fritz, J. C.: Availability of iron. J.A.O.A.C., *53*:791, 1970.

White, H. S.: Iron nutriture of girls and women—a review. J. Amer. Dietet. Assoc., *53*:563, 570, 1968.

Availability and Absorption

Apte, S. V., and Iyengar, L.: Absorption of dietary iron in pregnancy. Amer. J. Clin. Nutr., *23*:73, 1970.

Bing, F. C.: Assaying the availability of iron. J. Amer. Dietet. Assoc., *60*:114, 1972.

Crosby, W. H.: Intestinal response to the body's requirement for iron: Control of iron absorption. J. Amer. Med. Assoc., *208*:347, 1969.

Höglund, S., and Reizenstein, P.: Studies in iron absorption v. effect of gastrointestinal factors on iron absorption. Blood, *34*:496, 1969.

Kuhn, I. N., Monsen, E. R., Cook, J. D., and Finch, C. A.: Iron absorption in man. J. Lab. Clin. Med., *71*:715, 1968.

Lynch, S. R., et al.: Iron absorption in kwashiorkor. Amer. J. Clin. Nutr., *23*:792, 1970.

Mameesh, M. S., Aprahamian, S., Salji, J. P., and Cowan, J. W.: Availability of iron from labeled wheat, chickpea, broad bean, and okra in anemic blood donors. Amer. J. Clin. Nutr., *23*:1027, 1970.

Martinez-Torres, C., and Layrisse, M.: Effect of amino acids on iron absorption from a staple vegetable food. Blood, *35*:669, 1970; Iron absorption from veal muscle. Amer. J. Clin. Nutr., *24*:531, 1971.

Ranhotra, G. S., Hepburn, F. N., and Bradley, W. B.: Availability of iron in enriched bread. Cereal Chem., *48*:377, 1971.

Wheby, M. S., Suttle, G. E., and Ford, K. T. III: Intestinal absorption of hemoglobin iron. Gastroent., *58*:647, 1970.

Other References

Askoy, M.: Carbohydrate metabolism in severe and longstanding iron-deficiency anemia due to dietary and zinc deficiency. Amer. J. Clin. Nutr., *25*:262, 1972.

Beal, V. A., and Meyers, A. J.: Iron nutriture from infancy to adolescence. Amer. J. Pub. Health, *60*:666, 1970.

Bradfield, R. B., Jensen, M. V., Gonzales, L., and Garrayar, C.: Effect of low-level iron and vitamin supplementation on a tropical anemia. Amer. J. Clin. Nutr., *21*:57, 1968.

Burroughs, A. L., and Chan, J. J.: Iron content of some Mexican-American foods: Effect of cooking in iron, glass, or aluminum utensils. J. Amer. Dietet. Assoc., *60*:123, 1972.

Burroughs, A. L., and Huenemann, R. L.: Iron deficiency in rural infants and children. J. Amer. Dietet. Assoc., *57*:122, 1970.

Calloway, D. H., and McMullen, J. J.: Fecal excretion of iron and tin by men fed stored canned foods. Amer. J. Clin. Nutr., *18*:1, 1966.

Committee on Iron Deficiency: Iron deficiency in the United States. J. Amer. Med. Assoc., *203*:407, 1968.

Crichton, R. R.: Ferritin: Structure, synthesis and function. New Eng. J. Med., *284*:1413, 1971.

deCastro, F. J., and Miller, F. L.: Survey of differences in cost of diets of anemic and nonanemic children. Pub. Health Rep., *85*:1087, 1970.

Ericsson, P.: The effect of iron supplementation on the physical work capacity in the elderly. Acta Med. Scand., *188*:361, 1970.

Filer, L. J., Jr.: The USA today—is it free of public health nutrition problems? Anemia. Amer. J. Pub. Health, *59*:327, 1969.

Finch, C. A.: Iron metabolism. Nutr. Today, *4*:2, 1969.

Fox, H. M., et al.: Diets of preschool children in the North Central region. J. Amer. Dietet. Assoc., *59*:233, 1971.

Hegsted, D. M.: The recommended dietary allowances for iron. Amer. J. Pub. Health, *60*: 653, 1970.

Herbert, V. (ed.): Symposium: Iron deficiency and absorption. Amer. J. Clin. Nutr., *21*: 1138, 1968.

Hutcheson, R. H., Jr.: Iron deficiency anemia in Tennessee among rural poor children. Pub. Health Rep., *83*:939, 1968.

Lytton, D. G., Godbole, V. K., and Lovric, V. A.: Assessment of iron deficiency in children without anaemia. Pathology, *3*:87, 1971.

Pearson, H. A., McLean, F. W., and Brigety, R. E.: Anemia related to age: Study of a community of young black Americans. J. Amer. Med. Assoc., *215*:1982, 1971.

Scott, D. E., and Pritchard, J. A.: Iron deficiency in healthy young college women. J. Amer. Med. Assoc., *199*:147, 1967.

White, H. S.: Iron deficiency in young women. Amer. J. Pub. Health, *60*:659, 1970.

White, H. S., and Gynne, T. N.: Utilization of inorganic elements by young women eating iron-fortified foods. J. Amer. Dietet. Assoc., *59*:27, 1971.

Zee, P., Walters, T., and Mitchell, C.: Nutrition and poverty in preschool children: A nutritional survey of preschool children from impoverished black families, Memphis. J. Amer. Med. Assoc., *213*:739, 1970.

Nutrition Reviews

Iron deficiency and growth. *24*:330, 1966.

Symptoms of iron deficiency anemia. *25*:86, 1967.

Effect of phytate on iron absorption. *25*:218, 1967.

Iron deficiency anemia due to hookworm infection in man. *26*:47, 1968.

The prevalence of iron deficiency anemia. *26*:263, 1968.

Secondary effects of iron deficiency. *27*:41, 1969.

Fortification of bread with iron. *27*:138, 1969.

Iron deficiency and gastrointestinal lesions. *27*: 231, 1969.

Recommendation for increased iron levels in the American diet from the Food and Nutrition Board, NAS-NRC. *28*:108, 1970.

Anemia in children living in the tropics. *28*:289, 1970.

Absorption of dietary iron in man. *29*:113, 1971.

Availability of iron. *29*:234, 1971.

Anemia and iron intake. *29*:246, 1971.

Mobilization of liver iron by ferroxidase I (ceruloplasmin). *29*:250, 1971.

Available iron—*in vitro* or *in vivo*. *30*:62, 1972.

Iodine
(also see references 18–22)

General, History, and Reviews

Brush, B. E., and Altland, J. K.: Goiter prevention with iodized salt: Results of a thirty-year study. J. Clin. Endocrin. Metab., *12*:1380, 1952.

Follis, R. H.: Patterns of urinary iodine excretion in goitrous and nongoitrous areas. Amer. J. Clin. Nutr., *14*:253, 1964.

Kojima, N., and Brown, H. D.: The effects of iodized salt in processed fruits and vegetables. Food Tech., *9*:103, 1955.

Wayne, E. J., Koutras, D. A., and Alexander, W. D.: *Clinical Aspects of Iodine Metabolism.* Oxford, Blackwell, 1964.

Other References

Gillie, R. B.: Endemic goiter. Sci. Amer., *224*:93, 1971.

Gurevich, G. P.: Soil fertilization with coastal iodine sources as a prophylactic measure against endemic goiter. Fed. Proc., *23*: T511, 1964.

Koutras, D. A., Papapetrou, P. D., Yataganas, X., and Malamos, B.: Dietary sources of iodine in areas with and without iodine-deficiency goiter. Amer. J. Clin. Nutr., *23*:870, 1970.

Lowenstein, F. W.: Iodized salt in the prevention of endemic goiter: A world-wide survey of present programs. Amer. J. Pub. Health, *57*:1815, 1967.

Oddie, T. H., Fisher, D. A., McConahey, W. M., and Thompson, C. S.: Iodine intake in the United States: A reassessment. J. Clin. Endocrin., *30*:659, 1970.

Pharoah, P. O. D., Buttfield, I. H., and Hetzel, B. S.: Neurological damage to the fetus resulting from severe iodine deficiency during pregnancy. Lancet, *1*:308, 1971.

Staff Report: Iodized salt. Nutr. Today, *4*:22, 1969.

Thilly, C. H., Delange, F., and Ermans, A. M.: Further investigations of iodine deficiency in the etiology of endemic goiter. Amer. J. Clin. Nutr., *25*:30, 1972.

Wolff, J.: Iodide goiter and the pharmacologic effects of excess iodide. Amer. J. Med., *47*:101, 1969.

Nutrition Reviews

Goiter among Ceylonese and Nigerians. *26*:77, 1968.

Dietary iodine and goiter in Ceylon. *27*:108, 1969.

Iodine fortification and thyrotoxicosis. *28*:212, 1970.

Copper
(also see references 23–30)

General, History, and Reviews

Cartwright, G. E., and Wintrobe, M. M.: Copper metabolism in normal subjects. Amer. J. Clin. Nutr., *14*:224, 1964.

Elvehjem, C. A.: The biological significance of copper and its relation to iron metabolism. Physiol. Rev., *15*:471, 1935.

Leverton, R. M., and Binkley, E. S.: The copper metabolism and requirement of young women. J. Nutr., 27:43, 1944.

McElroy, W. D., and Glass, B. (eds.): *Copper Metabolism: A Symposium on Animal, Plant, and Soil Relationships.* Baltimore, The Johns Hopkins Press, 1950.

Peisach, J., Aisen, P., and Blumberg, W. E. (eds.): *The Biochemistry of Copper: Proceedings of the Symposium on Copper in Biological Systems.* New York, Academic Press, 1966.

Wintrobe, M. M., Cartwright, G. E., and Gubler, C. J.: Studies of the function and metabolism of copper. J. Nutr., 50:395, 1953.

Other References

Carlton, W. W., and Kelly, W. A.: Neural lesions in the offspring of female rats fed a copper-deficient diet. J. Nutr., 97:42, 1969.

Dowdy, R. P.: Copper metabolism. Amer. J. Clin. Nutr., 22:887, 1969.

Everson, G. J., Shrader, R. E., and Wang, T.: Chemical and morphological changes in the brains of copper-deficient guinea pigs. J. Nutr., 96:115, 1968.

Frieden, E.: The biochemistry of copper. Sci. Amer., 218:103, 1968.

Godette, L., and Warren, P. J.: The concentration of copper in the liver of African children with marasmus. Brit. J. Nutr., 21:419, 1967.

Gollan, J. L., Davis, P. S., and Deller, D. J.: Binding of copper by human alimentary secretions. Amer. J. Clin. Nutr., 24:1025, 1971.

Graham, G. G.: Human copper deficiency. New Eng. J. Med., 285:857, 1971.

Karpel, J., and Peden, V. H.: Copper deficiency in long-term parenteral nutrition. J. Pediat., 80:32, 1972.

Klevay, L. M.: Hair as a biopsy material. II. Assessment of copper nutriture. Amer. J. Clin. Nutr., 23:1194, 1970.

Walshe, J. M.: Copper: one man's meat is another man's poison. Proc. Nutr. Soc., 27:107, 1968.

Wolf, P., Enlander, D., Dalziel, J., and Swanson, J.: Green plasma in blood donors. New Eng. J. Med., 281:205, 1969.

Nutrition Reviews

Copper deficiency in malnourished infants. 23:164, 1965.

Copper toxicity. 24:305, 1966.

Cytochrome oxidase activity during treatment of copper deficiency. 26:246, 1968.

Copper deficiency in adult rats. 26:282, 1968.

A role of copper in elastin formation (by Hill, C. H.). 27:99, 1969.

Copper and the aorta. 27:325, 1969.

Adrenal control of copper mobilization and transport. 28:232, 1970.

Dietary copper and the melting point of pig adipose tissue. 28:244, 1970.

Plasma levels of apoceruloplasmin and holoceruloplasmin in copper-deficient and normocupremic rats. 28:291, 1970.

Manganese
(also see references 31–33)

General, History, and Reviews

Cotzias, G. C.: Manganese in health and disease. Physiol. Rev., 38:503, 1958.

Schroeder, H. A., Balassa, J. J., and Tipton, I. H.: Essential trace metals in man: Manganese. A study in homeostasis. J. Chron. Dis., 19:545, 1966.

Other References

Everson, G. J., and Shrader, R. E.: Abnormal glucose tolerance in manganese-deficient guinea pigs. J. Nutr., 94:89, 1968.

Lang, V. M., North, B. B., and Morse, L. M.: Manganese metabolism in college men consuming vegetarian diets. J. Nutr., 85:132, 1965.

McLeod, B. E., and Robinson, M. F.: Metabolic balance of manganese in young women; Dietary intake of manganese by New Zealand infants during the first six months of life. Brit. J. Nutr., 27:221, 229, 1972.

North, B. B., Leichsenring, J. M., and Norris, L. M.: Manganese metabolism in college women. J. Nutr., 72:217, 1960.

Tsai, H. C., and Everson, G. J.: Effect of manganese deficiency on the acid mucopolysaccharides in cartilage of guinea pigs. J. Nutr., 91:447, 1967.

Shrader, R. E., and Everson, G. J.: Pancreatic pathology in manganese-deficient guinea pigs. J. Nutr., 94:269, 1968.

Nutrition Reviews

Manganese balance in children. 23:236, 1965.
Manganese and glucose tolerance. 26:207, 1968.

Zinc
(also see references 34–47)

General, History, and Reviews

Luecke, R. W.: The significance of zinc in nutrition. Borden's Review of Nutrition Research, 26:45, 1965.

Miller, W. J.: Zinc nutrition of cattle: a review. J. Dairy Sci., 53:1123, 1970.

Prasad, A. S. (ed.): *Zinc Metabolism.* Springfield, Ill., Charles C Thomas, 1966.

Prasad, A. S. (ed.): Twelve papers on zinc metabolism, in Sept. and Oct. issues of Amer. J. Clin. Nutr., *22*:1215–1339, 1969.

Stern, A., Nalder, M., and Macy, I. G.: Zinc retention in childhood. J. Nutr., *21*:Suppl. 8, 1941.

Other References

Bradfield, R. B., Yee, T., and Baertl, J. M.: Hair zinc levels of Andean Indian children during protein-calorie malnutrition. Amer. J. Clin. Nutr., *22*:1349, 1969.

Caggiano, V., et al.: Zinc deficiency in a patient with retarded growth, hypogonadism, hypogammaglobulinemia and chronic infection. Amer. J. Med Sci., *257*:305, 1969.

Coble, Y. D., et al.: Zinc levels and blood enzymes in Egyptian male subjects with retarded growth and sexual development. Amer. J. Clin. Nutr., *19*:415, 1966.

Halsted, J. A., and Smith, J. C., Jr.: Plasma-zinc in health and disease. Lancet, *1*:322, 1970.

Lindeman, R. D., Bottomley, R. G., Cornelison, R. L., Jr., and Jacobs, L. A.: Influence of acute tissue injury on zinc metabolism in man. J. Lab. Clin. Med., *79*:452, 1972.

McBean, L. D., Dove, J. T., Halsted, J. A., and Smith, J. C., Jr.: Zinc concentration in human tissues. Amer. J. Clin. Nutr., *25*:672, 1972.

O'Dell, B. L., Burpo, C. E., and Savage, J. E.: Evaluation of zinc availability in foodstuffs of plant and animal origin. J. Nutr., *102*:653, 1972.

Sandstead, H. H.: Zinc: A metal to grow on. Nutr. Today, *3*:12, March 1968.

Sandstead, H. H., Lanier, V. C., Jr., Shephard, G. H., and Gillespie, D. D.: Zinc and wound healing: Effects of zinc deficiency and zinc supplementation. Amer. J. Clin. Nutr., *23*:514, 1970.

Sarram, M., et al.: Zinc nutrition in human pregnancy in Fars Province, Iran: Significance of geographic and socioeconomic factors. Amer. J. Clin. Nutr., *22*:726, 1969.

Sullivan, J. F., and Heaney, R. P.: Zinc metabolism in alcoholic liver disease. Amer. J. Clin. Nutr., *23*:170, 1970.

Nutrition Reviews

Zinc deficiency and congenital malformations in the rat. *25*:157, 1967.

Zinc, calcium, and phytate. *25*:215, 1967.

Zinc deficiency in ruminants. *26*:351, 1968.

Zinc and reproduction. *27*:16, 1969.

Zinc in relation to DNA and RNA synthesis in regenerating rat liver. *27*:211, 1969.

Zinc in hair as a measure of zinc nutriture in human beings. *28*:209, 1970.

Zinc homeostasis during pregnancy. *29*:253, 1971.

Fluorine
(also see references 38–43)

General, History, and Reviews

Doberenz, A. R., et al.: Effect of a minimal fluoride diet on rats. Proc. Soc. Expt. Biol. Med., *117*:689, 1964.

Ericsson, Y. (ed.): *Fluorides and Human Health.* WHO Monograph Series No. 59. Geneva, WHO, 1970.

Hodge, H. C., and Smith, F. A.: Fluorides and man. Ann. Rev. Pharmacol., *8*:395, 1968.

McClure, F. J.: A review of fluorine and its physiological effects. Physiol. Rev., *13*:277, 1933; *Water Fluoridation: The Search and the Victory.* Washington, D.C., Superintendent of Documents, 1970.

McClure, F. J. (ed.): *Fluoride in Drinking Waters.* Public Health Service Publication 825. Washington, D.C., Superintendent of Documents, 1962.

Simons, J. H. (ed.): *Fluorine Chemistry. IV. Biological Properties of Inorganic Fluorides and Effects of Fluorides on Bones and Teeth.* New York, Academic Press, 1965.

Sognnaes, R. F.: Fluoride protection of bones and teeth. Science, *150*:989, 1965.

Other References
(also see fluoridation references, Chap. 22)

Cohn, S. H., Dombroski, C. S., Hauser, W., and Atkins, H. L.: Effects of fluoride on calcium metabolism in osteoporosis. Amer. J. Clin. Nutr., *24*:20, 1971.

Committee on Nutrition: Fluoride as a nutrient. Pediatrics, *49*:456, 1972.

Englander, H. R., et al.: Incremental rates of dental caries after repeated topical sodium fluoride applications in children with lifelong consumption of fluoridated water. J. Amer. Dent. Assoc., *82*:354, 1971.

Ericsson, Y., and Ribelius, U.: Increased fluoride ingestion by bottle-fed infants and its effect. Acta Paediat. Scand., *59*:424, 1970.

Ferguson, D. B.: Effects of low doses of fluoride on serum proteins and a serum enzyme in man. Nature New Biol., *231*:159, 1971.

Henrikson, P., et al.: Fluoride and nutritional osteoporosis: Physicochemical data on bones from an experimental study in dogs. J. Nutr., *100*:631, 1970.

Knutson, J. W.: Water fluoridation after 25 years. J. Amer. Dent. Assoc., *80*:765, 1970.

Nutrition Reviews

Carbohydrate metabolism of rats consuming 450 ppm of fluoride. *24*:346, 1966.

Fluoride, bony structure, and aortic calcification. *25*:100, 1967.

Survey diagnosis of skeletal fluorosis. *25*:136, 1967.

Prenatal exposure to fluoride. *25*:330, 1967.

Fluoride concentration in enamel and bone. *26*: 75, 1968.

Physiological distribution of fluoride. *26*:103, 1968.

Cobalt
(also see references 44–45)

Ammerman, C. B.: Symposium: Trace minerals. Recent developments in cobalt and copper in ruminant nutrition: A review. J. Dairy Sci., *53*:1097, 1970.

Latt, S. A., and Vallee, B. L.: Spectral properties of cobalt carboxypeptidase. The effects of substrates and inhibitors. Biochem., *10*: 4263, 1971.

Northrop, D. B., and Wood, H. G.: Transcarboxylase. V. The presence of bound zinc and cobalt. J. Biol. Chem., *244*:5801, 1969.

Scriver, C. R.: Vitamin B_{12} dependency and cobalt-dependent metabolism. Pediatrics, *46*:493, 1970.

Smith, S. E., and Loosli, J. K.: Cobalt and vitamin B_{12} in ruminant nutrition: A review. J. Dairy Sci., *40*:1215, 1957.

Nutrition Reviews

Epidemic cardiac failure in beer drinkers. *26*: 173, 1968.

Synergism of cobalt and ethanol. *29*:43, 1971.

Molybdenum
(also see references 46–48)

Cohen, H. J., Fridovich, I., and Rajagopalan, K. V.: Hepatic sulfite oxidase. A functional role for molybdenum. J. Biol. Chem., *246*:374, 1971.

Dowdy, R. P., and Matrone, G.: Copper-molybdenum interaction in sheep and chicks. J. Nutr., *95*:191, 1968.

Mills, C. F., and Mitchell, R. L.: Copper and molybdenum in subcellular fractions of rat liver. Brit. J. Nutr., *26*:117, 1971.

Schroeder, H. A., Balassa, J. J., and Tipton, I. H.: Essential trace metals in man: Molybdenum. J. Chron. Dis., *23*:481, 1970.

Nutrition Reviews

Metals as constituents of enzymes. *29*:97, 1971.

Selenium
(also see references 49–53)

General, History, and Reviews

Muth, O. H. (ed.): *Symposium: Selenium in Biomedicine.* Westport, Conn., Avi Publishing Co., 1967.

Rosenfeld, I., and Beath, O. A.: *Selenium: Geobotany, Biochemistry, Toxicity, and Nutrition.* New York, Academic Press, 1964.

Smith, M. I., and Westfall, B. B.: Further field studies on the selenium problem in relation to public health. Pub. Health Rep., *52*: 1375, 1937.

Subcommittee on Selenium, Committee on Animal Nutrition: *Selenium in Nutrition.* Washington, D. C., National Academy of Sciences–National Research Council, 1971.

Other References

Ganther, H. E., et al.: Selenium: Relation to decreased toxicity of methylmercury added to diets containing tuna. Science, *175*: 1122, 1972.

Hurt, H. D., Cary, E. E., and Visek, W. J.: Growth, reproduction, and tissue concentrations of selenium in the selenium-depleted rat. J. Nutr., *101*:761, 1971.

Krehl, W. A.: Selenium: The maddening mineral. Nutr. Today, 5:26, Winter 1970.

Schroeder, H. A., Frost, D. V., and Balassa, J. J.: Essential trace metals in man: Selenium. J. Chron. Dis., *23*:227, 1970.

Nutrition Reviews

Selenium (letter to the editor by Draper, H. H.). *25*:127, 1967.

Selenium and cancer. *28*:75, 1970.

Chromium
(also see references 54–57)

Hambridge, K. M., and others: Three papers on hair chromium concentration. Amer. J. Clin. Nutr., *25*:376, 1972.

Levine, R. A., Streeten, D. H. P., and Doisy, R. J.: Effects of oral chromium supplementation on the glucose tolerance of elderly human subjects. Metabolism, *17*:114, 1968.

Mayer, J.: Chromium in medicine. Postgrad. Med., *49*:235, 1971.

Mertz, W.: Chromium occurrence and function in biological systems. Physiol. Rev., *49*: 163, 1969.

Morgan, J. M.: Hepatic chromium content in diabetic subjects. Metab., *21*:313, 1972.

Schroeder, H. A.: The role of chromium in mammalian nutrition. Amer. J. Clin. Nutr., *21*:230, 1968.

Nutrition Reviews

Trivalent chromium in human nutrition. *25*:49, 1967.

Intestinal absorption of chromium. *25*:76, 1967.

Idiopathic hemochromatosis: A specific disorder. *25*:318, 1967.

Dietary chromium and eye lesions. *26*:223, 1968.

Chromium and carbohydrate metabolism in infantile malnutrition. *26*:235, 1968.

Chromium and glucose tolerance. *26*:281, 1968.

Sugar, chromium, and serum cholesterol. *27*: 185, 1969.

Nickel

Anonymous: Studies show nickel could play major metabolic role. J. Amer. Med. Assoc., *214*:675, 1970.
Schroeder, H. A., Balassa, J. J., and Tipton, I. H.: Abnormal trace metals in man: Nickel. J. Chron. Dis., *15*:51, 1962.
Sunderman, F. W., Jr., et al.: Nickel deprivation in chicks. J. Nutr., *102*:259, 1972.

Tin

Benoy, G. J., Hooper, P. A., and Schneider, R.: The toxicity of tin in canned fruit juices and solid foods. Food Cosmet. Toxicol., *9*:645, 1971.
Farrow, R. P.: Research program on can detinning in canned food storage. Food Technol., *24*:44, 1969.
Schroeder, H. A., Kanisawa, M., Frost, D. V., and Mitchener, M.: Germanium, tin and arsenic in rats: Effects on growth, survival, pathological lesions and life span. J. Nutr., *96*:37, 1968.

Vanadium

Hopkins, L. L., Jr., and Tilton, B. E.: Metabolism of trace amounts of vanadium 48 in rat organs and liver subcellular particles. Amer. J. Physiol., *211*:169, 1966.
Schroeder, H. A., Balassa, J. J., and Tipton, I. H.: Abnormal trace metals in man—vanadium. J. Chron. Dis., *16*:1047, 1963.
Söremark, R.: Vanadium in some biological specimens. J. Nutr., *92*:183, 1967.
Voors, A. W.: Minerals in the municipal water and atherosclerotic heart death. Amer. J. Epidemiol., *93*:259, 1971.

Silicon

Archibald, J. G., and Fenner, H.: Silicon in cow's milk. J. Dairy Sci., *40*:703, 1957.
Carlisle, E. M.: Silicon: A possible factor in bone calcification. Science, *167*:279, 1970.
Lewin, J., and Reimann, B. E. F.: Silicon and plant growth. Ann. Rev. Plant Physiol., *20*: 289, 1969.

Nonessential Trace Elements

General, History, and Reviews

Flick, D. F., Kraybill, H. F., and Dimitroff, J. M.: Toxic effects of cadmium: A review. Environ. Res., *4*:71, 1971.

Friberg, L. T., Piscator, M., and Nordberg, G. F.: *Cadmium in the Environment.* Cleveland, Chemical Rubber Co., 1971.
Frost, D. V.: Arsenicals in biology—retrospect and prospect. Fed. Proc., *26*:194, 1967.
Lenihan, J. M. A., Loutit, J. F., and Martin, J. H. (eds.): *Strontium Metabolism.* New York, Academic Press, 1967.

Lead and Mercury

Chatterjee, P., and Gettman, J. H.: Lead poisoning: Subculture as a facilitating agent? Amer. J. Clin. Nutr., *25*:324, 1972.
Chisolm, J. J., Jr.: Lead poisoning. Sci. Amer., *224*:15, 1971.
Clarkson, T. W.: Epidemiological and experimental aspects of lead and mercury contamination of food. Food Cosmet. Toxicol., *9*:229, 1971.
D'Intri, F. M.: *The Environmental Mercury Problem.* Cleveland, Chemical Rubber Co., 1972.
Eyl, T. B.: Organic-mercury food poisoning. New Eng. J. Med., *284*:706, 1971.
Finkel, A. J.: Mercury residue blood levels and tolerance limits in fish eaters. J. Amer. Med. Assoc., *216*:1208, 1971.
Friberg, L. T.: *Mercury in the Environment.* Cleveland, Chemical Rubber Co., 1972.
Goyer, R. A.: Lead toxicity: A problem in environmental pathology. Amer. J. Pathol., *64*:167, 1971.
Hammond, A. L.: Mercury in the environment: Natural and human factors. Science, *171*: 788, 1971.
King, B. G.: Maximum daily intake of lead without excessive body lead-burden in children. Amer. J. Dis. Child., *122*:337, 1971.
Klein, M., Namer, R., Harpur, E., and Corbin, R.: Earthenware containers as a source of fatal lead poisoning. Case study and public health considerations. New Eng. J. Med., *283*:669, 1970.
Nelson, N. (chmn.): Hazards of mercury. Environ. Res., *4*:1, 1971.
Symposium: Lead poisoning. Amer. J. Med., *52*:283, 1972.
U.S. Public Health Service: Medical aspects of childhood lead poisoning. Pediatrics, *48*: 464, 1971 (also in HSMHA Health Rep., *86*:140, 1971).

Pica

Bruhn, C. M., and Pangborn, R. M.: Reported incidence of pica among migrant families. J. Amer. Dietet. Assoc., *58*:417, 1971.
Halsted, J. A.: Geophagia in man: Its nature and nutritional effects. Amer. J. Clin. Nutr., *21*:1384, 1968.
Neumann, H. H.: Pica—symptom or vestigial instinct? Pediatrics, *46*:441, 1970.
Roselle, H. A.: Association of laundry starch and clay ingestion with anemia in New York City. Arch. Int. Med., *125*:57, 1970.

Other References

Crampton, R. F., Elias, P. S., and Gangolli, S. D.: The bromine content of human tissue. Brit. J. Nutr., *25*:317, 1971.

Omdahl, J. L., and DeLuca, H. F.: Strontium induced rickets: Metabolic basis. Science, *174*:949, 1971.

Parsons, V., et al.: Aluminum in bone from patients with renal failure. Brit. Med. J., *4*:273, 1971.

Schroeder, H. A.: Cadmium as a factor in hypertension. J. Chron. Dis., *18*:647, 1965.

Schroeder, H. A., and Balassa, J. J.: Abnormal trace metals in man: Niobium. J. Chron. Dis., *18*:229, 1965; Arsenic. J. Chron. Dis., *19*:85, 1966; Germanium. J. Chron. Dis., *20*:211, 1967.

Schroeder, H. A., and Mitchener, M.: Toxic effects of trace elements on the reproduction of mice and rats. Arch Environ. Health, *23*:102, 1971.

Thompson, J. C., Jr., Alexander, R. R., and Comar, C. L.: Dietary ^{90}Sr reductions through food substitutions in the fruit and vegetable category. J. Nutr., *91*:375, 1967.

Voors, A. W.: Lithium in the drinking water and atherosclerotic heart death: Epidemiologic argument for protective effect. Amer. J. Epidemiol., *92*:164, 1970.

Woody, J. N., London, W. L., and Wilbanks, G. D., Jr.: Lithium toxicity in a newborn. Pediatrics, *47*:94, 1971.

Nutrition Reviews

Cadmium and cardiovascular disease. *25*:134, 1967.

Pagophagia and iron lack. *27*:244, 1969.

Pica and lead poisoning. *29*:267, 1971.

Hazards from lead. *30*:82, 1972.

Part Two

Food
Intake
and
Utilization

thirteen

Digestion and Absorption of Food

DIGESTION

Why Digestion Is Necessary

Digestion, which takes place in a series of organs known collectively as the alimentary tract, is the **process by which food is prepared for absorption** into the body proper. As eaten, most of the food materials are in the form of complex substances, which are either insoluble in water or of such a nature that they cannot diffuse through the membranes that line the digestive organs and cannot be absorbed into the blood.

Moreover, even if the material could get through the intestinal lining and into the blood stream, the **tissues could make no use of most of these complex substances,** for the cells are so constituted that they use in their life processes only simple substances.* Starch and the more complex sugars are all

---

*Tissues can use fat if it is injected into the blood stream, but food fat cannot cross the intestinal barrier without first being broken down into simpler substances.

compounds made by linking together simple sugars (p. 53); proteins are complex substances formed by linking together amino acids (p. 74); fats are made by the combination of fatty acids with the simple substance glycerol (p. 62). The process of digestion is chiefly concerned with breaking down these three classes of foodstuffs into simple *sugars, amino acids, fatty acids,* and *glycerol,* which are the forms in which **food materials** are **usable by the tissues,** either as energy or for tissue building.

The Alimentary Tract

The alimentary tract is best understood if it is considered as organized for its two sets of functions: namely, its **muscular** or motor apparatus, and its **secretory** apparatus. The first has the task of mixing the food mass with digestive juices and moving along partially digested material from one part of the alimentary tract to another. The second has the function of secreting the important digestive fluids which are responsible for bringing about the

307

chemical breakdown of foodstuffs. The arrangement of the various organs in series (mouth, esophagus, stomach, small intestine, large intestine) is familiar to almost everyone. This arrangement of the digestive organs forms a continuous hollow tube (sometimes called the alimentary canal), with widenings in certain sections (stomach, large intestine) which act as reservoirs where the contents may be held for longer periods. A diagram of the alimentary tract and glands which secrete digestive fluids into it is given in Figure 13–1. The digestive tract operates, somewhat like a railway system, by means of signals sent on ahead from one organ to the next in the series.

Motor Processes in Digestion

The **muscular apparatus** concerned in digestion may be briefly described as follows. First there are the muscles of the jaws and tongue which function in chewing and swallowing. More important are the muscular coats of the stomach and intestines by which the movements of these organs are carried out. The structure of the walls of the alimentary canal is essentially similar throughout its whole length—a so-called *mucous membrane* lining the cavity, two coats of *muscular tissue*, one consisting of *circular* and one of *longitudinal* muscle fibers, and a very thin membrane covering the outside of the tract.

The cells of the mucous membrane that lines the digestive tract are constantly renewed, much in the same way as are skin and hair. However, the turnover time of the lining of the small intestine is only about one and a half days, which means that this is one of the most rapidly growing tissues of the body. The aged cells are discharged into the digestive tract. These cells (as well as the digestive secretions) are largely recovered in the processes of digestion and absorption, and their constituents

are used again by the body just as are nutrients from the diet.

When the circular muscle fibers contract, as they do in small, separate segments, they exert a squeezing motion which presses the contents of the tube closely against its inner wall, churns them about and divides them into separate segments. When the longitudinal muscle fibers contract, the resulting motion pushes the food mass along the digestive tract. These contractions occur in regular waves that pass along the tract almost always in such a way as to propel the food ahead—that is, toward the rectum and its outlet, the anus. Such rhythmic, recurring waves of contraction are spoken of as **peristalsis**. In a few parts of the alimentary canal these waves of contraction in the muscle coat may travel in the opposite direction, thereby pushing the food backward in the tube. In this case the term *antiperistalsis* is applied to these waves of contraction. Emotional or digestive upsets may sometimes bring about antiperistaltic waves, resulting in *vomiting*.

The stomach has a slightly more complex system of muscular coats, in which there are diagonal as well as circular and longitudinal fibers, so that its movements are more varied though similar in general to the movements of the intestines. Active peristaltic waves begin about the middle of the stomach and travel downward. The esophagus and upper part of the stomach have less marked muscular coats and are relatively inactive muscularly.

Progress of Food Material Through Digestive Organs

In the **mouth,** food is more or less finely divided by *chewing* and is mixed with saliva, which moistens the food and also exerts a chemical action, and with mucus that assists in lubricating the food for swallowing. The swallowed food mass is carried down the esophagus by a muscular movement, a wave

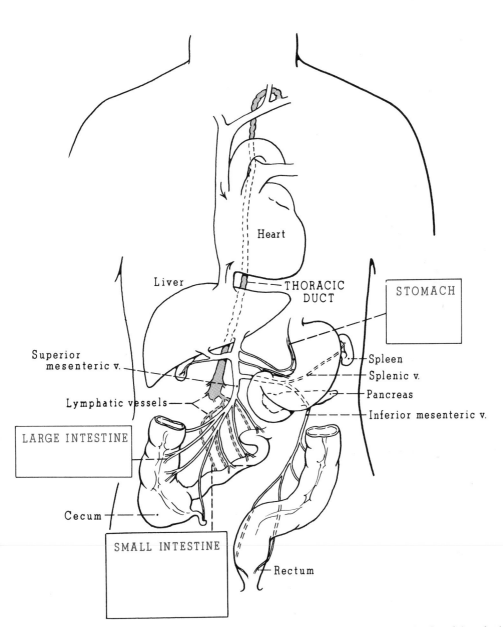

Figure 13–1. Schematic drawing of the gastrointestinal tract and the major blood and lymphatic vessels through which digested food materials are transported. (From Jacob, S. W., and Francone, C. A.: *Structure and Function in Man.* Philadelphia, W. B. Saunders Co., 1965, p. 397.)

of relaxation preceding the food and a wave of contraction following it.

In the **stomach,** swallowed food collects largely in the muscularly inactive upper part (cardiac end), which acts as a reservoir where food may remain for some time before it is gradually pushed along toward the outlet end (pyloric portion). The portion of the stomach adjoining the pylorus (a circular muscle that guards the opening into the intestine) is muscularly active, and in its wall are situated the glands that secrete the digestive fluid gastric juice. Here the food mass is mixed with gastric juice and churned about until, partly by mechanical means and partly by action of the digestive fluid, it is reduced to a semiliquid state (chyme). From time to time, the pylorus opens and a peristaltic wave sends a gush of the more fluid portion of the stomach contents into the first part of the intestine (duodenum); thus the stomach is gradually emptied. As it empties, the stomach contracts upon itself, so that it is relatively small and usually contains only a little fluid between meals. The rate at which the stomach empties is chiefly dependent on the type of foods that comprise the meal. Liquids leave the stomach relatively quickly; concentrated foods are retained longer. In general, carbohydrate-rich foods tend to pass out faster than foods high in protein, and these faster than fatty foods, while mixtures of proteins and fats leave the stomach more slowly than either alone. The healthy stomach usually empties in 1½ to 6 hours, depending on the quantity and nature of the meal taken. The average time for the stomach to discharge an ordinary meal is about 3 hours.

If the stomach is empty for a long period, strong rhythmic contractions occur, *hunger contractions.* The inclusion of some fat or fat and protein in a meal is useful to prevent hunger contractions before the next mealtime.

Food material which has been passed on from the stomach into the **duodenum** is well mixed with the digestive juices poured in at that point. It is then gradually pushed along into lower portions of the intestine by peristaltic contractions and by further discharges from the stomach. The largest part of the processes of digestion and absorption takes place in the small intestine. These processes are aided by contractions of the intestinal muscles — those of the circular muscle fibers, which divide intestinal segments, thus mixing the contents thoroughly and squeezing them against the intestinal walls; and those of the longitudinal fibers, whose peristaltic movements gradually pass the intestinal contents along toward the opening (ileocecal valve) into the large intestine. By the time the outlet to the large intestine is reached, food material is nearly completely *digested and absorbed.* The length of time required for food material to pass along the small intestine varies with the relative muscular activity of that organ in various persons. Irritating or toxic substances within the intestine, as well as some cathartics, stimulate peristalsis and are the usual cause of diarrhea, a condition in which food residues pass through the intestines so quickly as to be excreted in fluid condition.

The **large intestine** has about twice the diameter of the small intestine but is much shorter and less muscularly active. It acts as a reservoir in which food residues stay for some time and are concentrated by absorption of the large volume of water added in the digestive process. Propulsive motion moves the progressively drier mass into the descending colon and rectum. These propulsive waves are strongest after eating and are enhanced by physical activity. Final evacuation through the anus, an opening guarded by a double ring of circular muscle fibers is voluntarily controlled in healthy older children and adults and housebroken animals. Food residues and excretory material often remain in the colon 18 hours or more, and conditions for bacteria to grow are more favorable here than in any other part of the alimentary tract. Some of these bacteria are beneficial, such as those that manufacture vitamins; others form products that may be absorbed and must be detoxified elsewhere in the body.

Chemical Processes in Digestion

The chemical processes by which foodstuffs are broken down in preparation for absorption and use by the tissues constitute digestion in the narrower, correct use of the term.

In digestion, complex food materials are cleaved into simpler component parts. In the case of very complex substances like proteins and starch, this chemical breakdown takes place gradually, so that a good many intermediate compounds are formed in the process of digestion before the original material is reduced to its simplest components. The long chains of glucose radicals which constitute starch molecules are gradually broken down by splitting off two sugar groups at a time (maltose molecules), the intermediate compounds being dextrins with smaller-sized molecules. Eventually the dextrins are completely converted to maltose and the maltose is broken down into the simple sugar, glucose (Fig. 13–2). The very large molecules of proteins are likewise broken down in orderly fashion into those of gradually decreasing size (proteoses, peptones, polypeptides, tripeptides, dipeptides) until they are completely reduced to those amino acids from which they were originally built (as shown diagrammatically in Fig. 13–3).

Fats, although they have molecules much smaller and simpler than those of starch and protein and are acted upon by only one enzyme, are also broken down in a series of steps. The fatty acids are digested off one at a time, forming di- and monoglycerides, a good portion of which are absorbed

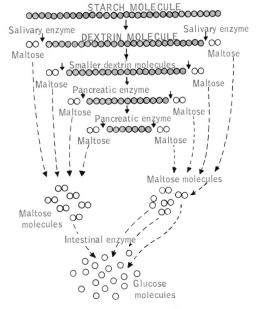

Figure 13–2. Gradual breaking down of large starch molecules by enzymes in digestion. The disaccharide maltose is split off by enzymes in the saliva and pancreatic juice, with smaller and smaller dextrin molecules formed as intermediate products, until the starch has been completely reduced to maltose. An intestinal enzyme then acts on the maltose molecules, splitting them into molecules of the monosaccharide, or simple sugar, glucose.

in this form. The remainder (usually representing 40 to 50 percent of the fat) is completely broken down into fatty acids and glycerol.

The disaccharides (sucrose, lactose, and maltose) are broken up at a single step into their components—the simple sugars (glucose, fructose, and galactose). The simplest constituents of the diet do not need to be broken down by digestion. This is true of simple sugars, alcohol, and water, which are absorbed in the form in which they are consumed.

The gradual chemical breakdown of proteins and of starch through various intermediate stages until they are finally reduced to their simplest units, and the simpler cleavage of fats and double sugars into their components during digestion, are summarized in word form on the bottom of page 312. The arrow

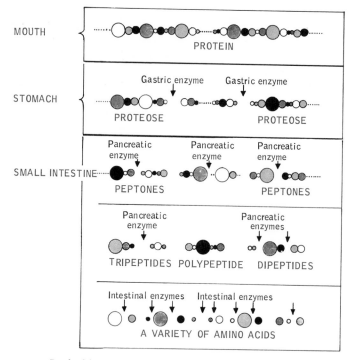

Figure 13–3. Gradual breaking down of the large molecules of protein into their constituent amino acids during digestion, with proteoses, peptones, and peptides as intermediate products. The molecules of protein, proteose, and peptones are too large to be portrayed in this diagram by more than small segments (as indicated by the dotted lines), but those of the smaller peptides (di- and tripeptides) are given in entirety. When digestion is complete, each huge protein molecule is completely broken down into the different amino acids of which it was composed.

in each instance represents the splitting of a larger molecule into a number of smaller ones by means of a chemical reaction with water—a process known as *hydrolysis*.

Digestive Enzymes

These chemical cleavages which constitute digestion are brought about through the agency of substances called **enzymes.** The same chemical changes take place if proteins, starch, fats, or disaccharides are subjected to prolonged heating with water and acid or alkali in the laboratory. The acid or alkali acts as a catalyst—that is, an agent that speeds up the chemical change merely by its presence. In the body, digestive enzymes bring about these chemical changes more rapidly and at

Proteins → proteoses → peptones → peptides → amino acids
Starch → dextrins → maltose → glucose
Fats → di- and monoglycerides, fatty acids, and glycerol
Maltose (malt sugar) → glucose and glucose ⎫
Sucrose (cane sugar) → glucose and fructose ⎬ simple sugars
Lactose (milk sugar) → glucose and galactose ⎭

lower temperatures than the catalysts mentioned above. They do not themselves take part in the chemical processes by which foodstuffs are broken down but their presence facilitates these processes. Enzymes are catalysts that are formed by living cells* and the digestive enzymes are formed by the secreting cells of the digestive tract.

Enzymes are typical **proteins**, although of relatively small molecular size. They are formed in the body from the amino acids brought to cells by the blood. Their enzymatic activity is lost if they are exposed to any chemical that renders protein insoluble, or to a degree of heat sufficient to coagulate protein. All enzymes are sensitive to heat and cold; they are destroyed by boiling temperatures and their activity is suspended by cold. The digestive enzymes all seem to work best at about the temperature of the body (37°C).

Enzymes are **specific** in that each one acts only on a certain type of substance (called a substrate) and brings about only one special chemical reaction. Thus, when a digestive fluid has the ability to act on two or more kinds of foodstuffs, we know that there must be separate enzymes in it for the performance of each of these chemical reactions. Nor are the enzymes in different digestive juices that act on the same kind of foodstuff identical—we know this because they require different

---

*Enzymes are formed in both plant and animal tissue cells and can facilitate many different types of chemical changes—oxidation, reduction, transfer of some chemical group from one compound to another, splitting off the amino or carboxy radicals, etc. Some, such as the digestive enzymes, catalyze reactions by which compounds are split by reaction with water (hydrolysis). Practically all chemical reactions in body tissues take place through the action of enzymes. We have seen that enzymes and coenzymes, in which various vitamins are incorporated, catalyze the important oxidation-reduction reactions in tissues by means of which foodstuffs yield energy for the body. Since (as catalysts) they are not used up in the reaction they bring about, a small amount of enzyme can act on a large amount of substance even at high dilutions.

working conditions. The enzyme in the gastric juice that acts on protein requires quite a high degree of acidity to be effective, whereas there is a protein-splitting enzyme in the pancreatic juice that works well in either a slightly acid or even an alkaline medium. Each of the digestive enzymes has some degree of acidity or alkalinity (optimum pH) at which it works best and a certain range outside of which it will not work at all. A prominent example of this is the starch-splitting enzyme in saliva, which acts only in neutral or slightly alkaline conditions such as found in the mouth and in the stomach before the food material is mixed with the acid gastric juice. As soon as the stomach contents become acid, the digestive activity of this enzyme is stopped.

In addition to optimum temperature and pH, two other conditions are required for the action of digestive enzymes. One is *surface contact* with the substance acted on, and for this reason intimate mixing of digestive juices with finely divided food material and getting the food material ultimately into solution or colloidal dispersion (as with fats) are important. Also important is the *removal of the products* formed by the reaction. Hence it is only in the small intestine, where the products of digestion are continuously removed by absorption, that conditions are favorable for digestive processes to run to completion.

Enzymes are usually named to indicate the substances on which they act. To this substrate root is added the suffix *-ase*, which indicates that it is an enzyme, and often an adjective is prefixed to show the source of the enzyme. Thus, all protein-splitting enzymes are called **proteases**; fat-splitting enzymes are **lipases** (from the word *lipids*, for fats); and starch-splitting enzymes are **amylases** (from the classical name *amylum*, for starch). To distinguish between the different enzymes, the starch-splitting enzyme found in saliva is called *salivary amylase* and the one secreted by the pancreas is known as *pancreatic amylase.* Although this system of naming is more descriptive, many enzymes have other names which had become well established before the system was introduced; some of the older names still persist. For instance, the salivary amylase is well known by the name of *ptyalin,* while almost everyone is familiar with the names of *pepsin* and *trypsin,* which are respectively the gastric and pancreatic proteases.

The best known digestive enzymes, with their names and the reactions they bring about, are listed in Table 13–1.

Enzymes secreted farther along in the alimentary canal carry on the digestive processes started by those in saliva and gastric juice. For the digestion of large molecules, such as starch and proteins, there are two or more enzymes so that any of the foodstuff that escapes digestion by the action of one enzyme is subjected to digestion by others secreted lower down in the digestive tract. This makes for very efficient utilization of carbohydrates and proteins.

Fats are insoluble in water and their digestion is almost entirely dependent on the action of pancreatic lipase (called steapsin). **Bile,** which is discharged from the gallbladder and liver into the intestine, is important for good digestion of fats, even though it contains no

Table 13–1. Summary of Digestion

	Material Acted on	Enzyme Acting	Products Formed	Absorbed
In *mouth* (continuing for time in stomach)	Starch	Ptyalin (salivary amylase)	Dextrins Maltose	
In *stomach*	Proteins	Pepsin (gastric protease)	Proteoses Peptones	
	Casein in milk	Rennin	Precipitates Ca paracaseinate	
	Emulsified fats	Gastric lipase	Glycerol Fatty acids (small amts.)	
In *intestine*	Proteins Proteoses Peptones	Trypsin Chymotrypsin	Polypeptides Dipeptides	
	Polypeptides Dipeptides }	Erepsin (3 enzymes—carboxypeptidase, aminopeptidase and dipeptidase)	Amino acids →	In blood to liver
	Starch Dextrins }	Amylopsin (pancreatic amylase)	Maltose	
	Maltose	Maltase (intestinal mucosa)	Glucose →	In blood to liver
	Sucrose	Sucrase (intestinal mucosa)	Glucose Fructose } →	In blood to liver
	Lactose	Lactase (intestinal mucosa)	Glucose Galactose } →	In blood to liver
	Fats	Steapsin (pancreatic lipase)	Simple glycerides Fatty acids Glycerol } →	Mostly in lymph Small amts. in blood

enzymes. Bile acts to emulsify fats and assists in the absorption of the fatty acids formed by digestion so that they are removed from the intestinal contents and digestion goes to completion.

Rennin is an enzyme contained in the gastric juice, which precipitates milk in solid form (curds). Heat-treated cow's milk and human milk form a finer, more easily digested curd than ordinary cow's milk. Rennin is especially abundant in gastric juice of babies and young animals fed on milk; it is less important in adults, when the hydrochloric acid content of the gastric juice is sufficient alone to coagulate milk.

Secretion of Digestive Fluids

The **glands** which secrete the digestive fluids are either situated in the mucosa, or mucous membrane that lines the alimentary tract, or they are located outside the digestive tract but pour their secretions into it through ducts.

The salivary glands, pancreas, and liver secrete digestive fluids (the saliva, pancreatic juice, and bile) into the alimentary tract. Glands located in the membrane lining the stomach secrete pepsin and the hydrochloric acid that acidifies the gastric juice. The columnar cells in the intestinal mucosa manufacture enzymes that complete the digestion of disaccharides to simple sugars, of peptides to amino acids (mono-, di-, and tripeptidases) and, in addition, secrete a substance that activates trypsin. The enzymes responsible for splitting disaccharides (maltose, sucrose, and lactose) to simple sugars remain in and produce their action in the columnar cells of the mucosa (Fig. 13–4).* These cells are also responsible

---

*The process by which the disaccharides enter the cell is uncertain, but it is theorized that another enzyme, called a *permease*, is responsible for the passage across the cell wall.

for the *active transport* of various nutrients across the mucosal membrane into the blood and lymph (see p. 317). Other cells, found in the mucous membrane throughout the whole course of the alimentary tract, secrete a slimy substance called *mucus*, which has no digestive powers, but serves to lubricate and protect the lining membrane.

Various factors **stimulate** or **inhibit** the secretion of digestive fluids. The secretion of saliva and gastric juice is largely controlled by **nervous stimuli** but the flow of digestive fluids in the lower part of the alimentary tract is relatively free from nervous control and is stimulated by chemical substances carried in the blood, specific **hormones.**

Small amounts of saliva and gastric juice are secreted all the time, but their flow is stimulated when food is present. Factors that stimulate the flow of saliva are chewing, and the taste, sight, smell, or even the thought of food. The latter type of stimulus causes what is known as **psychic secretion,** and the traditional "watering of the mouth" that occurs at odors or thoughts of appetizing food also causes the stomach to secrete more gastric juice in preparation for receiving food. **Appetite** (a psychic factor) thus initiates the secretion of digestive juices. Appetite is influenced in turn, either favorably or unfavorably, by one's state of mind, by companionship, and by the attractiveness of the table service and food, so that all these factors may have an influence on digestion. Fear, anger, worry, strong emotions, and fatigue all set in operation undesirable effects on the secretion of saliva and the flow of gastric juice, and have a strong effect on the muscular movements of the alimentary tract.

Although the secretion of gastric juice and the motility of the stomach are sensitive to nervous and psychic influences, by far the strongest stimulus to the secretion of **gastric juice** comes from the **presence of food in the stomach.** The formation of a hormone called *gastrin* in the pyloric glands of the stom-

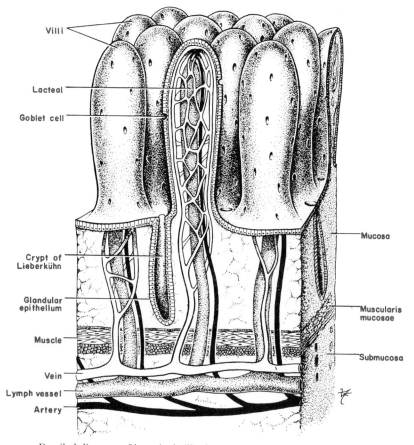

Villi

Lacteal

Goblet cell

Mucosa

Crypt of
Lieberkühn

Glandular
epithelium

Muscularis
mucosae

Muscle

Submucosa

Vein

Lymph vessel

Artery

Figure 13–4.   Detailed diagram of intestinal villi, showing their structure and blood and lymph supply.
Other features of the intestinal wall are indicated by labels at sides of the drawing. (From Villee, C. A.:
Biology, 4th Ed. Philadelphia, W. B. Saunders Co., 1962.)

ach (under influence of food present) stimulates the muscular activity of the stomach and the secretion of gastric juice. One of the stimuli to secretion is distention of the stomach with food or fluid. Some foods call forth a more copious secretion of gastric juice than others. Meats and meat extract (as in soups made from meat) and alcoholic beverages are thought to have an especially stimulating effect on gastric secretion.

The chief stimulus to the secretion of the ***pancreatic juice*** and ***bile*** comes from the ***hormone*** called ***secretin.*** This hormone is formed in the wall of the duodenum by interaction with sub-

stances present in the acid chyme discharged from the stomach into the duodenum. Carried by the blood to the various organs, it stimulates the flow of pancreatic juice, the secretion of bile, and gastric enzyme pepsin, but inhibits gastric acid secretion. Another hormone, cholecystokinin, formed when fatty chyme enters the duodenum, causes the emptying of stored bile from the gallbladder. The presence of fatty food residues and bile in the small intestine has a particularly delaying effect on gastric muscular and secretory activity. The mechanism of this effect is uncertain, but a hypothesized hormone, enterogastrone, has never been isolated.

ABSORPTION

Absorption is the process by which the *products of digestion* pass through the lining of the intestine **into the blood** and **lymph**.* Simple sugars, amino acids, and short-chain fatty acids are absorbed directly into the blood stream, but the products of fat digestion pass chiefly into the lymph, which is collected through tiny lymph vessels and finally emptied into the blood (via the thoracic duct in the neck; see Figure 13–1, page 309).

The **absorption** of food material **takes place almost entirely in the small intestine** and is favored by the fact that the inner surface of this part of the digestive tract is much increased by being thrown up into tiny projections called **villi** (Fig. 13–4). Each of these villi contains numerous small *blood vessels* and a *lymph space* and is covered with still smaller units (microvilli), so that both the blood and lymph are brought very close to the intestinal membrane. The muscular contractions of the intestine also serve to bring its contents into close contact with its wall and to "milk" blood and lymph into and out of the villi. Because chyme is emptied from the stomach gradually and the products of digestion are absorbed as they are formed, the intestine is not overwhelmed with a great surplus of food material to be absorbed at one time.

Anything which makes for either more intimate contact of the intestinal contents with the lining membrane or for slower passage of food through the small intestine favors more complete absorption. Incomplete absorption may be the result of an irritated, highly motile intestine which hurries food through too rapidly, of the formation of insoluble compounds in the intestine,

---

*Lymph is a straw-colored fluid that is the intermediary between the blood and the tissues, since the blood is enclosed in blood vessels and does not come directly in contact with the tissue cells.

or in the case of fat absorption, of lack of bile.

Water-soluble substances can be absorbed by the passive process of diffusion, but in most instances transport is carried out by active or facilitated processes. *Active transport* processes enable absorption of a large amount of nutrient in a much shorter time than would be possible by simple diffusion. In active transport, the absorbing cells perform metabolic work and require energy. Active transport mechanisms have been described for all essential and some nonessential amino acids, for most simple sugars, and for some micronutrients. For active transport of sugars and amino acids, sodium is required as well as oxygen, energy sources, and carrier substances within the cell.

The absorption of vitamin B-12 is carried out by a unique process in which *intrinsic factor*, a protein secreted in the stomach, facilitates absorption in the small intestine. Thus, if the glands that produce intrinsic factor are inactive (or if that portion of the stomach is removed surgically), the vitamin B-12 deficiency disease called pernicious anemia develops even though the diet contains as much vitamin as is normally required (see Chap. 7, p. 159). Absorption of some nutrients (calcium, for example) depends on the presence of specific carrier substances, usually proteins, in the intestinal wall.

Bile plays an essential role in enabling products of fat digestion and fat-soluble vitamins, which are insoluble in water, to pass through the membrane lining the intestine. Bile salts combine with monoglycerides formed during fat digestion to make compounds that are able to bind with both water and lipids, acting much in the same way as dishwashing detergents, which bind greasy food residues in dishwater. The short-chain fatty acids (ten carbons or less) may pass directly into the blood, but those with larger molecules (chains of 16 and 18 or more carbon atoms) pass preferentially into the lymph. Fatty acids of intermediate size may enter either system. Rather than being transported in the blood as free fatty acids, however, most fatty acids are reformed by the cells of the intestine into fats, which are then carried in loose combination with protein.

Normal amounts of mixed food fats are well digested and absorbed by healthy persons. In diseases with associated impairment of lipid digestion and absorption and in experimental studies, differences in the absorbability of various forms have been demonstrated. In general, short-chain fatty acids appear to be better absorbed than those of long-chain length, and unsaturated acids are absorbed better than saturated acids of the same length. Fatty acids may unite with calcium and magnesium ions to form insoluble compounds, resulting in failure to absorb both the mineral and the lipid. This is usually of little significance unless the diet contains very large amounts of hard fat or if digestion is impaired.

Absorption of both calcium and iron (and of some of the other minerals) is adversely affected when the diet includes *large* amounts of substances that form highly insoluble compounds with these metals. For example, iron and calcium form insoluble salts with phytic acid, which is found in whole-grain cereals; and calcium reacts with oxalic acid found in rhubarb, spinach, and beet tops to form the insoluble calcium oxalate (see Chap. 11). Normally, the diet does not contain enough of these interfering substances to impair nutrition, but these could assume importance if the diet provides only marginal amounts of the nutrients or if absorptive processes are impaired by disease.

Dietary factors can also influence absorption favorably. Iron is more readily absorbed in reduced (ferrous) state than when oxidized (ferric form). Thus, the presence in the diet of factors that promote reduction or prevent oxidation—such as vitamins C and E and antioxidants that are added to fats—favor absorption of iron. Calcium absorption depends on an adequate supply of vitamin D and is benefited when the milk sugar lactose is included in the diet.

Absorption is usually very efficient and *complete*; the **foodstuffs or energy nutrients (carbohydrates, fats, and proteins) are about 90 percent digested and absorbed** on a mixed diet and under normal conditions.

CONDITIONS WHICH AFFECT DIGESTION

The chief factors which affect digestion may be grouped in the following categories:

1. Nervous or psychological factors.
2. General nutritive factors.
3. Food factors.

Each of these factors acts either **by affecting the motor functions** of the digestive organs, **by exerting an influence on the flow of the digestive juices,** or **by altering the health of the digestive tract itself.** Different conditions exert a favorable or unfavorable influence on digestion, depending on whether they have a stimulating or inhibiting action.

Nervous Factors

Fear, worry, anger, irritation, and stress all exert **unfavorable** influences on secretion and motility. Prolonged tension and suppressed aggression or dependency needs are common in the life experiences of people who develop peptic ulcers. In these persons, emotionality is accompanied by increased acid secretion and gastric blood flow. Others react to fear or sadness with decreased acid production and blood flow.

The reverse conditions exert a **beneficial** influence on digestion through promoting good secretion of digestive fluids and proper muscular activity of the alimentary tract. Peace and quiet, cheerful companionship, appetizing food, and attractive surroundings all favor good digestion.

General Nutritive Factors

Because the lining of the digestive tract is continuously and rapidly being renewed, and because secretions and enzymes are formed constantly and in large volume, the digestive system is particularly susceptible to the effects of poor nutrition. Lack of thiamin is especially likely to be associated with lack of appetite, and diarrhea is one of the typical symptoms of pellagra, a niacin-deficiency disease. Inadequacy of iron intake and failure to secrete gastric acid occur together. Protein is needed for formation of digestive enzymes and intestinal cells, as are other vitamins and minerals. Through these effects on the digestive system, deficiency of one nutrient can impair the utilization of *virtually all* other nutrients. In fact, a person who is in **poor general nutritive condition,** whatever may be its cause, is likely to show the effects of this condition in a *poorly functioning alimentary tract.*

Food Factors

This category includes the factors to which the lay mind attributes most of the ills of digestion, but these factors are less important than is usually supposed. The healthy stomach and intestines can digest any ordinary food or combination of foods without trouble. A few people are unquestionably sensitive to certain foods and are made ill by them, but **food allergy** is not very common and needs to be confirmed by the tests of a physician. The reason many persons experience digestive distress when they eat foods or combinations of foods which they believe will give them trouble is that the *apprehension of harm* to come is sufficient in itself

to alter gastrointestinal motility and blood flow.

Some types of food are digested more slowly than others, and such foods are often spoken of as being "hard to digest." In general, liquids and finely divided foods are those most rapidly handled by the digestive tract. Fats and foods rich in fats (especially mixtures of proteins with fats), foods which are introduced into the stomach in large pieces (and especially in chunks coated with fat), and protein-rich foods which have been made tough in texture by overcooking are digested more slowly but not less completely than other foods.

The **influence of cooking** is more through making the food palatable and appetizing than through any effect on the nutritive properties or digestibility of the food. Most raw foods are well digested, but starchy foods and those that contain tough fiber need thorough cooking in order to rupture the starch granules and to soften the fiber so that the digestive juices can penetrate them. There is seldom more than 5 percent difference between the extent to which raw or poorly cooked foods are ultimately digested and absorbed, and the degree of utilization of the same foods when properly cooked.

Incomplete digestion is likely to result in the formation of *gases* (through bacterial action in the intestine), which may cause pain and distention of the intestines. The diet may be at fault, but the general condition of the individual, nervous or otherwise, is a contributing factor. Some foods, such as legumes, have carbohydrates that are not digested by human enzymes but that are used by bacteria, with formation of gas and other end-products. The intestinal bacteria will attack almost any foodstuff that is not absorbed in the small intestine, so gas formation and, in severe cases, cramping pain and diarrhea always accompany malabsorption. In recent years it has been discovered that many adults and some youngsters have little or no lactase enzyme in the intestine and experience flatulence and softening of stools when they drink **large** amounts of milk or other products containing the milk sugar, lactose. The incidence of this lactase deficiency is higher in Asiatic, Mediterranean, and African populations than in Caucasian Americans and Europeans. The incidence increases with age and also occurs temporarily or permanently as a result of severe protein malnutrition and of diseases that damage the intestine. People who have this problem can eat cheese without any distress, proving conclusively that sugar absorption is at fault.

Naturally, it is a matter of discretion to take only **small amounts** of the **easily digested foods** if a *digestive upset* or other *illness* has affected the gastrointestinal tract. This is the reason convalescents are given smaller amounts of food at shorter intervals.

Excretion Through the Intestine

The intestinal waste, feces, consists of:

1. *Indigestible undigested*, and *unabsorbed food residues;*
2. Residues from *digestive secretions, mucus,* and *cell debris* from the lining of the alimentary tract;
3. Small amounts of *material secreted* into the digestive tract;
4. *Bacteria* and the products of their action;
5. *Water.*

The **bulk of the feces** is made up of **water**, and **food and digestive residues.** Some *mineral salts* (notably salts of calcium and phosphorus) are excreted through the intestinal wall into the lower digestive tract; the main pathway for excretion of excess or unutilized calcium and iron is by way of the intestine. *Certain waste products are found in the bile,* which is secreted by the liver and empties into the duodenum; some

of these substances (e.g., bile salts) are partially reabsorbed and excreted in the urine. The *pigment* which gives the feces their brown color is formed from the bile pigment, which in turn comes from hemoglobin. Bile is the major excretory route for cholesterol.

Feces of ordinary semisolid consistency contain 60 to 70 percent **water,** but the water content is higher if the fecal material is hurried through the alimentary tract, and lower when its excretion is long delayed, owing to further absorption of water in the colon. About one-tenth to one-third of the feces consists of **bacteria** (both living and dead), and the number excreted per day has been estimated as varying between 50 and 500 billion. The presence of bacteria in the intestinal contents is entirely normal and some of them may even be beneficial in that they synthesize certain vitamins. (See Chapters 7 and 9.)

FACTORS WHICH AFFECT EXCRETION THROUGH THE INTESTINES. We have already discussed some ways in which the nature of the diet affects absorption of specific nutrients, the amount of unabsorbed material passed on to the large intestine, and the importance of good nutrition in maintaining the health and normal muscular tone of the digestive tract. In healthy persons, almost all the components of a normal diet are nearly completely digested and absorbed, leaving little residue.

The factor that most affects the *volume* of feces passed by normal persons is the amount of *water* retained in the feces. Indigestible substances consumed (chiefly cellulose and other complex carbohydrates) and the growth of intestinal bacteria contribute to *fecal dry matter.* A combination of these influences accounts for the slightly increased bulk of feces formed when the diet contains large quantities of vegetables and fruits, unrefined cereals, and milk, in contrast to large amounts of meat and refined cereals.

Some foods stimulate intestinal motility in the same way laxative drugs do. Prune juice is especially effective in this respect. Similar but less potent effects are produced by acid fruit juices and cooked pulp of dried fruits. Little information is available as to the active factors in these foods. Mineral oil softens the feces and is often used as a mild laxative, but its regular use is to be avoided because fat-soluble nutrients are also soluble in mineral oil and are excreted along with this nonabsorbable substance.

Stimuli to which the presence of feces in the rectum gives rise result in the desire and ability to defecate. *Psychic influences*, such as hurry and overanxiety to have a movement daily, have the effect of inhibiting these stimuli and preventing the normal reflex which causes the colon to contract and expel its contents. Thus, a good many people either have, or think they have, trouble in producing bowel movements with sufficient frequency or regularity. This problem may persist at intervals throughout life, and it is perhaps especially frequent among elderly persons. Constipation can usually be corrected by establishing a regular time for going to the toilet, preferably shortly after breakfast; drinking one or two glasses of water half an hour before breakfast; and increasing consumption of prunes, figs, fibrous vegetables, fruits, and unrefined cereals, as well as taking some brisk physical activity.

A given set of symptoms may have a variety of causes, and the treatment appropriate to one cause may be disadvantageous for another. If simple, short-term efforts fail to correct constipation, competent medical advice should be sought for diagnosis of the underlying disorder.

Diarrhea is another commonly encountered symptom that may be due to many causes: irritant substances or toxins in food, infectious disease, allergy, etc. Mild, transient cases of diarrhea usually respond favorably to severe restriction of dietary fat, fruits, and vegetables, and to increased consumption of tea in preference to coffee. The loss of fluids and minerals is potentially *very* dangerous, particularly in infants and children, so a physician should be consulted if the condition persists beyond a few hours in infants and more than a few days in adults, or if there are accompanying symptoms such as fever or vomiting.

QUESTIONS

1. What is digestion? Why is it necessary? Describe the alimentary tract and show how it is especially adapted for carrying out the process of digestion.

2. What are the end products of digestion of proteins, starch, cane sugar, and fats? Name the principal digestive fluids that bring about the chemical breakdown of these foodstuffs into their simplest components. Tell where each of these digestive fluids is formed, and give the main functions of each.

3. Chemical changes involved in digestion are brought about or facilitated by the presence of enzymes in the digestive fluids. What is an enzyme? What is meant by saying that enzymes are specific in their action? Name the different enzymes (and substances on which they act) in gastric juice and in pancreatic juice, and those formed in the intestinal mucosa. What is the chemical nature of enzymes, and why is their activity destroyed by boiling? What are the optimum conditions for activity of the enzymes in saliva, in gastric juice, and in the digestive fluids in the intestine?

4. What are the chief factors that stimulate or inhibit the secretion of saliva and gastric juice? Explain the action of hormones in stimulating the flow of the digestive fluids that act on food in the small intestine. What happens to food residues in the large intestine or colon?

5. Describe how absorption of amino

acids, simple sugars, and end products of fat digestion takes place in the intestine. What substances taken in food can be absorbed without being chemically changed in digestion? Explain how bile helps in the digestion and absorption of fats. What substances are found in the residues at the end of the digestive tract—the feces—and what factors alter the consistency and composition of the feces?

6. Discuss the effects of nervous factors, of the general nutritive condition of the individual, and of different types of food eaten, on the relative ease and comfort with which digestion is accomplished; upon the completeness of digestion.

7. What are the main constituents found in the feces? Which of these may be described as residues from the contents of the digestive tract? What waste products of metabolism are excreted through the intestine?

SUPPLEMENTARY READING

Alfin-Slater, R. B.: Absorption, digestion and metabolism of fats and related lipids. In *Modern Nutrition in Health and Disease* (Wohl, M. G., and Goodhart, R. S., eds.). 4th Ed. Philadelphia, Lea & Febiger, 1970.

Ballman, J. L.: The physiology of the gastrointestinal tract and its bearing on nutrition. In *Modern Nutrition in Health and Disease* (Wohl, M. G., and Goodhart, R. S., eds.). 4th Ed. Philadelphia, Lea & Febiger, 1970.

Barboriak, J. J., and Meade, R. C.: Effect of alcohol on gastric emptying in man. Amer. J. Clin. Nutr., 23:1151, 1970.

Bayless, T. M. (ed.): Symposium: Structure and function of the gut. Amer. J. Clin. Nutr., 24:44, 1971.

Booher, L. E., Behan, E., and McMeans, E.: Biologic utilizations of unmodified and modified food starches. J. Nutr., 45:75, 1951.

Code, C. F. (ed.): *Handbook of Physiology*, Section 6: Alimentary Canal. Vols. II-V, American Physiological Society. Baltimore, Williams & Wilkins Co., 1967-1968.

Curran, P. F.: Active transport of amino acids and sugars. Arch. Intern. Med., 129:258, 1972.

Draser, B. S., Shiner, M., and McLeod, G. M.: Studies on the intestinal flora. I. The bacterial flora of the gastrointestinal tract in healthy and achlorhydric persons. Gastroenterol., 56:71, 1969.

Floch, M. H. (ed.): Current concepts in intestinal absorption and malabsorption (Symposium). Amer. J. Clin. Nutr., 22:239, 1969.

Gardner, F. H.: Nutritional management of chronic diarrhea in adults. J. Amer. Med. Assoc., 179:69, 1962.

Gardner, J. D., Brown, M. S., and Laster, L.: The columnar epithelial cell of the small intestine: Digestion and transport. New Eng. J. Med., 283:1196, 1970.

Go, V. L. W., and Summerskill, W. H. J.: Digestion, maldigestion and the gastrointestinal hormones. Amer. J. Clin. Nutr., 24:160, 1971.

Guyton, A. C.: *Function of the Human Body*. 3rd Ed. Philadelphia, W. B. Saunders Co., 1969.

Holdstock, D. J., Misiewocz, J. J., Smith, T., Rowlands, E. N.: Propulsion (mass movements) in the human colon and its relationship to meals and somatic activity. Gut, 11:91, 1970.

Holter, H.: How things get into cells. Sci. Amer., 205:167, 1961.

Huang, S. S., and Bayless, T. M.: Milk and lactose intolerance in healthy Orientals. Science, 160:83, 1968.

Ingelfinger, F. J., et al.: Malabsorption: Nutrition Society Symposium. Fed. Proc., 26:1388, 1967.

Joint Committee of the American Dietetic Association and the American Medical Association: Diet as related to gastrointestinal function. J. Amer. Med. Assoc., 176:57, 1961.

Klipstein, F. A. (ed.): Symposium: Malabsorption and malnutrition in the tropics. Amer. J. Clin. Nutr., 21:939, 1968.

Laster, L., and Ingelfinger, F. J.: Intestinal absorption—aspects of structure, function and disease of the small-intestine mucosa. New Eng. J. Med., 264:1192, 1246, 1961.

Levy, G., and Hewitt, R. R.: Evidence in man for different specialized intestinal transport mechanisms for riboflavin and thiamin. Amer. J. Clin. Nutr., 24:401, 1971.

Mao, C. C., and Jacobson, E. D.: Intestinal absorption and blood flow. Amer. J. Clin. Nutr., 23:820, 1970.

Neurath, H.: Protein-digesting enzymes. Sci. Amer., 211:68, 1964.

Ockner, R. K., Pittman, J. P., and Yager, J. L.: Differences in the intestinal absorption of saturated and unsaturated long chain fatty acids. Gastroenterol., 62:981, 1972.

Phillips, S. F.: Absorption and secretion by the colon. Gastroenterol., 56:966, 1969.

Portman, O. W.: Importance of diet, species and intestinal flora in bile acid metabolism. Fed. Proc., 21:896, 1962.

Rehm, W. S.: Some aspects of the problem of gastric hydrochloric acid secretion. Arch. Intern. Med., 129:270, 1972.

Rosensweig, N. S., and Herman, R. H.: Diet and disaccharidases. Amer. J. Clin. Nutr., 22:99, 1969.

Saint-Hilaire, S., Lavers, M. K., Kennedy, J., and Code, C. F.: Gastric acid secretory value of different foods. Gastroenterol., *39*:1, 1960.

Saraya, A. K., Tandon, B. N., Ramachandran, K., and Saikia, B.: Intestinal structure and function in megaloblastic anemia in adults. Amer. J. Clin. Nutr., *24*:622, 1971.

Treadwell, C. R., Swell, L., and Vahouny, G. V.: Factors in sterol absorption. Fed. Proc., *21*: 903, 1962.

Watts, J. H., et al.: Fecal solids excreted by young men following the ingestion of dairy foods. Amer. J. Dig. Dis., *8*:364, 1963.

Williams, R. D., and Olmsted, W. H.: The manner in which food controls the bulk of the feces. Ann. Intern. Med., *10*:717, 1936.

Nutrition Reviews

Iron absorption. *24*:247, 1966.

Gastric function and structure in iron deficiency. *24*:326, 1966.

Gastric secretions before and after vagotomy. *24*:328, 1966.

Intestinal absorption of chromium. *25*:76, 1967.

Jejunal mucosa after kwashiorkor. *25*:140, 1967.

Immune globulins and the gastrointestinal tract. *25*:144, 1967.

Fat absorption: Physiology and biochemistry. *26*: 168, 1968.

Absorption of essential amino acids in man. *26*: 269, 1968.

Diet therapy of gastrointestinal disorders. *27*:49, 1969.

Malabsorption due to neomycin. *27*:102, 1969.

Raw soybean meal and pancreatic secretion. *27*: 116, 1969.

Lactase deficiency in Thailand. *27*:278, 1969.

Effect of vitamin D on absorption of calcium and the template activity of chromatin in intestines of rats and chicks. *28*:21, 1970.

Calcium and magnesium absorption in the germ-free rat. *28*:101, 1970.

Intestinal lactase—an inducable enzyme? *28*:138, 1970.

Lactase activity levels in Nigeria—genetic or acquired phenomena? *30*:156, 1972.

Background information on lactose and milk intolerance. *30*:175, 1972.

Intestinal absorption of folates. *30*:179, 1972.

fourteen

Metabolism and Excretion

Metabolism is a *general* term used to designate all the **chemical changes which occur in living matter in the course of its vital activities.** These changes are of two kinds—anabolic and catabolic. Anabolism includes all chemical changes by which the absorbed products of digestion are used to *replace* substances broken down during life processes or to build new tissues in growth. *Catabolism* refers to processes by which nutrients, reserve tissue material, and cellular substances are broken down into chemically simpler compounds with the liberation of energy. In catabolism, energy nutrients are oxidized gradually, ultimately yielding carbon dioxide and water (plus some nitrogen compounds, from protein catabolism). Part of the energy released by catabolism is used as the source of energy for anabolism, and the remainder is usually converted to heat.

Discussion in this chapter is limited to the metabolism of the three chief foodstuffs—proteins, carbohydrates, and fats. Intensive research in recent years has accumulated a mass of information about the intermediate compounds formed in the breaking down of these three types of nutrients, the enzymes and coenzymes involved in bringing about these chemical changes, and the ways in which intermediate products may be built interchangeably into one or another substance as needed by the body. This chapter presents a simplified version of this information.

It should be emphasized that the body constituents are in a *dynamic state*, with both diet and body tissues contributing to a common metabolic pool in which the contributions of each are functionally indistinguishable. Thus, when the fate of glucose is being discussed, for example, it should be taken to mean both glucose coming from the diet and that coming from the tissues. It is possible to prove the existence of this dynamic state and to measure the size and activity of the common metabolic pool by the use of isotopes—such as heavy or radioactive forms of carbon, hydrogen, and nitrogen.

Cells: Functional Units of Metabolism

All living matter is composed of cells and cell products. Metabolism of carbohydrate, fat, and amino acids takes place within the cells of the body. (See Fig. 14-1.)

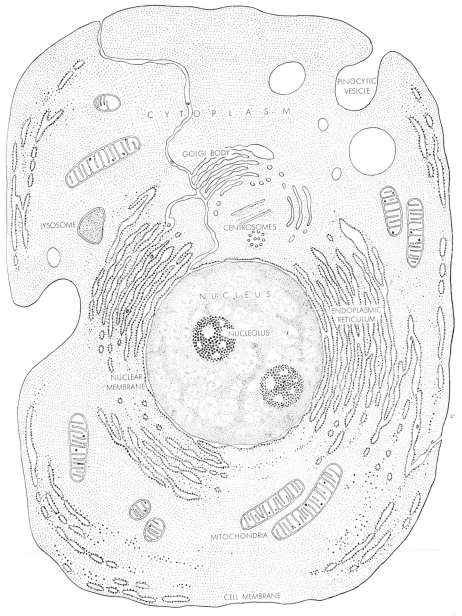

Figure 14–1. A typical cell. Cells are highly variable in structure and function. Within the human body there are many different cell types, such as the striated-muscle cell, the smooth muscle cell, the nerve cell, the liver cell, and the sperm cell. However, all cells have certain structural constituents in common, though they may vary in appearance and quantity. These similarities give rise to the concept of the typical cell. (From The Living Cell, by Jean Brachet. Copyright © 1961 by Scientific American, Inc. All rights reserved.)

Cells contain four interconnected membrane systems. The cell membrane acts to separate the cell from the external environment. It selectively controls the rate of movement of nutrient and waste material into and out of the cell. Generally, large molecules do not pass directly through the cell membrane; however, they may be taken into the cytoplasm by engulfing the molecule in a pinocytic vesicle. The endoplasmic reticulum allows transport of substances through the cell by a network of tubules. Frequently, it has numerous granules on the cytoplasmic side of its membranes. The granules are *ribosomes* which are the *sites of protein synthesis* in the cell. The Golgi body appears to aid secretion from the cell and absorption into the cell. The nuclear membrane consists of two membranes surrounding the nucleus of the cell. It contains pores that may function as sites of transfer for large molecules between the nucleus and the cytoplasm.

All the cell membranes (including those surrounding organelles) are composed of lipid and protein arranged in such a fashion that both water-soluble and lipid-soluble substances can pass through the membranes. An important feature of the membranes of the cell is that they subdivide the cell into compartments that enclose the aqueous phases of the cell. Often the membranes are the sites for chemical reactions involving enzymes located on the membranes.

Within the cell, the *nucleus plays a coordinating role* in the organization and perpetuation of the cell. The deoxyribonucleic acid (DNA) within the nucleus directs the synthesis of all cell proteins by means of ribonucleic acid (RNA) which carries the information to the ribosomes in the cytoplasm. As metabolic reactions require enzymes and enzymes are proteins, it is clear that the nucleus has the ability to control the fate of the cell. The DNA duplicates itself during cell division so that each cell of an organism contains identi-

cal genetic information in the form of DNA. The membrane-rich *mitochondria* are the *sites of the final oxidation of nutrients* into carbon dioxide and water. Approximately 40 per cent of the energy released can be used to synthesize the high-energy phosphate bond of adenosine triphosphate (ATP; see Fig. 14–2). The remainder of the energy is released as heat. The ATP formed provides energy for the anabolic reactions in the cell. The mitochondria are also the site of fatty acid breakdown in the cell. They contain, within a membrane, enzymes capable of splitting important complex compounds such as proteins, nucleic acids, and polysaccharides. Disruption of the membrane frees the enzymes and the cell digests itself. In the body, the death of individual cells and their replacement by young cells occur in the normal course of events.

THE FATE OF ENERGY NUTRIENTS IN THE CELL

The initial phases of carbohydrate, fat, and amino acid catabolism proceed more or less independently of each other to yield identical two- and three-carbon intermediates. From this common metabolic pool of intermediates, carbohydrate, fat, and protein can be synthesized or the intermediates can be further oxidized to carbon dioxide and hydrogen atoms by the citric acid cycle enzymes. It is the oxidation of the hydrogen atoms to water by a series of enzymes called the electron-transport system that is the primary source of ATP production for the cell.

Each metabolic reaction is catalyzed by an enzyme that, generally, is specific for that particular reaction. Often coenzymes are required for the reactions to proceed. These nonprotein substances usually act as carriers for the products of the reactions and are not specific for each reaction. The coenzymes frequently contain vitamins as

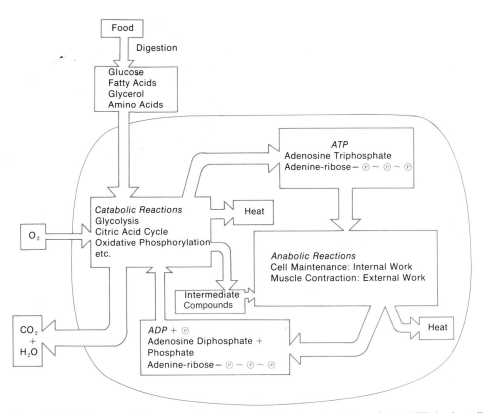

Figure 14–2. Diagrammatic interpretation of the role of adenosine triphosphate (ATP) in the cell. Whenever energy-producing reactions take place, such as the oxidation of glucose to carbon dioxide and water, some of the energy set free goes into forming ATP by the addition of a high-energy phosphate bond to adenosine diphosphate (ADP). The energy for anabolic reactions, whereby simpler groups or compounds are built into larger more complex molecules, is supplied by the splitting of a high-energy phosphate bond of ATP, leaving ADP plus a free phosphate group. Thus, in the cell ATP acts as a messenger between those reactions that supply energy and those that utilize energy. Heat is a by-product of metabolism; it warms the body but is of no value as a source of internal or external work.

part of their structure. Thus, deficiencies of the vitamins may profoundly change the course of metabolism. Mineral elements, such as iron, copper, and magnesium, are also contained in various metabolic enzymes and are necessary for their functioning (see Chaps. 11 and 12).

Carbohydrates

The products of digestion of carbohydrates, chiefly *glucose* with smaller amounts of fructose and galactose, are absorbed from the intestine into the blood, which passes directly to the liver.

The liver has the ability to remove excess glucose from the blood and to take up and metabolize fructose and galactose (since only glucose is found in significant amounts in the general circulation). Thus, after a meal rich in carbohydrates, a great deal of glucose appears in the **portal vein,** but the *glucose content of the blood* in circulation in the rest of the body is only slightly increased and soon returns to its remarkably *constant level.*

The **liver** is the *regulator of the blood sugar* and the main *storage house for carbohydrate* in the body. It takes the simple sugars brought to it from the intestine and combines them to form the more complex and less soluble carbohydrate, **glycogen** (see Chap. 3). This name, meaning "sugar former," was given to this compound because, whenever the body needs extra glucose the glycogen can be converted back into glucose again and released into the blood. In this way, the liver acts as a reservoir to keep the body from being flooded with glucose just after meals and from running short of it at other times. The role of blood glucose is to supply energy for current body needs. Tissues continually withdraw glucose from the blood for their own uses, and the glycogen in the liver must be reconverted to glucose to maintain blood glucose at the normal level.

The **muscles** also can store small amounts of glycogen. Even though muscle glycogen can be readily drawn on for the energy needed for muscular work, liver glycogen is the only reservoir from which the glucose of the blood can be replenished. The *amount of glycogen in the liver* and muscles naturally depends somewhat on whether the supply of carbohydrate (or of energy in other forms) in the diet has been *liberal* or *scanty*, but there is an *upper limit* beyond which no more glycogen is normally stored.

Dietary *carbohydrate* in excess of the relatively small amount which can be converted into glycogen *is stored as fat* in the fatty (adipose) tissues of the body. In the case of a lack of food, the glycogen stores are practically exhausted in *one to two days*, after which

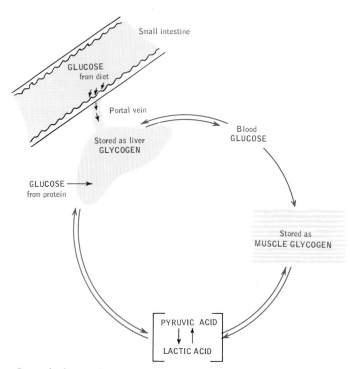

Figure 14–3. General scheme of anaerobic carbohydrate metabolism. This provides for the production of some ATP even though the oxygen supply to the body is limited. When the oxygen supply is adequate, pyruvic acid is oxidized completely via the citric acid cycle to provide energy for metabolism. The lactic acid that is produced during short-term oxygen shortage is largely (80 percent) converted to glycogen on restoration of an adequate oxygen supply.

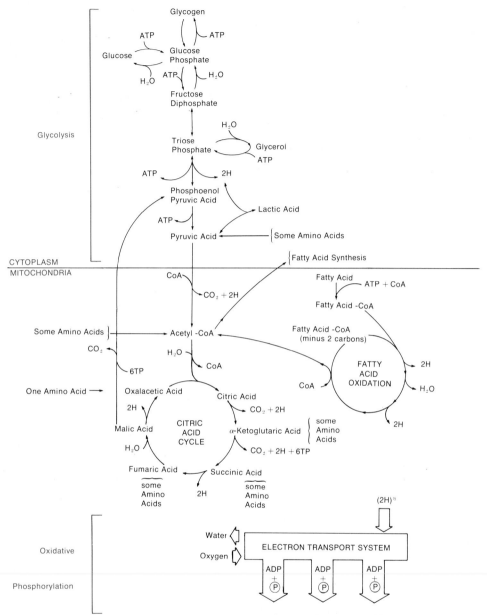

Figure 14–4. This is a simplified illustration of some of the interactions in carbohydrate, fat and protein metabolism. Acetyl-Co A (Co A contains the vitamin pantothenic acid) serves as an important central compound in the metabolism of these nutrients. ATP acts as an intermediary between the energy producing and the energy consuming reactions of the cell (See Fig. 14–2; the end products of the use and the precursors of the synthesis of ATP are not shown in order to simplify the diagram). GTP—guanosine triphosphate—is a compound with a high-energy phosphate bond similar to ATP. The hydrogen atoms (2H) produced in metabolism (these are carried by coenzymes containing riboflavin or niacin) are generally oxidized by the electron transport system, which is the major site of ATP production for the cell. Cell compartmentalization of the various sequences of reactions is essential for the life of the cell.

the body draws largely on its reserves of fat for energy. The limited stores of glycogen in liver and muscles serve *short-interval energy reserves,* while the main depots of extra fuel are the fat deposits in various parts of the body.

Within the tissue cells, the first phase of the breakdown of glucose takes place in the cytoplasm of the cell. This series of ten chemical reactions is known as *glycolysis,** the *anaerobic stage* of carbohydrate catabolism. It consists of the conversion of glycogen or glucose to pyruvic acid, which under conditions of adequate oxygen is converted to carbon dioxide and water. In anaerobic conditions (limited oxygen supply), the conversion of pyruvic acid to lactic acid is necessary for the regeneration of a niacin-containing coenzyme (NAD), so that glycolysis can continue to produce ATP. (See Fig. 14–3.)

During glycolysis only a small amount of the potential energy is set free, but enough to permit a muscle to operate temporarily when oxygen is not brought to it fast enough by the blood. When an adequate oxygen supply is restored, only about a fifth of the accumulated lactic acid is converted into pyruvic acid and then further catabolized by the citric acid cycle; the rest is conserved by resynthesis into glycogen.

The anabolic formation of glucose and glycogen from the intermediate compounds of metabolism is called *gluconeogenesis.* In addition to lactic acid, the glycerol moiety of fat and some of the amino acid intermediates can be used to make glucose and glycogen in the body (see Fig. 14–4).

---

*There are several other pathways through which carbohydrates may pass. The amount of traffic over a given pathway varies, depending on hormonal influences, tissue conditions, and the need for specific intermediate compounds. For example, glucose is oxidized to a variable extent by a shunt pathway in which pentoses are formed (such as ribose needed for building nucleic acids and ATP), as well as a coenzyme (containing niacin) required in several steps of fatty acid and steroid synthesis.

The Citric Acid Cycle and Oxidative Phosphorylation

The *citric acid cycle* is the *common final oxidative pathway* for the intermediate compounds of carbohydrate, fat, and protein catabolism. It is also known as the tricarboxylic acid cycle (because it involves acids with three carboxyl (–COOH) groups) or the Krebs cycle (named after the man who first worked it out). Pyruvic acid can enter the mitochondria where it must be converted to acetyl coenzyme A before entering the citric acid cycle. This complex reaction requires five different enzymes and five coenzymes, four of which each contain a different vitamin (pantothenic acid, thiamin, niacin, and riboflavin). The coenzyme A (Co A) contains pantothenic acid as part of its structure. The Co A is released when the two-carbon acetic acid combines with the four-carbon oxalacetic acid to begin the cycle with the formation of citric acid, a six-carbon compound.

The citric acid cycle is represented diagrammatically in Figure 14–4. A few intermediate substances are omitted, but all steps at which hydrogen atoms, carbon dioxide, or ATP are formed are included. The reactions by which carbohydrate, glycerol, fatty acids, and amino acids enter the cycle are shown in abbreviated form. The cycle moves only clockwise, starting with citric acid and ending with oxalacetic acid. Each revolution accomplishes the degradation of one molecule of acetic acid to carbon dioxide and water. At the end, a molecule of oxalacetic acid is left, free to combine with another acetyl-Co A to form citric acid and start the cycle again.

The hydrogen atoms formed in the citric acid cycle are transported as coenzymes (containing either niacin or riboflavin) to a nearby set of enzymes called the electron transport system. The hydrogen is oxidized to water with oxygen by this system of enzymes. Some of the energy released by the oxidation of a pair of hydrogen atoms can be used to synthesize three high-energy phosphate bonds of ATP. This process is referred to as *oxidative phosphorylation* and is the *major source of the ATP needed* as the driving force *in many anabolic reactions* in cells. The complete set of citric acid cycle enzymes are found in proximity to the electron transport enzymes within the mitochondria of the cell.

Fats

Fats, being insoluble in water, require a special system for transportation in blood, an aqueous medium. Triglycerides, phospholipids, and cholesterol are carried to the tissues combined with globulin proteins as lipoprotein complexes. Chylomicrons are the largest of the lipoprotein complexes and are basically large fat droplets covered with a very thin protein layer. After a meal rich in fats, plasma becomes turbid by the chylomicrons released from the lymphatic system, but this extra fat leaves the blood and passes into the tissues within a few hours. The liver is the primary site of synthesis of the other lipoproteins. These particles are the means of fat transport to the tissues from the liver; they are smaller than chylomicrons and contain varying amounts of protein, from 10 to 60 percent of their weight. A small amount of free fatty acids is always present in the blood and is bound to the albumin protein of the blood for transport from adipose tissue. Free fatty acids are thought to be the most active form of lipids involved in metabolism. Their concentration in the blood is affected by the mobilization of fat from fat depots and by the action of several hormones.

The liver and adipose tissue are the main sites for fat metabolism, but other tissues can also perform the same chemical transformations. Dietary fat is changed into various related fatty substances which the body cells either need for their structure or can readily use for energy production. Thus, some fat may be transformed into phospholipids; saturated fatty acids may be converted to unsaturated ones and vice versa; and fats not characteristic of the animal may be converted into the arrangement needed for storage in the tissues.

Most of the fat ingested is used as *body fuel*. Formerly it was thought that carbohydrate was the main source of energy used by the tissues, but it is now known that fat also performs this role. In fact, it is now known that even the brain and other nervous tissues are not totally dependent on glucose for energy. The final *end products of fat oxidation* are the same as formed by the complete oxidation of glucose—namely, *carbon dioxide* and *water*. The intermediate steps are very different and the amount of energy liberated is $2\frac{1}{4}$ times as great as would be produced by oxidizing an equal weight of glucose.

Initially, fats must be broken down into glycerol and fatty acids, which follow different chemical paths of catabolism. *Glycerol* is transformed in the cytoplasm of the cell into a triose (three-carbon sugar) phosphate intermediate of glycolysis. The triose phosphate can be used to make glucose, or it can be oxidized to carbon dioxide and water via the citric acid cycle (Fig. 14–4). The *fatty acids,* with their long chains of carbon atoms, are oxidized stepwise into two-carbon fragments in the form of acetyl-Co A, which is then metabolized by the citric acid cycle and the electron transport system in the manner described previously.

The breakdown of fatty acids takes place in the mitochondria of the cell. Initially, a molecule of ATP is required to supply energy to convert the two-carbon units of fatty acid to the coenzyme A intermediate necessary for further catabolism (Fig. 14–3). This reaction is followed sequentially by hydrogen removal (by means of a coenzyme containing riboflavin), addition of water, removal of another hydrogen (with a niacin-containing coenzyme), and finally the addition of another Co A. Acetyl-Co A is split off and a fatty acid (minus two carbons)-Co A is formed which then goes through the series of reactions again. For a fatty acid like stearic acid, which has a chain of 18 carbon atoms, this series of reactions would have to be repeated eight times in order to produce the nine two-carbon molecules of acetyl-Co A. The citric acid cycle completely oxidizes acetyl-Co A, so there is no net synthesis of glucose from fatty acid oxidation.

Acetyl-Co A may be used for building other substances, including new fatty acids and cholesterol. As acetyl-Co A is also formed during catabolism of both glucose and amino acids, it is easy to explain how fat can be synthesized from either carbohydrate or protein when these are eaten in excess of the body needs for energy. The deposit of fat in the tissues represents fuel taken in excess of the energy needs of the body, whether it is taken as fat or made from excess carbohydrate or protein.

Although adipose tissue was formerly thought to be rather inert, experiments with fatty acids tagged by containing an isotopic element indicate that there is a more active interchange of fatty acids between these tissues and the blood than was previously supposed. Stored fat can, of course, be withdrawn from adipose tissue and oxidized to provide energy, whenever energy intake is insufficient for current body needs.

Proteins

The products of protein digestion —*amino acids*—are absorbed into the blood and carried in this form to the tissues, which take them up rapidly from the blood. The amino acids that are absorbed by the tissues following a meal disappear within a few hours.

The primary and unique function of amino acids is to provide the components for synthesis of *tissue* proteins (including the important proteins of the blood) as needed for maintenance and *growth*, and to serve as precursors of antibodies, some hormones and a vitamin. (See Chap. 5.) Normally the body does not store protein, although small reserves of protein are accumulated in the liver and muscles by actual growth of the tissue. These and blood proteins can be used for more essential purposes when protein intake is inadequate.

Experiments with amino acids containing isotopic elements demonstrate that amino acids are very labile compounds capable of being converted one into another and into substances other than tissue proteins. The first step in this conversion is the loss of the nitrogen-containing amino group ($-NH_2$), called *deamination*. Deamination can occur by a reaction in which the amino group is transferred to an acceptor keto-acid ($R-C-COOH$), to form a new

$$\overset{\|}{O}$$

amino acid and leaving a new keto-acid. The enzymes catalyzing these reactions are called transaminases and usually require a vitamin B-6-containing coenzyme for activity. This is the way the body makes many of the amino acids described as nonessential, meaning that they do not have to be supplied by protein in the diet because they can be made in the body. The formation of ammonia and a keto-acid from amino acid is another type of deamination. The enzymes catalyzing these reactions, called amino acid oxidases, generally require riboflavin-containing enzymes for activity. Most deamination occurs in the liver, but the kidneys also have enzymes that can perform this function, if needed.

The keto-acid intermediates of amino acids are *subject to oxidation*, either directly or after transformation into other compounds, depending on the composition of the different amino acids (Fig.

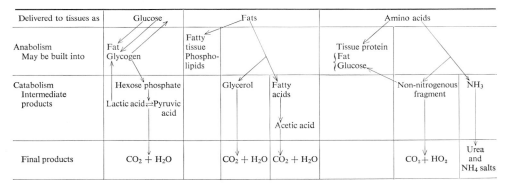

Delivered to tissues as	Glucose		Fats			Amino acids		
Anabolism May be built into	Fat Glycogen	Fatty tissue Phospho- lipids				Tissue protein {Fat {Glucose		
Catabolism Intermediate products	Hexose phosphate Lactic acid⇌Pyruvic acid		Glycerol	Fatty acids Acetic acid			Non-nitrogenous fragment	NH_3
Final products	$CO_2 + H_2O$		$CO_2 + H_2O$	$CO_2 + H_2O$			$CO_2 + HO_2$	Urea and NH_4 salts

Figure 14–5. Condensed summary of the metabolism of the three fuel foodstuffs—carbohydrates, fats, and proteins.

14–3). For instance, the simple amino acid alanine on deamination becomes pyruvic acid, which can readily be oxidized to carbon dioxide and water or used to synthesize glucose. Some amino acids, including alanine, are said to be *glucogenic* because the deaminized fragment may be converted into some intermediate of glucose synthesis. Other amino acids are said to be *ketogenic,* because on deamination compounds are produced which are oxidized like fatty acids. All of the deaminated intermediates can enter the citric acid cycle and be completely oxidized to carbon dioxide and water with ATP production by the electron transport system.

The fate of the **nitrogen-containing groups** split off from the amino acids presents a special metabolic problem. Most of this nitrogen (80 to 90 percent of the nitrogen excreted) is transformed into *urea* in the liver and **excreted in the urine,** since the body is unable to store protein or other nitrogen-containing substances to any considerable extent (except in growth).

One other fact needs to be pointed out. The amino acids that are deaminated and then oxidized of course yield energy, but the ones that are built into tissue protein yield no immediate energy to the body. If the diet supplies carbohydrate and fat in too small amounts to meet the body's energy needs and more of the amino acids from protein have to be burned for energy, the quota left for tissue building is reduced, or may even be wiped out. Hence, in growth, pregnancy, or recovery from wasting illness, when it is desirable to build up tissue protein in the body, sufficient food must be eaten so that protein will not be oxidized for energy but can instead be used for tissue protein synthesis.

A simplified summary of metabolism of the three energy nutrients is given in Figure 14–5. This diagram shows graphically that the final products of oxidation of all three are the same— carbon dioxide and water—with the exception of those substances formed from the nitrogen split off from the amino acids. If the food supplies energy in excess of body needs, the excess is built chiefly into glycogen or fat for storage. If the food supplies inadequate energy to meet body needs, the insufficiency is made up by destruction of some body materials—that is, by oxidizing first the stored glycogen and adipose tissue, and, finally the tissue proteins.

EXCRETION

Excretion is the process by which the body rids itself of **waste products.** True waste products fall into four general categories:

1. Materials that cannot be digested and absorbed.

2. Materials that, although absorbed, cannot be utilized.

3. Materials that are consumed or produced in the body in larger amounts than the body can use or is able to store.

4. The end products of the metabolism of foodstuffs, chiefly urea (and other nitrogen-containing substances) and excess carbon dioxide.

The *pathways* for the removal of waste products are also four in number —namely, the **lungs,** the **skin,** the **kidneys,** and the **intestine.** It should be obvious that material which has never been absorbed into the body proper passes out by the intestinal route, as discussed in the previous chapter. Substances of the second class (absorbed but not utilizable) are, if water-soluble, generally excreted by the kidney in the urine. An example of such materials is the artificial sweetener saccharine.

The third class of waste products is more common. They are useful to the body up to a certain level (which may vary according to circumstances) but are detrimental if allowed to accumulate. **Water** might be said to belong to this class, although technically it is not a waste product. Water is consumed in large amounts and is also an end product of the metabolism of foodstuffs. It is vital to the body welfare, yet the water balance in the body must be maintained. This usually calls for the excretion of a variable amount of excess water mostly through the kidneys but also by route of the skin, lungs, and feces. The excess of water-soluble vitamins, above the limited amounts that are needed or that can be held in the tissues, is also excreted in the urine.

Urea and other nitrogenous substances (end products of metabolism of protein and other nitrogen-containing substances) leave the body almost entirely through the kidneys. Excess **carbon dioxide** is excreted by the lungs.

Under the general heading of excretion it is sometimes helpful to consider all pathways of *ultimate loss* from the body, whether or not the substances removed are of any further utility. Dead cells and hair are constantly being lost from the body surface and, in a less conventional sense, may be thought of as waste products. Sometimes the excretion of one substance causes the unavoidable loss of another—for instance, water vapor (useful substance) is lost with carbon dioxide (waste product) in breathing. Likewise, where high environmental temperature causes profuse secretion of sweat for the useful purpose of cooling the body, the loss of sodium chloride may be excessive and require replacement (See Chap. 10).

Excretion Through the Lungs

Excess **carbon dioxide** passes into the blood from the tissues and is held in loose chemical and physical combinations in the circulating blood. When the blood reaches the lungs, it is brought into contact in the fine capillaries with air in the innumerable small air sacs of the lungs—that is, there is between the blood and air only a double membrane consisting of the very thin walls of the capillary and of the air sac, permitting the free exchange of gases. Accordingly, in passing through the lungs the blood loses about one-sixth of its carbon dioxide content in gaseous form to the carbon dioxide-poor air in the lungs and takes up from inspired air gaseous *oxygen,* which is carried to the tissues in loose chemical combination with the blood pigment, *hemoglobin.* Fresh air contains only 0.03 to 0.04 percent of carbon dioxide and about 20 percent of oxygen. The process of *respiration* in animals consists essentially of taking up 4 to 5 percent of oxygen from the inspired air and giving off 3 to 4 percent of carbon dioxide to the expired air. The inspired air becomes saturated with *water vapor* while in the lungs, which accounts for the considerable and constant loss of water through the lungs. Small amounts of other volatile substances present in the blood are also found in exhaled air (e.g., alcohol, ammonia, gases formed by intestinal bacteria); and gaseous substances present in inhaled air are absorbed into the blood (e.g., anesthetics, auto fumes).

Frequency of respiration is controlled by the *respiratory center* in the brain, this center in turn being chiefly affected by the *carbon dioxide content of the blood.* Thus, after exercise during which the production of carbon dioxide is more rapid, stimulation of the respiratory center causes an increased rate of breathing, with the result that the excess of carbon dioxide is removed from the body through the increased ventilation of the lungs. In ordinary shallow breathing only about one-sixth to one-fifth of the air contained in the lungs is involved, although the whole volume of air is probably fairly efficiently renewed at least twice every minute. Efficient respiration is an important factor in good health.

Excretion Through the Skin

Through the activity of the sweat glands in the skin, *water* is lost from the body in the perspiration, as well as salt, and small amounts of the diffusible substances present in plasma, such as urea, minerals, amino acids, and water-soluble vitamins. Under normal conditions, most people lose about a quart of water daily through the combined channels of the skin and lungs. The relative amount excreted by the skin is largely determined by the amount of perspiration needed to take care of ridding the body of excess heat—that is, under conditions in which *heat* is a waste product and must be removed for body temperature regulation. Solar radiation, *temperature* and *humidity* of the surrounding air, along with *exercise*, are the chief factors that most directly affect the amount of heat to

be removed and, therefore, the excretion of water from the skin.

Excretion by the Kidneys

The kidneys are *perfused by an exceptionally large amount of blood* from which they selectively remove waste products. The kidneys actively secrete other substances to form the final product—urine. Urine is secreted continuously (although more rapidly under certain stimuli), and is collected in the urinary bladder (Fig. 14–6).

The functional unit of the kidney is the *nephron,* in which blood enters a tuft, or network, of capillaries called the *glomerulus,* and is filtered through this into the surrounding double-walled, funnel-like *Bowman's capsule,* which leads to a tubule (Fig. 14–7). Only water-soluble substances of relatively low molecular weight can pass through the semipermeable membrane of the glomerulus and into the filtrate. These include salts, glucose, amino acids, vitamins, and limited amounts of simple proteins. Large protein molecules, lipids, and blood cells are retained in the blood stream unless the membrane is injured. It is the task of the cells that line the tubules to selectively reabsorb such useful substances as glucose and amino acids, along with large amounts of water, and to secrete certain other products into the urine, while efficiently removing waste products. Some substances are nearly completely reabsorbed by the tubule when their concentration in the blood plasma is at a normal level. For instance, glucose appears in the urine only when plasma concentration is high, as in diabetes, or when kidney tubular function is impaired. Other substances, such as sodium, potassium, and chloride, are either selectively reabsorbed or secreted, according to body needs. Waste products are reabsorbed only slightly or not at all. Both absorption and secretion are active processes requiring energy. That the work of the tubule

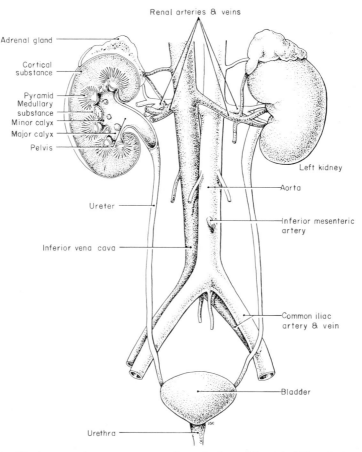

Figure 14-6. The human urinary system, seen from the front. The right kidney is shown cut open to reveal the internal structures. (From Villee, C. A.: *Biology,* 4th Ed. Philadelphia, W. B. Saunders Co., 1962.)

cells is very great may be appreciated from the fact that the volume of glomerular filtrate is 80 to 100 times larger than the final volume of urine excreted and is of vastly different composition.

Of the products excreted in the urine, *water* is by far the largest in quantity (urine is about 96 percent water). When an unusual amount of water is lost through the skin in hot weather, or during very active exercise, or through the alimentary tract during abnormal conditions (vomiting and diarrhea), the amount excreted by the kidneys is correspondingly less. Likewise, if the water intake is low, water is conserved in the body and the kidneys secrete a smaller volume of more concentrated urine.

The next most abundant constituents of urine are the *nitrogenous end products of protein metabolism* (see p. 84). One of these alone—*urea*—makes up about half the total solids of the urine and constitutes the form in which 80 to 90 percent of the nitrogen from metabolized proteins is excreted. Smaller amounts of *uric acid, creatinine,* and *ammonium salts* account for most of the remaining nitrogen in urine. These nitrogenous waste products can be eliminated from the body in significant amounts only through the activity of the kidneys.

Although some **mineral salts** are excreted by the intestine, the bulk of the salts leaves the body in the urine. *Sodium chloride* (common salt added to foods) is excreted largely in the urine. When the kidneys fail to function well, salt may accumulate in the blood and tissues, holding back sufficient water to dilute the salt to normal concentration in the tissues (see p. 229), thus causing the bloating or edema which often accompanies diseases of the kidneys. *Phosphates* and *sulfates* come chiefly from the metabolism of the proteins which contain phosphorus and sulfur. Other salts are largely those ingested in the food. There are a number of other substances which appear in the urine in only small amounts but which have important physiologic implications. Variable and usually minor constituents of the urine include pigments, hormones, vitamins and their derivatives, intermediate metabolic products, and detoxified substances.

FACTORS THAT AFFECT EXCRETION THROUGH THE KIDNEYS. For purposes of discussion, we may divide the factors which influence urinary excretion into two main groups: (1) physiologic fac-

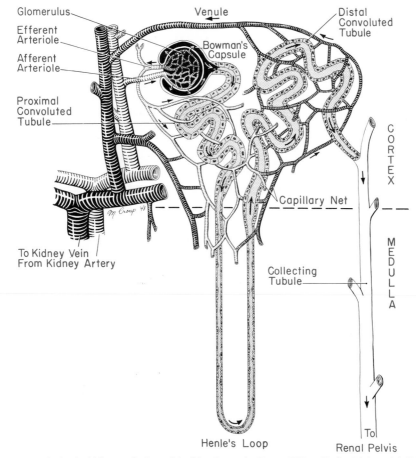

Figure 14–7. A single kidney tubule and its blood vessels (From Villee, C. A.: *Biology,* 4th Ed. Philadelphia, W. B. Saunders Co., 1962.)

tors—hormones, diuretics (substances which stimulate urine flow), and the amount of blood supply to the kidneys; and (2) dietary factors—that is, variations in the kinds and amounts of nutrients ingested, including water. The dietary factors are important, for they may alter the effectiveness of the kidneys in two of its most important roles:

1. Maintaining normal osmotic pressure and the concentration of electrolytes in body tissues and fluids—that is, the internal environment of body cells and organs;

2. Maintaining the acid-base balance of the body.

The pituitary gland secretes a hormone that decreases the volume of urine (an antidiuretic hormone), while the adrenal cortex elaborates hormones that affect mineral metabolism, especially the relative amounts of sodium and potassium excreted in the urine. Just as the respiratory center responds with increased activity to small increases in the carbon dioxide content of the blood, the secretion of these hormones by the pituitary and adrenal glands is triggered by small changes in osmotic pressure and by the composition and volume of body fluids, thus providing rapid response to alterations in amount of water and salts absorbed into or lost from the body.

The most common *diuretics* are coffee and tea. Both increase urine flow, owing to their content of caffeine (and related substances) which increase the rate of blood flow through the kidneys and alter the transport of salts and water by tubule cells. Another diuretic—alcohol—brings about increased urine flow by depressing the production of pituitary antidiuretic hormone.

A number of dietary factors may affect the *excretion of water* by direct effects on the kidneys. Healthy kidneys can concentrate substances dissolved in urine to a remarkable extent and can handle easily the salts (either ingested as such or arising from protein metabolism) and urea that need to be excreted

by a person on a normal, mixed diet. However, there is a limit to the extent of concentration the kidneys can achieve, and if such soluble substances are present in excessive quantities, additional water is required to dilute them to the point where they can be excreted. Normally, drinking more water can supply this need, but if the water supply is limited, the extra water needed is drawn from body fluids or tissues. This is why drinking sea water, which has such a high content of salts, takes water away from the body and thus is damaging to water-deprived castaways. Excretion of the large amounts of urea formed as a result of a very high protein intake may also require extra water. This may become important if water consumption is inadequate, if water loss from other routes is unusually large, or in some diseased states.

It is very generally recognized that drinking large amounts of water results in the excretion of a much increased volume of urine. This urine is very light in color and more dilute than usual in its content of dissolved solids. In other words, the amount of pigment and waste products excreted remains about the same, so that the extra water merely renders the urine more dilute.

The important part that the kidneys play in maintaining the normal level of electrolytes (chiefly ionized mineral salts) in the blood and tissue fluids, which in turn are largely responsible for normal conditions of *osmotic pressure*, should be apparent from much of the previous discussion.* The loss of sodium, potassium, and chloride from the body is regulated almost exclusively by the kidneys. Ordinarily the kidneys have no difficulty in keeping these substances at a normal level in blood and tissues by promptly excreting any excess amounts,

---

*The action of mineral salts in exchange of body fluids and in normal functioning of muscles and nerves was treated in Chapter 10 (pp. 228–229). Their role in maintenance of body neutrality was also discussed more fully in the same chapter (pp. 230–231).

and if losses from other routes are excessive (from sweat or diarrhea), urinary excretion may fall to very low values. In this way the constancy of amount of various mineral salts in the blood and extracellular fluids is safeguarded.

The kidneys play an important role in maintenance of body neutrality. Any increased level of acidic ions (chloride, sulfate, or phosphate) in the blood perfusing the kidneys is excreted as salts in the urine, after being balanced with ions of some fixed base (sodium, potassium, and to a much lesser extent calcium or magnesium). The kidneys conserve these basic elements and eliminate acidic groups, thus regulating the acid-base balance of the body. This is done by exchanging for basic elements hydrogen ions that are secreted by the tubular cells, shifting the form of phosphate eliminated from a more basic or a more acidic salt and forming a more acid urine. Under conditions in which there is a large excess of acidic products to be eliminated, the kidneys can produce ammonium groups and excrete some of the acid products as ammonium salts (see equations in footnote, p. 231).

Just as there is a limit to the degree to which soluble substances can be concentrated by the kidney, so there is a limit to the acid-base range within which urine can be excreted. Normally the acid-base balance of the diet is well within the functional range of the kidney. The chief acidic products of the diet are sulfates and phosphates formed in the process of protein metabolism. The organic acids found in most fruits and vegetables do not yield acid residues because they are oxidized in metabolism to carbon dioxide and water and are accompanied in the foods by large amounts of potassium and other basic elements. However, if very large amounts of organic acid (such as the 5 to 10 gm doses of ascorbic acid taken indiscriminately to counteract the common cold) are consumed, the urine will become acidic and extra minerals will be required for neutralization. The most frequently encountered instance in which large amounts of acidic substances must be excreted is when fat is incompletely oxidized in the body and acidic intermediate products of its metabolism (ketone bodies, see p. 524) accumulate, as in starvation and diabetes. Ingestion of extremely high-fat, low-carbohydrate diets has this same effect. Under these conditions, basic elements (chiefly sodium and potassium) are required for their neutralization, and thus they are lost from the body.

QUESTIONS

1. Define metabolism. Why is digestion not included in metabolism? What happens when the intake of energy is in excess of body needs? When it is inadequate for body needs?

2. Describe the metabolism of carbohydrate, covering the following points: the form in which it is absorbed from the intestine into the blood, the form in which it is carried in the blood to the tissues, the role of the liver in carbohydrate metabolism, the fate of glucose in the tissues (both that needed to supply energy and that in excess of immediate needs), and the final products of carbohydrate metabolism.

3. Describe the metabolism of fats, covering the same general points listed in Question 2 for carbohydrate metabolism. Describe the chemical changes that amino acids undergo in the tissues, including the fate of both the nitrogenous and non-nitrogenous parts of the molecule. What are the chief end products of the metabolism of the three fuel foodstuffs?

4. What common pathway do all three foodstuffs follow in the final stages of oxidation to carbon dioxide and water? Why is this route called a cycle? Why the citric or carboxylic acid cycle? What makes acetyl-coenzyme A such an important intermediate compound in the cycle? What are the advantages of

having a common pool of lower metabolites from all three foodstuffs?

5. What two products of metabolism are excreted through the lungs? When a man exercises, there is increased energy expenditure and hence increased production of carbon dioxide. How is this sudden excess of carbon dioxide excreted?

6. What is the chief substance excreted through the skin? What other substances are present in perspiration?

7. What waste products are excreted through the kidneys? In a normal person, what conditions cause an increased or a decreased output of each of the following in the urine — water, urea, sodium chloride, phosphates, and ammonium salts? Is urine normally acid or alkaline, and what may cause its reaction to vary?

SUPPLEMENTARY READING

Albanese, A. A., and Orto, L. A.: The proteins and amino acids. In Wohl, M. G., and Goodhart, R. S. (eds.): *Modern Nutrition in Health and Disease.* 4th Ed. Philadelphia, Lea & Febiger, 1968.

Alfin-Slater, R. B.: Absorption, digestion and metabolism of fats and related lipids. In Wohl, M. G., and Goodhart, R. S. (eds.): *Modern Nutrition in Health and Disease.* 4th Ed. Philadelphia, Lea & Febiger, 1968.

Calloway, D. H., Odell, A. C. F., and Margen, S.: Sweat and miscellaneous nitrogen losses in human balance studies. J. Nutr., *101*:775, 1971.

Devlin, T. M.: The relation of diet to oxidative enzymes. In Wohl, M. G., and Goodhart, R. S. (eds.): *Modern Nurtition in Health and Disease.* 4th Ed. Philadelphia, Lea & Febiger, 1968.

Eisenstein, A. B. (ed.): Gluconeogenesis: A symposium. Amer. J. Clin. Nutr., *23*:971, 1970.

Harper, H. A.: The metabolism of carbohydrates. In *Review of Physiological Chemistry.* 13th Ed. Los Altos, Calif., Lange Medical Publications, 1971.

Krebs, H. A.: The history of the tricarboxylic acid cycle. Perspectives Biol. Med., *14*:154, 1970.

Lennarz, W. J.: Lipid metabolism. Ann. Rev. Biochem., *39*:359, 1970.

Levine, R., and Haft, D. E.: Carbohydrate homeostasis. New Eng. J. Med., *283*:175, 1970.

Loewy, A. G., and Siekevitz, P.: The natural history of the cell. In *Cell Structure and Function.* San Francisco, Holt, Rinehart and Winston, Inc., 1969.

Mitchell, H. H., and Edman, M.: Nutritional significance of the dermal losses of nutrient in man, particularly of nitrogen and minerals. Amer. J. Clin. Nutr., *10*:163, 1962.

Pike, R. L., and Broen, M. L.: The cell. In *Nutrition: An Integrated Approach.* New York, John Wiley & Sons, Inc., 1967.

Nutrition Reviews

Human renal calculus formation and magnesium. *24*:43, 1966.

Formation of lipid-protein complexes. *24*:147, 1966.

Vitamin A and lysosomes. *24*:240, 1966.

Lipids and fat soluble vitamins in cellular metabolism. *24*:272, 1966.

Regulation of gluconeogenesis. *24*:347, 1966.

Dietary and hormonal influence on glycolytic and lipogenic enzymes of rats. *25*:315, 1967.

Renal failure in infantile malnutrition. *25*:350, 1967.

Dietary protein and acute renal failure. *26*:44, 1968.

Present knowledge of nutrition in inborn errors of metabolism (by Craig, J. W.). *26*:161, 1968.

Metabolism of fatty acids of the linoleate series. *26*:217, 1968.

Dialysis, renal failure, and vitamin homeostasis. *27*:75, 1969.

Mitochondria and cellular activity. *27*:154, 1969.

Nutrition in renal failure (by Berlyne, G. M.). *27*:219, 1969.

Diet and protein synthesis. *28*:25, 1970.

Glucose, free fatty acids, and insulin secretion. *28*:93, 1970.

Total protein turnover in animals and man. *28*:115, 1970.

fifteen

The Endocrine System and Regulation of Food Intake

The metabolism of the body is exceedingly complex. It is essential for the survival and proper functioning of the body that the multiplicity of individual chemical reactions be integrated and regulated in ways responsive to changing internal and external environmental conditions. There are two major coordinating systems in the body, the nervous system and the endocrine system. The nervous system is a complex system of fibers which deliver signals rapidly and repetitively to specific organs—muscles or glands.

The endocrine system consists of a number of small ductless glands scattered throughout the body. The glands use the blood circulating through them as a means of distributing their chemical messengers—hormones—in the body. Because hormones are very potent substances and are carried by the blood, small amounts are adequate to produce an effect on the cells of the target issues very soon after secretion by the gland.

The endocrine glands are interrelated and work together to regulate and coordinate the activities of the organism. Interaction of the endocrine system with the nervous system provides for the translation of external stimuli into signals to which the endocrine glands can respond. When the endocrine glands function normally, one is completely unaware of their existence and the metabolism of the body goes smoothly in all respects. When one or more of the glands become overactive or underactive, the normal equilibrium of the endocrine system is disturbed, leading to more or less grave abnormalities of metabolism, growth, sexual development, or body functioning.

INFLUENCE OF THE ENDOCRINE GLANDS ON METABOLISM

At least 30 hormones have been isolated and studied, and most of them can now be synthesized in the laboratory. Many are proteins (with relatively small molecules) and two are derivatives

341

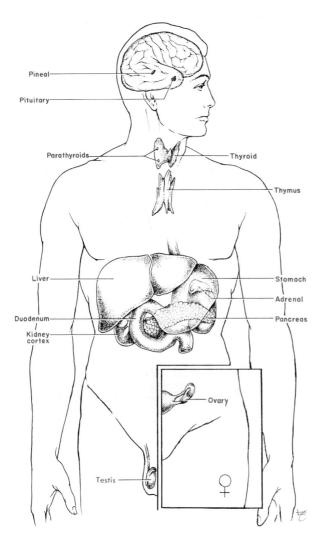

Figure 15–1. The approximate locations of the endocrine glands in man. Although the pineal body, thymus, and stomach are shown, they are not definitely known to secrete hormones. (From Villee, C. A.: *Biology.* 6th Ed. Philadelphia, W. B. Saunders Co., 1972.)

of amino acids; others are steroids, related to cholesterol. Comprehensive discussion of the endocrine glands, their numerous hormones, and the many effects of these secretions on the body is beyond the scope of this book. The discussion that follows is limited to the specific ways in which certain glands influence *metabolism and general nutrition.**

---

*We saw in the study of digestion (p. 315) that hormones are formed in the walls of the alimentary tract, and that they regulate motility of its organs and the flow of digestive juices.

Thyroid Gland

This gland consists of two lobes, located near the base of the neck, with a connecting isthmus across the trachea. Its chief function is to secrete an iodine-containing hormone, **thyroxine,** which has a powerful effect in regulating the *rate of oxidation processes* in the tissues (basal metabolism). As little as a single milligram of thyroxine raises basal metabolism 3 percent above normal. Apparently only about one-third of a milligram needs to be released daily from storage in the thyroid into the blood to keep basal metabolism at a normal level. Thyroxine is a derivative of the amino acid tyrosine, and has four iodine atoms in each molecule. As stored in the thyroid gland, it is part of a large protein molecule called thyroglobulin; it is slowly liberated into the blood as thyroxine, either free or combined with blood proteins. The thyroid hormone influences growth, mentality, and deposition of protein and fat in the body, as is evidenced by symptoms seen when the gland is abnormally under- or overactive.

When the thyroid is markedly *underactive* and secreting too little thyroxine, this is evidenced by *low basal metabolism* and sluggish mentality. A child who is born with the thyroid gland lacking or underdeveloped is called a **cretin** and is either a potbellied dwarf or a pudgy, stunted child with limited intelligence. Such a child may usually be made to grow and develop fairly normally by administration of thyroxine. Underactivity of the thyroid in later life results in a condition known as **myxedema,** because it is characterized by puffiness of the hands and face and thick, dry skin. Other symptoms are low basal metabolism, blunting of mental activity, sluggishness of body processes, and a tendency to put on weight. However, the commonly held belief that underactivity of the thyroid gland leads to fatness is erroneous. The greater proportion of weight gained is water held because of faulty tissue protein structure. Animals in which the thyroid gland is removed actually have a lower percentage of body fat than do normal animals. Basal metabolism may be markedly increased by giving thyroxine, which also induces improvement in the other symptoms.

Hyperthyroidism, or overactivity of the thyroid with secretion of thyroxine in too large amounts, is evidenced by an abnormally *high rate of basal metabolism*, emaciation, rapid heartbeat, nervousness, and frequently by protruding eyes. The energy need may be increased to two or three times normal, causing loss of weight in spite of increased consumption of food. The overactive gland usually becomes more or less enlarged, and such a condition is known as toxic or exophthalmic goiter (the latter name because of the eye involvement).

Simple goiter is a nutritional disease, brought about by an insufficient supply of iodine and is discussed in Chapter 12. The gland enlarges in an attempt to compensate by additional glandular tissue for the shortage of necessary material (iodine) for making its internal secretion (thyroxine). Basal metabolism may or may not be affected, depending on how successful the gland is in producing thyroxine under difficulties, but the symptoms of excessive thyroxine seen in toxic goiters are absent.

The thyroid gland secretes a second hormone, a small protein called *calcitonin.* This hormone lowers the calcium content of the blood and so acts antagonistically to the hormone secreted by the parathyroid gland (described below).

Parathyroid Glands

The parathyroid glands are minute structures, embedded in or closely associated with the thyroid gland, usually one pair to each lobe of the gland. These tiny glands were unrecognized for some time and so were removed along with the thyroid at surgery. When the parathyroids are completely removed, the amount of calcium circulating in the blood is so much reduced that **tetany** (rigid spasmodic contraction of the muscles) sets in, and death results. When they are underactive, blood calcium is below normal. In the rare cases wherein they are overactive, calcium is withdrawn from the bones, blood calcium is at a high level, and calcium and phosphorus are drained away in the urine. In **regulating the calcium content of the blood,** parathyroid hormone is intimately concerned in the metabolism of calcium, and it is the level of ionized calcium in the blood that regulates the secretion of this hormone.

Pancreas

The pancreas has both an exocrine secretion, pancreatic juice, which it pours into the digestive tract through a duct, and endocrine secretion, which it gives up to the blood. Pancreatic hormones are manufactured by special cells grouped throughout the ordinary glandular tissue. The pancreas secretes two hormones, both proteins, that affect carbohydrate metabolism—*insulin* and *glucagon. Diabetes mellitus* results from a *lack of insulin* activity. There is no known disorder related to faulty glucagon production or utilization.

Insulin is necessary to enable glucose to enter muscle and fat cells, hence to be utilized by the tissue cells. It also promotes the storage of glucose as *glycogen* in the liver and muscles. When the metabolism of carbohydrate is limited by lack of insulin, there is an increased burning of fats with production of the lower intermediates of fat metabolism (such as acetoacetic acid) in amounts greater than can be oxidized by the tissues. Protein metabolism is also deranged, with more amino acids converted to glucose than normal. The result of this condition is that glucose accumulates in the blood and is excreted in the urine, while if the condition is severe, acetoacetic acid and acetone also accumulate in the blood (acidosis) and are found in the urine.

In mild diabetes, the disease can often be held in check merely by *limiting the quantity of carbohydrate food eaten,* by reducing to or maintaining ideal body weight, and by taking more vigorous exercise. With only small amounts of sugars and starches to be broken down into glucose in the digestive tract, the amount of this substance carried to the tissues does not exceed what they can store or oxidize with the limited amount of insulin available. If more insulin is required to keep the patient in good nutritive condition, it must be injected because insulin, being a protein, will be destroyed by digestion if taken by mouth. Injection of suitable amounts of insulin causes the abnormally high blood sugar in diabetics to fall rapidly and return to normal. Slowly absorbed preparations of insulin are available which need to be given only once or twice a day.

When chromium is eliminated from the diet of rats, they have abnormalities of glucose utilization that resemble diabetes (Chap. 12). This observation has led to a search for evidence of chromium deficiency in older persons with diabetes, but an association has not been proved to date.

The second pancreatic hormone, **glucagon,** acts to increase blood sugar by increasing the rate of glycogen breakdown in the liver. Thus, the overall effect of glucagon is exactly opposite to the effect of insulin.

Adrenal Glands

The adrenal glands are two small glands located just above the kidneys. They are made up of two layers that have quite different endocrine functions—the interior portion, called the medulla; and an outer layer, called the cortex.

The major hormone secreted by the inner portion, known as *epinephrine (adrenalin),* is a derivative of the amino acid, tyrosine (phenylalanine). Ordinarily this potent hormone is released in very small amounts but under the influence of fear, anger, or other emotional states, extra quantities of epinephrine are poured into the blood and gear the whole body for the muscular action that would accompany such emotions under primitive conditions. The heartbeat is quickened, blood pressure rises, blood is shifted from the internal organs to the muscles, extra sugar is released from the liver into the blood, fat is mobilized, the blood content of free fatty acids rises, and oxidations in the tissues are temporarily speeded up.

The outer portion of the adrenal glands (cortex) secretes a number of hormones, all of which are steroids derived from cholesterol. All these hormones—but especially *aldosterone*—affect the metabolism of minerals and water by causing the retention of sodium and chloride and the excretion of potassium. When these hormones are lacking, there is increased excretion of sodium in the urine and subnormal sodium content of the blood. The concentration of potassium in the blood is abnormally high.

Four of the cortical hormones—including the well known *cortisone*—affect carbohydrate, protein, and fat metabolism in many ways antagonistic to insulin. They elevate blood glucose and increase production of glucose from protein breakdown. Their generally antianabolic influence on protein metabolism includes degradation of the protein matrix of bone with consequent loss of bone mineral. Among other effects, these hormones also stimulate the production of hydrochloric acid and pepsin by the stomach.

Under conditions of stress (such as injury, cold, and anxiety) epinephrine is secreted to meet the immediate emergency, but adjustment to living under stress is mediated by increased production of the cortical hormones. Excessive loss of nitrogen (protein) and calcium, elevated blood sugar, and ulcer formation (due in part to increased gastric acidity and enzyme activity) may thus accompany severe prolonged stress.

Cortisone also in some way acts to slow the growth of connective tissue cells and the formation of complex polysaccharides in these tissues. Injections of cortisone give relief from pain and crippling effects in some cases of rheumatoid arthritis. Continued administration of adrenal cortical hormones may be accompanied by undesirable side effects, which emphasizes the sensitivity of hormonal balance under normal conditions and the dangers of disturbing this balance.

Pituitary Gland

The pituitary gland, which lies in a groove at the base of the brain, is composed of two distinct parts called the anterior and posterior lobes. The smaller posterior lobe produces only one hormone of metabolic significance— the antidiuretic hormone that regulates conservation of water by the kidney. The anterior lobe, on the other hand, is often referred to as the *master gland* of the body because it secretes hormones that have a marked influence on the other endocrine glands and on total body growth.

The anterior pituitary hormones are called tropins—a term which indicates that they stimulate activity of other organs or glands. One of these hormones is said to be adrenocorticotropic, because it stimulates the adrenal cortex. This hormone, commonly referred to as ACTH, may be used for rheumatoid arthritis, because it produces indirectly the same general effect as giving one of the steroid hormones of the adrenal cortex (cortisone). The thyrotropic hormone stimulates the activity of the thyroid gland, and a group of tropins act on the reproductive glands. Frequently there is interaction between the anterior pituitary and one of the endocrine glands, which serves to regulate the amount of the hormone secreted by the target gland. For instance, a decline in the output of thyroxine causes the pituitary to secrete thyroid-stimulating hormone, while an increased output of thyroxine suppresses secretion of the thyroid stimulating hormone by the pituitary. Similar reciprocal relationships (called feedback mechanisms) exist with respect to the other tropic hormones and the specific organs on which they act.

The anterior pituitary also manufactures *growth hormone.* This hormone stimulates the growth of both long bones and soft tissues of the body and is anabolic, promoting retention of nitrogen, potassium, and phosphorus. It is one of the substances that contribute to the diabetogenic properties of pituitary secretion (inhibition of glucose oxidation and glycogen storage, effects directly opposite to those of insulin). ACTH also increases blood sugar and acts antagonistically to insulin.

It is clear that removal or destruction of the pituitary has profound effects on body development and endocrine function. If the pituitary is underactive in youth, marked dwarfing of growth results; in the adult there is lowered metabolism and increased sensitivity to insulin. Conversely, gigantism, or overgrowth of the long bones, occurs if pituitary hormone production is excessive.

PHYSIOLOGICAL REGULATION OF FOOD INTAKE[1]

All animals must eat to live during at least some stage of the life cycle, and all have some mechanism that directs them to take food. Behavior patterns are diverse, but in almost every case some control is exerted over the kind and amount of food that is taken. In some of the lower forms, food seeking and consuming behavior, presumably in response to a hunger signal, occupy most of their lifetime. Carnivores may eat enormously of a fresh kill and then not eat again for a long period; some insects eat but once between molts. Robins eat during the day, and mice mainly by night. Cats hunt optionally by day or night, depending on the relative abundance of robins and mice, or they may forego hunting in favor of a domestic bill of fare. Country cats are rarely fat, but the indulged household tabby very well may be. That is to say, basic inherent regulation of food intake exists in all species — regulation as to time, kind and amount of food — but can be abridged by environmental factors and learning.

Hunger and appetite are not synonymous terms. *Hunger* refers to the unpleasant group of sensations that are experienced when there is an urgent need for food. *Appetite,* on the other hand, means a desire for food whether or not the individual is hungry. Hunger is a physiologic condition, and while appetite has physiologic components, it is basically an affective state. *Satiety* refers to the set of conditions that exist when the individual stops eating because his hunger is satisfied, but it is recognized that hunger can be overcome without the food having satisfied the appetite fully. Most of us have taken a bit of sweet or a brandy after our true hunger has been satisfied; we are responding to a learned appetite directed according to the way our culture teaches a meal should be ended.

Regulation of Energy Balance

Most people maintain their weight reasonably well in spite of large day-to-day variations in physical activity and, thus, energy need. A person may sit in an office or classroom for the better part of five days a week and then spend almost the entire weekend in active recreation. Or a person may work in heavy construction all week and spend his weekend watching baseball in front of the television set. People do not necessarily eat sufficiently more food on days of increased activity, perhaps even the contrary, yet body weight shifts but little from week to week. Experiments with animals have shown that food intake is regulated each day, approximately according to the day's energy output. Superimposed on the daily regulation is a fine adjustment that corrects for small errors in the daily balance over a longer period of days or weeks. Humans show the same general regulatory pattern except that the daily regulation is less precise than in laboratory animals.

At very low levels of energy output, neither animals nor man are able to regulate energy balance precisely, with the result that both become fat. Similarly, at very high levels of forced work output, regulation of intake is inadequate to maintain body weight constant. Miraculously, over broad ranges of physical activity and food availability, input and output are nearly balanced. Average Americans gain about 20 pounds between ages 25 and 45, or about one pound a year. This yearly fat gain represents about 3600 kcal, which means that the error in balance is only 10 kcal per day or less than 0.5 percent of the requirement. Regulation is 99.5 percent accurate.

Gastrointestinal Factors

Hunger sensations occur simultaneously with contractions of the stomach. These contractions are forceful and recur in groups lasting for varying periods of time from a half hour to an hour and a half. A common experience is to feel hunger contractions which subside whether or not one eats, only to reappear later in greater intensity unless food is taken. Contractions are inhibited by a number of things, including simply tightening the belt (which probably gives rise to the use of that expression as denoting straitened financial circumstances). Eating food, of course, inhibits the contractions but so does tasting or chewing food without swallowing it, drinking cold water or alcoholic beverages, smoking, or experiencing the emotions of fear or hate. Contractions are enhanced by administration of insulin and inhibited by glucagon, hormones that respectively lower and raise the blood sugar level. Hunger contractions continue even when the main nerve to the stomach (the vagus nerve) is severed,* but the sensation,

the hunger pang, is no longer perceived. Severing the vagus nerve does not stop a person from eating the needed amount of food, so the awareness of hunger contractions is apparently not a necessary feature of food intake regulation.

Animals stop eating long before the full metabolic impact of a meal can be felt, so the gastrointestinal tract must participate in events that lead to cessation of eating. The act of eating and swallowing food is one possibility, but if food is prevented from reaching the stomach (by cutting through the esophagus), animals eat for a longer than normal period of time before stopping, and they begin eating again in a short period of time. If food is placed directly into the stomach by means of a tube (intragastrically), so that the animal does not taste, chew, or swallow the food, some lowering of oral intake occurs, depending on the volume of material administered by tube. In animals, intragastric volumes less than 20 percent of the normal intake are without effect on oral intake, but volumes in the order of 50 percent cause a compensatory reduction of intake. This happens no matter if the material given intragastrically is food or a bulk material without energy value. Young men also are reported to reduce their oral intake of a formula diet only if 40 percent or more of their usual oral energy intake was given intragastrically. Even then they consistently took more total energy (oral plus tube) during the days of combined feeding than when they ate only by mouth. However, when the men were not allowed any food by mouth and were required to administer their own intragastric feedings, they did consume an adequate amount of energy.[2]

Several stimuli are involved in the gastrointestinal contribution to cessation of eating. As the preceding discussion suggests, one is distention or stretch due to the presence of bulk which triggers neural responses. Nu-

---

*This nerve is sometimes cut surgically to stop acid secretion in persons with ulcers.

trient substances cause release of hormones that act to alter secretion in the alimentary tract (Chap. 13) and that also affect other hormonal systems, specifically insulin and glucagon. Thus, the gastrointestinal system anticipates and initiates the integrated mechanisms that ultimately stop one from eating.

The Hypothalamus

Attention was focused on a specific portion of the brain as containing a regulatory feeding center when French pathologists observed at autopsy that very obese people had lesions in that area (Fig. 15–2). Because of their anatomic proximity there was some question if the regulatory center was in the pituitary gland or in the hypothalamus, with which it is intimately connected. Development of an instrument capable of destroying a minute area in the brain of a living animal made possible experiments which proved that the center is in the hypothalamus. In the early 1940's Heatherington at Chicago and Brobeck at Yale reported that destruction of two small areas located in the central portion of the hypothalamus (the ventromedial portion) caused rats to eat voraciously and become obese.

That is, the rats became hyperphagic because the satiety center had been destroyed. Later, Anand and Brobeck discovered that destruction of two areas in the side region of the hypothalamus (the lateral portion) caused just the opposite effect: the rats refused water and food, and starved to death unless forcibly fed. This meant that they had destroyed the center that causes an animal to eat and drink. Mayer and his colleagues at Harvard proved that the failure of animals to eat after destruction of the lateral centers was not due to the failure to take in water, and subsequent research has shown that the eating and drinking centers are separate but quite near each other in the rat. Since then, lesions have been made in chickens, cats, dogs, monkeys, and goats, and all show similar anatomic locations and feeding responses. Electrical stimulation of the feeding and satiety centers causes the reactions that would be expected. Stimulation of the satiety center causes animals to stop eating, and stimulation of the feeding center causes them to eat. Precise location of the drinking center is easier in some animals than others—the goat, for instance—and stimulation of this area of the hypothalamus causes an animal to drink whether or not it is thirsty,

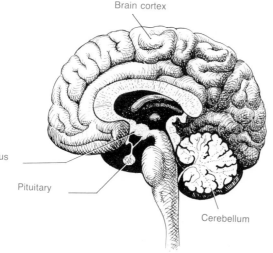

Figure 15–2. Located in the hypothalamus are centers that control eating and drinking. Note that the hypothalamus is adjacent to and exerts some control over the pituitary gland.

thus disproving an old adage; as Mayer has said, you can now lead a (goat) to water and you can make him drink.

Further study of the hypothalamic centers has shown that the satiety center is dominant in regulating eating behavior. It is thought to act like a brake on the feeding center. Arees and Mayer have succeeded in mapping the nerve fibers in the hypothalamus and have found connections between the two centers.[3] Once the control center was located, further research uncovered the signal to which it responds.

Glucostatic Theory of Regulation

The glucostatic theory of food intake regulation, put forward by Mayer, postulates that there are receptors in the satiety center that are especially sensitive to glucose and are activated according to the rate at which it is being utilized. When food is taken, blood sugar rises and the rate of glucose utilization in the tissues rises. The receptors are stimulated and the satiety center signals the responses to stop eating. Conversely, some hours later, blood glucose falls and the receptors detect low utilization rate; the brake is released and eating begins.

An important distinction is that the hypothalamic receptors are responsive to *utilization* of glucose rather than to the level of glucose in the blood. In the disease diabetes, appetite is high even though blood sugar levels are elevated. The normal fuel of the brain is glucose, and the brain is different from most other tissues in the body in that it does not require insulin in order to utilize glucose. With respect to glucose utilization the hypothalamus behaves in the same way as the other body tissues (muscle, fat, etc.). That is, unlike the rest of the brain of which it is a part, the hypothalamus is not able to use glucose without insulin. In diabetes, the message would be "food is needed," irrespective of the fact that the blood sugar level is high.

Animals with lesions in the hypothalamus have other alterations in behavior than simply those relating to the amount of food eaten. Operated rats are less active, have diminished libido, and have altered responses to test situations involving food. They are more encephalized. Placed in a situation where they must risk a shock to obtain food, they are less responsive to hunger than is the normal animal. The animal with a lesion is also more prone than the normal to reject food that has an unpleasant taste (for instance, with quinine added to it). Depending on how precisely placed the lesion is, animals may have deranged water intake, as noted earlier, and they may be unable adequately to regulate body temperature. All of this suggests that regulation of the most vital animal processes is even more complex and interrelated than we now appreciate and that there is participation of higher brain centers in all these functions.

Long-Term Regulation of Energy Balance

Little is known about the mechanism whereby the daily small errors in energy regulation are compensated so that body weight remains nearly constant, if that is appropriate; or so that weight is regained after an illness or period of food deprivation. A lipostatic theory of regulation is currently the most accepted. This theory requires that precise information on the current level of fat stores be relayed from the adipose tissue to the nervous control center. If the stores are filled, the animal is directed to stop eating; but if the stores are low, eating continues past the point at which the satiety center is usually activated. Several observations provide general support for this theory. One is that animals with lesions in the satiety center do not go on gaining indefinitely but stop at some degree of obesity. If the obese lesioned animal is then starved, when food is again available it regains its original obese weight, not some other degree of fatness. Also, when rats are made fat by forced feeding, they subsequently reduce their voluntary food intake until the excess weight is lost.

What this adipose tissue sensor might be is unknown, but an endocrine substance has been postulated. The probability of a humoral substance is suggested by an observation made in animals that are joined surgically, so that their blood interchanges but their organs remain separate (parabiotic preparation). If one member of the pair has the satiety center destroyed, it becomes obese; the other member of the pair becomes thin. Presumably this happens because some message is transmitted from the large adipose stores of the fat partner through the blood to the regulatory center of the normal pair member; energy intake of the normal partner is then reduced because excessive fat stores have been sensed.

REGULATION OF ESSENTIAL NUTRIENTS

Besides energy regulation, animals somehow must manage to select diets that are nutritionally adequate or they cannot live and reproduce. Adequacy could be coincidental to satisfaction of energy needs because, in nature, nutrients are not found singly. Food plants and animals are all mixtures of organic compounds and minerals, and animals come to occupy an ecologic niche where the food available to them matches their needs for energy and nutrients. However, animals do show specific hunger for isolated nutrients—salt is a familiar example—and to some extent they are able to choose the better of nutritional alternatives. Given a choice of mixed diets that are protein-free or

contain an adequate amount of protein, rats eat very little of the poorer one. Rats will also eat a reasonable balance of two diets that have widely different protein qualities, but they do not make very fine discriminations between proteins that are marginally different. When they are required to select among pure foodstuffs (pure protein, pure fat, and sugar), some animals are able to do so, but others within the same strain and age group are unable to do so. There is little information regarding human capability in this respect, but in one brief study men were unable to select a complete mixture of amino acids over one that was lacking a single essential amino acid.[4]

Specific Hunger

Specific hunger refers to the situation in which an animal is deficient in one nutrient and seeks out that specific nutrient. Some specific hunger is thought to be genetically determined in that animals can recognize a substance in which they are deficient and will go to it selectively, even if they have never before been deficient in that nutrient. Salt is thought to be in this class. Other specific hungers are learned, as illustrated in Harris'[5] classic experiments with rats deficient in B vitamins.

The general pattern of experiments was to deprive rats of the vitamin B complex or a single B vitamin, thiamin. The animals were then offered diets flavored with easily recognizable substances which were thought to mask the vitamin odor: Bovril (without B vitamin) or yeast or marmite, both containing B vitamin. The deficient rats reliably learned to select the diets containing the vitamin, but nondeficient rats showed no such preference among the diets. However, if animals made deficient were given a large number of diets (six to ten) only one of which contained the missing vitamin, they were unable to pick the correct one. The rats could be taught to choose the correct diet by giving them a training period when only that diet was given; later, when all the different diets were offered again, the rats would continue to choose the one they had learned contained the vitamin. If the vitamin was then removed from that diet and added to a diet with a different flavor, the rats continued to eat the previously learned, but now deficient, diet. They could be re-educated to accept the new flavor of diet by repeating the process of offering only one choice while they were in a deficient state. This indicates that the ingestion of the vitamin that had been lacking caused some reaction in the animal's body that provided a sufficient cue to establish learning. Additional experiments with pantothenic acid, which does not have a readily identifiable taste or odor (as thiamin does), showed that the rats did not seek out a vitamin per se, but rather a flavor because they were unable to find the vitamin unless a recognizable flavor was added to direct their choice of diet. Thus, the animals sense well-being, but there is nothing innate about vitamin recognition.

Ability to Choose a Balanced Diet

Perhaps nutritional food habits are formed by a comparable learning process. Animals that are deficient in one or more nutrients may try eating something in their environment, and if they feel better according to some internal cue, they learn that this is what animals should eat. That this mechanism is faulted is well known, because animals will eat things that they like to their detriment. Animals will founder in a corn field, birds eat fermented fruit to the point of drunkenness which shortens their life span if predators are handy, and people seem to prefer sweet, rich foods over the simpler ones, in spite of internal cues that signal satiety and intellectual awareness of too much body fat.

One famous experiment is usually cited as proof that man can choose his diet wisely. Davis[6] allowed three newly weaned infants to choose their own diets from among thirty common natural food materials. The choice was restricted to foods thought suitable for infants, and neither mixed dishes nor sweets were offered. Two of the infants were studied for six months and the other for a year. At first the babies tried anything in their mouths—inedible plates as well as edible foods—but they became selective and developed definite tastes. Their food preferences were erratic and unpredictable and their diets were not balanced within a day. Sometimes the babies would indulge in binges, eating many oranges a day for several days and then none, for instance. Some of the babies' choices did suggest specific selection. They ate salt only rarely and obviously did not enjoy it, even crying when they took it, but they did go back for more. Davis regarded her experiment as flawed, in retrospect, because she had limited the possible choices the babies might make to what her knowledge dictated they should have, and she thought the test might otherwise have failed. However, the infants did balance a diet from among 30 options daily, and their health and growth were acceptable by 1928 standards.

In sophisticated man, appetite seems to be a somewhat fickle guide to choosing an adequate diet. Some individuals are always found to have poor intakes in any group of people, in spite of abundant availability of nutritious foods. For this reason, guides are needed to good eating, based on scientific knowledge of nutrient requirements and accumulated human wisdom as to what constitutes suitable food.

QUESTIONS

1. What are the endocrine glands, and what is a hormone? What is the hormone secreted by the thyroid gland, and what unique constituent does it contain? How does the thyroid hormone influence metabolism, and what are the effects of oversecretion and undersecretion of this hormone?

2. What gland secretes insulin and what is its role in carbohydrate metabolism? In what disease is insulin activity deficient? What symptoms are indicative of insulin lack, and in what ways may the disease be treated?

3. For each of the following endocrine glands, tell what influence their hormone or hormones have on metabolism: adrenal cortex, parathyroids, and anterior lobe of the pituitary gland. Why is the pituitary gland called the master gland of the body?

4. Over what periods of time is energy balance regulated? Where is the regulatory center located? How was this proved to be the regulatory center? What change in the body causes the center to be activated? What mechanisms are involved in long-term regulation of energy balance? How does the gastrointestinal tract participate in regulation of energy balance?

5. What is meant by specific hunger? Is specific hunger genetic or learned? Do human beings have the ability to select an adequate diet? Justify your answer.

6. If you were a nutritionist or a physiologist, what question relating to food intake regulation would you wish to investigate? What factors do you think might affect a person's preference for specific foods other than the ones discussed in this chapter? What factors might affect his acceptance of food?

REFERENCES

1. Code C. F. (ed.): *Handbook of Physiology*, Section 6, Volume I: Food and Water Intake. Baltimore, Williams & Wilkins for Amer. Physiol. Soc., 1967. (All material in this section, unless otherwise noted.)

2. Jordan, H.: Voluntary intragastric feeding: oral and gastric contributions to food intake and hunger in man. J. Comp. Physiol. Psych., *68*:498, 1969.

3. Arees, E. A., and Mayer, J.: Anatomical connections between medial and lateral regions of the hypothalamus concerned with food intake. Science, *157*:1574, 1967.

4. Bowering, J., Margen, S., and Calloway, D. H.: Failure of men to select a balanced amino acid mixture. J. Nutr., *99*:58, 1969.

5. Harris, L. J., Clay, J., Hargreaves, F., and Ward, A.: Appetite and choice of diet. The ability of the vitamin B deficient rat to discriminate between diets containing and lacking the vitamin. Proc. Roy. Soc. Lond., Ser. B, *113*:161, 1933.

6. Davis, C. M.: Self-selection of diet by newly weaned infants. Amer. J. Dis. Child., *36*: 651, 1928.

SUPPLEMENTARY READING

Endocrine System

Arnaud, C., Glorieux, F., and Scriver, C. R.: Serum parathyroid hormone levels in acquired vitamin D deficiency of infancy. Pediatrics, *49*:837, 1972.

Bergström, S., Carlson, L. A., and Weeks, J. R.: The prostaglandins: A family of biologically active lipids. Pharm. Rev., *20*:1, 1968.

Catt, K. J.: ABC of endocrinology. Lancet, *1*: 763, 1970.

Delange, F., Camus, M., and Ermans, A. M.: Circulating thyroid hormones in endemic goiter. J. Clin. Endocrinol. Metab., *34*: 891, 1972.

Dyck, W. P., Texter, E. C., Lasater, J. M., and Hightower, N. C.: Influence of glucagon on pancreatic exocrine secretion in man. Gastroenterol., *58*:532, 1970.

Freedland, R. A., Murad, S., and Hurvitz, A. I.: Relationship of nutritional and hormonal influences on liver enzyme activity. Fed. Proc., *27*:1217, 1968.

Frye, B. E.: *Hormonal Control in Vertebrates.* New York, The Macmillan Company, 1967.

Gill, G. N.: Mechanism of ACTH action. Metab., *21*:571, 1972.

Hamwi, G. J., and Tzagournis, M.: Nutrition and diseases of the endocrine glands. Amer. J. Clin. Nutr., *23*:311, 1970.

Jennings, I. W.: *Vitamins in Endocrine Metabolism.* Springfield, Ill., Charles C Thomas, 1970.

Luhby, A. L., et al.: Vitamin B_6 metabolism in users of oral contraceptive agents. I. Abnormal urinary xanthurenic acid excretion and its correction by pyridoxine. Amer. J. Clin. Nutr., *24*:684, 1971.

Rose, D. P., and Braidman, I. P.: Excretion of tryptophan metabolites as affected by pregnancy, contraceptive steroids, and steroid hormones. Amer. J. Clin. Nutr., *24*:673, 1971.

Regulation of Food Intake

Ashworth, N., et al.: Effect of nightly food supplements on food intake in man. Lancet, 2:685, 1962.

Cabanac, M., and Duclaux, R.: Specificity of internal signals in producing satiety for taste stimuli. Nature, *227*:966, 1970.

Durnin, J. V. G. A.: "Appetite" and the relationships between expenditure and intake of calories in man. J. Physiol., *156*:294, 1961.

Hervey, G. R.: Regulation of energy balance. Nature, *222*:629, 1969.

Hoebel, B. G.: Feeding: Neural control of intake. Ann. Rev. Physiol., *33*:533, 1971.

Kekwick, A., and Pawan, G. L. S.: Body weight, food and energy. Lancet, *1*:822, 1969.

Leopold, A. C., and Ardrey, R.: Toxic substances in plants and the food habits of early man. Science, *176*:512, 1972.

McCance, R. A., chmn.: Symposium: The regulation of voluntary food intake. Proc. Nutr. Soc., *30*:103, 1971.

Peng, Y., and Harper, A. E.: Amino acid balance and food intake: Effect of different dietary amino acid patterns on the plasma amino acid pattern of rats. J. Nutr., *100*:429, 1970.

Yaksh, T. L., and Myers, R. D.: Neurohumoral substances released from hypothalamus of the monkey during hunger and satiety. Amer. J. Physiol., *222*:503, 1972.

Nutrition Reviews

Central nervous system centers and regulation of lipid mobilization. *24*:283, 1966.

Thyroid status and adipose tissue lipolysis. *25*:252, 1967.

Diet preferences and specificity of hungers in rats fed diets deficient in various vitamins and minerals. *26*:25, 1968.

The effect of gastric distension on activity of single neurons in the hypothalamus. *26*:87, 1968.

Plasma growth hormone in childhood. *26*:241, 1968.

Nicotinamide deficiency and adrenocortical steroids. *26*:343, 1968.

Cues affecting eating behavior and obesity. *27*:11, 1969.

Glucagon interaction in the pancreatic duodenal axis. *27*:90, 1969.

Malnutrition and the pancreas. *27*:100, 1969.

Transferable intestinal factor which depresses body weight. *27*:123, 1969.

Food intake and brain temperature. *28*:17, 1970.

Parathyroid mediation of magnesium-calcium interrelationships. *28*:129, 1970.

The feeding center and body weight regulation. *28*:216, 1970.

The hypothalamus and food intake regulation in response to amino acids and protein. *29*:20, 1971.

Parathyroid hormone effects on mineral absorption and excretion. *29*:257, 1971.

Metabolic actions of growth hormone. *30*:79, 1972.

Part Three

Applied Nutrition

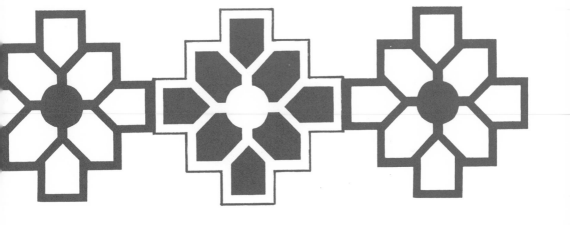

sixteen

Food Habits and Beliefs

Food is one of the basic needs of existence. In every society which has been studied, food plays a central part in beliefs of the people about life and health, and is included in some fashion in sacred rituals. Joy is celebrated in feasts, for which, whether it is an American Thanksgiving dinner or a European country wedding, special, more expensive foods are obtained and prepared. Ritual overeating may be practiced at such times. There is scarcely a group which does not express hospitality to a guest through an offer of food or drink, and through such customs a whole etiquette may evolve into a tradition.

The importance of food to life is recognized by its use in nonfood ways, especially among pretechnologic peoples, in magical rites, and in divination. Women guests at a Malay wedding are given hard-boiled eggs dyed red and formed into flowers, as a symbol of fertility. Guests at an American wedding throw rice at the departing bride and groom in a similar gesture. A form of punishment in or out of prisons has been reduction of food to bread and

water. Mothers sometimes withhold sweet desserts from a child for some infraction of their rules. Political or spiritual leaders go on hunger strikes to make a point or force an issue.

Food is a powerful force in society. It may truly be said that, while culture forms the diet, the food of a people also molds the kind of culture in which it is eaten. Nutrition is just one expression of this force.

Food habits and beliefs about properties and qualities of foods have a profound influence on nutritional status through their effect on the selection of diet by the individual who holds them. A classic case in point is the deficiency disease pellagra, discussed more fully in Chapter 7. It was highly prevalent among poorer people in the southern United States in the early years of this century when diets consisted of maize cornmeal, molasses, fatback, some greens, and very little meat or other foods of animal origin. This diet was chosen from what was economically and culturally available. Among corn eaters in Latin America, however, pellagra does not exist despite low animal protein intakes. This is due to the cultural practice of pounding cornmeal with limestone before making it into the flat-bread, tortilla. Laboratory research[2] showed that this indigenous practice, arrived at empirically, made the previously chemically bound niacin in the corn available to the consumer.

Food beliefs and food practices of different population groups have long been observed and documented by anthropologists and ethnographers, but the effect of these attitudes on nutritional status has been relatively little studied until recent years. One such study[3] demonstrated that Malay women's beliefs prohibiting foods considered "cold," or "cooling," to the body in the 40 days following childbirth resulted in deficiency, as measured in the blood, of folacin, vitamin A, and carotene. The foods defined as "cold" included nearly all fruits and vegetables. The women were afraid that if they ate them, air would enter their bodies and damage the tissues, causing them to bleed.

Food habits tend to persist among people entering another social group after other cultural differences are erased. Nutritionists and social scientists would like to know what causes changes in selection of types of foods people eat, and whether and how such changes might be directed. A good deal of research has been applied to these problems, which center around habits of choice of foods to eat. Food *habits* are often the result of economic pressures. *Beliefs* about food and its properties, on the other hand, are often more subtle and more resistant to efforts at alteration. Beliefs about food are usually woven into the fabric of a society or group; they are an integral part of the culture. To learn the reasons behind them we must often study the whole structure of the society for an explanation of their role. This kind of research has not been done so widely as have studies about food habits and their change.

NUTRITION AS A PART OF CULTURE

Eating is one of the fundamentals, essential to all life. But even for a Robinson Crusoe or a dedicated misanthrope, eating is done in a cultural setting. The ways of the group determine who is served first, who shall get which portions of which foods offered, how much may be eaten — Thais, for example, are reared to believe it is greedy to take more than the smallest morsel of the foods served with rice — and what utensils shall be used. In most American and European households, families eat together around a table, each from his own plate. Asians have separate bowls of rice and help themselves to side dishes with fingers, chopsticks, or spoons, often sitting or squatting on the floor (Fig. 16–1). Some Africans sit around and dip their fingers in the common pot. The choicest food, the most expensive cut of meat, is offered to a guest, or eaten by the men of the household. In many societies, women eat apart from or at a later time than the men. Children, too, often come at the end of the line of distribution of cooked food, with nutritional implications for reduction in availability and variety of foods and nutrients. And if father won't eat leftovers, a thrifty housewife often warms them over for herself, lowering their vitamin content in the process.

The culture or society defines a meal, both as to time and content. We would not call the usual coffee break, or the hot dog, potato chips, and popcorn eaten at a game, a meal. Americans tend to take tea when they are ill, or as an iced drink in hot weather. However, to a host of Britons and many other peoples, tea is a meal, small or large, which precedes (evening) dinner, and consists of a cup or more of hot tea and cakes, sandwiches or sometimes even more substantial food. Tea precedes breakfast in certain countries, British and others, sometimes accom-

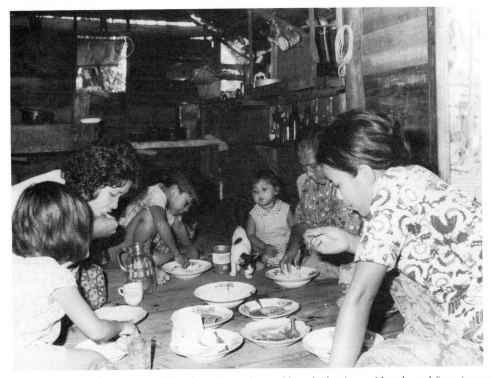

Figure 16–1. Eating customs differ throughout the world, and what is considered good form in one culture may be unacceptable in another. Even within a culture, accepted modes may vary from one social group to another. In this Malay family, the traditional food service of the fishing village is used, in which each member serves himself from communal bowls placed on the floor and eats his own food with fingers. (Courtesy of Dr. C. Wilson, University of California.)

panied by fruit or bread. Western people like to complete a meal by serving a sweet dessert. Continental Europeans prefer cheese and fruit. Many Americans like to start the day with fruit. In other parts of the world as far apart as South America and Southeast Asia fruit is never eaten save as a snack food, picked from the trees in passing, or brought home from market for immediate consumption, as though it were candy or chewing gum.

Just as we buy jars and cans of foods especially prepared for babies, so other groups. define certain foods as "children's foods." Often, these are fruits. There are also people who delimit consumption of some foods to women only, or prohibit them to girls who have not yet reached maturity.

Most cultures have a staple food which they believe is fundamental to existence. Around this food, beliefs, rituals, and traditions have sprung up. Jelliffe[4] has called them "cultural superfoods." Thus to that large portion of the world which subsists on rice, a meal is usually defined as a time when rice is taken. A morning meal of other foods is considered a snack. For many Asians, a customary greeting is, "Have you taken rice?" If the answer is affirmative, it is considered that all is well with the speaker. The Indians of the Americas revered the maize corn, and much of their cultural activities related to its cultivation and propagation. Rice among Malays is imbued with a spirit which is both respected and perpetuated through rituals. We ourselves speak of "the staff of life," while admitting "man does not live by bread alone," thus defining our basic staple.

Diet Patterns — How They Come About

Despite the coast-to-coast dispersal of certain restaurant companies selling hamburgers and soft drinks, and of national food store chains, there are still regional as well as ethnic differences in the kinds of foods eaten in this country. New England has its baked beans and codfish cakes on Saturday night. Southerners like cornmeal whether served as spoonbread or hush puppies, a "mess" of greens and other components now classed as "soul food." Black-eyed peas are not readily available in all markets out of the South, and one finds more tacos, enchiladas, and refried beans in areas of large concentrations of Mexican-Americans. An order for fried eggs for breakfast in the South will be served accompanied with hominy grits. In New England and parts of the Midwest the plate will include fried potatoes instead.

The reasons for these differences are several. Some components of diets are chosen due to local availability of foods, what grows well, or what is easily obtained. Now that we have refrigerated storage and transport country-wide, our theoretical choice is very large indeed. Out-of-season foods and scarce gourmet items can be ours at any time, provided we are only able and willing to pay the price. But this situation is relatively new, and diet habits, once established, tend to persist. Current diets thus reflect to some extent what was available at periods in the past.

It should be noted that no group of people which has been studied thus far ever eats all the potential edible commodities available to it. For various cultural or other reasons some things are still not defined as food, though they may safely be eaten.

It is probable that taste, physiologic reactions subsequent to eating a particular item (whether a food was toxic or not), and local climatic, environmental, and economic conditions determined what foods made up the diet of pretechnologic man. Traditional diets under which people have lived satisfactorily for long periods, and which have been studied for their nutritive value, have been shown to meet the known requirements of the population. Thus empirical trial and error over time produced a diet suited to the individual from potential foods he was free to choose.

Foods that could be kept well for long periods under prevailing living conditions would be selected for storage for later consumption in areas where food could not be raised the year round. Many American farm families used to have root cellars to keep carrots, onions, potatoes, turnips, and other food for winter consumption. The Eskimo still uses the permanently frozen ground as his storage area for berries and similar foods. Africans, South Americans, and some Southeast Asians who depend upon tapioca (cassava or manioc) roots as a carbohydrate source often leave them in the ground until the need for them arises. Grains traditionally have been kept in large dry containers, such as elevators in the American midwest. Asians dry fish or make fermented fish products for later consumption. In a like way, South Americans dry beef, and cheese and other milk products are altered for longer useful nutrient life.

There have always been some people who do not store any food. Thus New Guineans eat all their fish catch at once. One of the functions of feasts among traditional people when an animal or animals are killed is probably the very practical one of disposing of all the meat while it is still in excellent condition so far as nutrient content and taste are concerned. From such activities, when observed by technologically oriented people, may have come the long-held view of eating patterns of traditional peoples as "a feast or a famine."

Different national groups who have settled our country brought with them many different cuisines which have persisted, though sometimes in altered form. However, other forces have had far more profound influence on the American diet in the last generation. We are all aware that advertising in newspapers, magazines, radio, and television, and food industry innovations such as convenience foods, frozen specialties and frozen complete dinners, "instant" drinks, and "instant" almost everything else edible have introduced new foods and new ways of eating. The U.S. Department of Agriculture, which regularly keeps track of these things, has found that the foods we are now buying or being persuaded to buy provide us less of the nutrients that the National Research Council recommends we take every day than was true 10 years earlier. The U.S. Department of Agriculture 1965–6 Household Consumption Survey showed that diets which met these recommended daily nutrient intakes dropped from 60 percent of those studied in 1955 to 50 percent in 1965. In the same time, diets considered "poor," that is, meeting less than two-thirds of the recommended dietary allowances, rose from 15 to 20 percent of the families studied.

Parrish has presented the reasons for these changes.[5] Most could be considered cultural as well as nutritional. Families now raise only a little of their own food compared with 30 years ago, and prepare much less food at home. Snacking has increased as a general food habit, and people prefer their snacks to be convenience foods. More meals are eaten away from home, and more people are skipping meals. Increasingly parents don't fix breakfast for children who claim they are "not hungry" anyway. Food now uses a relatively smaller amount of the family budget. With this decline in dollar value, time and interest given to food

have lessened. Prices of individual food items have changed over time. While the price of eggs and chicken has dropped 7 to 10 percent, those of fruits and vegetables have risen 22 to 50 percent higher than they were 10 years earlier. It is not hard to see why families are now buying less of the latter. People are increasingly following dieting and health food fads. Among other effects, dieting limits the selection of foods one can eat. Finally, Parrish cites present preferences for convenience foods, which are particularly low in vitamins A and C.

Whoever goes out to obtain the foods and prepare them for the family's consumption is usually the final arbiter of what is served at family meals. This is true whether all foods are bought from the nearest supermarket, selected at a peasant village market and brought home on foot in a shopping basket, or gathered in the fields and carried on the head of a tribeswoman. Children may act as friendly persuaders, with more or less success depending on the leniency of the mother or the culture. And the personal preferences of the male household head are usually considered. But, leaving aside gifts, or a producing farmer or fisherman, it is the homemaker who decides what foods will enter the home. For this reason, efforts in nutrition education are primarily directed to homemakers.

In this country, as indicated by Parrish's report, the cultural patterns of eating have been changed drastically by changes in economic patterns. More mothers have full-time jobs outside the home. Much less time is spent on meal preparation at home. More meals are eaten out, including children's lunches at school. Margaret Mead, commenting on the North American diet pattern in 1943,[6] remarked, ". . . father presides over meat and fish, the mother over milk, vegetables, fruit juices and liver, while adolescents . . . demonstrate their independence by refusing to eat what is good for them." Perhaps only the description of the teenager is as true and applicable today as it was a quarter century ago.

While the quality of the diet of the average present-day American concerns nutritionists, we do still have a wide potential choice of foods from which to select all the nutrient sources we need, using our knowledge of nutrition and a little intelligent thought. However, a number of subgroups or cults with widely different diets from the norm have sprung up among us. Most of these people have little basic nutritional information. These groups, in attempting to attain perfection through a "natural" diet, have many proscriptions and taboos. Some of them are good; we could all learn from some of their simplifications of diet. However, the zeal with which these people have limited their potential food choices has also eliminated some needed nutrients. Erhard has recently described some of these food cults, from personal observations and study.[7]

All those studied were Caucasians and all were vegetarians. Diet is the focus of their philosophy and their living habits. Some of them will eat milk, cheese, and eggs; some omit eggs; others, vegans or pure vegetarians, spurn all animal foods, including seafoods, eggs, and dairy products. Those who follow Zen Buddhism are influenced by the Chinese philosophy of *yin* and *yang*, and try to achieve a balance between the two by adjusting amounts of *yin* foods (relaxing ones) and *yang* foods (activating ones), eaten together. Meat is too *yang* and hence is discouraged, though not strictly prohibited. Fruitarians (who eat only raw or dried fruits, nuts, honey, and olive oil), and others who eat only organic foods observe fasts as part of their regimen. One group observed an "acid fast" by drinking only citrus or tomato juice one day a week to "clean out the system." These people treat all diseases by herbs, special manipulations of allowed foods, and proprietary vitamin preparations. Those who condemn animal products need to plan very carefully to obtain enough nutrients from the foods they allow themselves to eat (see Chapter 18). Erhard found that, all too often, they do not have the knowledge to do so.

Another subgroup whose food habits are often deleterious to nutritional status are dieters (see Chapter 23). The faulty food habits which led to overweight in the first place are frequently replaced by others which may shed pounds and deplete nutrient stores at the same time.

Food Beliefs—Prescriptions and Proscriptions, Preferences and Aversions

The folklore of food of the United States population has been studied far less than it has for many other cultures. Examination of food beliefs and rituals is the province of the social scientist, ethnographer, anthropologist, or psychologist rather than the nutritionist. Thus, although we have a large body of published material on food habits which is potentially relevant to nutritional status—what people eat in different cultural groups in this country, how prepared and when—we have far less written information on what American people believe about foods. What is available is chiefly part of studies by anthropologists of various ethnic groups in specific localities. Most ethnographic studies—descriptions of the lives and customs of a particular population group—include a section on usual diet and beliefs and rituals concerning foods.

However, though they have not yet been compiled in a readily available resource, there is a body of food ideology in the culture of the United States. Consider, for example, the long-held belief that fish is brain food. Or that eating red meat is strengthening, especially for athletes. Cannibalism arose originally, it is said,[8] because man wanted to destroy the ghost of his killed enemy or relative, and acquire his courage. Although the views in the two last sentences are not too far apart, not eating our fellow is Western man's foremost taboo. One does not hear so much now of the dangers of combining certain foods at the same meal. Fish and ice cream if consumed together were once believed by many Americans to cause "ptomaine" poisoning. We still eat oysters when they "R" in season. Some fallacious food beliefs held by people in the United States are presented, with refutations, in Table 16–1.

There seem always to have been superstitions and false theories about food in this country. It is possible that the present ideas are echoes of the food beliefs of our more traditional forefathers.[9, 10] Some of these current beliefs or fads are exploited by "health food" manufacturers and quack "doctors" at considerable profit to themselves. Fad foods are big business. It has been estimated that at least 10 million people spend well over half a billion dollars a year on special foods, food supplements, and "health" lectures or literature. Many persons who are without adequate scientific nutrition information can be readily persuaded to try fad foods, especially if their pur-

veyor makes exciting promises and tells a likely story which jibes with the individual's own folklore. Many of these health foods sell for higher prices than regular foods. People believe that raw sugar, wheat germ, honey, and alfalfa sprouts have health-giving properties superior to those of the ordinary wholesome food in the grocery stores.

Some food fads may do little harm except to relieve one of money that might be spent more profitably. Sometimes the suggestion and belief that benefit will be derived is sufficiently strong to be a force that makes for improved health (if the cult is a relatively harmless one). If the special diet is administered at a sanatorium, improvement in health may also be induced by baths, outdoor life, and more exercise. Often a fake diet may give a false sense of security or hope of relief to a person suffering from a disease or disorder for which it promises a "sure cure," thus causing him to forego consulting a doctor for proper diagnosis and treatment. The quack will claim success in curing diseases for which medicine has yet to find a cure. Patients who suffer from severe and chronic disease conditions not only obtain no relief but may delay seeing a doctor until it is too late.

Table 16–1. Refuting Erroneous Ideas About Foods

Fallacies	Facts
About certain foods Onions—cure a cold. Fish—is a brain food. Celery—is a nerve tonic. Oysters—increase sexual potency.	Foods in the same food group are more or less interchangeable, and the different tissues take up whatever nutritive elements they need from the blood stream, to which common reservoir of body-building materials all foods have contributed when they were absorbed after digestion. Special foods do not build special tissues.
Lemons—aid digestion. Oranges—cause acid stomach.	Acid fruits are supposed by some to be a cure for dyspepsia and by others to cause acid stomach. The stomach secretes a digestive fluid that contains hydrochloric acid, which is many times more strongly acid than lemons. If we did not have an acid stomach, conditions would be very abnormal and unfavorable for digestion.

Table continued.

Table 16–1. Refuting Erroneous Ideas About Foods (Continued)

Fallacies	Facts
Meats — necessary to build muscle and red blood. — extra amounts needed for muscular work. — poison the system.	Meats, especially organ meats, are excellent sources of iron, protein, and B vitamins, which are important for regeneration of red blood cells and plasma proteins. However, other foods, such as eggs and leafy vegetables, also furnish these nutrients. The energy for muscular work comes mostly from oxidation of carbohydrate and fat. If meats are inspected (free of bacteria and spoilage), kept refrigerated, and well cooked, they can have no harmful effects.
Combinations of foods Some food combinations are to be feared or shunned (fish and ice cream, tomatoes and milk).	Fear of certain foods or food combinations is psychologically bad and may lead to one-sided diets which do not provide essential nutrients in adequate quantity. When eaten in moderate amounts and under proper conditions, there are no foods that are incompatible. Selection of foods from all food groups, in the suggested number and size of servings, furnishes a better balanced diet, and thus one that is better for building health.
Nature cults Foods should be eaten in their natural state, mostly raw.	It is good to eat some foods raw, but others (such as whole grains and meats) are usually cooked to soften fiber, develop flavor, and promote their digestibility. If properly cooked, the loss of minerals and vitamins is moderate.
Natural sugars, such as honey and raw sugar, are better for one than refined sugar.	Although one may enjoy honey or raw sugar for the traces of impurities which give them flavor, they are no better as body fuel than refined sugar (cane or beet). The small amounts of minerals and vitamins in the unrefined products do not add appreciably to the whole days quota, which must be furnished chiefly by other types of food.
Opposition to use of Iodized salt	Adding small amounts of iodide to refined sea salt is simply replacing the iodine lost in the refining process. Use of iodized salt has proved a safe and effective way of preventing simple goiter in regions where both the water and soil are iodine-poor.
Fluoridated water	Addition of fluorine compounds to city water supplies in areas where water has less than normal amounts of this element represents regulating the naturally low fluorine content to a level that is entirely safe but sufficient to effectively reduce dental caries.
Pasteurized milk	Pasteurization of milk gives important protection against harmful bacteria and does insignificant damage to the nutrients in milk, except for some loss of vitamin C. The normal content of this vitamin in milk is too low and undependable to be counted on in the diet, so that it must be supplemented anyway by one or more rich sources of this vitamin.

Table 16–1. Refuting Erroneous Ideas About Foods (Continued)

Fallacies	Facts
Highly milled grains — should never be used	Either whole or highly milled grains are good sources of energy and furnish some protein. However, the removal of the embryo and outer coats of the grain in milling involves loss of a relatively large proportion of the original content of higher-quality protein, of minerals, B vitamins, and all the vitamin E (in the embryo). Whole-grain products tend not to keep as well in storage, and thus the highly milled products are favored by millers and bakers. If bread and cereals made with highly milled grain are used, they should be of the "enriched" variety — with several B complex vitamins and iron added to replace amounts lost in milling, and other rich sources of the missing nutrients must be included in the diet. Although whole grains have a higher content of minerals and vitamins, bread and cereals made either from the whole grains or from highly milled ones, when enriched, are good food. White (patent) flour is not rendered poisonous by bleaching, as the faddists claim.
Devitalization by overprocessing The American food supply is devitalized by overprocessing.	Some processes do result in lowered nutrient content. Commercial firms take care to protect food flavor, color, and texture. This requires use of techniques that coincidentally tend to conserve nutrients better than home preservation does. Factories for canning or quick-freezing are located in the midst of areas where special crops are produced. Foods are canned in sealed tins from which air has been evacuated before the sterilization process. Dehydrated foods are processed at relatively low temperatures, under conditions (such as in vacuum) in which water is lost quickly. Special packaging also helps conserve vitamin content of foods before they reach the consumer.
Food additives are poisons.	Substances added to foods must pass rigid tests that the foods themselves were never required to do, and the probability is that most are safer than some substances in casual food use (cassava, nutmeg etc.). Some common additives are nutrients (vitamin C to prevent browning) and another can substitute for a vitamin (the antioxidant BHT for vitamin E).
Vitamin and mineral concentrates — Are needed by most persons.	The federal Food and Drug Administration has stated: "According to the subclinical deficiency myth, anyone who has 'that tired feeling,' or an ache or pain in almost any part of the body, is probably suffering a 'subclinical deficiency' and needs to supplement his diet with some concoction. . . . Of course, no normal person can go through even a small part of his life without experiencing some of these symptoms. There is no basis for believing that they are usually due to subclinical deficiencies."

The food quacks of today probably take the place of the medicine man of traditional cultures, and of the vendors of patent medicines in the United States of an earlier era.

We are all familiar with some religious fiats concerning foods. Few would need to be reminded that Hindus keep the cow sacred and uneaten, and that Muslims and Jews have stringent dietary rules forbidding consumption of a wide variety of protein sources. Roman Catholics used to substitute fish for other flesh foods in order to fast on Friday. Many Western people would feel they were committing cannibalism if they were to eat either dog or horse meat. They would perhaps experience a physical revulsion at the idea of dining off their animal friends. Yet dog is relished by some Africans, and the Chinese have long considered dog flesh a delicacy. Horse meat was reintroduced at times of scarcity in Europe in the eighteenth and nineteenth centuries, and is still eaten in some Western countries and by some Western peoples to this day. Indeed, it has been a popular menu item at the Harvard Club in Boston for many years! During the food shortages of World War II it is probable that many people in the United States ate horse meat without being aware of it.

Many theories have been put forth to explain the Biblical food prohibitions against the meat of pigs and other animals that do not chew the cud or cleave the hoof, first presented to the Israelites in Leviticus xi, 27. Douglas, writing recently, suggests that these prohibitions may have been only an attempt by the priests to restrict animals eaten to those meeting their definition of perfection as part of the worship and sacrifice in the Temple, rather than a codification of the dangers of eating undercooked pork.[11]

Chicken used to be a food reserved for special occasions in the United states. When chicken rearing moved from the back yard to big batteries of broiler and egg factories, prices went down and chicken became one of our best meat buys. However, chicken and their eggs are avoided by some social groups. They have been traditionally important in divination for many societies, both the eggs and the entrails and bones of the chicken. To some Southeast Asian tribes, cocks are sacred. To others, cockfighting is a highly popular sport. Simoons, who has detailed avoidances and uses of animals as food throughout the Old World,[12] suggests that chickens, which were domesticated in Asia, were probably initially bred from the wild for their role in religious rites rather than as food.

Food beliefs and all traditional medical systems are rather closely entwined. This is particularly true of the Ayurvedic (traditional Hindu) and Chinese medical systems. This fact is being demonstrated repeatedly in a new discipline called medical anthropology. A few generations ago the arrival of spring was the signal for a dose of "sulfur and molasses," or eating a boiled-up mess of dandelion greens. Some people still "feed a cold and starve a fever." Folk medicine survives among subgroups or in out-of-the-way areas in our own country. Not so many years ago a Vermont doctor made a bit of money selling honey and vinegar as a twentieth century cure-all, and even published a book about it.

Latin Americans, including Mexicans who have emigrated to our country, ascribe to most foods an assumed physiologic "heating" or "cooling" effect. These beliefs about innate characteristics of food that can be transferred to those eating them are found throughout a large part of the world. Latin Americans obtained them from the colonizing Spaniards, who in turn probably received them from the Moors. They were spread by the Arabs along with Islam to Southeast Asia, including Indonesia, the Philippines, and the Malay Peninsula. Mainland Chinese hold similar beliefs.[13] The ultimate origin of these beliefs that foods are of themselves "cold" or "hot" is not yet known with certainty. We find an echo of it in our own saying, "cool as a cucumber." These categorizations have nothing to do with temperatures of the foods, nor does "hot" mean the peppery hotness of red chilis.

To most persons holding these views other things besides foods, including illnesses, have "hot" or "cold" properties. The assignment of the quality of "hot" or "cold" is not, however, consistent from one population group to another, or even among the people within the group who have these beliefs. Thus, some societies will define an illness as "hot" and try to bring the body into balance by treating it with food or medicine having "cooling" properties, or vice versa. Some cultural groups try to "balance" the diet by setting "hot" foods against "cold" ones at the same meal. This practice is observed by the Chinese and many Latin Americans. Others, like Malays, allow only people culturally defined as quite healthy to eat "cold" foods. Clark, while studying a Mexican community in California, found that women who wish to conceive, as well as those who have just given birth, must avoid "cold" foods, fruit juices, tomatoes, and most vegetables as "too cold" for the stomach.[14] Pork, ordinarily defined by most people in the community as "hot," is also to be avoided by the lying-in woman. If she eats them, she will get varicose veins of the leg. Like the Malay woman,[3] the Mexican women in this California community observed the dietary proscriptions against "cold" foods for 40 days. Those more traditionally oriented continued them until the child was weaned, which at the time of the research was anywhere from 6 to 8 weeks to a year or 18 months.

We have numerous subgroups in the United States with their own distinctive diets and cuisines, not yet wholly altered by contact with supermarkets and advertising. Puerto Ricans, Seventh Day Adventists, Amish, American Indians, health food advocates and Southern Negroes, to name a few scarcely considered in this chapter, are all peoples who for various cultural reasons (such as religion, economics, or habitual choice) eat differently from Anglo-Americans. Though their food habits may be known, little study has been made of their beliefs about food and its properties, to see how far they may deviate from present-day scientific knowledge, or what effect their beliefs may have upon nutrient intakes of the groups in question. Much more needs to be done in this area.

It should be emphasized that food beliefs and practices which differ from our own are not all deleterious. Again and again, as Mead[15] points out, traditional groups have been found to have an adequate diet either because they ate parts of plants or animals discarded elsewhere (such things as eyes, or adrenals, for instance, sources of riboflavin or ascorbic acid, respectively), or combined various kinds of food in proper proportions for a good balance of vitamins, amino acids and other known nutrient needs. Problems arise with such diets when they are changed in some ways by the groups eating them coming in contact with other types of foods which seem more desirable but are not balanced nutritionally.

Lee[16] has described an extreme example of nutritional adaptation to a rather harsh environment in his study of the Bushmen of the Kalahari Desert. Their diet consists solely of edible items available in the area. They have various reserve foods used in emergencies when climatic conditions interfere with the usual food supply. The diet is nutritionally adequate, and they do not suffer in periods of shortage of their usual staple, a local nut.

One other aspect of beliefs about food which can influence nutrient intake is the relative status which certain foods are accorded. Sometimes prestige is attached to scarce, high-priced items, making them sought after. We can think immediately of white flour and white bread, which replaced natural "black" bread in Europe in the last century. These same products have been considered prestigious and hence have been much sought after when introduced to peoples in developing regions of the globe, despite higher prices than those of the indigenous foods for which they substituted. The same has been true for polished white rice, sweetened canned condensed milk, biscuits (sweet cookies), and other foods once reserved for the upper social strata. Sometimes low status foods are good nutrient sources, and their consumption ought to be encouraged rather than looked down on. Many cultures consider local indigenous greens "emergency" or "poor folks" foods, and although they may eat them they are most reluctant to allow outsiders to know of it. The Indians of the high Andes of South America have low regard for the local grain *quinoa,* which grows only in this region, despite its being one of their staples. Chemical examination has showed it to be high in protein, calcium, phosphorus, iron, and niacin.[17] Seacoast Southeast Asians who dry their surplus fish catch for times of scarcity consider dried fish far less desirable than fresh.

There are foods classed by different groups as unfit for human consumption, despite their being as nutritious as the usual dietary components. Efforts to introduce sorghum to one country were futile because the people considered it donkey food. Recommendations to add sweet potatoes to the rations of troops of another country deficient in vitamin A were rejected because sweet potatoes were usual food for swine. Maize corn has been grown in Europe for centuries, but except for Eastern Europe and the Iberian peninsula it is used as animal feed. Its fairly recent introduction to Southeast Asian countries for this latter purpose has had a reverse side influence: it is sold by

shops and sidewalk vendors, boiled on the cob, as a snack food.

Changing Food Habits

Authorities agree that food habits are one of the most difficult things to try to change. Especially in countries where problems of malnutrition have reached serious proportions, government authorities would like to know how to alter traditional patterns of feeding that nutritionists have shown to be deleterious, or how to induce new, more nutritious foods. But food habits do change spontaneously, all the time, and new foods are constantly being introduced. The potato, maize corn, chocolate, cassava, tomato and cashew are just a few foods which were taken by the Spanish conquerors of the New World back to Europe, from which they have spread worldwide. Latter-day conquerors of a different sort have caused refined flour and sugar and cola and other soft drinks to be available in nearly every corner of the globe.

The problems that changing food habits present are indeed complex, and there do not appear to be any simple answers, although knowledge has progressed beyond an earlier attitude that people would change their "bad" food habits if only they were told how to do so. During the Second World War the U.S. National Research Council established a Committee on Food Habits which examined some of the cultural and psychologic aspects of eating and made some concrete suggestions for improving diets.[6, 18] The Committee was created, among other reasons, to help encourage consumption of less familiar foods among the population at home when much that was customary had been diverted for troop feeding abroad.[19] Diet improvements included introduction of substitutes resembling familiar foods, and enrichment. Research supported by the Committee showed the importance of emotional and cultural components of attitudes about food in choice of diet.

Problems of food habits that are changing undesirably or of undesirable ones that should be changed are important everywhere now in the developing world where sudden changes in the social and economic environment are taking place. An international conference on malnutrition and food habits in 1960 stated the situation that still exists, and suggested some ways to work toward solutions.[17]

New foods may be accepted if they resemble some already-liked item in taste or texture. Foods already eaten by leaders or other prestigious persons, or foods with a money value, are also more likely to be incorporated into diets. It is far more difficult to eradicate undesirable food habits. And it seems likely that, once people have begun to change, it would be futile to try to hold them back to the more traditional way of eating that they are trying to abandon. When attempts are made to change food habits it has always to be remembered that what is really being changed is part of the culture. When changes in the culture go along with the changes in food practices in ways which help reinforce and encourage the latter, both have a better chance of success.

Burgess and Dean[17] have emphasized that food habits which are learned very early in life in a pleasurable home environment are most resistant and difficult to change. Other workers have found that the food habits of some people do change more readily when they move to a very different cultural setting. At present there are no formulas that would permit prediction in advance as to whether or not a particular habit or group of attitudes will respond to efforts to guide or direct changes.

Because an individual's choices of food are affected by so many variables, such as climate, availability, religion, emotions, taste, economics, local agricultural practices, and customary traditions, many factors must be studied

and considered before attempts at change are made. Many disciplines are combining to contribute further to knowledge about this area. Much still remains to be done.

QUESTIONS AND PROBLEMS

1. Make a list of any prejudices that you may have against the eating of certain foods or combinations of foods. Are these prejudices warranted in the light of facts? Are you inclined to indulge in certain well liked foods or classes of food to the exclusion of other food groups that are needed for proper nutrition? Have you any dietary fads or fancies?

2. Talk with several other persons, and make a list of any superstitions about food, prejudices against or in favor of certain foods, or practice of dietary fads, which you may find among these people. Which of these may have some basis in fact and which are not based on reason? Give reasons for your conclusions.

3. Discuss causes—physical, economic, psychological, or emotional—why persons develop and persist in faulty food habits or take up with food fads. Make suggestions on ways to induce such persons to alter their food habits.

REFERENCES

1. Harris, R. S.: The nutrition problem of Mexico. J. Amer. Dietet. Assoc., 22:974, 1946.
2. Laguna, J., and Carpenter, K. J.: Raw versus processed corn in niacin-deficient diets. J. Nutr., 45:21, 1951.
3. Wilson, C. S.: Food beliefs affect nutritional status of Malay fisherfolk. J. Nutr. Educ., 2:96, 1971.
4. Jelliffe, D. B.: *The Assessment of the Nutritional Status of the Community.* WHO Monograph Series No. 53, Geneva, World Health Organization, 1966.
5. Parrish, J. B.: Implications of changing food habits for nutrition educators. J. Nutr. Educ., 2:140, 1971.
6. Mead, M.: The Problem of Changing Food

Habits. Washington, D.C., National Academy of Sciences–National Research Council Bulletin 108, 1943.

7. Erhard, D.: Nutrition education for the "now" generation. J. Nutr. Educ., 2:135, 1971.

8. Wagner, P. M.: Food as ritual. In *Food and Civilization, A Symposium.* Springfield, Ill., Charles C Thomas, 1966.

9. Deutsch, R. M.: Who's to blame for nutrition nonsense? Today's Health, *May*:66, 1967.

10. Stare, F. J., and Nelson, P.: Don't fall for fads. Family Health, 2:41, 1970.

11. Douglas, M.: *Purity and Danger. An Analysis of Concepts of Pollution and Taboo.* Harmondsworth, England, Penguin, 1970.

12. Simoons, F.: *Eat Not This Flesh. Food Avoidances in the Old World.* Madison, University of Wisconsin Press, 1967.

13. Hart, D. V.: *Bisayan Filipino and Malayan Humoral Pathologies: Folk Medicine and Ethnohistory in Southeast Asia.* Data Paper No. 76. Ithaca, New York, Southeast Asia Program, Cornell University, 1969.

14. Clark, M.: *Health in the Mexican-American Culture.* Berkeley, University of California Press, 1970.

15. Mead, M. (ed.): Nutrition. In *Cultural Patterns and Technical Change.* New York, United Nations Educational Scientific and Cultural Organization, New American Library, 1955.

16. Lee, R. B., and DeVore, I. (eds.): *Man, The Hunter.* Chicago, Aldine, 1968.

17. Burgess, A., and Dean, R. F. A.: *Malnutrition and Food Habits.* New York, Macmillan, 1962.

18. National Reasearch Council: *Manual for the Study of Food Habits.* Washington, D.C., National Academy of Sciences–National Research Council Bulletin 111, 1945.

19. Mead, M.: *Food Habits Research: Problems of the 1960's.* Washington, D.C., National Academy of Sciences–National Research Council Publication 1225, 1964.

SUPPLEMENTARY READING

Blix, G. (ed.): *Food Cultism and Nutrition Quackery.* Symposia of the Swedish Nutrition Foundation VIII, 1970.

Bruhn, C. M., and Pangborn, R. M.: Reported incidence of pica among migrant families. J. Amer. Dietet. Assoc., 58:417, 1971.

Caron, H. S., and Roth, H. P.: Popular beliefs about the peptic ulcer diet. J. Amer. Dietet. Assoc., 60:306, 1972.

DeGarine, I.: Food is not just something to eat. Ceres, 4:46, 1971.

Deutsch, R. M.: *The Nuts Among the Berries.* New York, Ballantine, 1961.

Dubois, C.: Attitudes toward food and hunger in Alor. In Spier, L., Hallowell, A. I., and Newman, S. S. (eds.): *Language, Culture and Personality.* Menasha, Wisconsin, Sapir Memorial Publication Fund, 1941.

Gelfand, M.: *Diet and Tradition in an African Culture.* Baltimore, Williams & Wilkins Co., 1971.

Haag, W. G.: Aborigine influence on the southern diet. Pub. Health Rep., 70:920, 1955.

Harwood, A.: The hot-cold theory of disease. J. Amer. Med. Assoc., 216:1153, 1971.

Knutsson, K. E., and Selinus, R.: Fasting in Ethiopia. An anthropological and nutritional study. Amer. J. Clin. Nutr., 23:956, 1970.

Nobmann, E. D., and Adams, S.: Survey of changes in food habits during pregnancy. Pub. Health Rep., 85:1121, 1970.

Oddy, D. J.: Food in nineteenth century England: Nutrition in the first urban society. Proc. Nutr. Soc. (Gt. Brit.), 29:150, 1970.

Rappaport, R. A.: *Pigs for the Ancestors: Ritual in the Ecology of a New Guinea People.* New Haven, Yale University Press, 1968.

Renner, H. D.: *The Origin of Food Habits.* London, Faber & Faber, 1944.

Richards, A. I.: *Hunger and Work in a Savage Tribe. A Functional Study of Nutrition Among the Southern Bantu.* Glencoe, Illinois, Free Press, 1948.

Richards, A. I.: *Land, Labour and Diet in Northern Rhodesia. An Economic Study of the Bemba Tribe.* London, Oxford University Press, 1951.

Sakr, A. H.: Dietary regulations and food habits of Muslims. J. Amer. Dietet. Assoc., 58:123, 1971.

Seshadri, S., and Harrill, I.: Nutrient intake of college students from India in the United States. Nutr. Rep. Int'l., 3:159, 1971.

Sherlock, P., and Rothschild, E. O.: Scurvy produced by a Zen macrobiotic diet. J. Amer. Med. Assoc., 199:794, 1967.

Simoons, F. J.: Primary adult lactose intolerance and the milking habit: A problem in biological and cultural interrelations. I. Review of medical research. Amer. J. Digest. Dis., 14:819, 1969.

Stasch, A. R., Johnson, M. M., and Spangler, G. J.: Food practices and preferences of some college students. J. Amer. Dietet. Assoc., 57:523, 1970.

Wellin, E.: Maternal and infant feeding practices in a Peruvian village. J. Amer. Dietet. Assoc., 31:889, 1955.

Wolff, R. J.: Meanings of food. Trop. Geogr. Med., 17:45, 1965.

Yudkin, J., and McKenzie, J. C. (eds.): *Changing Food Habits.* London, MacGibbon & Kee, 1964.

Nutrition Reviews

Diets of the people on Tristan da Cunha. *25*:104, 1967.

Sociological techniques in nutrition studies. *26*:297, 1968.

Nutritional science and society (by Gordon, J. E.). *27*:331, 1969.

Food technology and society (by Pyke, M.). *28*:31, 1970.

seventeen

Food: From the Producer to the Consumer

In the preceding chapters, you have learned about the individual nutrients (water, proteins, carbohydrates, fats, vitamins, and minerals) and their functions in the body. In nature these nutrients are the chemical structures which comprise almost all of the plant, animal, or human body. Life has been sustained for short periods on highly purified mixtures containing only these nutrients. However, since not enough is yet known about man's requirements, it would be highly risky to attempt to live on nutrients isolated from any source or synthesized in the laboratory.

Not only would it be risky; it would probably be unpleasant and monotonous. Can you imagine sitting down to dinner to find your plate laden with a string of peptides, a scoop of triglycerides, a serving of polysaccharides, a salad of ascorbic acid and carotene, a sprinkling of nicotinamide and a pinch of alpha-tocopherol? These are some of the essential nutrients you take in when you eat a juicy steak, baked potato, and tossed green salad; a pizza; or a hamburger, noodles, and green beans. The nutrients essential for life are incorporated in the *food* you eat.

Food, while serving as a vehicle for bringing man his nutrients, also fulfills the need for variety, sensory pleasure, and social identification (see Chap. 16).

Thus, nutritionists who are concerned with nutrients in the body are also concerned with how to get these vital factors into the body. This chapter will deal with the channels through which nutrients travel to reach your body, from the production, processing, and distribution of food to the planning and preparation of meals.

PRODUCING, PROCESSING, AND DISTRIBUTING FOOD

In the United States, as in most countries, over 96 percent of our food is derived directly or indirectly from the land. Those who farm the land are responsible not only for growing the cereals, fruits, and vegetables man eats, but also for growing the grains to feed the animals which man eventually eats. From the land, farmers and ranchers raise crops, breed fish and poultry, and herd cattle. But food ultimately leaves the farm—in the form of plants, milk, eggs, or animals—in order to benefit the bulk of the population. Man must seek out food in order to obtain the energy and the essential nutrients present.

The Marketing Economy

Some primitive peoples in various parts of the world gather what food is growing nearby, but for most of the world's population, this process of getting food means going to some kind of market. Markets have arisen to fill wants or needs for such things as salt, spices, and other condiments not available locally, as well as for luxury goods and nonfood articles such as metal cooking pots, cups and glasses, and other utensils.

At its simplest, a market can be someone sitting by a roadside selling surplus fruits he has raised or eggs to passing neighbors. Food on an American breakfast table is there as a result of a very complex market system. It might include melon grown in Texas, toast made from wheat grown in Kansas and made into bread in a large city bakery nearby, coffee from Central America or Brazil, sugar grown in Louisiana or Hawaii and refined in California or Boston, bacon from hogs raised in Iowa or Tennessee, and marmalade made in Scotland from bitter oranges grown in Spain. All this food reached the family down a long chain of middlemen—food brokers, food industries, shippers, and truckers—until it reached the shops or supermarkets where it was bought and brought home to serve.

In a simpler society, a very different breakfast could still have reached the consumer by similar routes, though from differing origins. As an example, in rural Southeast Asia some peasant women add to the family income by making small cakes, the usual breakfast food, to be sold to other women via shops or to be peddled from house to house. These cakes may be either of

rice or of wheat flour. Sometimes the rice is home grown. More likely, it was bought from a local shop, as was the wheat, imported from Europe, North America, or Australia. The tea or coffee which accompanies the breakfast cake may be grown in the country, but it, too, reached the consumer via a line of middlemen before it reached the shop from which it was purchased. The sugar with which the drink was sweetened was probably grown and refined in another country, such as Taiwan, and shipped by sea to the country of the consumer.

The existence of markets and the middlemen who supply them means that some kind of organization has taken place in the production of food, so that a steady supply may be depended upon as much as climate, soil fertility, and other geographic conditions will permit. Regular cultivation of crops and domestication of plants and animals go back far into man's past. Perhaps occasional surpluses, and a system of barter to dispose of them, may have brought about the most primitive form of marketing.

Improvements in technology and transportation have long since made many products available world-wide on a year-round basis for much of the technically advanced world, and even in more cosmopolitan centers of developing countries. Income permitting, one can find fresh strawberries in winter, French truffles in New York, American turkey in Singapore, and frozen peas in a host of cities in between. Despite our highly complex marketing system, which depends on a sophisticated food technology industry along with a large, highly developed and integrated network of transportation, the modern market still can be reduced to the same fundamental components as the earliest and most primitive market: ultimately there is a producer—a farmer, herder, or fisherman—and a consumer. They interact, however many intermediates stand between them, and this interaction of consumer and producer influences what the middleman offers for sale. Consumers want products and producers seek profit; thus whether a food appears in a market depends on what price the consumer is willing to pay.

The economy — what can be produced and marketed while showing a profit — probably has as much influence on what foods are available as consumer preferences and growing conditions for the producer. Cheaply raised foods which have no local means for preserving them or storing them for long periods without deterioration (so that they cannot be transported to distant markets) will not be bought by middlemen for later sales elsewhere. A producer in a money economy will be discouraged from raising such crops, despite the ultimate consumer's interest in the goods. In many agricultural communities, including here in the United States, it has long been more profitable, often, to raise nonfood crops for cash — tobacco, hemp, cotton, flax — than food crops. This removes land from producing food and makes the producer join other consumers to bargain for and purchase his food in the market place.

In the United States and a number of other Western countries today, agriculture has become so highly specialized that one farmer can feed about 45 other people.* The converse of this situation still holds in many parts of the developing world, where up to 70 percent or more of the adult population must work in agriculture in order to feed the population. In many parts of the world, especially in warm climates, one still finds peasants using the primitive methods of agriculture employed by their ancestors (wooden plows, water

wheels to irrigate turned by camels or manpower, primitive methods of threshing). Naturally the yields per acre may be scanty under such conditions. When conditions favor a more efficiently run agriculture, larger numbers of people are freed to do other things than produce food. When one man can grow enough to feed several others, that culture in which he produces can afford for others to become priests, artisans, teachers, and scientists. In this way, civilizations began, through specialization made possible by more effective agricultural production, the products of which could be economically marketed.

In pre-Columbian America, food was obtained by hunting and gathering, or by subsistence agriculture. With European colonization, a prosperous economy developed in which the farm homes and small towns were mostly self-sufficient in food supplies and crafts needed for making other necessities of life (cloth, soap, tools, household utensils, carpentry and wood carving products). As the population grew, new lands were used for cultivation, resulting in less intensive farming. Industrialization and the resultant migration to cities came somewhat later here than in Europe, but it developed from the early 1800's, with increasing rapidity during the 50 years between 1880 and 1930. Following the American Civil War, the founding of the land-grant colleges gave stimulus to scientific agriculture (including mechanization of farms). However, it took World War II (with the necessity to export foods to allies overseas) to give initiative to increased food production by increasing the yield per acre (fertilization, crop rotation, better strains of seed, pesticides), as well as promotion of improved breeds of animals and more efficient production of meats, eggs, and milk.

Another result of more efficient agriculture is a reduction of total land under cultivation, while yields from each

---

*However, many middlemen are necessary to accomplish this feat. Some furnish the equipment, supplies, and research which allow one farmer to grow enough for 45 people. Others are the shippers, processors, inspectors, wholesalers, and retailers who facilitate distribution of the food.

acre rise. In the United States fewer farmers produce more food on less land. Former farm or pasture land is being subdivided for housing developments near larger centers, or converted to parks or golf courses or paved over for highways.

Food gets to markets in as many ways as there are styles of transportation. We think immediately of refrigerated trailer trucks and box cars, freighters and planes. But around the world food also reaches markets on heads, bicycles, bullock carts, donkeys, camels, horses, and other draft animals, and by canoe, river steamer, or coastal sailer. Transportation is vital for marketing of fresh food, even if it must be carried on foot. Highway systems, paved all-weather roads, ports, and suitably dredged waterways are thus important contr butors to improvements in marketing.

Most of the food on America's tables is routed from the farmer by way of various middlemen to processors for cann ng, freezing, or drying, packaging, or other types of food preparation such as the making of biscuits, noodles, bread, cakes, sauces, and condiments. Then, by way of other middlemen, it reaches wholesalers, including food chain warehouses, from which it is shipped again to retail stores and supermarkets.

Methods of Processing and Preserving Food

Even food which we buy in its "natural" state, such as eggs, fresh fruits, and vegetables, is usually routed through various middlemen and undergoes processing such as cleaning and sorting. Such processing ensures digestible, safe, and clean products. Inedible portions of the food, such as husks and pods, are removed. Naturally occurring toxins are inactivated. Filth and impurities such as twigs, pebbles, and dirt are washed out. Other processing operations are performed to preserve food products so that they can remain free of microbial spoilage, rancidity, flavor loss, enzyme destruction, and other types of deterioration over the period of time necessary for transportation and storage.

HEATING. Canning has probably contributed more than any other form of food processing to the maintenance of an adequate food supply throughout the year. The industry had its beginning in the United States in 1819, but gained in volume steadily after the introduction (in 1874) of steam pressure processing in sealed tins. Under steam pressure, processing is accomplished at higher temperatures, in a much shorter time, and results in a better quality product. For many foods (including some that have been concentrated by removal of water), it offers the most convenient method for transportation and storage without refrigeration. Pasteurization is another process employing heat.

DEHYDRATION. Dehydration (removal of most or all of the water) is still one of the best ways of preserving foods and reducing transportation costs. Technological advances have made possible products of much-improved quality at lower cost. New methods include quick drying at lower temperatures under vacuum or reduced pressure, with controlled temperature and fans for removal of the water vapor. If the product is in liquid form, it may be blown in small droplets into a heated chamber, where it dries almost instantly to a fine powder, which has excellent keeping qualities and which can later be "reconstituted" by the addition of water. This process has given us the very useful dried milk, which is the least expensive and most transportable form of milk solids. Some milk powders are "instantized" to make them more readily dispersible in cold water. Partial dehydration (condensed or evaporated milks) has long been in use, but now antioxidants may be added, or an inert gas (nitrogen or carbon dioxide) is used to displace air (containing oxygen) in the package.

Other products made by spray-drying are cream substitutes for use in coffee, citrus products, other fruit beverages, and instant coffee, all of which are ready for use merely by adding suitable amounts of water. Foods may also be dehydrated by cutting in thin slices which are passed on a conveyor belt through a specially designed oven, or may be finely mashed and placed on a perforated tray or mat. A current of heated air is blown up through the perforations. Such processes have been successfully used in drying fruits (for use in prepared cereals), vegetables (for casserole dishes), and soup mixes.

Dehydrated foods, precooked or raw, have been developed for the military forces, which require light weight foods (for individual carrying or air drop) that keep without refrigeration over long periods and can be reconstituted with the mere addition of water (hot or cold as the food requires). With special packaging, such foods can be readily adapted for space travel.

FREEZING. Frozen foods first came into wide use some years ago, when deep-freeze refrigerator compartments and separate units for quantity storage became available in the home. Meats, fish, and vegetables were the foods most commonly preserved by this process. When frozen in a single solid block, they took considerable time for defrosting, and it was difficult to divide a block for use at separate meals. Now a variety of products are frozen in smaller units, so that it is possible to remove only the amount desired. The variety and quality of frozen foods continue to improve, and one can purchase them in packages with quantities to suit the size of the family. Because of their excellent flavor and the saving of labor in preparation, frozen vegetables are strong competitors with the fresh varieties in popular favor. Frozen fruits re-

tain their fresh flavor and nutritive value better than canned ones. Such items are especially valuable for variety in the diet during the seasons when fresh fruits and vegetables are scarce or high in price.

FREEZE-DRYING. Foods may be frozen raw or precooked and may be partially dehydrated either before or after the freezing process. In the latter process (known as freeze-drying), raw food is quickly frozen, then passed into a special vacuum chamber, where the moisture is removed from the food by sublimation—that is, ice crystals go directly into the vapor state without passing through the liquid state. Freeze-dried foods have a spongy texture but retain their shape and flavor, require no refrigeration in storage, and can be reconstituted readily by placing in warm water. The reconstituted product looks and tastes very much like its fresh counterpart. Many products, including coffee, onions, chives, and vegetables, are freeze-dried.

Most frozen foods must be kept constantly refrigerated in storage, in transport, and finally in the grocer's display counter, all of which adds to their cost. Those frozen foods that sell in very large volume are competitive in price with fresh products, or they may even be cheaper (e.g., frozen, concentrated orange juice usually is cheaper than fresh orange juice). Other frozen foods that entail considerable labor in preparation and expense in packaging and refrigeration tend to be luxury items, which the consumer may buy, regardless of cost, in order to save time and labor in preparing meals.

RADIATION. Radiation preservation is being tested as a means to decrease product spoilage by bombarding the product with radioactive isotopes. In the United States, the Atomic Energy Commission and the Food and Drug Administration are involved in long-term studies to determine the nutritional losses and safety of this method.

Increased Use of Convenience
Foods

Probably the most important change in American dietary habits over the past several decades has been the great shift from more conventional types of food to so-called "convenience" foods: for example, meal-in-one dishes; mixes for soups, dressings, sauces, and desserts; frozen entrées; minute rice, instant mashed potatoes, and precooked cereals. These foods, either processed from natural foods or created *de novo*, have increased the quantity and variety of foods available in this country. Some new products are of questionable nutritional value—for example, imitation milk. Some processed foods, such as quick-frozen vegetables, are essentially equivalent nutritionally to their fresh counterparts. However, some foods lose a large proportion of their nutrients through refining (see Table 17–1) or exposure to water, heat, light, or oxygen during processing (refer to Chaps. 7

through 12 for effects on specific nutrients). The extent of the loss depends on the food, the severity of processing, and the food particle size. If these foods are the exclusive source of the lost nutrient, there is cause for concern. However, if other foods of the mixed diet can provide these nutrients, the advantages of processing may outweigh the disadvantages. For example, a small loss of vitamin C from milk during pasteurization is not so important, because milk is a poor source of vitamin C anyway. However, a population which depends on potatoes for vitamin C will not get enough of the nutrient from dehydrated potato flakes.

The *advantages* of by-passing some of the more tedious processes in the preparation and cooking of foods are evident, and a good many foods that formerly were made in the home are now given over almost entirely to commercial production—for example, making bread, baking beans, making pickles, jams, and jellies. The wide variety of ready-to-cook frozen vegetables also relieves the homemaker of labor, and as bought, they are free from waste. In certain foods and under certain circumstances, the convenience of buying specially prepared foods may well be worth the price; in others it may not—facts which everyone must decide for himself.

Not all convenience foods are more expensive than their home-prepared equivalents. In general, meat products, bakery goods, and desserts are more expensive as convenience items, but some fruit and vegetables cost less when frozen or canned than when fresh.[1] The cost of time saved and the quality of the product would have to be considered in deciding whether the fresh or processed product was a better buy.

A few *precautions* should be mentioned for the benefit of those who are inclined to be heavy users of specially prepared and precooked foods. While most Americans enjoy sufficient intakes of most nutrients, those citizens with borderline intakes of one or more nu-

Table 17–1. *Losses of Nutrients in the Refining of Wheat**

Nutrient	Wheat μg/gm	White Flour μg/gm	Loss in White Flour, %
Percent of wheat	100	72	28.0
Thiamin	3.5	0.8	77.1
Riboflavin	1.5	0.3	80.0
Niacin	50	9.5	80.8
Vitamin B$_6$	1.7	0.5	71.8
Pantothenic acid	10	5	50.0
Folacin	0.3	0.1	66.7
α-Tocopherol	16	2.2	86.3
Betaine	844	650	22.8
Choline	1089	767	29.5
Calcium, %	0.045	0.018	60.0
Phosphorus, %	0.433	0.126	70.9
Magnesium, %	0.183	0.028	84.7
Potassium, %	0.454	0.105	77.0
Manganese, ppm	46	6.5	85.8
Iron, ppm	43	10.5	75.6
Zinc, ppm	35	7.8	77.7

*Adapted from Schroeder, H. A.: Amer. J. Clin. Nutr., *24*:562, 1971.

trients cannot afford to trade nutrients for convenience. Also, there is still need for meal planning to make sure that the family receives the recommended number of servings of the four food groups to ensure an adequate intake of all nutrients each day. A hastily assembled dinner, with no beforehand planning, may not supplement the other two meals of the day properly. The meal-in-one dishes tend to be high in carbohydrate and of lower protein content. The ready assembled entrée courses are often a little skimpy on meat, and the vegetables used are almost always the ones high in carbohydrates (peas, corn, succotash, lima beans, or mixed vegetables).

Food Additives: Intentional and Incidental

Many convenience foods are made possible by the use of *intentional food additives,* added to food to improve the appearance, texture, taste, nutritional value, or stability of the food. For example, food coloring may make a packaged pie more attractive, a flavoring compound may be added to ice cream, emulsifiers may keep a salad dressing from separating, antioxidants may prevent rancidity development in potato chips, and calcium propionate may retard staling in bread. By 1980, more than half the foods sold will contain additives. Currently they are used at a yearly rate of 5 lb per person in the United States.[2]

The 1958 Food Additives Amendment to the Food, Drug and Cosmetic Act of 1938 was enacted to ensure the safety of additives by requiring industry testing of new additives. About 580 substances were excluded from this requirement, because through years of use they were Generally Recognized As Safe (GRAS).[3] Since then, some GRAS items (for example, monosodium glutamate and cyclamates) have been found to be questionable for indiscriminate use, and have been removed from the GRAS list.

Control over food coloring is covered in a separate amendment of 1960, and the Miller Pesticide Amendment (1954) establishes the procedure for setting tolerances on pesticide residues allowed to remain on fresh agricultural commodities shipped interstate.

Nonfood substances not purposely added to food are legally known as *incidental additives.* These contaminants or "defects" are present in the final product as a result of some phase of cultivating, processing, or packaging. Pesticides and grease from conveyor belts, if present in a food, are two incidental additives. Mold, insect fragments, or rodent hairs are other examples. Both the food industry and regulatory agencies try to control these contaminants of serious concern.

Our phenomenal agricultural production would be impossible without pesticides. Even with these chemicals, crop losses are estimated to amount to eight billion dollars a year in the United States. Using these plus preservation techniques and additives, the food industry has been able to offer the consumer exotic, convenient, or out-of-season foods, and the consumer has eagerly accepted them. Not many in the United States would trade today's free choices of 8000 attractive items on the grocery shelves for the specter of rancid, stale, moldy, insect-infested products.

Fortification and Enrichment

Often, food additives are nutrients. Vitamins, minerals, and amino acids may be added to foods if they were removed during processing, if they were present in the food in limited supply, or if the product replaces a food in the diet which contains the nutrient. Addition of nutrients to food is called fortification or enrichment. These terms are used interchangeably here (although the term "enrichment" is often limited, under legal standards, to the addition of nutrients to bread and cereals—see pp. 398–399).

OBJECTIVES. Food fortification is carried out as a public health measure. Sometimes a population or members of a subgroup are deficient in a nutrient. They may suffer gross deficiency symptoms (as goiter in iodine deficiency), or exhibit clinical signs of deficiency (as low hemoglobin levels in iron deficiency), or change their food habits and thus eliminate a source of nutrients.

With fortification, diets can be nutritionally improved without changing food habits. This is important, it can be argued, because people are generally averse to changing their habits to improve their nutrient intake. Nutritionists need to respect eating habits and preferences, be they culturally or individually determined. Food is viewed in many ways, only one of which is its role as a vehicle for nutrients. To provide a person with a food which is highly nutritious but totally unfamiliar, unpalatable, unattractive, or inconvenient (if he seeks convenience), is not only a waste of food; it leaves unsolved the problem of poor nutrient intake. Thus, fortification of foods already in the diet ensures acceptance of the nutrients in short supply. Today, many traditional foods are being replaced or interchanged in the diet by manufactured foods. To keep the population's nutrient intake at an acceptable level, manufactured food may be fortified. For example, with the public's switch from the use of butter to the use of margarine, it became necessary to fortify margarine with the vitamin A found in butter.

Nutrients may be added to foods for reasons of preservation rather than improvement of nutrient composition. For example, ascorbic acid (as a color preservative) and α-tocopherol (as an antioxidant) can prolong the shelf life of products to which they are added.

TECHNICAL CONSIDERATIONS. Once fortification is deemed necessary, decisions must be made concerning which foods should carry the nutrient in question. This is determined, in part, by who is in the target group. The food consumption habits of those in this group, the ones thought to be deficient, must be known, for the food supplying the nutrient must be consumed in sufficient quantity to make a contribution to the diet. For example, in the United States, bread may soon have larger amounts of iron added, because surveys have found women and children to be iron deficient. But whether bread is the best vehicle for bringing iron to women and children remains to be seen. Some have suggested fortifying milk with iron, in the belief that milk is consumed in more substantial amounts than bread by women and children.

A second technical consideration is the chemical form in which the nutrient is added. It is important that the nutrient be physiologically available. In addition, it should not change the appearance, flavor, odor, or keeping qualities of the food. For example, food technologists had to contend with the unfamiliar yellow color which riboflavin imparted to rice. Adding the fat-soluble vitamins A and D to nonfat milk also posed a challenging technical problem. In order to keep bread volume high in protein-fortified loaves, dough conditioners and emulsifiers have been added along with the protein.[4] The manner in which food will be prepared must also be considered. Coating rice with water-soluble vitamins, when the rice is cooked in water which is then discarded, does not increase the nutrient intake of the population. A more useful method of fortification of rice is the addition of a white rice-shaped vitamin-mineral preparation in a ratio of one to 200 rice grains.

WHICH NUTRIENTS IN WHICH PRODUCTS? Nutrients found to be low in the diet of a population can be added to almost any product which is used widely. Staples such as wheat, rice, and corn have served as vehicles for niacin, riboflavin, thiamin, iron, calcium, and vitamin D. Salt is fortified with iodine in the United States. In India, locally produced salt is used by almost everyone, and it is being tested as a product for calcium and iron fortification. Tea is also drunk in quantity in India, even by youngsters, and thus it, too, is being considered for fortification.[5]

Many developing countries depend on cereal and vegetable products as their protein sources. Worldwide, cereal contributes 60 percent more protein to the diet than animal sources provide. Legumes offer about half as much protein as animal products do.[6] However, the protein quality of cereals and legumes is generally below that of meat products because they are low in one or more essential amino acids. The protein quality of vegetables and cereals can be raised by adding these limiting amino acids in an amount which will create a more balanced protein. For instance, wheat and rice are improved with the addition of lysine; methionine added to legumes and seeds increases the quality of their protein (see Chap. 5).

Other fortified foods include milk with vitamin D; fruit juices with vitamin C; salt with iodine; and drinking water with fluoride.

PROBLEMS POSED BY FORTIFICATION. Fortifying foods allows a quick and easy solution to a pressing problem. It is less trouble to add nutrients to food than to change food habits, educate consumers, or implement long-range agricultural programs. Fortification is based on the premise that since people will not change their food habits, public health officials must look out for their welfare to protect them from themselves. Aside from the reluctance of some to accept these principles, there are some practical problems with fortification.

As people's eating habits change, so do their nutrient intakes. Constantly adjusting fortification levels to meet changing trends would be cumbersome,

but not doing so would defeat the public health objective of fortification. In the United States, bread enrichment standards were established over 30 years ago to provide thiamin, riboflavin, niacin, and iron because the population was deficient in these nutrients (see later section of this chapter). But with today's decreased bread consumption, the population is not receiving the amounts of these nutrients as planned. Also, additional nutrients have been shown to be low in our diets, namely calcium, iron, and folic acid. Our needs have changed, but fortification levels remain stable.

The idea of fortifying a food to make it self-sufficient presents another problem. No food but human milk for the infant is the "perfect" food. Each food needs to be complemented by other, different foods to make an adequate diet. Dependence on one so-called complete food would be foolhardy at this stage of our knowledge.

Other drawbacks to indiscriminate fortification will be considered later in the chapter (see page 386).

Cost and Demand

Our food supplies on the whole are less expensive today than they would be without present preservation methods. But in some cases, services built into a product add to the price the consumer pays for the food. The advertising necessary to make consumers aware of the availability of new products also adds to the price. The top 20 food company advertisers in the United States now spend almost one billion dollars in advertising, or an average of about 5 percent of their sales.[7] For each dollar the consumer spends in the market, the farmer receives just 39 cents. Processing, packaging, and distribution account for the other 61 cents. The farmer's share varies with the product (see Fig. 17–1).

Many marketing factors affect the cost of food. Foods that are scarce or out-of-season are often relatively

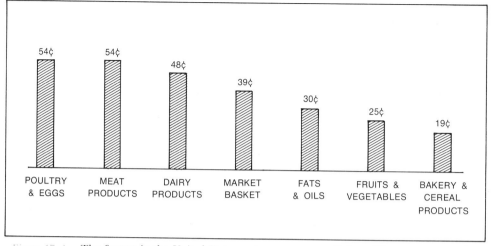

Figure 17–1. The farmer in the United States makes an average of about 39 cents on every dollar spent in the market. His share varies with the product. (From U.S.D.A. Economic Research Service. Published in 1971 Handbook of Agricultural Charts, Agriculture Handbook No. 423, U.S.D.A.)

higher priced. Those that are staples, have good storage life, and are in constant demand are cheaper. Choice cuts of meat are higher priced because the amount of them is small in proportion to the whole carcass. Red meats are usually relatively high-priced food because it costs a good deal to raise and feed animals. Production costs also influence the prices for eggs and milk. To these must be added the cost of transportation and getting the food to the consumer in good condition (refrigeration of perishable foods as well as frozen foods). Peaches and apples from Oregon or lettuce from Georgia often cost more in New York City than the same foods locally produced. Precooked and fancily packaged foods (especially in small packages) are usually more expensive. Advertised brands are no assurance of a higher quality than brands produced by smaller firms that do not advertise widely. "Cash and carry" groceries may sell at lower prices than the same items purchased at stores which make deliveries or extend credit. Large chain stores often package and market their own brands of staple foods at economy prices, and all stores offer special bargain days for certain foods they wish to "move" in quantity or for

"loss leader" items, which serve to draw people into their stores.

At present, two other factors affect the cost of food and the resulting amount necessary for an adequate diet. One factor is the *fluctuating purchasing power, or value, of the dollar,* which reflects the degree of inflation. The food dollar now buys less than half as much as its average purchasing power in the 1935 to 1939 period. Other items in the budget, such as transportation, housing, and services, have increased at the same ratio or at an even greater rate.

In spite of these increased costs, American families as a rule are living more comfortably and the food budget accounts for less of the disposable income than ever before—about 16 percent (see Fig. 17–2).* This seems para-

*This average figure excludes alcoholic beverages, which when included would add significantly to some food budgets. Also, the percentage of income spent on food varies widely according to area of the country, number in the family, and income level (see pp. 403–405). The lower the income, the greater is the proportion of it spent on food. For example, the Bureau of Labor Statistics reports that an urban family of four living on $7000 a year devotes 34 percent of its budget to food, whereas the same family with a $16,000 a year budget allots 27 percent to food expenditures.

doxical in light of the foregoing statements, but one must consider the fact that the *hourly wage* buys more food today than it did 35 years ago. Thus, while the market price for foods (and other items) has increased, family income has also increased. In addition, today than it did 35 years ago. Thus, advantage of new and more efficient techniques in food handling, preservation, and marketing, as well as to purchase a greater variety and a better quality-controlled product than 35 years ago.

Because it is impossible to tell how much foods will cost at any given time, it is imperative that a discussion of food costs should be on a *relative cost basis.* Even if the general level of prices goes up or down, certain *kinds* or *classes* of food are always less expensive than others. Then we have to take into account what return in nutritive essentials is obtained by equal amounts of money spent for different types of food.

What appears on the grocery shelf is generally in response to consumer *demand.* But in modern marketing, this "demand" is often a created one. The chain of events usually sees a new product created, promoted through advertising campaigns, and then put to the test of consumer *acceptance.* According to a home economist for a large advertising agency, for example, the change in preference from home preparation of cakes and pastries to the use of packaged mixes "has come about primarily as a result of advertising."[8] Thus, consumers are constantly being urged to try new products. Those the consumer likes and continues to buy survive. The others join the several thousand new food products doomed to failure each year. It is the consumer's vote in the marketplace which determines the long-time success of any food product or new convenience.

Uneven Distribution of Food Supplies in Proportion to Population Density

In the United States, we are concerned with the details of food production and distribution, such as price changes and market "specials." Our highly productive agricultural economy and well-organized distribution system allow most of us this luxury. But in parts of this country and over the entire world, food is not evenly distributed in relation to the population. More than half the world's population goes hungry and lives under substandard conditions, while more favored nations have plentiful rations, higher living standards, and greater life expectancy. These inequities are graphically illustrated in Figure 17–3. The areas of greatest population density (the Far

Figure 17–2. Americans are spending more money for food than they used to, but their incomes are increasing at an even faster rate. Thus, the percentage of income spent on food is decreasing. (From U.S.D.A. Econ. Res. Serv. Published in 1971 Handbook of Agricultural Charts.)

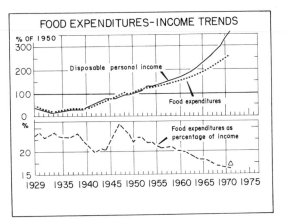

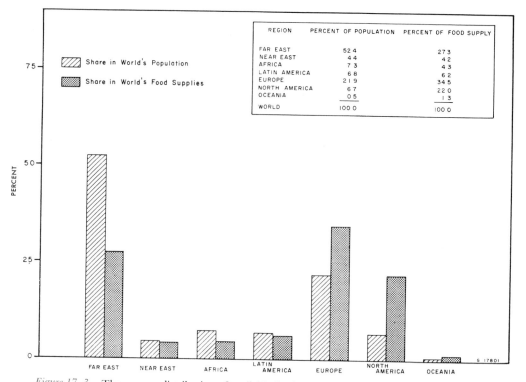

REGION	PERCENT OF POPULATION	PERCENT OF FOOD SUPPLY
FAR EAST	52 4	27 3
NEAR EAST	4 4	4 2
AFRICA	7 3	4 3
LATIN AMERICA	6 8	6 2
EUROPE	21 9	34 5
NORTH AMERICA	6 7	22 0
OCEANIA	0 5	1 3
WORLD	100 0	100 0

Figure 17–3. The uneven distribution of available foods (including grains for farm animals) in different parts of the world is graphically shown in this chart. The Far Eastern countries, with more than half the world's population, have only a little more than one-fourth the world's food supplies. North America, with 6.7 percent of the world's population, enjoys 22 percent of the world's food supplies; Europe accounts for 22 percent of the world's population and has about one-third of the world's food supplies. The rest of the world's population is left with only 16 percent of the total food supply. Thus, there is a surfeit of food in North America, while great numbers of people in Asia, the Near East, Africa, and Latin America go hungry. (From Guating Institute, FAO and UNESCO: *The World Must Eat.* Dobbs Ferry, N.Y., Oceana Publication, Inc., 1962.)

East and much of the Near East, Africa, and Latin America) have available far less of the total food supplies than do the countries of North America, the United Kingdom, and Europe. There are now over 3.6 billion people in the world to be fed, and by the year 2000 it is estimated that the world's population will be close to six billion. The situation now is that, as the food supply of a developing nation is gradually increased, the number of mouths to be fed increases faster and no real betterment of diet and living standards can be brought about (see Fig. 17–4).

In developing countries, where 74 percent of the world's population lives,

the diet may furnish only 1700 kcal or less per day (contrasted with an average 3000 kcal intake in Europe and North America). The protein intake is usually well below 50 gm kcal daily compared to an intake of 90 to 100 gm in more favored countries, and is furnished mostly by grains (rice, corn, millet, or wheat, which carry proteins deficient in one or more of the essential amino acids), with almost minute quantities of the high-quality animal proteins (as low as 5 percent or less up to 20 percent animal protein). This exceedingly large "food gap" between the types of diet available to peoples living in privileged and underprivileged nations has be-

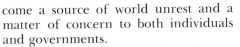

WORLD AGRICULTURAL PRODUCTION

Figure 17–4. Agriculture in developing countries can barely keep ahead of population growth. Increasing food production without curbing population growth cannot solve the problem of world hunger. (From U.S.D.A. Econ. Res. Serv. Published in 1971 Handbook of Agricultural Charts.)

come a source of world unrest and a matter of concern to both individuals and governments.

What happens to people who are forced to subsist on diets that supply less energy, protein, and essential amino acids than are required for body needs? Children born of poorly fed mothers and up to four years of age suffer the most. György has stated that the mortality rates among children one to four years of age in developing countries are

Figure 17–5. Two year old African girl found to be suffering from both kwashiorkor and rickets. Adult food given too soon after weaning and a one-sided diet cause severe malnutrition among young children in this tribe of nomadic fishermen, although sufficient quantities of food seem available. (Courtesy of the World Health Organization, United Nations.)

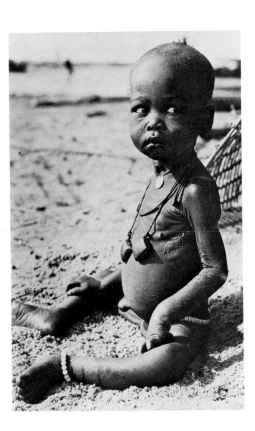

from 10 to 40 times higher than the comparable rates among children of the same age in affluent countries.[9]

Such a high mortality rate encourages more pregnancies, in an effort to guarantee that some offspring will live to maturity. But the nutrition of pregnant and lactating women in developing countries is of major concern. Burgess and Dean, in a study of pregnant women in South India, found that their daily energy intake was only about 1750 kcal and their average weight was 93 lb[10] (about standard for an 11 to 12 year old girl in the United States). Thus the malnourished pregnant and lactating women produce unhealthy children, who either die because of their weak start or live marginal lives.

World population growth must be brought under control, and one way in which people will learn to limit their families is to be assured that their food supplies are sufficient to keep the existing family members in optimal health. Experience has shown that increased standards of living bring a fall in birth rate. The industrialized nations have an average population growth rate of less than 1 percent per year, while the developing countries grow at rates of 2.5 to 3.5 percent per year.[11]

WAYS OF INCREASING FOOD SUPPLIES. It is obvious that we cannot equalize available food supplies by moving the people around; nor can we do much for the less favored countries by exporting our food surpluses to them. The latter process serves only in emergencies and does little to permanently

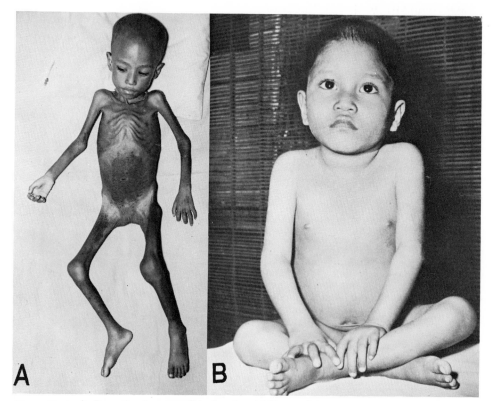

Figure 17-6. **A,** Starvation is responsible for the pitiable condition of this three year old girl found abandoned in the streets of Rangoon, Burma. **B,** Same little girl after three months' treatment at the Rangoon General Hospital. She was adopted later by the doctor who took care of her. (Courtesy of the World Health Organization, United Nations.)

build up these countries. As many of these countries emerge from colonialism and become independent nations, they are anxious to better the living conditions of their people, but this cannot be accomplished without some outside help. Most developing countries still have a primitive agriculture in which a large proportion of the people are occupied, and yet this is still not able to supply enough food. There are few raw materials or industrial products for export, by which money could be obtained to augment their food supply through imports. Moderate increases in the amount of available foods are "swallowed up" by increasing population, so that it is difficult to raise the standard of living. To break this vicious cycle requires mass education (including training of scientists, engineers, and other leaders from the native population), capital, expert assistance from the more developed countries, and stable governments within the developing countries. Although there must be assistance from outside, the major part of selecting and carrying out development plans must come from the cooperation and effort of the peoples themselves.

The time-honored ways of increasing agricultural production are (1) bringing more land under cultivation, and (2) increasing the yield per acre (by improved seed, fertilizer, pest control, and introduction of some farm machinery).

During the so-called current "Green Revolution," sparked by the development of high-yielding varieties of wheat and rice, food production has increased phenomenally. But the new grains are a stopgap measure, a way of buying time until, hopefully, we reduce population growth. Also, the success of the Green Revolution may be only temporary, and can be partially traced to the luck of good weather and adequate rainfall, as well as to the use of irrigation and fertilizers. The availability of these last two assets is restricted in poor areas, where farmers have no capital

and countries have no credit structure.

Many seemingly simple solutions to meeting the crisis of food shortages fail to take into account the lack of capital resources in developing countries and the lack of acceptance of unfamiliar products. Central processing, transportation, and distribution systems are essential to any large-scale food operation. For example, green leaves theoretically could be an important source of protein, but transport of the bulky raw material to the processing plant, protection from spoilage, and the unacceptable green color and taste of the final concentrate have proved major obstacles to their use.[12] Developing the resources of the sea likewise requires capital and major changes in food habits.

In many developing countries there is great disparity between the rich and the poor, while the instability of governments and extremely large land holdings by a few have held back the development of both agriculture and industries. There are large tracts of undeveloped land, but in many areas, roads are few and it is difficult to reclaim land from the jungle. Much remains to be done in Asia and South America, and in Africa, where conditions for development are even more adverse, before the educational level and standards of living can be raised to even a half-way satisfactory point. These countries are clamoring for help in development, and the matter is urgent.

It is impossible to predict what scientific discoveries of the coming years may contribute to the solution of these problems. Biochemists are working on the production of protein by microorganisms, which can be grown in pure cultures under controlled conditions. Perhaps the simplest of these are *yeasts*, which contain a fairly high amount of good-quality protein, and can be incorporated in other foods in dried form. Production of protein foods by *bacteria, algae* or *fungi* is also being investigated. One of the algae—*chlorella*—has a higher protein content than either *dried* yeast, beef, soy meal, or skim milk; the protein formed contains all essential amino acids. Certain fungi synthesize protein from sugar in considerable amounts, but it is still a long step to presenting these products in palatable form for human consumption.

We already have found it possible to develop low-cost mixtures of locally available vegetable foods which, added in small amounts to the diet, provide enough of the essential amino acids missing in the grain proteins to avoid protein malnutrition and deficiency disease. Another possibility is the direct reinforcement of different cereal grains with the lacking amino acids, which can be made synthetically. All the common cereals are deficient in lysine (wheat, rice, rye, oats, and barley), and the small content of methionine limits the efficiency of legumes (peas, beans, soy beans, peanuts, etc.). But there are severe problems with fortification programs (see page 379). The interaction of nutrients requires much more study before we can claim complete understanding. We know now that increased consumption of protein, for example, creates a greater requirement for vitamin B-6 (see Chap. 7); yet, protein-fortified foods do not have this vitamin added.

However, in the face of starvation, creation of nutrient imbalances might be of less concern. Certainly, fortification is an efficient means of quickly improving the nutrient content of diets. Unfortunately, here again, the wealthier segments of the developing nations are the ones benefiting most from fortification. In India, "Modern Bread," fortified with lysine, reaches only 1 to 2 percent of the population. For the rest of the people, bread itself is too expensive. Another problem with fortification is that in order to deliver the nutrients into the food supply, the food must pass through some sort of central processing. Currently in developing countries, food finds its way from the farm directly to the market, leaving no opportunity for fortification steps.

Perhaps the greatest problem with fortification is that the procedure might mushroom from a stopgap measure to the sole means of coping with malnutrition. In its growth, it could well stifle efforts of nations to implement long-range agricultural and nutrition improvement programs. There is the danger that an expedient fortification program will give a false security when conducted at the expense of slower but more farsighted measures. In addition to protein, developing nations also need calories, along with a well-balanced mixture of all 14 vitamins and nearly 20 minerals and trace elements. These come from *food*, and are impossible to provide through fortification alone.

Whether the solution to the present situation of inadequate food supplies for a large proportion of the world's people will be accomplished by more efficient agriculture, by totally new forms of food, by some form of birth control, or by a combination of such methods, remains for the future to determine. Certainly the present situation is sufficiently acute to constitute a challenge, which will engage the best efforts of men and nations, both for humanitarian reasons and for the sake of world peace, for a long time to come.

PURCHASING FOOD AND PLANNING THE MENU

The objective of production and marketing processes is to bring food to the consumer. Wise buying of groceries calls for budgeting the family income and planning nutritious, appealing meals within the family's purchasing power. Even when money is not scarce, good planning is essential to ensure the purchase of foods which make up a nutritious diet. Figure 17–7 shows how distribution of the food dollar in an average family may affect the nutritive value of the diet.

Classification of Food by Groups

To facilitate planning menus and purchasing food, it is useful to consider food in groups of similar products. Since 1956, most nutrition educators in the United States have been using the U.S.D.A. "Basic Four Food Groups" plan, which provides a nutritious diet and which encourages the use of foods from each of the following basic groups: *milk, meat or equivalent, fruits and vegetables,* and *grains.* These broad categories were designated on the basis of the nutrient composition of the foods within that group. For example, foods in the "meat" group—such as beef, pork, poultry, eggs, fish, beans, legumes, and nuts—are considered together because they all supply significant amounts of protein, minerals, and vitamins. The milk group also provides protein, but is considered separately because its distinguishing feature is that it is a primary source of calcium, as well as of other important minerals and vitamins.

Designation of *four* groups of food is just one of many satisfactory ways of distinguishing different types of foods. For example, before 1956, foods were divided into *seven* groups by the U.S.D.A. In Puerto Rico, food is divided into the four groups of milk; meat, fish, eggs, and beans; fruits; and vegetables.[13] Grains, a staple in the diet, are considered, along with coffee, tea, and butter, to be eaten by everyone routinely, and therefore not in need of emphasis in a separate food group. In West Africa, many people are taught the *three* food groups: Group 1 provides protein for body building and maintenance and includes milk along with meat, poultry, fish, eggs, and legumes. Group 2 provides calories, or energy, and includes fats, cereals, roots, and tubers. Group 3 provides vitamins and minerals to ensure proper functioning of the body, and includes fruits and vegetables.[14] (See Chaps. 1 and 18 for more discussion on the Four Food Groups.) Following is a detailed description of each of the foods in the U.S. Four Food Group plan.

MILK AND MILK PRODUCTS. Milk is especially important in the diet for its outstanding contributions of (1) *high-quality protein,* (2) *calcium,* and (3) *riboflavin.* In addition, it provides some of practically all other essential nutrients in well balanced amounts and in easily assimilated forms.

The chief *proteins* in milk are casein and lactalbumin. Together they form a protein mixture which is so rich in the essential amino acids required for tissue building that it is more efficient in promoting growth than any other combination of proteins except those in eggs. Milk proteins supplement the incomplete proteins found in the grains better than any other food proteins and

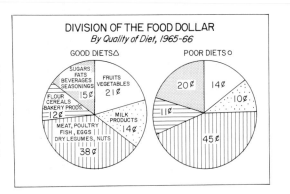

Figure 17–7. Two U.S. families spending the same amount of money—in this case an amount above the national average—can buy diets which differ widely in nutrient composition. In good diets, more of the food dollar is spent on fruits, vegetables, and milk products, and less on sugars, fats, beverages, and the meat group than in poor diets. (From U.S.D.A. Agricultural Service.)

are a fairly economical source of protein. Only cereals and dried legumes furnish protein at less cost, and their proteins are not of as high a biological value as those of milk and eggs.

In most American dietaries, milk is usually the mainstay for calcium and riboflavin. No other common food except its product, cheese, approaches it for richness in *calcium*, and it is extremely difficult to plan a dietary that provides the recommended allowance of this element without use of a moderate amount of milk (or cheese and ice cream). Two cups (one pint) of milk furnishes 66 percent of the total daily calcium allowance for an adult. The remainder usually can be provided in other foods, and the recommended allowance is sufficiently more than the minimal need that a slightly lower intake does not result in any deficiency for the average adult. The calcium requirement is increased in periods of rapid growth, pregnancy, and lactation, and it is added protection under these conditions to have most of the calcium allowance furnished by milk, which also carries high-quality proteins and other important nutrients. The quantities of milk* needed to provide the total recommended daily calcium allowances for these special periods are:

3 cups—full calcium allowance for child 2 to 6 years.
4 cups—full calcium allowance for child 6 to 12 years.
5 cups—full calcium allowance for teenager 12 to 18 years and for pregnant or lactating woman.
6 cups—full calcium allowance for pregnant or lactating young (teen-age) woman.

*In countries where milk and milk products are scarce or not a traditional part of the diet, or if one does not wish to consume so much milk, the burden of furnishing needed calcium can be allotted to other sources, such as soft fish bones, added lime water or ashes, leafy vegetables, legumes, sesame seed, whole grains, and eggs.

Along with calcium, milk provides high levels of *phosphorus* needed for building strong bones and teeth, and together these two mineral elements are present in a ratio to each other that favors excellent utilization. Milk's contribution of *riboflavin* is almost as outstanding as that of calcium among the minerals. In a recent survey of American diets, the food group of milk, cheese, and ice cream accounted for 13 percent of the average food expenditure, while it furnished 76 percent of the calcium and 42 percent of the riboflavin (see Table 17-2 and Fig. 17-8). Because these two nutrients are among those most likely to be supplied in less than optimal quantities, and because a goodly surplus of these nutrients is conducive to better health, it is obvious that liberal use of milk in the diet, whenever possible, is a wise procedure.

Milk is a good "buy" for other nutrients besides calcium and riboflavin. It is a dilute food—87 percent water. Whole milk's 13 percent of solids is fairly evenly distributed between proteins, fat, and milk sugar (lactose), and these nutrient substances supply considerable energy (630 kcal per quart). Skim milk contains more water than whole milk, and about 0.1 percent or less of fat, compared with 3.5 percent of fat in whole milk. It provides 350 kcal per qt. The product known as 2 percent milk contains 2 percent fat and offers 590 kcal per qt. The proteins, as stated, are of particularly high quality and are useful for supplementing other proteins which may be low or lacking in certain of the essential amino acids. The fat (and the vitamin A it carries) is in finely divided or emulsified condition, which favors its digestion and absorption. People on low-fat diets can benefit from the nutrients in milk by drinking fortified skim milk. The presence of *lactose* in the intestines favors the absorption of certain minerals. Milk is precipitated in "curds" in the stomach by the enzyme rennin and by the hydrochloric acid of the gastric juice, which keeps it from passing out of the

TABLE 17–2. Approximate Sources of Nutrients in the Average United States Diet*

Food Groups	Food Energy	Protein	Fat	Carbo-hydrate	Calcium	Phos-phorus	Iron	Magne-sium	Vitamin A Value	Thiamin	Ribo-flavin	Niacin	Vitamin B-6	Vitamin B-12	Vitamin C
	PERCENT	PERCENT	PERCENT	PERCENT	PERCENT	PERCENT	PERCENT	PERCENT	PERCENT	PERCENT	PERCENT	PERCENT	PERCENT	PERCENT	PERCENT
Meat (including pork fat cuts), poultry, and fish	21.1	42.0	36.0	0.1	3.7	26.7	31.4	14.1	23.8	31.2	25.9	47.7	47.6	70.4	1.1
Eggs	2.2	5.8	3.2	0.1	2.6	6.0	6.0	1.4	6.8	2.5	5.8	0.1	2.2	9.2	0
Dairy products, excluding butter	11.2	22.2	12.3	7.0	76.1	36.1	2.3	22.1	11.2	9.5	42.4	1.7	9.4	20.4	4.4
Fats and oils, including butter	17.7	0.1	41.6	†	0.4	0.2	0	0.4	8.5	0	0	0	0.1	0	0
Citrus fruits	0.8	0.4	0.1	1.8	0.9	0.7	0.8	2.0	1.4	2.6	0.5	0.8	1.2	0	25.3
Other fruits	2.3	0.6	0.3	5.0	1.2	1.1	3.6	4.0	6.3	1.9	1.6	1.8	5.7	0	11.6
Potatoes and sweet potatoes	2.8	2.4	0.1	5.6	0.9	4.0	4.7	7.4	5.0	6.6	1.8	7.5	12.1	0	20.3
Dark green and deep yellow vegetables	0.2	0.4	†	0.5	1.5	0.6	1.6	2.0	21.1	0.8	1.1	0.6	1.7	0	8.2
Other vegetables, including tomatoes	2.4	3.2	0.4	4.7	4.8	4.8	9.2	10.3	15.4	6.9	4.5	6.0	9.2	0	29.1
Dry beans and peas, nuts, soya flour	2.8	4.7	3.5	1.9	2.5	5.4	5.9	10.4	†	5.1	1.7	6.7	3.9	0	†
Flour and cereal products	19.3	17.7	1.3	35.6	3.3	12.3	26.2	17.9	0.4	32.8	14.1	22.2	6.8	0	0
Sugars and other sweeteners	16.4	†	0.0	37.2	1.1	0.2	5.7		0	†	†	†	0	0	†
Coffee and cocoa‡	0.7	0.4	1.2	0.6	1.0	1.8	2.5	7.7	†	0.1	0.7	4.9	0.1	0	0
Totals§	100.0	100.0	100.0	100.0	100.0	100.0	100.0	100.0	100.0	100.0	100.0	100.0	100.0	100.0	100.0

*From National Food Situation. Washington, D.C., U.S.D.A., November 1971. Percentages were derived from nutrient data which include quantities of iron, thiamin, and riboflavin added to flour and cereal products; quantities of vitamin A value added to margarine and milk of all types; and quantities of vitamin C added to fruit juices and drinks.

†Less than 0.05 percent.
‡Chocolate liquor equivalent of cocoa beans.
§Components may not add to total due to rounding.

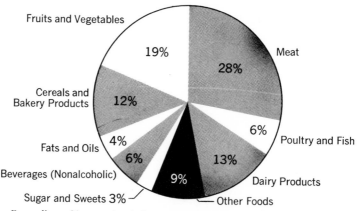

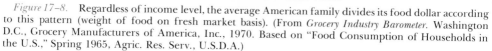

Figure 17–8. Regardless of income level, the average American family divides its food dollar according to this pattern (weight of food on fresh market basis). (From *Grocery Industry Barometer*. Washington D.C., Grocery Manufacturers of America, Inc., 1970. Based on "Food Consumption of Households in the U.S.," Spring 1965, Agric. Res. Serv., U.S.D.A.)

stomach too quickly and favors its digestion.

The function of milk in nature is to serve as the sole food for young animals, and milk contains all the vitamins and minerals needed for this purpose. Both *carotene* and *vitamin A* are found in the fat globules, varying somewhat with the feed of the cow, and variable amounts of vitamin D are also present. (In the United States, milk is generally fortified with 400 IU of vitamin D per quart.) The water-soluble vitamins are carried in the whey. Milk contains only about one-sixth as much thiamin as riboflavin, but all the B vitamins are present, including B-12. The value of milk as a source of niacin is augmented by the amino acid tryptophan in its proteins. Although fresh milk contains moderate amounts of vitamin C, much of this may be lost in handling, storage, and pasteurization, so it is not to be depended on for this vitamin. The content of iron and copper in milk is rather low, but what iron is present is well assimilated.

Per capita milk production and consumption in this country have been declining for the past 25 years. Between 1957–59 and 1971, consumption dropped 24 percent.[15] Nearly half the milk produced is used in the manufacture of dairy products (butter, canned milks, cheese, and ice cream).

Many people prefer to consume at least part of their milk allowance in the form of milk products rather than as fluid milk. These products all share the nutritive properties of milk, in greater or less degree, but lack of space prevents little more than their enumeration here.

Cream. Light cream has only slightly less protein than fresh milk and six times its fat content. Heavy cream carries about ten times as much fat as whole fresh milk. Cream is a luxury food and is not a substitute for milk, for the content of protein, calcium, and riboflavin is decreased as the fat content goes up.

Processed Milks. In all these products, much of the water and/or fat is removed. Water is evaporated off in a partial vacuum at fairly low temperatures, with little resultant loss of vitamins other than vitamin C, except in the production of dry skim milk, in which vitamin A is removed along with the fat in processing.

Condensed milks keep because of added sugar (about 50 percent of final product).

Evaporated milks keep because they are sterilized in the can—no sugar is added but about half the water is removed.

Dried skim milk powders keep because of low water content (only 3.5 percent), and because fat has been removed.

Filled milks may be fresh, dried, condensed, or evaporated. They contain the nonfat milk solids, but with nondairy fat substituted for the butterfat.

Canned milks meet the need for a concentrated preserved milk which is economical to transport. Evaporated milk is used in infant feeding because of its softer, finer curd, in comparison with that formed by raw milk. Condensed milk is a good substitute for cream in coffee and will keep for long periods in an opened can if properly refrigerated. Dried milk powders are much used in commercial bakeries, as well as in home cooking. Dried skim milk is the cheapest form in which to purchase milk; it may be reconstituted or used dry in cooking processes. Dried milk in which much of the fat has been retained has a creamier taste and a higher energy value and probably has some antioxidant added to insure keeping quality. The use of dried milk powder (or granules) in breads, cream sauces, casseroles, and soups is an excellent way to reinforce the diet with protein, calcium, and riboflavin.

Filled milk* has the same protein and other nutrients as whole fresh milk, and the number of calories per serving is the same. If the fat which replaces the butterfat is high in polyunsaturates, filled milk can be used, as skim milk, for fat-modified diets. However, if coconut oil, which is higher in saturated fat than is butterfat, is used, filled milk

*Filled milk, by this name, is illegal in some states in the United States on the basis that it is no longer "milk." In other states, such as California, the legal name is "imitation milk," a term which in most other places describes a product looking like milk but with few of its nutritional properties.

cannot be used on a fat-modified diet. The source of fat should be mentioned on the label.

Cheeses. Cheeses vary considerably as to water content (hard and soft cheeses) and in fat content, depending on whether they are made from whole or skim milk. They contain all of the casein and fat of the milk from which they were made, but usually some of the lactalbumin and calcium are lost in the whey that separates from the curd used for the cheese. In ripened cheeses, the protein has been partially digested and rendered more soluble by bacterial action. American (Cheddar) cheese is a hard cheese (37 percent water), so is a concentrated source of all milk solids. Cottage cheese (as made from skim milk) is low in fat and high in protein, but has only about one-eighth of the calcium content of American (Cheddar) cheese. Cream cheese differs from other soft cheeses in having more fat and less protein. A number of commercial cheese products, such as cheese spreads, have recently come into popular use. They are soft enough to be stirred into batters or sauces or to be spread on crackers, and they are packaged so they do not dry out or spoil.

Ice Cream. Ice cream is a popular form in which to take part of one's milk quota. Ice creams vary widely in composition, depending on substances added. Most "ice milks" contain about 4 to 5 percent fat, and regular ice creams from 10 to 16 percent fat (the "richer" the ice cream, the greater the amount of fat). Most ice creams are, in effect, a frozen mixture of milk and cream with some added table sugar (about 16 percent of the final product on a weight basis—or about 1²/₃ tablespoons of sucrose per cup of final product) plus various flavors, fruits, stabilizers, and often egg. Ice cream, before freezing, contains about 63 percent water and has up to 100 percent air beaten into it during the freezing process. This improves the texture and taste for most people.

Fermented Milks. Fermented milks may be either from fat-free milk (buttermilk) or whole milk (koumiss, yogurt, acidophilus milk, etc.). They are made by fermentation with various strains of bacilli that convert the lactose to lactic acid or alcohol. Yogurt is a very nutritious food, but offers no magical promise of good health or longevity beyond milk itself. Because much of its lactose has been split in its manufacture, fermented milks are often used by persons who have difficulty digesting lactose.

MEATS AND OTHER PROTEIN FOODS. The outstanding contributions of these foods to the diet are (1) high-quality *protein* in concentrated form, (2) *B vitamins,* especially riboflavin and niacin, and (3) *iron.* The proteins of meat are somewhat similar to those of milk and eggs in their amino acid make-up and, therefore, in the efficiency with which they supplement those of the cereal grains and some other vegetable proteins. Only in protein do meats supplement grains, for both grains and meats are poor in calcium and in vitamins A and C. Whole grains and meats contain fair amounts of phosphorus and iron and are good sources of the B vitamins, and both are acid-forming in the body.

Meats, Fish, and Poultry. Meats are well-liked foods and give the feeling of satiety. They are usually consumed in larger amounts if the economic level permits and have come to be associated psychologically with prosperity and with a higher standard of living. With the exception of zinc, their place in the diet can be entirely met by the use of milk, cheese, and eggs. Judicious use of legume seeds (beans), as often happens in the diet of vegetarians (see Chap. 18) is acceptable if vitamin B-12 needs are met. In countries where grazing land is plentiful (United States, Canada, Australia, New Zealand, and Argentina), meat production and consumption are high. In populous countries (such as in Asia), where land is at a premium and must be used for field crops in order to get enough food for humans, very little

meat is available. Only when cattle and sheep are raised on grazing lands does meat production represent the most economical use of national resources.

An average American buys about 250 pounds of meat, fish, and poultry per year. This is an average of 11 oz per day per person[15] (though nearly one half of this is bone, skin, and unconsumed fat). Average expenditure for this food group amounts to 34 cents of every dollar spent for food (see Fig. 17–8). Consumption of meat and poultry is increasing rapidly in the United States (see Fig. 17–9).

Meat is an excellent food, containing good protein in concentrated form, but it should not be consumed to the extent that other protective foods, rich in minerals and vitamins, are excluded. It takes only $1\frac{1}{2}$ pints of milk or three eggs to provide approximately as much protein as an average ($3\frac{1}{2}$ oz) serving of meat. One medium-sized serving of meat daily is a great help in securing an adequate protein intake. One should not lose sight of the fact that the same amount of meat may be purchased for less money if the cheaper cuts are chosen and cooked in an appetizing manner.

The flesh of all animals (mammals, birds, fish, or shellfish) is essentially the same. The difference in composition in flesh from different portions of the same animal is sometimes greater than the usual variation between the flesh of different animals. Variations in composition are due chiefly to differences in *water* or *fat* content. These are largely dependent on the species—for example, fish is usually higher in moisture content than beef or lamb; salmon is relatively high in fat, compared with cod or flounder; and pork is richer in fat than most other meats. The fat content also varies in different cuts of meat and according to previous feeding. Fat that is in layers surrounding the lean portion is usually discarded and should not be counted in the caloric value of the meat eaten. Fat may also be lost in the drippings during cooking. In pork,

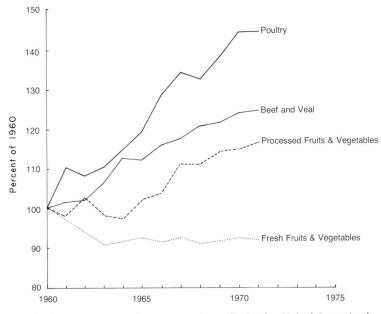

Figure 17-9. Poultry consumption has increased rapidly in the United States in the past decade. Americans are also buying more beef and veal. Processed fruit and vegetable sales are increasing, while sales of fresh fruits and vegetables are decreasing. (Drawn from data in the 1971 Handbook of Agricultural Charts, U.S.D.A.)

considerable fat is located between the muscle fibers, which adds to the fuel value of pork and pork products (such as sausages) and also slows down digestion. Lean muscle meats may be described as consisting of approximately one-fifth protein, three-fourths water, and one-hundredth ash (with varying small amounts of fat). They also contain small amounts of connective tissue, which holds the muscle fibers together, and of extractives, which give the flavor to meat soups.

There are some variations in mineral elements and vitamins. Pork is many times higher in thiamin (vitamin B-1) than other muscle meats. Fatty fish (e.g., canned salmon) has a good content of vitamin D. The glandular organs, such as liver and kidneys, are especially rich in vitamin A, the B vitamins, and iron. All lean meats are good sources of phosphorus. Marine fish and shellfish are good sources of iodine, which is a scarce element in most foods.

The effect of cooking on the vitamin content of meats also deserves mention. Meats contain little vitamin C (ascorbic acid), even in the raw state, and practically none after cooking. The vitamin A contained in meat fats is usually in the discarded trimmings or in the drippings from the cooking. The loss of B vitamins in cooking depends on the specific B vitamin and on the method of cooking. Thiamin (the most heat-labile B vitamin) may be lost to the extent of 50 to 75 percent in stewing or braising, 30 to 50 percent in roasting or broiling, and only 10 to 15 percent in quick frying.

Eggs. The general composition of eggs is roughly three-fourths water, one-eighth protein, and one-eighth fat. The protein is about equally divided between the white and the yolk, but all the fat, as well as the mineral elements and vitamins (except riboflavin), is in the yolk. The proteins of eggs are as efficient for promoting growth and supplementing deficient vegetable proteins as are those of milk, and egg fat like milk fat is finely divided or emulsified, making it easily and fully digested.

Egg yolk (like milk) serves as food for young, growing animals and contains practically all the essential minerals and vitamins, some in higher concentration than others. It is rich in phosphorus, sulfur, iron, and vitamin A plus carotene; it is a fair source of the B vitamins. Eggs are completely lacking in ascorbic acid. In mineral elements and vitamins, eggs supplement milk in respect to certain constituents, and in respect to others they supplement meats. All three of these protein foods need to be supplemented with the vitamin C in fruits and vegetables.

Eggs are easily cooked in a variety of ways so that they form an acceptable meat substitute. Their ease of digestion and high content of tissue-building nutrients make them a valuable food for growing children or convalescents. They are especially useful in cookery, where they serve the purposes of thickening (as in custards) or stiffening and lightening texture (as in batters and doughs). Our consumption of eggs is about six per person per week, including those used in home cookery and in commercial bakery products.[15] Eggs are a rich source of dietary cholesterol (about 270 mg per egg), which is a cause of much conflicting dietary advice. We believe that one or two eggs per day are nutritionally very useful in most people's diets. There are some persons who have difficulty handling cholesterol in the diet, probably less than 5 percent of the American population. Such persons can generally be identified by physicians on the basis of lipid analysis of the blood or other symptoms (see Chap. 23).

Legumes and Nuts. Legumes are seeds and nuts, although technically they are hard-shelled fruits and are similar to seeds in composition. This food group resembles the grains more than any other group, but is characterized by having almost twice as much protein as grains. The dried legumes (beans, grams, peas, lentils, and cowpeas), because of their low moisture content, are as much as 60 percent carbohydrate (starch) and 22 percent protein—figures that may be misleading because in the state in which we eat them, fresh or cooked dried ones, their protein content ranges from only about 6 to 8 percent. Although they are often classed as "meat substitutes," an average serving of a legume furnishes probably only about one-third as much protein as an average ($3\frac{1}{2}$ oz) serving of meat. The quality of their proteins tends to be inferior to that of animal foods, except for the proteins of the peanut and soybean, which are of good biological value. However, legume proteins do supplement in satisfactory manner the proteins of cereal grains, and this is particularly true of the proteins of peanuts ("groundnuts"), soybeans, and peas, when combined with wheat. The addition of small amounts of peanut or soybean flour improves the nutritive quality of white (wheat) bread. The digestibility of legume proteins is improved by cooking. Dried legumes and soybeans require long, slow cooking, and the undigestible carbohydrates in beans may lead to intestinal fermentation and flatulence. Dried legumes have considerable use in thick soups (purées) and canned bean products (pork and beans, beans with tomato sauce, chili con carne, etc.). In the southern sections of the United States, cowpeas and chickpeas are well liked and widely used.

Nuts also have a relatively high protein content (7 to 18 percent), but, instead of being rich in starch as are legumes, they have high fat content (roughly 50 to 70 percent). Soybeans and peanuts (which are legumes) have both high protein and fat, being more like nuts in this respect than like legumes. Being low in water and high in fat, nuts have a relatively high energy value, and they are apt to be avoided by calorie-conscious individuals. The proteins of nuts are apt to be deficient in one or more of the essential amino acids but excellently supplement other proteins. In a survey by the U.S. Department of Agriculture, dried legumes and nuts accounted for only 1 percent of the food money, and for this outlay they furnished 5 percent of the protein, 6 percent of the iron, and 5 percent of the thiamin of the total diet (see Table 17–2, p. 389).

In the discussion of food sources of mineral elements and B complex vitamins, it may be recalled that legumes (especially dried) and nuts usually rank high in the list of such sources. They are excellent sources of *phosphorus, iron,* and *thiamin* (vitamin B-1) and are fair sources of calcium and riboflavin (vitamin B-2). Unfortunately, they are practically entirely *lacking in vitamins A and C.*

Peanuts and peanut butter enjoy wide popularity (especially with children and teenagers), either alone or spread on crackers, and if consumed in sufficient quantity, they can reinforce the dietary protein, calcium, iron, and thiamin (vitamin B-1), for which the requirement is high during periods of growth. They are an excellent source of niacin.

VEGETABLES AND FRUITS. Fruits and vegetables are of value in the diet for their laxative and base-forming properties, and as carriers of mineral elements and vitamins. Together with milk, they supplement those foods on which we depend largely for meeting our energy and protein needs—highly milled cereals, sugar, fats, and meats. Thus, even though they furnish little energy and protein, fruits and vegetables are very important for the sake of other nutrients which they carry. Increasing the quantity and variety of fruits and vegetables in the diet usually improves its quality.

We are dependent almost entirely on fruits and vegetables for *vitamin C,* and all of them carry some of this vitamin, especially if eaten raw. Canned fruits carry smaller amounts of vitamin C, and in dried fruits it has been almost completely destroyed. Dried fruits are rich in mineral elements, especially iron in apricots, peaches, prunes, and raisins. Most fruits are poor in vitamin A value; exceptions are apricots, yellow peaches, prunes, avocados, and cantaloupe, which are good sources of vitamin A. Because most fruits and vegetables consist of 75 to 95 percent water (and some fiber), the B complex vitamins and mineral elements are usually present in dilute conditions, so that a considerable quantity of them would have to be consumed if they were to add appreciably to the intake of these nutrients.

Potatoes and Sweet Potatoes. White potatoes and sweet potatoes are not related botanically, but both are bland foods, furnish energy at low cost, and are high in carbohydrate. The white potato has 17 percent starch, while the carbohydrate content of the sweet potato (26 percent) includes 5 to 8 percent simple sugar. Because they are approximately three-fourths water, their mineral and vitamin content does not look impressive, but when eaten in quantity, they may make considerable contribution to safeguard the diet in these respects. These two foods furnish more than their quota of iron and thiamin but are low in calcium. The valuable contribution of vitamin C which potatoes make to the diet has been noted under the discussion of scurvy prevention. Retention of their mineral and vitamin content requires due care in cooking procedures. The protein of potatoes, although low in amount, is of good nutritive value. White potatoes have almost no vitamin A value but sweet potatoes show a vitamin A value of 600 to 10,000 IU per 100 gm, varying with the depth of color in different varieties, but the main variety has a value around 8000 IU. If sweet potatoes were more commonly used, they would bolster the ordinary vitamin A intake.

It may be well to call attention to the fact that potatoes and sweet potatoes are not the only vegetables high in starch. Such vegetables as lima beans, green peas, and sweet corn are also starchy, while beets and carrots contain sugar. If starchy vegetables are consumed too freely, they contribute to the problem of excess body weight. In certain European countries, potatoes have a larger place in the diet than in the United States.

Green and Yellow Vegetables. Green and yellow vegetables are grouped together because they contain *carotenes*, which are the precursors of *vitamin A*; they constitute our vegetable sources of this vitamin. They may be subdivided into the leafy vegetables, other green vegetables, and yellow vegetables, because of differences in their contributions to the diet other than vitamin A activity.

Leafy vegetables: Leaves are the most active parts of a plant, the chemical laboratories in which (with the aid of sunlight and chlorophyll) are built various substances necessary for the life of the plant. Hence, they are richer in mineral elements and vitamins than are other parts of the plant. They are especially rich in *calcium* and *iron*, in *provitamins A, ascorbic acid (C), and riboflavin* with a good content of other B vitamins. They supplement grain products, especially as to calcium and vitamin A value. The calcium in a few leafy vegetables is at least partially nonabsorbable, because it is bound in insoluble combination with oxalic acid, but these vegetables nevertheless are valuable sources of iron and many vitamins. Leafy vegetables with bound calcium include spinach, chard, sorrel, parsley, and beet greens. In other leafy vegetables, the calcium is in forms available to the body. Both in calcium and in vitamin A value, they rank next to milk as important sources. The vitamin C level is so high in broccoli, Brussels sprouts, collards, kale, mustard greens, and turnip greens (97 to 186 mg per 100 gm) that, if cooked for a short time in small amounts of water, these vegetables will still be richer in vitamin C than citrus fruits. Their iron content, fairly well utilized, is a

valuable contribution to the diet. Their energy and protein values are negligible.

The greener the leaf, the richer it is in vitamins and minerals. The blanched inner leaves of lettuce, cabbage, or celery are no richer in mineral salts and vitamins than are the stalks or roots of some other plants used as food.

Other green vegetables: These are usually stalks, stems, or green pods. Young shoots (such as green asparagus tips) are high in vitamin A value and similar in other composition to green leaves. Broccoli and cauliflower (which consist of flowerets with some leaves) contain only slightly less of certain minerals and vitamins than leafy vegetables do. Green string beans and peppers represent pod vegetables, which are intermediate between the green leaves and roots in minerals and vitamins. Loose leaf lettuce and cabbage rank much lower in vitamin A value than do vegetables with dark green leaves. Head lettuce (iceberg), along with blanched celery and asparagus, has little vitamin A value.

Yellow vegetables: This category includes fleshy roots (carrots, sweet potatoes, and rutabagas), fruit parts of plants (pumpkin, winter squash, cantaloupe, and other yellow fruits), and yellow corn. The vitamin A value varies with the depth of yellow color, but in deep-colored varieties, it is of almost the same magnitude as that of dark green leaves. These vegetables contribute relatively small amounts of the other vitamins and mineral elements, although in quantity they may be counted on to supply some of these nutrients.

Citrus Fruits and Tomatoes. These are grouped together as relatively rich sources of vitamin C, and they are reasonably inexpensive and well enough liked to be consumed in quantity. They also hold their vitamin C content well on cooking or canning. Grapefruit, lemons, and oranges have higher vitamin C contents (38 to 53 mg per 100

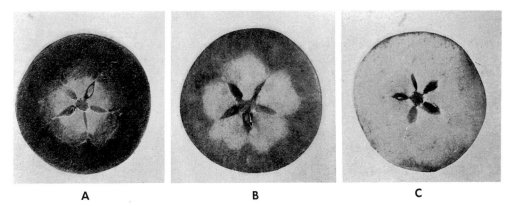

A   **B**   **C**

Figure 17–10. Apples cut in half and stained with iodine (black) to show the decrease of starch with ripening of the apple. **A** and **B,** Condition in apples as usually picked for market. **C,** Thoroughly ripened apple in which nearly all starch has been converted into sugar. (From Sherman, H. C.: *Food Products.* New York, Macmillan Co., 1948.)

gm) than do tomatoes (23 mg). Other than their vitamin C content, citrus fruits contain about 10 percent of readily assimilable sugar along with some calcium and thiamin. Tomatoes have considerable vitamin A activity (900 IU per 100 gm).

In planning an adequate diet, it should be remembered that there are other foods whose vitamin C content equals or exceeds that of citrus fruits and tomatoes. We have previously called attention to such green vegetables as broccoli, kale, turnip greens, and sweet green peppers, for high vitamin C value. Green peppers contain vitamin C in the same magnitude (70 to 90 mg per 100 gm, cooked), while fresh strawberries and raw cabbage contain amounts (59 and 47 mg per 100 gm, respectively) comparable to that of citrus fruits. If one of these foods is used in the day's meals, it would not be necessary to include citrus fruit or tomatoes. Also, if tomatoes are chosen as the vitamin C-rich food of the day, it takes more than twice as large a quantity to furnish the daily quota as it would if orange juice were used. The cheapest readily available food sources of vitamin C are canned orange or grapefruit juice.

BREAD AND CEREAL GROUP. This group includes the cereal grains and all foods that consist wholly or largely of grain in some form. This includes not only bread, rolls, biscuits, and breakfast cereals (both ready-to-eat and cooked), but also spaghetti, macaroni, noodles, hominy grits, crackers, cookies, cakes, and puddings which contain bread crumbs, rice, tapioca, sago, and flour or cornstarch used as thickening agents.

The importance of this food group in the diet is that they furnish *food energy* and some *protein* at relatively low cost and at the same time make worthwhile contributions of minerals and vitamins, especially when used in quantity. This holds true, however, only if the grains have not been subjected to a high degree of milling in which part of the protein and most of the minerals and vitamins have been removed. For this reason, directions for planning the diet on the basis of four food groups specify that the bread and cereals should be either whole-grain, enriched, or restored by addition of some of the vitamins and minerals removed in milling (see later section). Although whole grains make a many-sided contribution as to vitamins and minerals, perhaps the nutrients most missed when enriched products are not used are iron and thiamin, because these are furnished rather scantily by the milk group and by most fruits and vegetables.

Cereal grains are seeds of grasses. From the beginning of agriculture, grains have been the chief reliance of all peoples for their food supply. They are easily cultivated and stored and can be relatively simply made into palatable, wholesome, economical foods. Grains are usually crushed into a fine meal or flour and made into bread, which is often leavened by yeast. Bread has been for centuries literally "the staff of life" of many nations, especially of Europe and America.

The principal grains are *rice, wheat, rye, barley, oats,* and *corn.* Rice, grown in moist tropical or semitropical climates, has the largest consumption of any of the grains because of its very important place in the diet of the populous eastern countries. Wheat comes next in total amount produced and consumed, largely because its higher content of gluten (a protein) makes it the preferred grain for making yeast breads. Rye is grown in northern climates, and rye bread is commonly used in Germany and the Scandinavian countries. Barley thrives in more arid sections. In the United States, it is used as pearl barley in soups and as barley flour for infant foods. Oats must be combined with another cereal (usually wheat) if used in making bread. In Scotland and Sweden oats are consumed chiefly in the form of oat cakes, or scones, and cooked oatmeal (porridge). Cooked oatmeal is a breakfast food also common to Americans. In amount produced, corn is the main grain product of the United States, but most of it is used for feeding animals. Only 10 to 15 percent of the corn crop is used for human consumption, and much of this is used for the manufacture of corn syrup (glucose) and corn starch, rather than being consumed directly as hominy grits or corn meal (chiefly in the southern part of the United States). In Central and South American countries, as well as in parts of Africa and the Near East, corn is the chief grain used in the diet.

In preparation for human food, all grains must be *milled,* and the extent of this milling process determines how much of the original nutrients in the whole grain are left for human consumption. The reason for this is clear once one understands the distribution of the various constituents in the cereal grains (Fig. 17–11). Each kernel consists of (1) the outer husks, or bran; (2) the brownish outer part of the kernel, or aleurone layer; (3) the inner main portion, or endosperm; and (4) the small germ at one end of the kernel. Most of the vitamins and minerals, and much of the protein, are in the aleurone layer and germ. The inner part of the kernel consists chiefly of starch, with some protein. Usually, the harsh bran and the germ are removed in milling, the former to promote digestibility and the latter to improve the keeping qualities of the product. If, in addition, most of the aleurone layer is removed, as in milling of a high degree, very little of the original vitamin and mineral content of the grain is left. Thus, about 75 percent of the thiamin and a large part of the protein, iron, other B complex vitamins, and many minerals are lost in the process of making white wheat flour.[16] Much the same situation occurs when rice or corn is highly milled. The by-products (containing the germ and outer coats of the grain) are generally used for animal feed.

To meet possible deficiencies in the diet, the United States Government launched (in 1941) a program to enrich white bread by the addition of thiamin, riboflavin, niacin, and iron. Soon after, different manufacturers of breakfast cereals began to enrich highly milled products by addition of these nutrients approximately up to the level found in whole grains. More than 30 states (also Puerto Rico, Canada, and numerous other countries) now have laws that all white bread sold must be

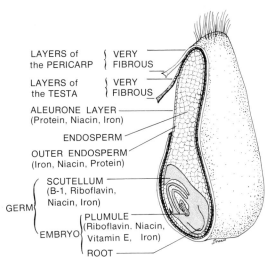

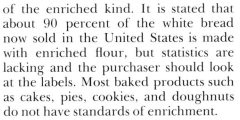

Figure 17–11. The distribution of nutrients in the wheat grain. (Courtesy of Sir J. Drummond, Dr. T. Moran, and *The Lancet.*)

of the enriched kind. It is stated that about 90 percent of the white bread now sold in the United States is made with enriched flour, but statistics are lacking and the purchaser should look at the labels. Most baked products such as cakes, pies, cookies, and doughnuts do not have standards of enrichment.

The legal standards of enrichment bring the levels of thiamin, riboflavin, niacin, and iron approximately up to the levels found in whole-wheat bread (see Table 17–3), but other B complex vitamins and minerals other than iron

Table 17–3. Comparison of Three B Vitamins and Iron in Pound Loaves of Wheat Bread*

Wheat Bread	Thiamin mg	Riboflavin mg	Niacin mg	Iron mg
Unenriched	0.40	0.36	5.6	3.2
Enriched†	1.1–1.8	0.7–1.6	10–15	8.0–12.5
Whole-Wheat	1.17	0.56	12.9	10.4

*From Bread Standards, Code of Federal Regulations, U. S. Food and Drug Administration, Title 21, Chap. 1, Section 17, April 22, 1964; and U. S. Department of Agriculture: *Handbook 8.*

†Enriched bread may also furnish, as an optional ingredient, vitamin D in such quantity that each pound of the finished bread contains not less than 150 IU and not more than 750 IU. It may also contain added calcium salts (including milk solids) in such quantity that each pound of the finished bread contains not less than 300 mg and not more than 800 mg of calcium. Higher levels of enrichment were proposed in 1972.

are also removed by high milling and they are not replaced. Nevertheless, the enrichment program has considerably increased the amount of the three added vitamins and iron in the American diet, varying in individual cases with the quantities of bread and cereal products which one eats. Families which depend more heavily on these carbohydrate foods benefit most. For average families at all income levels, it has been estimated that the percentage of the total nutrient in the diet added by enrichment of white flour is: thiamin, 16 percent; riboflavin, 3 percent; niacin, 13 percent; and iron, 12 percent. It costs less than one-tenth of 1 cent to enrich a loaf of bread.[17]

But even with widespread enrichment, surveys have shown below adequate iron intakes for women and low or deficient hemoglobin levels for children and the elderly, especially from low income groups. This phenomenon exists partly because the consumption of enriched flour and bread has decreased, while consumption of bakery products and confections, which are not enriched, has increased. In the last decade, per capita consumption of bread products has dropped 6 percent while consumption of other baked goods rose 67 percent.[18] Recommendations for increasing iron levels in bread and cereal products are currently being debated, however, and the question requires further study.

Other means, besides the official enrichment of white flour or the use of whole-grain products, may be used to increase the amount of thiamin, riboflavin, niacin, and iron carried by bread and cereal foods. Peanut butter, soy grits, and dried skim milk are all excellent sources of thiamin; any of these may be incorporated in home-baked breads, muffins, or cookies. Baking companies sometimes improve the nutritive quality of bread by adding dried skim milk, dried brewer's yeast,* or wheat germ.

The problem of replacing the B vitamins and minerals removed in milling grains is much more acute in many parts of the world other than in America. In this country, meat serves as a main source for iron, and most of the population enjoys a varied diet. But more than half the world's population use rice as their staple food, and the poorer classes often have almost nothing else to eat. Polished rice is still preferred to "brown" rice. It may be "enriched" by steeping it in an infusion of the nutrients lost in milling or (more commonly now) by coating with a mixture of thiamin, niacin, and iron, in amounts of one part to each 200 parts of rice. A new process now also permits the addition of riboflavin without discoloration of the grains. Rice so treated is said to be "processed" or "converted," and is gradually coming into wider use in the Orient. Where it has been used exclusively, as in the experiment of Burch, Salcedo, and associates[19] in the province of Bataan, Philippines, the mortality from beriberi dropped quickly, and the disease was virtually wiped out in about two years.

In addition, many people (in Africa, Central and South America, and the southern part of the United States) use corn as their chief grain food and, if it is highly milled and degerminated, there is likely to be a deficiency of B vitamins and minerals, as well as of other nutrients, in their diets. Many states are now considering making enrichment of all cereal grains mandatory (including corn meal, grits, and rice) as was pioneered by South Carolina.

All grain products (highly milled or otherwise) are characterized nutritionally by their high content of starch (nearly 70 to 80 percent) and moderate content of protein (ranging from 7.5 to 14 percent). Hence they serve as *economical sources of energy* and of some *protein*. The protein content is somewhat higher and of better quality if only the coarsest bran has been discarded and some outer coats and the embryo are retained. Likewise, the highly milled product contributes little in minerals and vitamins unless they are enriched (in which case at least iron and three B vitamins are present in suitable levels). In addition, grain products are readily handled in large amounts by the digestive tract and make for favorable texture of food residues.

Nutrients that grains *do not supply* in any considerable amounts are calcium, vitamins A (except for yellow corn) and C, and riboflavin. Also, to be satisfactory for growth and reproduction, the proteins in grains need to be supplemented (to a moderate extent) by some protein richer in the essential amino acids lysine and tryptophan. Milk or some other animal protein would meet this need. There are now available many breads that have been improved in their calcium and protein content by incorporating in the dough one or more of the following: milk solids (at a 4 to 6 percent level), soybean or peanut flour, wheat germ, or dried yeast. Of course the supplementation may be accomplished by foods taken separately, such as the fresh milk, meats, or eggs in the

---

*Brewer's yeast is 8 to 10 times richer in thiamin than is baker's yeast. It should be dried and ground to kill the living yeast cells if used as a dietary source of thiamin.

ordinary mixed diet, with citrus fruits or other fresh fruits for vitamin C.

In various surveys of American dietary habits, grain products were found to account for about 12 percent of the total cost of food, and for this outlay they contributed 19 percent of the total energy value and 18 percent of the protein of the diet (see Table 17–2 and Fig. 17–8). When most of the grain products were whole grain or enriched, they also contributed more than their quota of iron and thiamin. The per capita consumption of bread has decreased in the United States in recent years, but there is still wide use of grains in such foods as breakfast cereals, macaroni and similar products, crackers, cookies, and so on.

A recent estimate has placed the number of pounds of flour, cereals, and baked goods purchased per person per week at 2½ lb,[15] proving that the cereal group still occupies a prominent place in the American diet.

FOODS OUTSIDE THE BASIC FOUR. The four food groups encompass those foods that serve as good sources of particular nutrients. But most of us eat many foods, outlined below, which do not belong to one of these food groups. Such foods do not constitute separate food groups because they provide few, if any, essential nutrients.

Fats. Fats are essential in the diet to provide linoleic acid, which the body cannot manufacture (see Chap. 4). Fats also provide a concentrated source of fuel, improve the flavor and satiety value of food, and carry the fat-soluble vitamins. As to their energy value, weight for weight all pure fats are alike, whether solid, fluid, or of animal or vegetable origin. Butter and margarine are good sources of vitamin A (and, if enriched, of vitamin D). Most vegetable oils contribute vitamin E, and abundant amounts of the essential unsaturated fatty acid that is characteristic of low-melting-point fats.

All fats are *one-sided foods*. They lack protein, mineral elements, and all water-soluble vitamins. Hence, they must be supplemented in the diet by other foods that provide these nutrients essential for good nutrition. In order to assure a well balanced diet, it is generally stated that not more than 25 to 35 percent of the fuel value of the diet should come from fats. Because fats are such a concentrated fuel food, only a relatively small bulk of fat is needed daily. In the United States, fats supply slightly over 40 percent of the calories in the average diet. In Oriental diets, fats often furnish no more than 10 percent of the calories, but western peoples seem to want more fat in the diet both for flavor and satiety value. While the consumption of fat has been steadily increasing in the United States, there has been a definite shift from the use of animal fats to the use of vegetable fats. This has resulted in an increased intake of polyunsaturated fatty acids and a decrease of saturated fat in the American diet.[20]

Fats vary widely in cost, and economic considerations may cause people to alter the amount or kinds of fats consumed. Relatively cheap fats, such as lard and salt pork, may furnish inexpensive fuel in low-cost diets. Olive oil is now so expensive that people make use of refined cottonseed, peanut, or corn oil instead for salad dressings. The popular demand for margarine as a substitute for butter has given rise to its fortification with vitamin A up to the average level of butter. Most margarines are now made from vegetable oils (by hydrogenation) and contain a considerable proportion of linoleic acid.

Sugar and Concentrated Sweets. These foods furnish *energy* in relatively inexpensive, readily digested, and quickly available form; they also are useful for *flavor* and have some satiety value. They are practically completely *devoid of protein, minerals, and vitamins.* Except as an energy source, they are not considered nutritious foods.

We use sugar chiefly as refined cane

sugar or beet sugar (sucrose). Corn syrup, a concentrated solution of glucose, has considerable commercial use in making candies, jams, and bakery products. Including sugar consumed in candies, syrups, jams, and jellies, as well as for table use and in cooking, sugar consumption in the United States amounts to more than 100 pounds per person yearly, or about ¼ pound each day for every person in the country. Our annual candy bill is nearly two billion dollars and has increased over 1000 percent in the last 65 years. We spend over five billion dollars a year on soft drinks in the United States, which are made solely from carbonated water, sugar, and flavoring. This buys about 30 gallons of soda drinks per year for an average American. Our soft drink intake surpasses our intake of alcoholic beverages, tea, juices, and milk. Since soft drink consumption is increasing while coffee's is decreasing, the soft drink may soon be our number one national beverage.[21]

Sugar is one of the cheaper forms in which to buy energy, although the price of sugar has increased considerably in recent years. The content of essential nutrients in sugar and honey is negligible. If such a one-sided food is allowed too prominent a place in the diet, there would be a shortage of the essential proteins, mineral elements, and vitamins. Sugar and other sweets should be used chiefly as flavoring materials in fruits or desserts that contain milk, eggs, nuts, and so forth, and after all nutrient needs are met. Also, a large amount of sugar in the diet is a contributing factor in tooth decay and overweight. (See Chaps. 22 and 23.) For all of these reasons, it is recommended that not more than 5 to 10 percent of the energy intake come from sugar and other concentrated sweets, about half of the current contribution (16.4 percent).

Figure 17–12 shows what a large proportion of the diet (on a dry basis) is made up of sugars and other refined foods.

Other Foods. Coffee, tea, and alcohol (in various forms) are common adult foods in many countries, with the common characteristic of having significant drug action. They are carriers of small amounts of nutrients, and alcohol provides metabolizable energy (though no argument can be made for distilled spirits, nutritionally speaking). Some spices and condiments also provide nutrients (see Chap. 18).

Increasing numbers of Americans are eating *manufactured* or *fabricated foods.* These sometimes resemble, and are substituted for, traditional foods. For example, imitation milk might replace whole milk as a *food* in the diet, but its *nutrient* content does not compare favorably with whole milk's. Imitation milk, consisting of water, sugar, vegetable fat, emulsifiers, stabilizers, and a source of protein (casein or soy), is nutritionally inferior to milk.[22]

Similarly, coffee whiteners, whipped toppings, breakfast drinks, desserts, and meat substitutes may imitate the appearance, but not the nutrient content, of the foods they replace. These foods are gaining in popularity for a number of reasons: (1) They are convenient, requiring minimum storage and preparation. This is important in a nation where more and more women hold jobs outside the home. Also, more Americans are eating out, and the restaurants which want to attract their patronage are cutting labor costs by increasing their use of convenience foods. (2) They are attractive: formulated topping holds up better during transportation than does whipped cream. (3) They fill specific needs; for example, vegetarians use textured vegetable protein rather than meat.

In a recent policy statement, the Council on Foods and Nutrition of the American Medical Association noted, "The composition of an imitation or a new food becomes especially important when it contributes 10 percent or more of the recommended daily intake of any essential nutrient, including calories. The imitation or fabricated

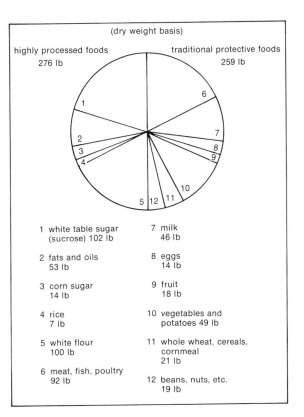

(dry weight basis)

highly processed foods
276 lb

traditional protective foods
259 lb

Figure 17–12. On a dry weight basis, the average American consumption of highly processed foods exceeds the consumption of traditional foods from the four food groups. (From the 1972 Britannica Yearbook of Science and the Future, p. 252.)

1 white table sugar
(sucrose) 102 lb

2 fats and oils
53 lb

3 corn sugar
14 lb

4 rice
7 lb

5 white flour
100 lb

6 meat, fish, poultry
92 lb

7 milk
46 lb

8 eggs
14 lb

9 fruit
18 lb

10 vegetables and
potatoes 49 lb

11 whole wheat, cereals,
cornmeal
21 lb

12 beans, nuts, etc.
19 lb

food should contain on a caloric basis at least the variety and the amounts of the important nutrients contained in the food which it replaces."[23]

Total dependence on fabricated products would not be wise nutritional practice (nor would total dependence on *any* single food item). We do not know enough about the composition of natural foods or the nutritional requirements of man to manufacture a food entirely from pure chemicals.

The consumer must depend on informative nutrient and ingredient labeling to know what substances are in a fabricated food. Labeling becomes most critical when a product appears to be one thing but actually is something different. Consumers who for years have depended on certain foods to provide particular nutrients naturally assume that substitute foods will provide the same nutrients, which they often do not.

Planning the Budget

The exact nature of the family food budget depends on a number of factors, among which are:

1. Overall income and eligibility for food stamps or commodities.

2. The availability of free or low cost school food service programs.

3. The number of members in the family and their food habits.

4. Where the family lives and how conveniently located the shopping areas are.

5. The amount of food produced or preserved at home.

6. Special dietary needs, as in pregnancy and disease states.

WHAT PROPORTION OF THE INCOME SHOULD BE SPENT FOR FOOD? In general, the *less the income, the greater the proportion of it that must be spent for food in order to secure a nutritionally adequate diet.* While the "average" American spends 16 percent of his disposable income on food, an American family at a low income level may have to spend over half, in some cases, of their total income for food in order to obtain a "*minimum-cost adequate diet.*" At very low income levels, even the most necessary expenditures for clothing and housing may rob a food budget that is already low, making it inadequate to maintain health over long periods. A mass of statistics proves that among such families are higher death rates (especially among young children and pregnant women), more sickness and absences from work or school, and smaller relative growth of children, than are found in families at higher income levels. In the 1965 dietary survey of United States households, a greater proportion of low-income families' diets, compared to high-income families' diets, were rated "poor" (see Fig. 17–13). However, low income families squeezed out a better nutritional return for each dollar spent (see Table 17–4). In most states, low-income families can participate in the United States Department of Agriculture's food stamp, commodity, or school lunch programs, all of which stretch the food dollar and help these families meet their nutritional requirements.

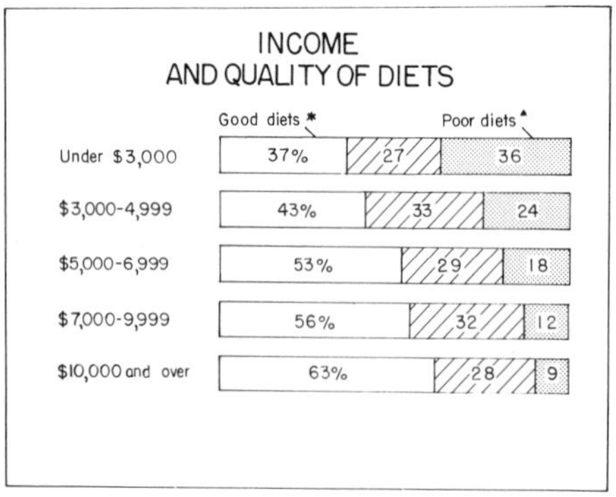

As the income level rises, the family may purchase a more "liberal diet." The student of nutrition recognizes, of course, that this does not mean more liberal as to calories (since overeating as to calories carries a penalty), but it does imply that certain foods of relatively higher cost (most of which carry nutritional values) may be provided more freely. These foods include the so-called "protective foods" — milk, eggs, fruits, vegetables, and probably either more or higher-cost meats. The greater freedom of choice ensures a better diet nutritionally only if wisely exercised, for the higher-cost foods are not necessarily those best for health. A so-called "luxury consumption" of meats, rich foods, and sweets does not make for health, and some cases of malnutrition still occur in families in which there is plenty of money for food. However, there is certainly less cause or chance of malnutrition and its resultant ill health when the money spent for food is liberal than when it is scanty.

Overall income is not the only determinant of the food budget. It is obvious that it costs more to feed four persons than one or two. A family of two adults usually has the most leeway on the amount to be spent for food, while the larger family, especially if there are several growing children, must spend not only a larger amount but also a greater proportion of its income for food. Young children and rapidly growing teen-agers need a larger allowance of certain foods that are relatively more expensive (such as fresh whole milk, meat and eggs for good quality protein; and fruits and vegetables for minerals and vitamins). In certain sections of the country (North Atlantic, Midwestern, and Pacific Coast states), the cost of living is higher than in other parts (especially the Southern states). City food costs vary more than

INCOME AND QUALITY OF DIETS

	Good diets *		Poor diets ▲
Under $3,000	37%	27	36
$3,000-4,999	43%	33	24
$5,000-6,999	53%	29	18
$7,000-9,999	56%	32	12
$10,000 and over	63%	28	9

Figure 17–13. Low-income families have a greater proportion of poor diets than high income families, because lack of money makes it difficult to buy the required nutrients. Having money does not ensure proper selection of nutrients, however, as can be seen from the percentage of poor diets in the upper income groups. (From Agric. Res. Serv., U.S.D.A., 1965.)

Table 17–4

Income	FOOD ENERGY	PROTEIN	CALCIUM	VITAMIN A VALUE	VITAMIN C
	A Dollar's Worth of Food Provided:				
	kcal	gm	mg	IU	mg
Under $3000	3150	99	1090	6860	85
$3000 to $4999	2860	92	970	6320	80
$5000 to $6999	2570	85	890	5990	81
$7000 to $9999	2380	79	830	5320	80
$10,000 and over	2100	72	750	5180	82

Low-income families bought more nutrients with their money than did high-income families. The reason their diets were rated "poor" is that they did not have enough money, not that they did not spend it wisely. (from Eagles, J. A.: talk at the 46th Annual Agricultural Outlook Conference, Washington, D.C., Feb. 19, 1969. Source: *Agric. Res. Service.*)

in small towns, and when one lives on a farm and can produce part of the family food supply, the money spent for food is naturally less. If the food is produced locally and the homemaker has the time, equipment, and storage facilities, then home freezing, canning, drying, or other methods of preserving foods plentiful only in certain seasons may prove economical in the long run.

The three main *ways of reducing the cost of an adequate diet* are:

1. Use a larger proportion of the less expensive food groups.
2. Substitute cheaper for more expensive foods within the same food group.
3. Eliminate waste in buying, storing, cooking, or serving foods.

USING MORE OF THE LEAST EXPENSIVE FOODS. Most of us do not need to subsist on a minimum-cost diet, but for those who do the problem is how to make such a diet adequate for body needs. One of the main problems is to get enough calories to satisfy hunger, to provide energy for work, and to keep warm. In Figure 17–14, the top graph shows the types of food that furnish the largest number of calories for a given amount of money ($1). Obviously, the best buys from the standpoint of energy yield are fats and oils, cereal products, potatoes, sugar, and dried

legumes. The group of dairy products, although excellent sources of other nutrients, furnish only about 35 percent as much energy per dollar spent as do cereal products and potatoes. The cheaper sources of food energy necessarily occupy a prominent place in low-cost diets, and as much as two-thirds the total amount of energy is sometimes furnished by this type of food in very low-cost diets.

Cereal products and starchy vegetables may be used more safely in large quantities than sugar or fats, because sugar and fats are mainly energy foods and they provide a one-sided diet. When a large percentage of cereal products are in the diet, it is important that whole-grain or enriched products be used, since these carry a valuable bonus in minerals and vitamins, which the highly milled products do not provide.

Obviously, adequate amounts of energy sources alone do not suffice to maintain health. The necessary quota of all essential nutrients must also be met. Table 17–5 shows inexpensive sources of various nutrients.

SUBSTITUTING PRODUCTS IN THE SAME FOOD GROUP. Substitution of cheaper for more expensive foods within the same group is another way to reduce food costs and is the *best program to follow when only moderate reduction of food expense is required*, because none of the

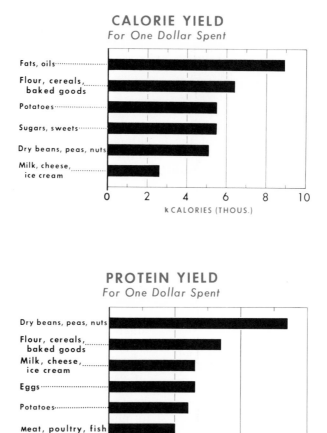

Figure 17–14. Relative economy of foods in different food groups as sources of (*top*) calories, and (*bottom*) protein. (From U.S. Department of Agriculture, *Family Food Plans and Food Costs.* Home Economics Research Report No. 20, 1962.)

Table 17–5. Inexpensive Sources of Various Nutrients

Nutrients	Food Sources
Energy	Fats, oils, flour, cereals, breads, potatoes, sugar, dried beans or peas, and peanut butter.
Protein	Dried beans or peas, peanut butter, whole-grain cereals or breads, milk (especially dried skim milk), cheaper cheeses, eggs, poultry, and less expensive meats and fish.
Calcium	Milk (especially dried skim milk), ice milk (dessert), cheese, dark green leafy vegetables, whole-grain products, and legumes.
Iron	Dried beans or peas, liver, whole-grain or enriched breads or cereals, dark green leafy vegetables, eggs, less expensive meats, potatoes and sweet potatoes, and prunes.
Vitamin A	Dark green and deep yellow vegetables, liver, fortified margarine, canned tomatoes, prunes, and less expensive cheeses.
Vitamin C	Canned or frozen citrus fruit juices, canned tomatoes, raw cabbage, some dark green and leafy vegetables, and potatoes.
Thiamin	Dried legumes, whole-grain or enriched bread and cereals, liver, inexpensive cuts of pork, and potatoes.
Riboflavin	Milk, ice milk (dessert), cheese, whole-grain or enriched breads, eggs, dried legumes, and dark green and leafy vegetables.
Niacin	Dried beans or peas, peanuts or peanut butter, whole-grain and enriched cereal products, meat, poultry, fish, some dark green, leafy vegetables.

nutritive advantages of the higher cost diet are sacrificed. For example, one can have the advantages of using fruits and vegetables *liberally* but keep down cost by selecting only the least expensive *kinds* of fruits and vegetables. In a moderate cost diet, the relative *amounts* of milk, fats, meats, and eggs can remain practically the same as in the high-cost diet. Considerable reductions in costs may be made, however, by using cheaper substitutes for the more expensive foods in the same group. How this kind of food economy may be effected is outlined in Table 17–6.

There are wide differences in costs within the different food groups. The cost difference depends considerably on whether one buys fat in the form of cottonseed oil or olive oil, and protein in the form of dried skim milk, dried legumes and whole grain cereals, or eggs and beef steak. Even among the meat group, there is a wide variation in costs ranging from ground beef through poultry (moderate cost) to filet mignon.

From Table 17–5, it is apparent why the free use of whole-grain bread and cereals, potatoes, leafy and yellow vegetables, legumes, cheese, and milk is recommended for the low-cost diet. Dried skim milk is useful as a beverage or in cooking to provide animal protein, calcium, and B complex vitamins at very low cost. Evaporated or concentrated whole milk is cheaper than fresh whole milk and has the same food value. Because meat is usually the most expensive item of the diet, low-income families are advised to serve cheaper cuts (such as chuck, breast of veal, shoulder of lamb, and ground, organ, and stew meats) only three or four

Table 17-6.   Economy from Substituting Cheaper Foods in Same Food Group

Grain products – Even in this relatively inexpensive food group some foods are cheaper than others.
Corn and *rice* are usually cheaper than wheat.
The processed, fancy *ready-to-serve cereals* are relatively expensive.
Uncooked cereals bought in large quantity are usually cheaper than in small packages.
Oatmeal and *whole-wheat cereals* give especially good value because of their higher content of protein, mineral salts, and B complex vitamins.
Homemade *breadstuffs* are cheaper than some bakery products, and plain breads are cheaper than those with special flavor appeal. Crackers, sweet buns, cake, cookies, and doughnuts are expensive when purchased at the store.

Sweets – *Sugar* is one of the cheapest fuel foods but should not furnish more than 5 to 10 percent of total calories.
Granulated white sugar and *brown* sugar are cheapest; *powdered* sugar, *loaf* sugar, and *maple* sugar are considerably more expensive.
Molasses, corn syrup, and *cane* syrups are inexpensive; blended syrups are of moderate cost; maple syrup and strained honey are expensive. Molasses and open-kettle sugar-cane syrup have a *mineral content* especially valuable in a low-cost diet.
Jellies, jams, marmalades, and preserves are relatively expensive, but may be useful to render bread and other inexpensive starchy foods more acceptable. Homemade jams and jellies are least expensive.
Candy, except for simple hard candies, is an expensive form of sweets.

Fats – *Meat fats, vegetable shortenings* (from cottonseed, corn, or peanut oils), and *margarines* are relatively inexpensive; *butter* and *cream* are relatively expensive. *Butter* and *olive oil* are the most expensive fats.

Protein-rich foods – Cereal grains and legumes are the cheapest sources of protein, but should not be the only protein-bearing foods in the diet. Nuts are an excellent source, but except for peanuts and peanut butter, are now high-cost foods. American (Cheddar) cheese, milk (dried milk is one of the cheapest sources of complete protein) and *fresh* or *canned fish* provide excellent quality protein at moderate cost. Eggs are a more economical protein source than most cuts of meat. Meats, fish, or shellfish, and poultry are usually the most expensive of the protein-rich foods.

Flesh foods – Within this group cost levels differ greatly. Certain *fatty meats* may be relatively inexpensive, next come the *cheaper cuts* of red meats and the less expensive *fish,* next the more *tender cuts* of lean meats and cuts that involve considerable waste, along with the more expensive forms of sea food such as shellfish. *Poultry* is usually moderately priced the year round. *Dried or canned fish* may offer good protein at low cost; canned *salmon* is valuable for vitamins A and D, and costs less than fresh salmon. *Frozen fish* are of excellent quality and have little waste.

Fruits – *Dried fruits* (raisins, dates, figs, apricots, prunes, peaches, and apples), an excellent source of minerals and some vitamins, were formerly inexpensive but have recently become high-cost. Any of them that are relatively inexpensive (e.g., prunes) should be used in the low-cost dietary. *Canned* or frozen *fruits* are usually less expensive than fresh, but they may not be when a fresh fruit is in season and plentiful. Of the *fresh fruits, apples, bananas* and *oranges* are apt to be the least expensive, though some of the others may be relatively cheap at the height of their season. The *citrus fruits* and *tomatoes* are especially valuable for their vitamin C content. Canned or frozen orange and grapefruit juices are usually the least expensive sources of vitamin C. Most expensive are the less common fruits and fresh fruits which are out of season.

Vegetables – *Potatoes* and the *root vegetables* are usually the least expensive.
Cabbage and some of the other *leafy vegetables* in their season are relatively inexpensive.
Leafy, green and *yellow vegetables* have the highest vitamin A value.
Dried legumes are relatively inexpensive. *Canned vegetables* are often moderately priced, and *canned tomatoes* are especially useful to add flavor and vitamins to a low-cost diet.
Frozen vegetables (and fruits) afford variety in moderate cost diets. They are without the waste and with full nutritive value of fresh vegetables.
Most *fresh vegetables* (especially the succulent ones) are at least fairly expensive, except at the height of their season.
The *less used vegetables* and those that are out of season are the most expensive of all.

times a week, and to use fish, legumes, and an egg or cheese dish on the other three or four days.

EFFICIENT BUYING AND PREPARATION OF FOOD. Efficient buying and preparation of food are the most satisfactory means of all to reduce food costs, because they *involve no diminution in the variety, attractiveness, or nutritive value* of the menu. By merely "stopping the leaks," enough saving may be effected to provide a better diet at less cost. Such waste can occur in the course of buying, storing, preparing, or serving foods. Sometimes one's carelessness enriches food merchants, or allows nutrients to be thrown away in cooking water or disappear in an overflowing garbage pail.

Considerable money savings can be effected by *thrifty marketing.* Some factors which cause higher costs for foods are discussed in the preceding section. In general, buying in larger quantities, watching for special bargains on certain foods, going to the market to select perishable foods that are of good quality, and selecting less expensive types or brands of food when these are suitable, all result in lowering the food bill. One should plan to use some of the cheaper cuts of meat as often as feasible, for they are just as nutritious as more expensive ones and may be made very palatable if properly cooked. Plan to use occasionally the organ meats, fish, or legumes or cheese in place of meat. Also smaller amounts of meat may be "extended" by combining with a starchy food, such as bread crumbs, noodles, or rice.

Read package labels to know what you are paying for. Ingredients are listed in descending order of amount present. Look for the total contents in canned foods. Often a can with twice the quantity does not cost very much more than the smaller one. With fruits and vegetables, higher price is usually based on appearance and those of lower quality and price may well be suited for one's use, such as small, tart apples for applesauce.

Waste in the kitchen may occur in many ways, some of the chief ones being: (1) discarding portions of food which have nutritive value (vegetable trimmings, meat trimmings, cooking water, liquid from canned vegetables) which are suitable for cooking, (2) burning foods or careless scraping of them from cooking utensils in serving, or (3) failure to utilize leftover foods properly, (4) food wasted at the table by taking too large individual portions or, in one way or another, rendering what is not eaten unfit to serve again, and (5) spoilage of food through improper care in storage.

There is no sense in purchasing fruits and vegetables chiefly for the minerals and vitamins and allowing most of these nutrients to be lost before the food reaches the table. The main losses occur through exposure to air or sunlight (either at room temperatures or the higher temperatures used in cooking), and through solution in water.

Some rules for minimizing the loss of nutrients in home storage and preparation are as follows:

1. Store perishables in a cool, dark place; buy no more than can be used.

2. Prepare perishables as short a time as possible before serving.

3. Save the water used in cooking vegetables, and use it for soup stock.

4. Cook vegetables in a small amount of water, or steam them until just tender. To shorten cooking time, add the vegetables to boiling water.

5. Leave on skins. Small pieces cook faster (reducing nutrient loss), but expose more surface area (increasing nutrient loss), so compromise.

Planning the Menu

Planning the menu ahead will help ensure more efficient marketing. Keep in mind family food habits, preferences, and needs, and design meals which you know will be enjoyed. The nutrients in food and the food in the market are of no value to you and your family if the food you buy and prepare is not eaten.

PLAN FOR THE DAY. The three meals of the day should always be considered as a whole, planned in advance, and arranged to supplement each other. This not only is more economical of time and money, but also ensures better balanced and more attractive meals, and it is the *only way of being sure to get in the full amount of essential foods each day.*

For some rules on menu-planning, see Table 17–8. It is best to keep the meals *simple* and to a somewhat standardized pattern based on the four food groups. When fewer foods are used, it is easier to secure variety from day to day. In general, *the greater variety of foods used from day to day, the better for health.* The staple foods in which one

does not crave variety are available for use as the appetite and energy needs of different members of the family dictate; for example, bread and butter or margarine, not listed in menus—may be added to the meal as needed. The too liberal use of relishes, jams, condiments, and spices is not advised, because it blunts the taste for the true flavor of raw or well cooked foods, and also may induce overeating. Garnishes and relishes are not specified in menus, but most homemakers will wish to add such touches to make meals more attractive and appetizing.

Having a general pattern for the three meals of the day is helpful in planning, and it avoids a dearth at one meal and a glut at another. Of course, the pattern must be adapted to the

Table 17–7.   Menus at Three Cost Levels

Low	Moderate	High
Breakfast		
½ grapefruit	Frozen orange juice	½ cantaloupe
Wheatena, with milk and sugar	French toast, with corn syrup	Puffed wheat, with cream
Toast	Margarine	Scrambled eggs and bacon
Margarine	Milk for children	Coffee cake
Milk for children	Coffee (adults)	Butter
Coffee (adults)		Milk for children
		Coffee (adults)
Luncheon		
Mixed vegetable salad, on lettuce	Bouillon	Cream of tomato soup
Peanut butter sandwiches, enriched bread	Spinach ring, with creamed eggs	Grapefruit and avocado salad, French dressing
Milk	Baking powder biscuits, with honey	Toasted cheese crackers
	Applesauce	Chocolate éclair
	Milk	Milk for children
		Tea
Dinner		
Casserole of rice, chopped meat, tomato, and green pepper	Meat loaf, with tomato sauce	Celery hearts and carrot sticks
Carrots	Baked potato	Roast prime ribs of beef
Shredded cabbage, raw, with vinaigrette dressing	Lima beans	Browned potatoes
Prunes	Mixed green salad, French dressing	Broccoli
Molasses cookies	Caramel custard	Endive salad, Roquefort cheese dressing
Milk	Cookies	Ice cream, topped with frozen raspberries
	Milk for children	Cake
	Coffee (adults)	Milk for children
		Coffee (adults)

Table 17–8. Some Guidelines in Menu Planning

GENERAL RULES

1. Use the *whole day as a unit* rather than the individual meal. Make breakfast relatively simple and standardized, then plan dinner, and lastly plan luncheon (or supper) so as to supplement the other two meals.

2. Use some foods from *each of the food groups* (carbohydrate foods, protein-rich foods, fatty foods, fruits, and vegetables) daily and usually in each meal.

3. Use some *raw* food at least once a day.

4. Plan to have in every meal at least one food which has *staying quality* or high satiety value, at least one food which requires *chewing*, one which contains *roughage*, and generally some *hot* food or drink.

5. Combine (or alternate) *bland* foods with those of more pronounced *flavor.*

6. Combine (or alternate) *soft* foods with those *crisp* in texture.

7. Have *variety* in *color, form,* and *arrangement* of foods.

8. Alternate *simple* and less nutritious dishes with those which are of higher protein and/or fat content, and hence slow down digestion in, and emptying of, the stomach.

9. When more foods are served at one meal, decrease the size of the portions and use fewer rich foods. When a more simple meal is desired, use a few nutritious, easily digested foods, and serve larger portions.

DON'TS

1. Avoid using the *same food twice in one day* without *varying the form* in which it is served, except staples such as bread, butter, and milk.

2. Do not use the same food twice in the same meal, even in different forms.

3. Do not use the same foods too constantly, even from day to day.

4. Avoid *monotony* of *color, texture,* etc., in any one meal or in the daily dietary.

---

physical needs, as well as to the likes and living habits of the individual or family. If one or more members have lunch away from home, the two other meals may need to provide more food and more hot foods than would otherwise be the case. If a packaged lunch is prepared, it should be planned as a meal, and the meals taken at home should supplement it. Some people like a light breakfast, but if there is a teenage boy or a man who does heavy labor in the family, he may want and need to have some substantial hot dish or dishes at breakfast. If breakfast is light, the other meals of the day should be heavier. Going without breakfast is not a good practice, because midmorning fatigue is likely to be experienced, and it is difficult to get in all the essential foods when only two meals are taken.

Breakfast. The pattern for breakfast may vary from light to moderately heavy, according to the physical activity of the persons concerned. Most Americans are sufficiently sedentary that their needs are well served with a light breakfast, and the old-fashioned breakfast, which included meat and potato, pie, or doughnuts, is a thing of the past. The practice of beginning the meal with fruit or fruit juice is beneficial both as an appetizer, a laxative, and a way of securing extra vitamins (especially C). A beverage (usually milk or coffee or both) is also helpful to most people in starting the day. Hence, it is customary to include fruit, a protein source, and a beverage in the breakfast menu.

Luncheon (or Supper). The size and character of this meal vary with different individuals and families. If breakfast has been light, a more substantial lunch is indicated (rather than making up by too heavy a dinner). If breakfast has been a fairly substantial meal, the luncheon should be light in order to avoid excessive calorie intake for the day. Sedentary persons need to avoid taking a meal at noon that is a second dinner, or overweight may result. Persons who do a good deal of muscular work need a substantial meal at midday.

For young children, invalids, and elderly people, the heaviest meal is best taken at midday and a supper of simple, easily digested foods taken in the evening. Much the same kind of menu is suitable for supper as for luncheon.

Luncheon (or supper) is usually accounted the most difficult meal to plan. It is best, in planning the day's meals, to plan breakfast and dinner first, then to make lunch a meal that will carry the rest of the day's quota of essential foods. It is the meal *par excellence* for using up leftovers and for securing pleasing variety in salads.

Dinner. Dinner is the *social* meal of the day, and as such it is best taken in a relaxed manner after the day's work is over. It tends to be a slightly more formal meal. However, there is a tendency toward less formality than formerly (including meal-in-one dishes, buffet service, and barbecued meats). The elaborate, many-course dinner is seldom served now in homes, except sometimes at banquets.

A very simple dinner consists of meat and vegetables (which may be combined in a single dish if desired), bread and butter, salad, a beverage, and dessert. An appetizer may be served at the start of the meal; for example, a fruit cup, carrot and celery sticks, or a light salad.

PLAN FOR THE WEEK. It is a great advantage to plan meals for the week, except for last-minute alterations. This facilitates efficient marketing, in which leftovers are planned to cover the week's meals. Planning by the week can also result in economy of labor in preparing meals. The family may also profit nutritionally from more evenly planned meals. Planning oven-cooked (slower) meals for two days of the week, with left-overs which can be used for assembling a quick dinner on other nights, saves time and labor.

Many women combine a job with homemaking, and for them careful planning ahead is especially important, if their families are not to suffer from hastily prepared, inadequate, or monotonous meals. They, and other homemakers, find that buying in larger quantities and keeping foods ahead in a freezer is economical, saves trips to the market, and is useful in assembling a meal quickly. Ready-prepared, frozen vegetables are also a great convenience, as are baking and pudding mixes, but mass-produced, ready-to-serve meals (such as TV dinners) are to be recommended only for very occasional use. The homemaker who makes them a mainstay is losing an opportunity to provide more flavorful, nutritious, and appetizing foods—meals that can be adapted to the individual tastes of the family, with little suprises and attractive combinations of foods that add zest to a meal.

The use of leftover foods is no disgrace; in fact, it indicates good planning for economy of money, time, and labor. With modern refrigeration, there need be little question of spoilage if foods are kept in covered dishes or plastic bags, or are otherwise kept from drying out (aluminum foil wrapping) in the refrigerator. If a day is allowed to intervene and they are presented in some quite different dish, they are often better liked at the second than at the first serving. Roast beef may be used in sandwiches, served in cold slices, as a quick stew by warming with gravy, or ground in patties. Leftover chicken may be served cold, as pot-pie, in salad, or in a nourishing chowder. Potatoes need not be cooked for each dinner but are relished in numerous warmed-up forms. Fresh vegetables, however, are best cooked only in quantities eaten at one meal, for they lose vitamins when stored and reheated. Americans throw away much food which should be saved and utilized—scraps of bread or bread crumbs that could be used in casserole dishes or puddings, meat and vegetable trimmings good for soups, and so on.

The introduction of variety in the planning of menus is the phase that is most troublesome to the average homemaker. Our great-grandmothers might have been excused on this score, because at some seasons of the year fresh fruits and vegetables were unobtainable and other foods were in scant supply. They used great ingenuity in making the limited variety of foods into many and quite different dishes. Trips to the modern supermarkets, with their enormous range of fresh, canned, and frozen meats, vegetables, and fruits, as well as ready-to-heat packaged foods, would seem to be enough to stimulate the imagination of the modern homemaker. Perhaps from force of habit, some still go on using only the same five meats and six vegetables they have been using for years. It does not seem to occur to them to buy broccoli instead of string beans, yellow squash instead of carrots, or ground veal for veal loaf instead of ground beef for hamburgers. Pleasing variety also may be obtained by different ways of cooking and serving the same food. Celery, which is usually served raw, can also be boiled and served with cream sauce, or can lend flavor to a dish of chop suey. Apples are one thing raw and crisp, and quite different in applesauce, in Brown Betty pudding, or in apple pie. There are said to be a hundred ways of cooking and serving chicken. So the modern homemaker not only needs to keep her eyes open in the grocery store but might also profit by collecting and keeping a file of new recipes.

PLANNING FOR THE SEASON. This includes two phases of meal planning: (1) using foods that are especially plentiful and relatively inexpensive at certain times of the year, and (2) making certain diet adaptations to suit hot or cold weather.

Foods that are *plentiful only at certain seasons* are chiefly the fresh fruits and vegetables, although eggs and certain meats may be scarcer and more expensive at some times of the year. In the large cities, one can often get out-of-season fruits and vegetables almost the

year round, but at fancy prices because they are either hothouse grown or must be brought from long distances. Oranges, apples, bananas, tomatoes, lettuce, and certain other green vegetables are staples which can be obtained the year round, but even so there are seasons when they are cheaper and of better quality. If we do not take advantage of fresh berries, peaches, pears, grapes, and melons in season, we are likely to have to fall back on canned ones or do without. When fresh foods are in the market in abundance one may well use them freely. Because they are seasonal, there is little danger of our tiring of them even if they appear on the menu daily or even twice a day for a time.

Nutrients must travel a long road before they reach the body. Food, which carries the nutrients, must be grown or raised on the farm, and then distributed, processed, and marketed through complex economic channels. It must then be bought at a store and prepared into appetizing meals. At every link of the chain, the nutrients in the food are subject to extinction or reduction. Careful processing, handling, and preparation of food, with an eye to the instability and value of the nutrients within, can help ensure that the money spent on foods buys the nutrients necessary for a healthy life.

QUESTIONS AND PROBLEMS

1. What types of food supply and level of civilization are characteristic of the following different stages of development in a country or region?

   a. Tribal organization, hunting, primitive agriculture, or herding of animals as main occupations.

   b. Larger area under central government, most people engaged in agriculture, and agricultural methods still primitive.

c. Smaller proportion of people engaged in agriculture, with more working in industries or other pursuits.

d. High degree of industrialization, more efficient agriculture which produces more food with labor of fewer people, and rise of cities and large towns.

Can you name two countries (or areas) which are at present representative of each of these stages of development?

2. What motivated the development of so many new, processed foods since 1945? Name five methods of food preservation or processing that are now commonly used and two food products prepared by each type of processing. To what extent has the introduction of "convenience foods" changed our food habits and/or the consumption of different food groups? What are the advantages and disadvantages of extensive use of ready-to-serve and pre-cooked foods?

3. Make a list of ten food additives you have found on the labels of foods. For each additive, describe the food in which it was found, give the purpose of the additive, and discuss its safety.

4. Name four factors that influence the cost of foods. Name four factors, other than food prices, that affect the amount which a family must spend to be adequately fed.

5. What countries or areas of the world now have food supplies adequate to, or in excess of, the needs of their population? In which countries are food supplies inadequate to supply the nutritional needs of the population? In respect to what nutrients is the diet in these areas most likely to be inadequate? What special groups among the people are most apt to be adversely affected by these dietary deficiencies?

6. What methods are being instituted to increase the food supplies in these regions, to increase the amount and quality of protein in the diet? Why have these efforts been successful in some countries and not in others?

7. In respect to what nutrients does milk make an outstanding contribution to the diet? What other nutrients does it furnish in lesser amounts? Is it low or lacking in any essential nutrients, and if so which ones? In respect to what nutrients does it supplement the grains? The legumes? Lean muscle meats? Name some of the milk products that may, at least in part, be substituted for fresh whole milk in the diet. What is the least expensive product in which one can buy milk solids?

8. For what reasons are meats, fish, poultry meat, and eggs especially valuable in the diet? In respect to the nutritive essentials that they provide, how do lean meats resemble and how do they differ from milk? How do eggs differ from meats and from milk in these respects? From the point of view of cost to the national resources, which of these types of food is most costly and which is most economical to produce— grains, milk, eggs, beef? Is this reflected in their market cost?

9. Are legumes and nuts good sources of protein? Inexpensive sources? Do any or all of them furnish protein mixtures that are complete as to essential amino acid content? Which ones are especially good for supplementing the proteins of wheat? Why? Are legumes and nuts "alternates" or complete "substitutes" for meats in the diet? Explain why. What mineral elements and vitamins are found in good or high quantities in legumes and nuts?

10. For what vitamin are we almost entirely dependent upon fruits and vegetables? For what other reasons are these classes of foods needed in the diet? What are the special nutritive contributions made by each of the following sub-groups: potatoes and sweet potatoes? green and yellow vegetables? leafy vegetables? citrus fruit and tomatoes?

11. What are the chief contributions of grains and their products (bread, breakfast cereals, etc.) to the diet? In what nutritive factors are they rich and in which ones are they lacking? In what

ways nutritionally do highly milled grains differ from whole grains, and why? Is enriched white bread nutritionally equivalent to bread made from whole grain?

12. Of what value are fats and sugar in the diet? What are their shortcomings as foods? To how great an extent may they safely be included in the diet? What dangers may be associated with too high consumption of fats, of concentrated sweets?

13. Give the three principal ways in which economies in the food budget may be effected. Which are especially useful for families of low income, moderate income, and high income? Why?

14. Why is menu-planning important? What should be the unit for planning menus—the meal, the day, or the week? Why?

15. Tell in what respects the following factors affect the type of meals planned:

a. Size of family and occupation and habits of family members.
b. Individual likes and dislikes of family members, regional or racial food habits.
c. Age differences of family members.
d. Cost and availability of different foods.
e. Storage facilities available in the home.

16. Why is use of a wide variety of foods from day to day, or week to week, good nutritional practice? How can sufficient variety be made consistent with the use of leftover foods?

17. Plan a day's menus for a moderately active college student, who should have a fairly hearty breakfast, a moderate lunch, and a hearty dinner.

18. Make a day's menus for a young married couple, both of whom work and eat lunch away from home. Plan for a moderate breakfast and a fairly hearty dinner, both of which are quickly prepared. Keep food costs as moderate as is consistent with providing adequately for their nutritional needs.

19. Suppose that this couple has invited two other couples for dinner. For this occasion, they may buy some more expensive foods or some that are ready to serve. Plan a menu for such a dinner, assuming the party takes place on a hot summer evening. Make another dinner menu suitable for a cold night in winter.

REFERENCES

1. Harp, H. H., and Dunham, D. F.: *Comparative Costs to Consumers of Convenience Foods and Home-Prepared Foods.* Marketing Res. Rep. No. 609. Washington, D.C., U. S. Department of Agriculture, 1963.
2. Hadsell, R. M.: Chem. Engin. News, Aug. 23, 1971, p. 17.
3. Sanders, H. J.: Chem. Engin. News, Oct. 10, 1966, p. 100.
4. Anonymous: Chem. Engin. News, Oct. 12, 1970, p. 11.
5. Berg, A. D.: Amer. J. Clin. Nutr., 23:1396, 1970.
6. Parman, G. K.: J. Agr. Food Chem., 16:168, 1968.
7. Anonymous: Weekly Digest, Sept. 18, 1971, p. 8.
8. Holden, P. M.: Food & Nutr., 28:102, 1971.
9. György, P., et al.: Amer. J. Clin. Nutr., 14:65, 1964.
10. Burgess, A., and Dean, R. F. A.: *Malnutrition and Food Habits.* London, Tavistock Publications, 1963.
11. Draper, W. M., Jr.: War on Hunger (AID), 2:1, 1968.
12. Anonymous: Chem Engin. News, Aug. 10, 1970, p. 36.
13. Sanjur, D.: *Alimentos Para Tu Salud.* New York, Cornell University Cooperative Extension, 1970.
14. Dupin, H. and M.: *Our Foods: A Handbook for Educationists in West Africa.* Paris, Editions Sociales Françaises, 1962.
15. Economic Research Service: National Food Situation. Washington, D.C., U.S. Department of Agriculture, November 1971.
16. Czerniejewski, C. P., et al.: Cereal Chem., 41:65, 1964.
17. Harris, R. S.: J. Agr. Food Chem., 16:149, 1968.
18. Senti, F. R.: Cereal Science Today, 16:92, 1971.
19. Burch, G. B., et al.: J. Nutr., 42:9, 1950; 46:239, 1952.
20. Friend, B.: Amer. J. Clin. Nutr., 20:907, 1967.
21. Anonymous: Weekly Digest, Apr. 17, 1971, p. 6; Nov. 27, 1971, p. 5.
22. Council on Foods and Nutrition: J. Amer. Med. Assoc., 208:1686, 1969.
23. Council on Foods and Nutrition: J. Amer. Med. Assoc., 205:160, 1968.

SUPPLEMENTARY READING

General

Agricultural Research Service: Household Food Consumption Survey, 1965-66. Washington D.C., U.S. Department of Agriculture, 1969.

Darrah, L. B.: *Food Marketing.* New York, Ronald Press Co., 1967.

Marion, B. W., Simonds, L. A., and Moore, D. E.: *Food Marketing in Low Income Areas.* Columbus, Cooperative Extension Service, Ohio State University, 1970.

Popkin, B., and Lidman, R.: Economics as an aid to nutritional change. Amer. J. Clin. Nutr., 25:331, 1972.

Tinklin, G. L., Fogg, N. E., and Wakefield, L. M.: Convenience foods: Factors affecting their use where household diets are poor. J. Home Econ., 64:26, 1972.

Food Processing and Additives

Anonymous: Food Additives: What They Are, How They Are Used. Washington, D. C., Manufacturing Chemists' Assoc., Inc., 1971.

Bender, A. E.: Nutritional effects of food processing. J. Food Tech., 1:261, 1966.

Goldblith, S. A.: Radiation preservation of food—the current status. J. Food Tech., 5:103, 1970; Thermal processing of foods: A review. World Rev. Nutr. Dietet., 13:165, 1971.

Goodwin, R. W. L. (ed.): *A Symposium on Chemical Additives in Food.* Boston, Little, Brown and Co., 1967.

Harris, R. S., and Von Loesecke, H. (eds.): *Nutritional Evaluation of Food Processing.* New York, Wiley, 1960.

Hellendoorn, E. W., et al.: Nutritive value of canned meals. J. Amer. Dietet. Assoc., 58:434, 1971.

Joint FAO/WHO Expert Committee on Food Additives: *Evaluation of Food Additives.* Rome, FAO, 1971.

Joslyn, M. A., and Heid, J. L.: *Food Processing Operations* (2 vols.). Connecticut, Avi Publishing Company, 1963.

Kermode, G. O.: Food additives. Sci. Amer., 226: 15, 1972.

Lang, K.: Influence of cooking on foodstuffs. World Rev. Nutr. Dietet., 12:266, 1970.

Schroeder, H. A.: Losses of vitamins and trace minerals resulting from processing and preservation of foods. Amer. J. Clin. Nutr., 24:562, 1971.

Sweeney, J. P., and Marsh, A. C.: Effect of processing on provitamin A in vegetables. J. Amer. Dietet. Assoc., 59:238, 1971.

Tressler, D. K., Van Arsedel, W. B., and Copley, M. J.: *Freezing Preservation of Foods* (4 vols.) Connecticut, Avi Publishing Company, 1968.

Van Arsedel, W. B., and Copley, M. J.: Food Dehydration (2 vols.). Connecticut, Avi Publishing Company, 1964.

Fortification and Enrichment

Baertl, J. M., Morales, E., Verastegui, G., and Graham, G. G.: Diet supplementation for entire communities. Amer. J. Clin. Nutr., 23:707, 1970.

Butterworth, C. E., Jr.: Iron "undercontamination"? J. Amer. Med. Assoc., 220:581, 1972.

Council on Foods and Nutrition: Iron in enriched wheat flour, farina, bread, buns, and rolls. J. Amer. Med. Assoc., 220:855, 1972.

Finch, C. A., and Monsen, E. R.: Iron nutrition and the fortification of food with iron. J. Amer. Med. Assoc., 219:1462, 1972.

Gounelle, H.: Amino acid fortification and the protein problem. Amer. J. Clin. Nutr., 22:4, 1969.

Kato, J., and Muramatsu, N.: Amino acid supplementation of grain. J. Org. Amer. Oil Chem., 48:415, 1971.

Milner, M. (ed.): *Protein-Enriched Cereal Foods for World Needs.* Minnesota, Amer. Assoc. Cereal Chemists, 1969.

Swaminathan, M., and Daniel, V. A.: Enrichment and fortification of foods with nutrients as a means for overcoming malnutrition in developing countries. J. Nutr. Dietet. (Indian), 5:316, 1968.

Symposium (eight papers): Enrichment and fortification of food with nutrients. J. Agr. Food Chem., 16:149, 1968.

Symposium: Iron enrichment controversy. Nutr. Today, 7:entire issue, March/April 1972.

Uneven World Distribution of Food Supplies

Borgstrom, G.: *The Hungry Planet.* New York, Collier Books, 1967.

Borlaug, N. E.: Genetic improvement of crop foods. Nutr. Today, 7:20, January/February 1972.

Chopra, J. G., Camacho, R., Kevany, J., and Thomson, A. M.: Maternal nutrition and family planning. Amer. J. Clin. Nutr., 23:1043, 1970.

Department of Economic and Social Affairs: Strategy statement on action to avert the protein crisis in the developing countries. New York, United Nations, 1971.

Goldsmith, G. A.: More food for more people. Amer. J. Pub. Health, 59:694, 1969.

Howe, E. E.: Prevention of malnutrition in the developing countries. Nutr. Rep. Internat., 4:315, 1971.

Hutchinson, J. (ed.): *Population and Food Supply: Essays on Human Needs and Agricultural*

Prospects. London, Cambridge University Press, 1969.

Marshall, C. L., Brown, R. E., and Goodrich, C. H.: Improved nutrition vs. public health services as major determinants of world population growth. Clin. Pediat., *10*:363, 1971.

May, J. M., and Lemons, H.: The ecology of malnutrition. J. Amer. Med. Assoc., *207*:2401, 1969.

Pollack, H., and Sheldon, D. R.: The factor of disease in the world food problems. J. Amer. Med. Assoc.,*212*:598,1970.

Rasmussen, C. L.: Man and his food: 2000 a.d.: Economics, supply and morality. Food Tech., *23*:56, 1969.

Ruffin, M., Calloway, D. H., and Margen, S.: Nutritional status of preschool children of Marin County welfare recipients. Amer. J. Clin. Nutr., *25*:74, 1972.

Woodham, A. A.: The world protein shortage: Prevention and cure. World Rev. Nutr. Dietet., *13*:1, 1971.

Government Publications

(These publications are available from the Superintendent of Documents. Government Printing Office, Washington, D.C., 20402.)

Beef and veal in family meals. Home and Garden Bulletin No. 118, 1970.

Cereals and pasta in family meals. Home and Garden Bulletin No. 150, 1968.

Cheese in family meals. Home and Garden Bulletin No. 112, 1966.

Composition of foods—raw, processed, prepared. Agriculture Handbook No. 8, 1963 ($2).

Conserving the nutritive values in foods. Home and Garden Bulletin No. 90, 1971.

Eat a good breakfast to start a good day. Leaflet No. 268, 1969.

Eggs in family meals. Home and Garden Bulletin No. 103, 1971.

Family fare: Food management and recipes. Home and Garden Bulletin No. 1, 1970.

Family food budgeting . . . for good meals and good nutrition. Home and Garden Bulletin No. 94, 1969.

Food for fitness: A daily food guide. Leaflet No. 424, 1967.

Food for the young couple. Home and Garden Bulletin No. 85, 1971.

Fruits in family meals. Home and Garden Bulletin No. 125, 1970.

How to buy cheddar cheese. Home and Garden Bulletin No. 128, 1967.

How to buy beef roasts. Home and Garden Bulletin No. 146, 1968.

How to buy beef steaks. Home and Garden Bulletin No. 145, 1968.

How to buy butter. Home and Garden Bulletin No. 148, 1968.

How to buy dry beans, peas, and lentils. Home and Garden Bulletin No. 177, 1970.

How to buy eggs. Home and Garden Bulletin No. 144, 1968.

How to buy fresh fruits. Home and Garden Bulletin No. 141, 1967.

How to buy fresh vegetables. Home and Garden Bulletin No. 143, 1967.

How to buy instant nonfat dry milk. Home and Garden Bulletin No. 140, 1967.

How to buy poultry. Home and Garden Bulletin No. 157, 1968.

Lamb in family meals. Home and Garden Bulletin No. 124, 1971.

Milk in family meals. Home and Garden Bulletin No. 127, 1967.

Money-saving main dishes. Home and Garden Bulletin No. 43, 1970.

Nuts in family meals. Home and Garden Bulletin No. 176, 1970.

Pork in family meals. Home and Garden Bulletin No. 160, 1969.

Poultry in family meals. Home and Garden Bulletin No. 110, 1967.

Vegetables in family meals. Home and Garden Bulletin No. 105, 1971.

Your money's worth in foods. Home and Garden Bulletin No. 183, 1970.

Nutrition Reviews

Nutrients in wheat, flour, and bread. 25:118, 1967.

Some observations relating to applied nutrition programs supported by the U.N. agencies (by Latham, M. C.). 25:193, 1967.

Studies of algae as a human food source. 25:272, 1967.

A blue-green alga as a human food source. 26: 182, 1968.

New wheat foods (by Pence, J. W.). 26:291, 1968.

Evaluation of high protein supplements containing oilseed flours. 26:333, 1968.

The economics of malnutrition. 27:39, 1969.

The green revolution. 27:133, 1969.

Fortification of bread with iron. 27:138, 1969.

Corn-soy-milk, a nutritional supplement. 27:156, 1969.

Malnutrition and mental behaviour. 27:191, 1969.

Agricultural planning and nutrient availability (by Smith, V. E.). 28:143, 1970.

Size and nature of the protein gap (by Sukhatme, P. V.). 28:223, 1970.

Considerations in agricultural planning (by Gurney, J. M.). 29:59, 1971.

The long-term consequences of protein-calorie malnutrition (by Cravioto, J., and DeLicardie, E. R.). 29:107, 1971.

The case for the proposed increase in iron enrichment of flour and wheat products (by Darby, W. J.). 30:98, 1972.

eighteen

Adequate Diets for Healthy People

We usually detect malnutrition by certain outward signs which are the effects produced by that condition. It would seem to be an easy matter to tell whether a person is well or ill nourished, and it is true that to the trained eye such differences in nutritive condition seem obvious and are quickly noted. However, it must be remembered that there are all degrees of malnutrition, and that the average individual is not apt to look at himself or his own child with unprejudiced eyes.

Often the parent assumes that the child is all right because he has no high standard of what a healthy child should be. For this reason, a list of some of the more striking **characteristics** of the **well nourished** individual, contrasted with those usually found in **undernourished** individuals, is given (Table 18–1).

Nowadays, physicians are trained also to look for signs of deficiency of any specific vitamin. They observe the eyes

carefully for inflammation about the cornea that may be the result of riboflavin deficiency, and they ask if there is difficulty in seeing in dim light (result of vitamin A deficiency). They look carefully at the mucous membranes of the mouth and at the tongue for signs of deficiency of niacin or riboflavin. They inquire as to appetite, and test nerve reflexes as a clue to deficiency of thiamin. They sometimes take x-ray pictures of bones to see whether ossification has been or is taking place satisfactorily (especially in the ends of bones). An unsatisfactory picture indicates lack of enough vitamin D or calcium, or both.

These are the visible signs, but we can go even further in order to detect milder grades of malnutrition. Chemical analyses of the blood may be made to determine whether a low level of any certain vitamin in blood points to insufficient supply of one or several vitamins. Excretion of the vitamin in the urine can be determined after giving a test dose of it. Excretion of an abnormally small proportion of the vita-

Table 18-1.   Characteristics of Good Nutrition and Poor Nutrition

Good Nutrition	Poor Nutrition
Well developed *body*	Body may be undersized, or show poor development or physical defects
About average *weight* for height	Usually thin (underweight 10 percent or more), but may be normal or overweight (fat and flabby)
Muscles well developed and firm	Muscles small and flabby
Skin turgid and of healthy color	Skin loose and pale, waxy, or sallow
Good layer *subcutaneous fat*	Subcutaneous fat usually lacking (or in excess)
Mucous membranes of eyelids and and mouth reddish pink	Mucous membranes pale
Hair smooth and glossy	Hair often rough and without luster
Eyes clear	Dark hollows or circles under eyes or puffiness; eyes reddened
Good natured and full of life	Irritable, overactive, fatigues easily *or* Phlegmatic, listless, fails to concentrate
Appetite good	Appetite poor
General health excellent	Susceptible to infections
	Lacks endurance and vigor

min given indicates that it has been taken up instead by the blood and tissues which had too low a supply because of previous lack of that vitamin in the diet.

The estimation of the amount of malnutrition that exists in the country depends on the standards set for good nutrition. If one takes only those who are markedly underweight or show gross signs of poor physical condition, the numbers may be reassuringly few. If one goes to the other extreme and classes everyone as undernourished in whom chemical tests show that the body is not saturated with certain vitamins, a lot of apparently healthy people will be included and the numbers will be alarmingly large.

Conditions of nutrition vary in different sections of the country, at different economic levels, and according to the standards used in judging malnutrition. When surveys are made of foods consumed by individuals (dietary records), and the results are judged by comparison with the yardstick of recommended allowances of the U.S. National Research Council's Food and Nutrition Board, the conclusions may be misleading.

Use of Recommended Allowances

Obviously there are wide differences in energy requirements, according to sex, age, size, and especially the amount of physical activity. The protein requirement also varies with body weight and the need to build new tissues. The recommended energy and protein allowances are given in terms of average or reference adults and are meant to be adapted to individual needs. Criteria for adjusting the mineral and vitamin allowances are not usually indicated except for the obvious scaling of some of the B vitamin allowances to energy expenditure. However, we know there are differences between individuals in the efficiency with which they utilize these nutrients, so that some function well on smaller amounts while others require larger amounts to meet body needs. The United States National Research Council's Recommended Dietary Allowances (RDA),[1] based on the average requirement plus a 30 to 50 percent surplus, are placed at a high level with the idea that this covers the needs of even those with especially high requirements. Allowances set for the United Kingdom are also intended to be "sufficient or more than sufficient for the nutritional needs of practically all healthy persons in a population."[2] Canadian standards are "proposed as adequate for the maintenance of health among the majority of Canadians," without allowing for extremes within the population.[3]

Because we know that the majority of the population have their nutritive requirements met by lesser amounts than the United States' RDA's, it is a mistake to assume that anyone whose intake falls below these levels is necessarily getting an inadequate diet. The body has some ability to adjust to less than optimum levels of various nutrients. Adults have been maintained satisfactorily over long periods on as little as 40 gm of protein, 0.4 to 0.6 gm of calcium, and only a few milligrams of iron per day, although a surplus is unquestionably needed by pregnant and lactating women and by children. In considering the world population as a whole, the World Health Organization (WHO) and Food and Agricultural Organization (FAO) have established somewhat lower standards than has the U. S. National Research Council's Food and Nutrition Board. For example, the calcium allowance is 400 to 500 mg per day in contrast to the U.S. allowance of 800 mg. FAO–WHO standards, however, conform to the expectation of smaller body size and a limited degree of adaptation to habitually lower intakes.

Nutritionists in this country believe that a substantial margin of protein, minerals, and vitamins over actual needs will probably promote better health for all individuals of our varied population, although this is by no means proved as far as some nutrients are concerned. Recommended allowances are revised as new information comes to light, and diets judged adequate or below standard on the basis of 1958 figures may be rated differently when measured against 1968 allowances. (For instance, 12 mg of iron daily was recommended for adult women in 1958, 15 mg in 1963, and 18 mg in 1968.) A person whose diet meets the lower British standard for vitamin C might be judged poorly nourished if the U.S. Food and Nutrition Board allowances were used as the standard. Thus, final evaluation of the nutritional status of an *individual* must be determined by the condition of the person consuming the diet, not by comparison of calculated nutrient intake against standards intended for population groups and not necessarily applicable to an individual whose needs may vary from the norm.

Recommended allowances are intended to be a help in planning well balanced diets for *groups of people*. They should not be regarded as a rigid standard to which the diet must measure up every single day. Slight shortages or surpluses even up from day to day. However, over a span of several days the diet should conform to accepted nutritional standards. The RDA should be met to prevent any continued shortage of protein, minerals, or vitamins. The energy intake must be adjusted to individual needs, for even a slight excess, if long continued, leads to overweight.

Malnutrition is most apt to occur in growing children, and the proper nutrition of our children is a matter of great concern. Surveys of school children in poverty areas have indicated that such symptoms of undernutrition may be found in 15 to 25 percent of the children observed. Taking the population as a whole (both adults and children), the 1965 dietary surveys of the Department of Agriculture indicate that the nutritive value of diets has been declining rather than improving in the last 10 or 15 years.[4] About one-fifth of the diets provided less than two-thirds of the RDA for one or more nutrients and were rated "poor". Even in households with incomes over $10,000, more than one third of the diets were below the RDA in one or more nutrients.

The **underlying causes** of faulty nutrition in children have been stated to be *ingorance, lack of home control, poverty, and disease.* These are the home or community conditions responsible for the factors that cause undernutrition. Left to their own discretion, inadequately informed and motivated, children often spend their lunch money on "Coke," French-fried potatoes, and sweets (or spend it for other purposes entirely), in preference to a more adequate but less socially acceptable school or home-packed lunch. Disorganized households in which full meals are rarely prepared and the family does not eat together provide no protection against poor eating behavior outside the home and offer no guidance in food selection by parental example. If one doesn't have the money to buy enough food or to provide more expensive but essential foods such as milk, fruits, and vegetables, it is impossible to prevent undernutrition.

PLANNING THE FAMILY DIET

It would be an almost impossible task to calculate and balance the diet with respect to 40 or more nutrients every day (not to mention flavor, cost, and availability considerations) without access to sophisticated computer programs. For this reason, one needs some general rule or set of rules which assure adequacy if followed in planning the diet.

The most commonly accepted plan is one sponsored many years ago by the Home Economics Research Division of the U. S. Department of Agriculture,[5] and which most children have been taught in elementary school, the "Basic Four Food Groups." This plan specifies the inclusion in the diet each day of definite amounts of foods from each of four food groups—milk, meat, cereals, vegetables and fruit—in a basal or foundation diet (see Chap. 17). The basal diet is intended to provide practically the full allowances of all nutritive essentials except energy.

Weakness of the Basic Four Food Groups Plan

This simple plan based on four food groups is by no means foolproof even for populations whose preferred style of eating fits the categories specified. It is quite easy to defeat the system by consistently making poorer choices within the group alternatives, by skimping on serving sizes and by cooking or processing a food in such a way that its nutrient content is substantially lowered. This latter problem becomes increasingly important with the development of substitute foods that mimic but do not match the original.

Any simplified eating plan is based on the assumptions that (1) there are a *few key nutrients* that *must be monitored* out of the 40-plus possible; and (2) the *nutrients not being monitored inevitably follow* in the variety of foods selected for the key or index nutrients. The Basic Four has oversimplified the indices. For example, legumes are accepted alternatives in the protein-index "Meat" Group of the Basic Four food plan. Almost the only thing these foods do have in common is protein of good quality. But there are differences. To name a few, meats contain vitamin B-12 and beans do not; most legumes are rich in folacin and most meats are only fair. Even the "meats" are not alike; marine fish provide iodine, but cattle and poultry flesh contribute very little of this nutrient. The consequences of these differences in composition depend upon all the other choices one makes. The absence of vitamin B-12 from the "Meat" Group alternative is irrelevant if the person selects the Milk Group as specified. The iodine in fish is of no importance to the inlander who uses iodized salt. On the other hand, a person who is allergic to milk or one who wishes to forego all animal food might carefully provide for his calcium needs elsewhere (remembering that calcium is the key nutrient in the Milk Group), but conclude by having a diet deficient in vitamin B-12. Similarly, the person who has no marine food, whose native soil is low in iodine, and who does not use iodized or sea salt may develop a goiter.

Substitute foods are even more likely to defeat an index system. Vitamin C-fortified, orange-flavored sugar is a far cry from a fresh orange, both as to vitamin and, especially, mineral content. Again, the consequences of its use will vary. The impact will be minimal if all the rest of the diet is of high quality; the juice-substitute might be an improvement if it replaced a sugared drink without any vitamins at all or if the diet were lacking in vitamin C and nothing else. In a poor quality diet, the substitution could be the final poor choice that changes a diet from marginal to deficient.

In time, food technologists could probably develop substitute foods that more nearly match the natural counterpart, provided that nutritionists were well able to give advice about which nutrients to add and in what amounts. Unfortunately, knowledge is not this far advanced. Several of the B vitamins were scarcely recognized at the time the original legislation on enrichment of refined cereals was drafted, and they are not, to this date, restored in milled grains and their products. We are rapidly expanding our knowledge of trace minerals but have not yet reached the point of certain qualification of essentiality of some of them, putting aside quantification of the amount needed. As you have learned in earlier chapters, in some instances the risk of too much is as great as the hazard of too little of a nutrient and the balance between some of them is critical. Under these circumstances, food fabrication is difficult and carries a high nutritional risk.

We cannot plan for what we do not recognize or know to be essential. This has been a weakness in all food plans proposed thus far. The Basic Four made no certain provision for vitamin E, folacin, magnesium, or zinc, and with reason. When the plan was devised there was no adequate information on the amount that should be included in the diet of all age groups, nor was there knowledge of the distribution of these nutrients in foods. The situation is not a great deal improved today as regards two of those four nutrients and we have added new ones to the list.

The only reasonable alternative to some sort of scientifically designed plan of family feeding is reliance on the accumulated wisdom of a cultural group whose children grow well, who reproduce successfully, and who live healthily into a spry old age. Some primitive groups fit these criteria, and their diets must have been adequate if the traditional patterns were followed *exactly*. Oftentimes some seemingly minor component of the diet or some method of food preparation was absolutely essential for adequacy of the total diet. Consumption of the stomach contents and all the organs and soft bones of fish and aquatic mammals provided the calcium and vitamin C needed in the primitive Eskimo diet, as one example. The common experience is that introduction of sophisticated diets has worked to the disadvantage of primitive peoples who cling to some of the old practices and adopt only some of the new, showing the importance of adherence to *all* the old traditions without picking and choosing among them. (Sometimes this primitive wisdom is not so wise as it should be, and a native practice or taboo interferes with good nutrition. See Chapter 16.)

What the Basic Four attempts to do is combine scientific knowledge with Western cultural wisdom and, faulted though it is, there is not now an equally simple, equally workable alternative plan for Western food patterns. Our goal, then, will be to add to the scientific basis of the Four Food Groups, making finer discriminations among the group alternatives based on newer knowledge of nutrients and the foods in which they occur. Ways to modify the Basic Four Food Groups Plan to suit other preferred patterns of eating will be considered. The one rule to be emphasized is that the family diet should include a wide variety of natural foods chosen from among a number of food classes.

Basic Four Food Groups Foundation Diet

Table 18–2 presents an evaluation of some of the nutrients provided by a conventional American Basic Four Plan diet compared to the total amounts specified as the recommended allowance. The nutrients tabulated are the well-studied ones around which the Basic Four Food Groups plan was designed. The foundation diet is intended to be supplemented by other foods but does in itself provide almost enough of most of the listed nutrients to meet the recommended allowances, except in energy, in iron for women, and in thiamin for men. (Although 30 percent low in pre-formed niacin, it probably meets the need for this vitamin by synthesis from tryptophan in the protein.) Because the foundation diet furnishes only about 1250 kcal, both diets need supplementary food for energy—for the man a considerable amount, 1550 kcal, and for the woman perhaps 750 kcal. The final quality of the diet will depend heavily on the food choices made to provide the extra energy. To understand this better, let us consider a typical American menu that might be devised from the foods listed in Table 18–2. The menu given in Table 18–3 allows for a lunch carried from home and includes more servings from the Vegetable-Fruit Group than the plan demands. Listed below this are the foods typically added to the foundation diet. Except for larger servings of some of the basic foods, most of the usual supplements add little in the way of essential nutrients. It is small wonder, then, that iron deficiency is a common finding in women and girls, who are

likely to forego the increased portions of ordinary foods to "save calories" for desserts and sweets. Men, with their higher energy requirements, are able to eat both larger servings and the high-energy foods of little other nutritive value and so may be better nourished than women.

Even the man's nutritional status may still be in jeopardy with this diet. Table 18–4 compares the content of lesser-studied nutrients in the typical menu plan with the allowances for them. With the exception of phosphorus, in which the diet is disproportionately high, this menu provides one-half to two-thirds, or less, of the recommended allowances. For some of the nutrients tabulated, especially folacin, the compositional data are not as reliable as one would like, but the discrepancies between content and recommended intake are so sizable that this does not negate the conclusions that must be drawn. Either the Basic Four Food Groups plan diet is marginal to inadequate *as commonly followed*, or allowances are unrealistically high, or both.

Improvement of the Basic Four Food Plan

How might these deficits be rectified? In part, the missing nutrients can be added by selecting different foods from within the categories and taking larger servings of some of them. Others are best handled by adding more servings or different types of foods.

Had liver been chosen instead of chicken, the contribution of one serving from the Meat Group would have been: iron, 8.8 mg; vitamin A, 53,400 IU; thiamin, 0.26 mg; riboflavin 4.19 mg; niacin, 16.5 mg; ascorbic acid, 27 mg; vitamin E, 1.62 IU; folacin, 294 mcg; vitamin B-6, 0.8 mg; vitamin B-12, 80 mcg; and pantothenic acid, 7.7 mg. (Amounts of the other nutrients tabulated would not differ appreciably, but there would be major added contribu-

Table 18–2.   Well-Known Nutrients in a Diet Planned According to the Basic Four Food Groups

	Grams	Approximate Measure	Energy (kcal)	Protein (gm)	Calcium (mg)	Iron (mg)	Vitamin A (IU)	Thiamin (mg)	Riboflavin (mg)	Niacin (mg)	Vitamin C (mg)
Milk Group											
Milk or equivalent	488	16 oz or two 8 oz glasses (1 pint)	330	17	570	0.4	740	0.14	0.82	0.4	4
Meat Group*											
Meat, fish, or poultry	100	1 avg. serving, cooked, lean only	295	24	11	2.2	178	0.16	0.21	6.0	2
Egg	50	1 medium	80	6.5	27	1.2	590	0.06	0.15	0.1	0
Vegetable and Fruit Group											
Vegetables:											
Deep green or yellow†	100	½ cup, cooked	29	2.0	5	1.1	3900	0.07	0.11	0.6	29
Potato	100	1 medium, baked	93	2.6	9	0.7	Trace	0.10	0.04	1.7	20
Other‡	100	½ cup, cooked	42	2.1	22	0.8	220	0.07	0.06	0.7	13

Compositional data are all from reference 2.

*Average of ten 100 gm servings of lean, edible portion of meats, including beef, lamb, pork, poultry, and fish.

†Average of ten 100 gm servings, one each of asparagus, broccoli, Brussels sprouts, carrots, green snap beans, green lettuce and romaine, spinach, yellow (winter) squash, and sweet potato.

‡Other vegetables: average of ten 100 gm servings of beets, cauliflower, celery, corn, green peas, lima beans, onions, summer squash, turnip, and zucchini.

Table 18–2. *Well-Known Nutrients in a Diet Planned According to the Basic Four Food Groups* (Continued)

	Grams	Approximate Measure	Energy (kcal)	Protein (gm)	Calcium (mg)	Iron (mg)	Vitamin A (IU)	Thiamin (mg)	Riboflavin (mg)	Niacin (mg)	Vitamin C (mg)
Fruits:											
Citrus or tomato§	185	6 oz juice	55	1.1	20	0.7	519	0.09	0.04	0.7	50
Other¶	100	1 avg. serving	75	0.7	13	0.7	550	0.04	0.05	0.5	11
Cereal Group											
Bread, white, enriched	70	3 slices	180	6.0	57	1.8	Trace	0.18	0.15	1.8	Trace
Cereal, whole-grain or enriched	30 dry wt.	⅔ cup flakes	70	1.8	5	0.6	Trace	0.09	0.03	0.6	0
Total nutrients in foundation diet			1250	64	740	10.2	6700	1.00	1.66	13.1	130
Recommended allowances:									Niacin Equiva-lents** mg		
Man, 70 kg, mod. active, 22–25 yrs.			2800	65	800	10	5000	1.4	1.7	18	60
Woman, 58 kg, mod. active 22–25 yrs.			2000	55	800	18	5000	1.0	1.5	13	55

§Daily average based on three servings of orange juice, two servings of grapefruit juice, three servings of tomato juice, and two servings of fresh raw tomatoes.

¶Other fruits: daily average based on one average serving each of fresh apple, banana, peach, pear; one serving each of canned apple sauce, apricots, peaches, and pineapple, plus one serving of dried or stewed prunes.

**Includes niacin as such and from tryptophan conversion.

Table 18–3. Typical American Menu for the Basic Four Food Groups Diet in Table 18–2

Breakfast	Carried Lunch	Dinner	Snacks
Foundation Diet, 1250 kcal			
Small glass orange juice Corn flakes with milk	Egg sandwich on white bread Raw tomato	Small chicken breast Baked potato Yellow summer squash Pickled green beans Hot bread or roll	Raw apple and cheese
Typical Supplements, 750–1550 kcal			
Coffee, tea, or chocolate Larger serving of juice Sugar for coffee, cereal Cream in lieu of milk Toast, butter, jam	Coffee or tea Butter and/or mayonnaise on sandwich Cookies Potato chips Soft drink	Larger serving of chicken Butter for potato, roll, and squash Sweet dessert Coffee or tea Alcoholic beverages Sugar in coffee More rolls and butter	Coffee or tea Sugar in coffee Soft drink or alcoholic beverages Candy

tions of copper, zinc, molybdenum, manganese, and all other substances that are stored in the liver.) The *difference* in iron yields a 12 percent improvement in the *daily average intake* if the liver were eaten only once weekly. Vitamin A content would meet the full allowance for ten days. Liver would add a two-week supply of vitamin B-12 and a full two-day allotment of riboflavin. Half of a daily allowance of folacin, vitamin B-6, and ascorbic acid would be provided, the latter being a characteristic in which liver is almost unique among animal foods. (Fish roe is also high in vitamin C, and breast milk, while not high in this nutrient, contains enough to meet all the needs of an infant.) Not everyone will eat liver, liver sausage, or paté de foie gras, but liver can be ground and added to other ground meats, in a proportion of 1 to 4 or 5 without imparting a flavor objectionable to most people.

A great improvement can be made in the diet from a few simple changes that are perhaps easier to practice on a day-to-day basis than is force-feeding liver. (Considering the relative amounts of muscle and liver in a carcass, it is evident that the whole population could not have liver every day in any case.) Substitution of whole grain cereals for refined milled ones, in our example three slices of whole wheat bread and a serving of oatmeal instead of enriched white bread and corn flakes, would increase the magnesium contribution from the Cereal Group five-fold and triple the amount of folacin, vitamin B-6, and pantothenate derived from this group. Vitamin E content is ten times higher in the whole grains. Note that potato is quite a good food and contributes nutrients that suggest it could well be classified with the Cereal Group with vitamin C as a bonus.

Another key change is to include larger and more frequent servings of dark leafy green vegetables. Products such as mustard and turnip greens, kale, dandelion greens, and collards all have about one-third more of all the essential nutrients than do the substitutes presently allowed (other green and yellow vegetables). A 100-gm serving of mustard or other greens meets almost the entire daily allowance of ascorbic acid and about half the vitamin E allowance. Addition of a gen-

Table 18–4. *Lesser-Studied Nutrients* in a Menu Based on Pattern of Four Food Groups in Table 18–3*

Food	Grams	Phosphorus (mg)	Sodium (mg)	Potassium (mg)	Magnesium (mg)	Zinc (mg)	Vitamin E (IU)	Folacin (mcg)	Vitamin B-6 (mg)	Vitamin B-12 (mcg)	Pantothenic acid (mg)
Milk Group											
Milk	244	227	122	352	32	1.0	0.1	36†	0.10	1.0	0.83
Cheddar Cheese	30	143	210	25	14	0.9	0.1	3	0.02	0.3	0.15
Meat Group											
Chicken	100	257	78	381	20	1.8	0.4	7	0.30	0.4	0.90
Egg	50	102	61	64	6	0.7	0.2	50†	0.06	1.0	0.80
Vegetable and Fruit Group											
Green beans	100	32	1	152	20	0.2	0.1	5(11)	0.07	0	0.14
Summer squash	100	25	1	141	16	0.1	<0.1	2(10)	0.06	0	0.17
Potato	100	65	4	503	20	0.3	<0.1	12(29)	0.09	0	0.32
Tomato	100	18	3	227	10	0.2	1.0	26	0.10	0	0.25
Orange juice	100	16	1	186	10	0.1	<0.1	66†	0.03	0	0.16
Apple	100	10	1	110	8	0.1	0.31	2	0.03	0	0.10
Cereal Group											
Bread, enriched, white	70	68	355‡	73	15	0.5	0.1	30†	0.03	trace§	0.30
Corn flakes	30	14	300‡	36	5	0.1	<0.1	5	0.02	0	0.06
TOTAL		977	1137‡	2250	176	6	2–3	240–280	1	3	4
Recommended allowance											
Men		800	¶	¶	350	¶	30	400	2	5	¶
Women		800	¶	¶	300	¶	25	400	2	5	¶

*Compositional data for these nutrients (except for phosphorus and potassium) are not as reliable as one would wish and are tabulated only to indicate the order of magnitude of a nutrient. Methods are poor for the vitamins, and minerals vary by a factor of 10 to 100 depending on soil composition and processing contaminants. Entries for minerals except zinc are from reference 6; vitamins B-6, B-12 and pantothenic acid from reference 7; vitamin E from reference 8. Folacin values marked with a dagger (†) are from reference 11; others are from various literature sources as compiled in unpublished tables of S. Cohenour and J. King, University of California, Berkeley; values in parentheses are for the raw food. Zinc data are from a published review: Schlettwein-Gsell, D., and Mommsen-Straub, S., Internat. J. Vit. Forschung, 40:659, 1970 (in German).

‡Sodium added to these cereal products in manufacture. Other foods would have salt added in cooking. The expected daily total would be about 5 gm of sodium, with these additions and use of salted butter or margarine.

§Vitamin B-12 due to added milk in recipe.

¶Recommended daily allowances of these have not been established. The probable need is about 10 mg of pantothenic acid and 10 to 15 mg of zinc. Potassium need is in the order of 2.5 gm a day, and a ratio of about 1:1 of sodium to potassium and of calcium to phosphorus is desirable.

erous serving of a *raw* leafy green, such as romaine, cos, or leaf lettuce, will go far toward guaranteeing the adequacy of folacin in the diet. These vegetables also contribute a large amount of calcium with relatively little phosphorus, a direction in which we wish to improve the diet. Many of the greens are as good a source of calcium as is milk on a gram-for-gram basis. Fruits are generally a more expensive source than are vegetables of the key nutrients, vitamins A and C, for which we rely on the Vegetable-Fruit Group, and many are lower in content of B vitamins. Note, however, that fresh or frozen orange juice contributes folacin and so do bananas.

It is worth considering addition of a third serving of food from the Meat Group every day and for this serving, choosing frequently fish (for iodine and other trace minerals) and dry beans or nuts (for more thiamin and folacin). This change would have the effect of increasing the spectrum of foods and thereby increasing the probability of including the nutrients we know very little about today. Meats, but not the alternative legumes or nuts, are the only recognized good source of zinc in the American diet.

The Milk Group contributes most of the calcium in the typical American diet and makes good contributions of protein and B vitamins. Since calcium is the key nutrient in this group, cheese is an accepted substitute for milk. However, the bulk of the water-soluble nutrients present in milk are lost in the whey, so cheese compares unfavorably with milk with respect to all the B vitamins, magnesium, and potassium. Some persons experience intestinal gas or softening of the stools when they drink milk due to the lactose present (Chapter 13). Cheese, which lacks the offending sugar, will be a good source of calcium for them, but lactose-intolerant persons may also be able to tolerate yogurt or soured milk in which lactose content is reduced by the action of bacteria. Other calcium sources do exist, of course. The dark leafy greens are one (excepting those that are high in oxalic acid, Chapter 11), and they provide as much riboflavin as does cheese. Fish bones eaten in sardines, smelt, salmon, or dried fishes are another. Another source commonly used in the Near and Middle East is whole sesame seed or sesame seed paste, the tahini of Egyptian cookery and a basic ingredient in the Oriental candy halvah. The plant sources of calcium are lacking in vitamin B-12 which will need to be added from an animal food.

To raise the vitamin E content of the diet to anything like the presently recommended allowance, it is necessary to turn to another food group, fats and oils. A few foods such as peanuts and soybeans are high in vitamin E, and oil expressed from these foods is a still more concentrated source of this fat-soluble vitamin.[8] Peanuts contain about 7 mg of alpha-tocopherol per 100 gm of nuts or 14 mg per 100 gm of crude fat. Potato chips, because they are fried in vegetable oil, have about the same concentration of this vitamin as peanuts do. Salad oils and mayonnaise which is made from vegetable oil have 5 to 40 mg of vitamin E per 100 gm, depending on which oil is used. The amount taken with a salad, about one tablespoon (15 gm), would provide about 1 to 6 mg of vitamin E. Margarines have about 13 mg of vitamin E per 100 gm and butter only 1 mg.

Vitamin D is not found in popular American foods in significant amounts, except for fatty marine fish (Chapter 9). Vitamin D adequacy is assured by the use of fortified milk and exposure to sunlight. Iodine nutrition is approached in the same way, by selection of salt fortified with iodine or use of sea salt. We know little about the trace minerals, and their concentrations in foods will surely depend on the soil conditions where the vegetables and fruits, cereals, and legumes are grown.

After the needs for essential fatty acids and vitamin E are met, which can be accomplished with one tablespoon of oil and a good diet, there is no reason to add more energy in the form of fat. There is no nutritional basis for use of sugar and alcohol except as alternative energy sources. How much of these fats, sugars, and alcohols the diet can tolerate depends on how well the other items are selected and prepared in the home and how much energy the individual needs. A reasonable plan is to take at least the first 1600 kcal (6700 kJ) from the natural foods listed above to provide a margin of safety for variation in food composition and preparatory losses.

If sugar is added, brown sugar is a better choice than white. Honey, the only animal sweetener, has very small amounts of essential nutrients, and its physiological properties are not superior to other sugars. Sweet desserts containing milk (puddings or ice cream) or milk and eggs (custard-filled pastries, cakes) or fruits and nuts (compote, fruit pastries) have obvious advantages over those that are mainly whipped cream or sugar. If alcohol is used, beer is the best choice, because it contains appreciable amounts of B vitamins and minerals; wine is second choice. Distilled spirits are a very poor last choice in terms of nutritive value.

Other Dietary Components

Some foods usually classed as non-nutritive substances are included in diets the world over. Tea is the favored beverage throughout the Orient and in the British Isles, while coffee and cocoa are more widely used in Europe and the Americas. These beverages do contain minerals because they are extracts of plant materials, but the steps through which they are processed leaves them without significant amounts of vitamins, except for some niacin in coffee (about 0.5 mg in a 6-ounce cup). All three beverages add 15 to 20 mg of magnesium per cup of fluid and 45 to 65 mg of potassium. Tea makes a significant contribution of fluoride (0.3 to 0.5 mg per cup). By themselves they yield no energy, but each *level* teaspoon of sugar used with them adds 16 kcal (67 kJ) and each tablespoon of light cream about 32 kcal (134 kJ). Dry cream substitutes may contain some cream or only a substitute fat, usually coconut oil which has a higher percentage of saturated fatty acids than does milk fat; the other usual ingredients are isolated milk protein (casein) or nonfat milk solids, corn syrup solids, and chemical additives. At equal "whiteness" in the beverage, cream substitutes may have negligibly lower energy yield than does light cream. Cocoa powder may be mixed with water or milk, and the total nutritional content of the beverage will vary accordingly. These contributions from beverages are not trivial in view of the large amount taken in the day. A not uncommon intake of five servings of beverage would add about 100 mg of magnesium, a nutrient in which diets tend to be low, plus whatever minerals are present in the local water.

Coffee, tea, and cocoa all contain a related group of stimulants, the one highest in concentration in each being caffeine, theophylline, and theobromine, respectively. Caffeine is added to most cola-flavored beverages. Caffeine is the most active of the three compounds and when taken in excess may cause sleeplessness. It has also been reported to increase the levels of glucose[9] and fatty acids[10] in the blood, particularly of persons with diminished or diabetic-like tolerance for glucose. Caffeine is a weak diuretic (Chapter 14). Tea also contains tannins that have astringent properties. All these beverages are taken without apparent untoward side effects in most healthy people, but tea is usually much better tolerated than coffee when there are digestive upsets.

Herbs, spices, and condiments are plant material and do contain nutrients; the significance of these depends on the amounts used. Chili peppers are high in vitamins C and A, and enough chili is used to make a real difference in Spanish-American and Oriental cookery. Kim-chee, a Korean condiment, is also a rich source of vitamin C. Dried kelp and other seaweeds used in Asiatic cookery are high in calcium, magnesium, iodine, and other minerals found in sea water.

Other substances quite casually added in cookery or preserving foods can make important differences in the diet. About half of the folacin in home-baked bread comes from yeast added for leavening[11] and the yeast and other bread ingredients add more B vitamins, an array of minerals, and some protein. Baking powders add substantial amounts of sodium (potassium tartrate type is an exception) and usually phosphate or sulfate and calcium, but no vitamins. All but about $1/2$ gm of the sodium present in the diet is there because it has been added as salt or one of the other sodium-containing compounds used in preserving or cooking the food, such as sodium nitrite in corning beef, brine for pickles, salt in butter, monosodium glutamate (MSG), and soy sauce in cooking.

Effects of Cooking on Nutritive Values

Some foods can be eaten raw, but most require cooking to improve their digestibility and to insure food safety. Providing that sanitary methods of fertilization and watering are practiced (unprocessed fecal matter harbors bacteria, amebae, and other parasites), most vegetables and fruits can be eaten raw after thorough washing in clean water. Potatoes, cereals, and legumes all should be cooked in order to improve digestibility of the starch, and the legumes to destroy anti-digestive and potentially toxic materials as well. Meats, fish, and poultry can be eaten raw but are better cooked if there is the least question of parasitic, bacterial, or viral

infections. Fish, pork, and beef muscle may carry parasites which may be killed during prolonged storage at home freezer temperatures; but for absolute certainty of kill, the muscle should reach an internal temperature of 180° F (82.2° C). Mollusks pick up hepatitis virus from infected water, and poultry and eggs are subject to salmonella infection. Milk must be pasteurized for safety, and this has little effect on nutritive values.

If foods are to be cooked in water, loss of water-soluble nutrients will be lessened if the food is left in large pieces and cooked quickly in a small amount of water. However, traditional Chinese and Japanese cookery sets another excellent example, in which vegetables are stir-fried for a short period of time and all the juices are included in the final product. Another way of coping with the problem of loss of nutrients in cooking water, especially good for coarse vegetables that require a fairly long period of cooking, such as collards and other greens, is to use the cooking water as a soup or soup base. "Pot liquor" from greens is a standard item of diet in the rural southern part of the United States; and in northern Chinese cookery, small bits of food are cooked in broth at the table and the cooking broth is eaten last, as a soup. Dry heat is also detrimental to many vitamins, and there is some damage to protein if such treatment is excessive. Well-controlled roasting, broiling, and frying, according to the directions in any good cookery text, will cause only modest losses. Again, juices should be salvaged and used in soup and gravy stock, but unless energy needs are large it is prudent to skim off and discard the rendered fat.

Some nutrients are susceptible to oxidation, but this is more a problem in commercial food processing than in home preparation. However, unsaturated fatty acids and vitamin E deteriorate when oils are opened to the air and the products become rancid.

Even in frozen storage, prepared foods lose much of their vitamin E content through oxidative changes that occur at these low temperatures. Little vitamin E or unsaturated fatty acid is lost in deep-fat frying in fresh oil, but there is substantial loss of vitamin content on storage.[8] When fats are heated to very high temperatures (250° C) or when oils are reused for long periods of time, damaged and potentially toxic products are formed.[12] Thus both palatability and nutritional considerations dictate that only fresh fats should be used in food preparation.

The only common home food preparation in the United States that involves fermentation with microorganisms is yeast leavening of doughs, to which we have referred earlier. Various bacterial and mold processes are employed quite commonly in Africa and Asia, such as manufacture of oggi from cassava, kefir and yogurt from milk, and tempeh from soybeans. Microorganisms are able to synthesize many nutrients that man requires in the diet, but some have a definite requirement for vitamins that are essential to man. For this reason it is difficult to guess what the net effect of a fermentation process will be in terms of vitamin and amino acid content of the food. Generally, food processing organisms add more vitamins than they use up in their growth and some bacteria and molds, but not yeast, even make the "animal" vitamin, B-12.[13]

Dill pickles are often cited as a good source of iron (about 1 mg per large pickle), which seems odd because cucumbers are not a good source of iron. The extra iron in pickles was present adventitiously, as a contaminant due to processing in metal equipment. Pickles packed at home in earthenware crocks would not have much iron. Unintentionally, we used to add iron in the home by slowly cooking foods such as tomato sauces or greens in iron pots. Also, we made extensive use of foods packed in tinned containers that often took up tin and iron by corrosion of the can on long-term storage.* With the introduction of frozen and ready-to-eat foods, and aluminum, stainless steel, and Teflon-coated pots and pans, these beneficial additions of iron have been lost. Zinc is also taken up from galvanized containers,* and such contamination probably accounts for the high concentration of zinc in maple syrup. The mineral content of household water depends not only on the composition of the main water supply, but upon the kinds of pipes and softening systems through which it flows.

The food that finally reaches the table reflects a host of factors: soil, water, harvesting, processing, transportation, and storage, as well as personal selection and home preparation. No amount of care in the household can make up for damage that has occurred in other steps of the food distribution chain. These other factors are discussed in Chapter 17.

Vegetarian Diets

A diet that avoids animal flesh but that does include milk and eggs poses no serious nutritional problems.[10] One simply changes the source from which protein is derived by adding more cheese, eggs, milk, dry beans, peas, and nuts. A reasonable menu plan might have an eggnog (1 egg + 1 cup milk; 14 gm protein); a peanut butter (2 tbsp) sandwich and a glass of milk (20 gm protein); and 1 cup cooked lentils and 1 oz cheese (23 gm protein) in addition to the needed amounts of fruits and vegetables, cereals, oils, and other energy sources. Some caution will be required in selection of iron- and zinc-rich alternative foods (Chapter 12).

Nutritional planning becomes virtu-

---

*Zinc and probably tin are essential nutrients, but both are toxic at high levels. For this reason storage of acid products in open tinned or galvanized containers is very hazardous. Poisoning has occurred from party punches made ahead and stored in metal pails.

ally impossible if all animal products are eliminated from the diet, especially for people accustomed to Western styles of food preparation. Such a diet has no vitamin B-12 and a limited spectrum of calcium sources in addition to the problem areas just mentioned. Traditional cultures that have maintained themselves on strict vegetarian diets have found a source of vitamin B-12 because this is a universal requirement of man. Some possibilities for synthesis may be found in microbial processes applied to foods and unintentional contamination with animal matter, such as insects or their eggs, or with soil microorganisms. There is perhaps some intestinal synthesis of this vitamin, but is is not certain enough to be relied upon, for ample evidence of vitamin B-12 deficiency has been found in strict vegans.[15]

Vitamin Supplements

Vitamin pills will not be needed by people who regularly eat a good diet, except under very unusual conditions. A person who has been well-nourished in the past will have ample reserves of vitamins in the liver and other tissues that will carry him through the ordinary minor illnesses and occasional periods of dietary indiscretion. Supplements will be needed if intestinal absorption is impaired by disease and sometimes during and after prolonged illness.

If a daily supplement is to be taken, it should contain the same balance of water-soluble vitamins as one would wish to have in the regular diet, that is, *all* of the vitamin B complex and ascorbic acid in amounts suggested in the recommended daily allowances. Only for therapeutic purposes and under competent medical advice should a pharmaceutical vitamin preparation be taken that exceeds the recommended allowances.

The fat-soluble vitamins must be treated cautiously, for vitamins D and

A are toxic at high dosages (Chapter 9). If the diet includes vitamin D-fortified milk, as it should, then no other supplement of this vitamin should be taken by normal persons. Quite commonly vitamins D and A are added to products such as ready-to-eat cereals, flavoring agents for milk, and "instant" meals, so there is some risk of increasing the intake unduly.

If a person suspects that his diet may not be adequate, his best procedure is to improve the diet, because if vitamins are low chances are that minerals will be inadequate also. There is no sensible way to prepare an all-round mineral supplement at the present stage of knowledge. However, a modest, well-balanced vitamin supplement will do no harm unless the practice of taking it tempts one to ignore the necessity for choosing foods wisely.

Meal Spacing

The times at which meals are eaten and the intervals between them are usually determined by the convenience of the family and the accepted pattern of a culture. All patterns have been utilized, from a very large number of very small meals (a nibbling pattern) to a single large meal daily. The body's metabolic machinery adapts to any habitual pattern so that we are able to cope with a flood of nutrients at one time and maintain critical functions in the intervals, or vice versa. However, in both human studies and animal experiments, a pattern of frequent small meals leads to more satisfactory levels of blood lipids and deposition of more lean and less fat in the body than if one or two large meals are fed daily.[16]

Other investigations of the effect of omitting meals have centered on (1) the maintenance of blood sugar level as a physiological parameter indicating homeostasis, or (2) the efficiency with which some mental or physical work is performed. Studies of American youth and older persons accustomed to eating three or more meals a day have shown that blood sugar begins to fall about 2½ to 3 hours after breakfast and the fall occurs somewhat later if protein-rich foods are included in the meal;[17, 18] blood sugar continues to fall unless a second meal is given about that time.[19] There was evidence of lessened efficiency that coincided with the blood sugar changes.[18] However, these subjects were not habituated to skipping meals and so were ill-adapted to this pattern of eating. Similar studies have not been made of persons who take fewer meals habitually.

People do seem to prefer a nibbling pattern, at least early in life. Infants eat at two to three hour intervals for the first days or weeks of life and only gradually are accustomed to long periods of sleep between bouts of eating. We think that a three-meals-a-day pattern is reached ultimately, but this is not quite true. Most people have two or three main meals a day interspersed with two to four small ones (morning and afternoon coffee or tea, snacks in the evening, the odd bit of fruit or candy, etc.). The pattern of large infrequent meals is customary in countries where food is in short supply and obesity is infrequent. In richer parts of the world, a larger number of small meals, five or six a day, seems to be preferred and physiologically desirable. However, nibbling is a good practice only if all the food forms part of a well-balanced diet. A mid-morning small meal of juice or milk is an asset, but one of a doughnut and black coffee is probably not. Table 18–5 indicates one way in which an American-style food pattern can be adapted to a frequent meal schedule without sacrificing nutritional value.

Equally important is the need to arrange mealtimes, at whatever frequency, so that the family or living group eat together at least once and preferably twice a day. Disorganization in the household and lack of commensality contribute heavily toward development

Table 18–5.   Menu Plan for Increased Meal Frequency*

Meal 1	Egg or cheese
	Whole grain bread
Meal 2	Fresh or dried fruit
	Milk
Meal 3	Vegetable or cream type soup
	Green salad with vegetable oil–
	vinegar dressing
Meal 4	Fish, meat, or nut butter sandwich
	Milk, fruit or vegetable juice
Meal 5	Meat, fish, poultry, or cheese
	Potato or whole grain cereal product
	Leafy green vegetable
	Other vegetables
Meal 6	Fruit
	Yogurt or ice cream

*Condiments, beverages, and more servings of cereals, fruits, vegetables, fats, and oils to be added as needed to meet energy requirements.

and practice of the poor food habits that lead to poor nutritional status.

ADOLESCENTS AND YOUNG ADULTS

Adolescence is a period of great physical, biological, and emotional adjustment. The teen-ager may exhibit immature judgment and uncertain behavior. The demand for independence may lead to abandonment of dietary practices taught in the family and acceptance of fad diets and food patterns decreed by the peer group.

The teen-age spurt in growth varies in intensity and duration from one person to another. For boys it takes place generally between 12 and 17 years. In girls, the spurt in height begins about two years earlier and lasts a shorter time than for boys. All skeletal and muscular dimensions of the body appear to participate in this adolescent development, although not at the same speed.

When girls and boys reach this period, their needs for energy and for most other nutrients increase sharply. Teen-age girls need 2300 to 2400 kcal and teen-age boys need 2800 to 3000 kcal, according to the United States RDA's. Canadian boys and girls engaged in their usual school activities are thought to require 3100 and 2600 kcal, respectively, between ages 13 and 15. Between 16 and 19, girls are thought to become less active and to have reached adult size, whereas boys continue to grow and engage in very active sports.[3] The Canadian allowances for this age span are for boys 3700 to 3800 kcal, which is 113 percent of the adult male value; and for girls, 2400 kcal, or 104 percent of the women's allowance. Protein, mineral, and vitamin needs will reach adult values during this same interval, including for girls the increased need for iron coincident with menarche.

School, work, and social activities take teen-agers away from home a great deal, with the result that food habits, frequently not good before, become even poorer. Young people living continuously on diets providing suboptimal amounts of nutrients are in poor condition to withstand the stresses and strains of their hectic life. They cannot afford to skip breakfast, grab a soft drink and a bag of potato chips for lunch, and skimp on dinner. A survey of 6200 teen-agers in North Carolina[20] revealed that although the majority ate breakfast, 15 percent had missed at least one meal in the 24-hour period. Dietary studies in the United States show that intakes of calcium, iron, and possibly vitamins C and A may fall far short of the probable needs of many teen-agers.[21] An Australian survey[22] found poorer dietary intakes of 16- to 19-year-old youths who were employed than of those who remained in school, particularly the girls. The diets of only 3 percent of employed 16-year-old girls and 33 percent of the boys met Australian standards for all of eight nutrients tabulated.

Usually, boys offer less of a problem than girls because their appetite is excellent and their energy need is large so they can afford to eat more. Girls of this age frequently have a finicky appetite, preferring sweets and highly flavored foods, and if they develop a phobia about remaining slender, it is difficult to get them to take all the protective foods they need.

The less food eaten, the more important it is to make all of it count. Foods with "empty calories" (i.e., little or no minerals or vitamins but plenty of energy) often replace foods with important nutrients. For teen-agers especially, foods high in sugar and fat often replace those with more needed protein, minerals, and vitamins.

The family meal pattern is satisfactory for the teen-ager, with an increase in the size of servings, if needed to provide additional protein, iron, and energy. However, the teen-ager is often away from home during some of the family meals, which places on him the responsibility of knowing how to select nutritious foods away from home.

Snacks often account for one-fourth the teen-ager's energy intake and so should furnish one-fourth the day's nutrients. If attractive, nutritious snacks are available at home, the teen-ager is able to select what he wants and still get food that contributes to his daily nutritive requirement. Even when eating away from home, there are many nutritious snacks available. Suggested snacks that make a contribution to the health of teen-agers include:

Fresh fruits	Peanut butter and
Fruit juices	crackers
Dried fruits	Fresh vegetable pieces
Cheese	Nuts
Milk beverages	Leftover meats or
Ice cream	sausages

Many young people are troubled by acne, a skin condition ascribed to effects of sex hormones on the sebaceous glands. There is no proved association of this disorder with nutritional deficiency or with specific foods, but physicians often suggest elimination of chocolate and cola beverages from the diet and reduction of fat intake. The net effect of such instruction, if followed, would be to reduce the amount of poor quality foods and increase the intake of other good foods to keep energy intake constant. Such an improved diet could benefit overall health, irrespective of its relevance to the skin disorder.

Obesity is a common finding in teenagers. A study in California[23] found 14 percent of high school seniors, both boys and girls, to be obese as judged by body weight and anthropometric measurements. A key factor in juvenile obesity is inactivity (Chapter 23), and the problem is better prevented or treated by increased energy expenditure than by food restriction at a stressful time of life. Participation in sports is to be recommended strongly for this reason and to establish habits that promote lifelong health (Chapter 21).

NUTRITION OF OLDER ADULTS

A marked change in life style often occurs at about 65 years of age or with retirement from business. The bodily condition known as "old age" (it almost invariably develops sooner or later) is not the inevitable result of living a certain number of years, and it may be long postponed by the right dietary regimen and manner of living. On the other hand, a poor diet or the wrong mode of living may bring on premature senility. Some people are "older" in body at 40 than others are at 80. Those who succeed in retaining their youthful vigor in the later years of life are usually not inactive people but, on the contrary, are those who are active mentally and moderately active physically.

The fundamental cause of aging relates to energetics of the biological system.[24] Currently held concepts suggest that aging begins early in life and that procedures to alter the rate of decline need to begin equally early. However, most people are little concerned about aging until they themselves reach the middle years of life when processes are well underway. Evidence from human populations is always epidemiologic and retrospective because the life span of an investigator is no longer than the subject he needs to examine. Thus, animal systems provide our only model for research into methods to interrupt the processes of senile change. Current nutritional research relates to two hypotheses: (1) that aging is due to oxidative changes that can be modified by increased dosages of vitamin E and other antioxidants;[25] and (2) that delayed growth and maturation rate brought about by restriction of dietary energy early in life lead to a longer life span.[26] There is no adequate proof of the antioxidant theory to date. Investigators found that rats which received a lower energy intake in the early postweaning period lived longer than those that were liberally fed.[26] However, there is no evidence that the same results would be true for humans, for in parts of the world where food intake is chronically low, average life span is shorter than in richer countries with more generous food supplies but also better public health practices. A diet which provides energy in *excess* of human needs, resulting in overweight, is definitely known to be associated with an increased incidence of heart and circulatory diseases, diabetes, and earlier mortality (Chapter 23). When the overweight person reduces to normal or even slightly below normal weight, the risk of heart disease decreases. In many cases, adult diabetes may also be controlled simply by reducing body weight to normal, together with moderate restrictions of dietary carbohydrate and judicious exercise.

A long-standing faulty diet may also be associated with osteoporosis, another disorder commonly seen in aged individuals. This disorder, in which there is thinning of the skeleton and lack of bone matrix, occurs especially frequently in old women, and it may lead to spontaneous fracture of the spinal column and loss of height. The princi-

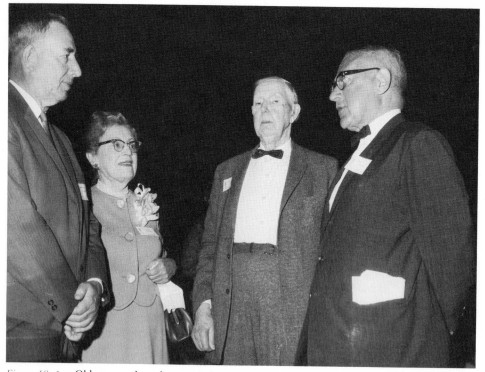

Figure 18–1. Old age need not be a period of isolation and boredom. Shown in this photograph are four famous nutritionists whose active careers extended well past the usual period of diminished productivity. At the time this picture was taken their ages were (left to right): W. H. Griffith, 70; Agnes Fay Morgan, 81; E. V. McCollum, 89; and Paul György, 72. (Photo courtesy of Ralph N. Smith, A.E.S., University of California, Berkeley.)

pal causes of osteoporosis are thought to be inactivity, lack of hormones, and perhaps decreased ability to absorb calcium from the intestine, coupled with chronic low intake of calcium and vitamin D.[27]

In the later years of life the ability of the body to handle an excess of food is diminished. First, the loss of teeth frequently results in inability to masticate hard or coarse foods. Inadequately chewed foods may cause digestive discomfort, while the omission of all coarse foods from the diet may lead to a diet of poorer quality. Blood flow to the alimentary tract, secretion of digestive juices, and intestinal absorption are diminished. There are fewer active cells in the body, and various organs and tissues are either less active or less able to do extra work. The oxidative proc-

esses by which foods are utilized in the tissues go on more slowly and sometimes less completely, while the excretion of excessive waste products is more difficult.

Nutritional needs of the older person vary from those of the younger adult, but not to the extent of a sparse and abstemious diet. The idea of such a diet for later life has gone out of style, and for good reason. The same nutritive essentials (energy, protein, mineral salts, and vitamins) are required in adequate quantities to nourish the body throughout life, and an insufficiency of any of them does harm at any age.

The most significant change in the diets of aging persons is that energy nutrients are needed in smaller quantities, so that principal curtailment should be in the intake of foods that supply only or chiefly energy. The energy requirement of older adults is materially reduced for two reasons:

1. Less energy is used in muscular activity.
2. The basal metabolism is lowered.

It is estimated that the resting metabolic rate between ages 60 and 70 is about 10 percent less than formerly, 20 percent less from 70 to 90, and about 25 percent less after 90 years of age. Thus, a man of average weight and in middle life requires about 1600 to 1700 kcal per day for maintenance when at rest. Requirements of the same man for maintenance alone at 60 to 70 years would be about 1440 to 1530 kcal, and at 70 to 80 years, 1280 to 1360 kcal. These differences in energy needs may be at least partially accounted for by changes in body composition during aging—an increased percentage of fat and a lesser amount of lean muscle tissue in the body.[28] Few men in their seventies do enough muscular work to raise their total energy requirement to more than 2400 kcal a day. Small, aged women may have surprisingly low energy needs.

It is thus apparent that the total amount of food—especially foods of high caloric value—should be somewhat curtailed after reaching 60 years (slightly so even at 40 to 60 years of age), and considerably reduced after 70. The Food and Nutrition Board has recommended that energy allowances be reduced by 3 percent per decade between ages 35 and 55, by 5 percent per decade from 55 to 75, and by an additional 7 percent for age 75 and beyond.[1] A Baltimore study[29] of 252 men, age 20 to 99 years and from upper income groups, found that energy intake declined from about 2700 kcal for ages 20 to 44, to 2300 kcal for ages 55 to 74 and 2100 kcal over age 75. Body weight was 74 kg for ages 20 to 34, 77 to 78 kg for ages 35 to 74, and only 71 kg for men who lived beyond that age. If the weight factor is taken into account, the sharpest drop in energy intake occurred

at about age 60. Over the total age range, energy intake fell by 12.4 kcal per day per year and the decrease in measured basal metabolism was 5.23 kcal per day per year. The remainder would be due to diminished activity and altered body composition.

Another variation in the needs of older adults as compared to younger persons may be in protein requirement. Some studies with amino acid diets have indicated that the requirement for essential amino acids is higher in men over 50 years of age than in younger adult males.[30] However, in another study, in which the ratios of essential amino acids were somewhat different, no such age difference was apparent.[31] While it is true that whole proteins do not behave exactly as do mixtures of amino acids (retention by the body is better with proteins than with amino acids) and that experimental findings differ, in no case is there any suggestion of a decreased protein requirement with increasing age.

Surveys of the diets of old people have indicated inadequate intake of vitamins and minerals. A British study[32] of 60 women living alone found inadequate intakes of protein, vitamins C and D, calcium, and iron. Such findings are typical of experience in Australia, New Zealand, and the United States. Although old people living alone are often in reduced financial circumstances, partially disabled, and without sufficient motivation to prepare foods for their solitary meals, residence in a care center does not guarantee an adequate intake of nutrients. A small group of women in an Australian hostel[33] had unsatisfactory levels of vitamin C in the blood even though the diet was calculated to contain enough of this nutrient; analysis of the food as served showed that 99 percent of the vitamin C had been lost because of poor institutional food practices. Food transported to old people in their homes ("Meals on Wheels") is also prepared in quantity and held warm for some time in the trucks, leading to excessive loss of vitamin C and other heat-sensitive vitamins, thiamin and folacin. Unacceptable blood levels of thiamin[34] and folacin[35] have been found frequently in old people, in addition to ascorbic acid as noted above.

In planning diets for the aged person, all aspects of his limited functional capability should be considered. Meals should be evenly spaced with perhaps smaller amounts of food taken at more frequent intervals in view of diminished digestive and absorptive capacity. Adjustment of energy intake to achieve desirable body weight relieves the strain imposed on the heart and on arthritic joints and an osteoporotic skeleton. The following physical conditions may impair the physical capability to ingest an adequate diet unless it is suitably prepared:

1. Crippling joint disease
2. Muscular tremor
3. Poor vision
4. Missing teeth, badly fitting dentures
5. Reduced senses of smell and taste
6. Difficulties in swallowing

Many workers in the field of geriatrics believe that lack of useful work or ways in which to fill their leisure hours and isolation from other people are the two most prominent factors that lead older people to take an inadequate amount of food. Other factors that have been found to influence food consumption of this group are:

1. Social situation
2. Income
3. Cooking and refrigeration facilities
4. Food faddism
5. Long-standing erroneous concepts of good nutrition

Planning a diet that is not too high in energy value, yet that at the same time furnishes plenty of high-quality protein, minerals, and vitamins, may at times be difficult. The daily food intake should consist mainly of milk, meats, eggs, whole-grain or enriched bread or cereals (in moderation), vegetables, and fruits, with restricted amounts of con-

centrated sweets and fats. Some raw fruits and vegetables should be included because of the question of nutrient loss in holding food for service. If the old person cannot chew these, fresh juices can be made from them. At this age in life, vitamin supplements may be advantageous, but at least one study[36] indicated that old people who took supplements regularly were the least likely to need them, having otherwise good diets.

Foods included in the menu should be chosen from well liked foods and presented in attractive, appetizing forms. Many old people have little to anticipate with pleasure in the day except their meals. They should not be deprived of this simple enjoyment by arbitrary insistence on fixed rules of food selection.

A word may be in order concerning the place of mild stimulants such as tea and coffee or the moderate use of alcoholic beverages. Most elderly persons experience comfort and cheer from hot drinks, and hot coffee or tea slightly stimulates the motility of the digestive tract. Their stimulating effect may be welcome to those whose bodily processes are slow. They also help to keep up fluid intake. Except in certain abnormal conditions, there is no reason to forbid their use. Much the same may be said of alcoholic beverages. Alcohol dilates the capillary blood vessels and thus may improve circulation temporarily. The abuse of alcoholic beverages by some persons should not rule out their proper uses by others.

QUESTIONS AND PROBLEMS

1. Plan a day's menu using the tables of Nutritive Values of Foods in the Appendix (pp. 546 to 574) and, as far as possible, foods that you commonly use. Estimate how much of each essential nutrient is furnished by the foods in your menus. Compare the total with the recommended daily allowance of

Complete

needs for one of your sex, body weight, and degree of physical activity. What changes would be needed to adapt this diet for a boy of 16? A woman of 70?

2. Consult Table 18–2, which gives the nutritive evaluation of the foundation diet; determine for each of the individual nutrients listed what proportion of the total values for nutrients in the basal diet comes from certain classes of foods? What are the strengths and weaknesses of the Basic Four Food Groups pattern of menu planning? How may adequacy of lesser-studied vitamins and minerals be assured?

3. Outline briefly the types of dietary pattern characteristic of the following countries – Italy, India, China, and Ethiopia. In each case, what nutrients might be provided in insufficient amounts and what foods are in use or could be used to reinforce the diet in respect to those nutrients?

4. If the diet does not furnish the full amount of the allowance recommended by the United States Food and Nutrition Board (National Academy of Sciences), does it necessarily indicate that a person will suffer a deficiency of the nutritive essential which is provided in less than this quantity? Explain your answer. Why may an intake of certain nutrients in excess of the nutrients needed by the body be desirable, and if so, under what circumstances?

5. What are the main factors affecting the physiological aging process? How is nutrition related to the problem of aging? What are the most common causes of death after 55 and how may their incidence be related to nutritional status? When should a diet for retarding the aging process begin? What special dietary factors may influence health in the later years of life?

6. According to the Food and Nutrition Board, how much should the total caloric intake of a 60 year old man be reduced below that recommended for him at 30 years of age? Are protein needs of older people also reduced? What is the evidence?

7. What factors i[...] ment of elderly pec[...] the consumption of [...] if finances are ade[...] menu for a bedridc[...] with artificial teet[...] foods given be ac[...] special disabilities [...] as between-meal nourishment?

REFERENCES

1. *Recommended Dietary Allowances.* 7th Edition. Publ. No. 1694. Washington, National Academy of Sciences, 1968.
2. Recommended intakes of nutrients for the United Kingdom. Repts. on Pub. Health and Med. Subj., no. 120, London, 1969.
3. Dietary standard for Canada. Canad. Bull. Nutr., 6:No. 1, 1964.
4. U.S.D.A. Dietary Levels of Households in the United States, Spring 1965. Household Food Consumption Survey 1965–66, Rept. No. 6, Agr. Res. Serv., 1969.
5. Page, L., and Phippard, E. F.: *Essentials of Nutrition.* Home Economic Research Report No. 3. Washington, D.C., Government Printing Office, 1957.
6. Watt, B. K., and Merrill, A. L.: *Composition of foods: Raw, processed and prepared.* Agric. Handbook No. 8, Washington, U.S. Department of Agriculture, 1963.
7. Orr, M. L.: *Pantothenic acid, vitamin B_6 and vitamin B_{12} in foods.* Home Econ. Res. Rept. No. 36, Washington, U.S. Department of Agriculture, 1969.
8. Bunnell, R. H., Keating, J., Quaresimo, A., and Parman, G. K.: Alpha-tocopherol content of foods. Amer. J. Clin. Nutr., 17:1, 1965.
9. Jankelson, O. M., Beaser, S. B., Howard, F. M., and Mayer, J.: Effect of coffee on glucose tolerance and circulating insulin in men with maturity-onset diabetes. Lancet, 1:527, 1967.
10. Bellet, S., Kershbaum, A., and Finck, E. M.: The response of free fatty acids to coffee and caffeine. Metabolism, 17:702, 1968.
11. Butterfield, S., and Calloway, D. H.: Folacin in wheat and selected foods. J. Amer. Dietet. Assoc., 60:310, 1972.
12. Nolan, G. A., Alexander, J. C., and Artman, N. R.: Long-term rat feeding study with used frying fats. J. Nutr., 93:337, 1967.
13. vanVeen, A. G., and Steinkraus, K. H.: Nutritive value and wholesomeness of fermented foods. J. Agr. Food Chem., 18: 576, 1970.
14. Hardinge, M. G., and Crooks, H.: Non-flesh

440

dietaries. III. Adequate and inadequate. J. Amer. Dietet. Assoc., *45*:537, 1964.

15. Kurtha, A. N., and Ellis, F. R.: Investigation into the causation of the electroencephalogram abnormality in vegans. Pl. Fds. Hum. Nutr., *2*:53, 1971.

16. Fábry, P.: Metabolic consequences of the pattern of food intake. In Code, C. F. (ed.): *Handbook of Physiology*, Section 6. Baltimore, Williams & Wilkins for Am. Physiol. Soc., 1967.

17. Thornton, R., and Horvath, S. M.: Blood sugar levels after eating and after omitting breakfast. Studies with teen-agers and young adults. J. Amer. Dietet. Assoc., *47*:474, 1965.

18. Tuttle, W. W., et al.: Effect on school boys of omitting breakfast. Physiologic responses, attitudes, and scholastic attainments. J. Amer. Dietet. Assoc., *30*:674, 1954.

19. Thornton, R. H., and Horvath, S. M.: Blood glucose as influenced by either one or two meals. J. Amer. Dietet. Assoc., *52*:214, 1968.

20. Edwards, C. H., Hogan, G., and Spahr, S.: Nutrition survey of 6200 teen-age youth. J. Amer. Dietet. Assoc., *45*:543, 1964.

21. Hueneman, R. L., Shapiro, L. R., Hampton, M. C., and Mitchell, B. W.: Food and eating practices of teen-agers. J. Amer. Dietet. Assoc., *53*:17, 1968.

22. McNaughton, J. W., and Cahn, A. J.: A study of the food intake and activity of a group of urban adolescents. Brit. J. Nutr., *24*:331, 1970.

23. Huenemann, R. L., Hampton, M. C., Shapiro, L. R., and Behnke, A. R.: Adolescent food practices associated with obesity. Fed. Proc., *25*:4, 1966.

24. Calloway, N. O.: The senescent sequences of normal processes. J. Amer. Geriat. Soc., *14*:1048, 1966.

25. Tappel, A. L.: Where old age begins. Nutr. Today, *2*:2, December 1967.

26. McCay, C. M.: J. Nutr., *18*:1, 1939; Riesen, W. H., et al.: Amer. J. Physiol., *148*:614, 1947; Berg, B. N., and Simms, H. S.: J. Nutr., *74*:23, 1961.

27. Nordin, B. E. C.: Clinical significance and pathogenesis of osteoporosis. Brit. Med. J., *1*:571, 1971.

28. Forbes, G. B., and Reina, J. C.: Adult lean body mass declines with age: Some longitudinal observations. Metab., *19*:653, 1970.

29. McGandy, R. B., et al.: Nutrient intakes and energy expenditures in men of different ages. J. Gerontol., *21*:581, 1966.

30. Tuttle, S. G., et al.: Further observations on the amino acid requirements of older men. II. Methionine and lysine. Amer. J. Clin. Nutr., *16*:229, 1965.

31. Watts, J. H., et al.: Nitrogen balances of men over 65 fed the FAO and milk patterns of essential amino acids. J. Gerontol., *19*:370, 1964.

32. Exton-Smith, A. N., and Stanton, B. R.: *Report of an Investigation into the Dietary of Elderly Women Living Alone.* London, King Edward's Hospital Fund, 1965.

33. Woodhill, J. M., Nobile, S. R. V., and Perkins, K. W.: Dietary surveys of small groups of elderly people: Eight women living in a hostel. Food Nutr. Notes Rev., *27*:51, 1970.

34. Griffiths, L. L., et al.: Gerontol. Clin. (Basel), *9*:1, 1967.

35. Girdwood, R. H.: Folate depletion in old age. Amer. J. Clin. Nutr., *22*:234, 1969.

36. Steinkamp, R. C., Cohen, M. L., and Walsh, H. E.: Resurvey of an aging population—fourteen year follow-up. J. Amer. Dietet. Assoc., *46*:103, 1965.

SUPPLEMENTARY READING

Allen, D. E., Patterson, Z. J., and Warren, G. L.: Nutrition, family commensality, and academic performance among high school youth. J. Home Econ., *62*:333, 1970.

Anonymous: Selected aspects of geriatric nutrition. Dairy Council Digest, *43*:7, 1972.

Bebb, H. T., et al.: Calorie and nutrient contribution of alcoholic beverages to the usual diets of 155 adults. Amer. J. Clin. Nutr., *24*:1042, 1971.

Durnin, J. V. G. A., et al.: Food intake and energy expenditure of elderly women with varying-sized families. Brit. J. Nutr., *15*:73, 1961.

Esposito, S. J., Vinton, P. W., and Rapuano, J. A.: Nutrition in the aged: Review of the literature. J. Amer. Geriat. Soc., *17*:790, 1969.

Hardinge, M. G., and Crooks, H.: Non-flesh dietaries. III. Adequate and inadequate. J. Amer. Dietet. Assoc., *45*:537, 1964.

Harris, W. H.: A survey of breakfasts eaten by high school students. J. School Health, *40*:323, 1970.

Hartcroft, W. S., et al.: Symposium: Alcohol, metabolism and liver disease. Fed. Proc., *26*:1432, 1967.

Holmes, D.: Nutrition and health-screening services for the elderly. J. Amer. Dietet. Assoc., *60*:301, 1972.

Hunter, R. : Why Popeye took spinach. Lancet, *1*:746, 1971.

Kurtha, A. N., and Ellis, F. R.: The nutritional, clinical and economic aspects of vegan diets. Pl. Fds. Hum. Nutr., *2*:13, 1970.

Miller, D. S., and Mumford, P.: Diet assessment and formulation in human nutrition. Proc. Nutr. Soc. (Gt. Brit.), *29*:116, 1970.

Murdock, H. R., Jr.: Blood glucose and alcohol levels after administration of wine to human subjects. Amer. J. Clin. Nutr., *24*:394, 1971.

Pelacovits, J.: Nutrition for older Americans. J. Amer. Dietet. Assoc., *58*:17, 1971; *60*:297, 1972.

Shock, N. W.: Physiologic aspects of aging. J. Amer. Dietet. Assoc., *56*:491, 1970.

Sinclair, D.: Canadian food and nutrition statistics, 1935 to 1965. Canad. Nutr. Notes, *25*:109, 1969.

Tuttle, W. W., and Herbert, E.: Work capacity with no breakfast and a mid-morning break. J. Amer. Dietet. Assoc., *37*:137, 1960.

USDA Agric. Res. Serv.: Dietary levels of households in the United States, Spring 1965. A preliminary report. ARS-17, Jan. 1968.

Walker, M. A., and Hill, M. M.: *Food Guide for Older Folks.* Home and Garden Bulletin No. 17, Washington, D.C., U.S.D.A., 1971.

Williams, R. J.: We abnormal normals. Nutr. Today, *2*:19, December 1967.

Nutrition Reviews

Availability of vitamins and minerals in tablet form. *24*:101, 1966.

On meeting certain recommended dietary allowances in the elderly and the indolent. *24*:319, 1966.

The effect of ethanol ingestion on liver dehydrogenases in various vitamin deficiencies. *25*:22, 1967.

Nutrition and metabolic bone disease in the elderly. *25*:71, 1967.

Effects of feeding frequency on fat and protein deposition in pigs. *25*:313, 1967.

Malnutrition and hunger in the U.S.A. (by Stare, F. J.). *26*:227, 1968.

Effects of caffeine in man. *28*:38, 1970.

Vitamin supplements for older people. *28*:260, 1970.

nineteen

Nutrition During Pregnancy and Lactation

For pregnant and nursing mothers, diet is of extra importance because the mother is nourishing the child through her own body, either in the uterus before birth or through the milk she secretes for the baby. Although both are entirely normal physiological processes, they do subject the body to special strain. The nutrients needed for the child must be furnished in the mother's food or they may be drawn to some extent from her own tissues. Pregnancy in teen-age girls presents a situation of particular stress, because the needs of the developing infant are superimposed on the mother's own needs for adequate growth and development. Maternal and infant complications occur about twice as frequently among early teen-age mothers as among mature women.[1] Pregnancy hazards are also higher in American nonwhite populations than in white and higher in women from lower socioeconomic groups.[1]

A young woman who has good food habits and is well nourished when she becomes pregnant has little cause for concern. She will need to alter her diet only by increasing intake of some of the foods she is accustomed to eating. Unfortunately, too many young women have not formed good food habits and thus come into pregnancy in a poorly nourished condition. Any borderline deficiency may become apparent at this time. If previous intake of iron or folacin has been low, anemia may develop during pregnancy, because of the extra demands of the fetus. In goitrous regions, pregnancy is one of the times when latent iodine deficiency is likely to be manifested by enlargement of the thyroid gland.

Nutritional Status of Women of Child-Bearing Age

In the United States, adolescent girls usually have the poorest diets in families from all socioeconomic strata, and those in the lowest socioeconomic group tend to have lower nutrient intakes than others.[2] After menarche, monthly blood losses increase the girl's need for iron. The iron loss in menstrual flow averages 15 to 30 mg, or 0.5 to 1.0 mg per day over the monthly cycle. Because only

442

10 to 20 percent of dietary iron is absorbed, iron intake should be increased by 5 to 10 mg per day after menarche, yet older girls and women usually take less iron in the diet than do boys and men (see Chapter 12). Thus, anemia and undesirably low iron stores are common in women.[3]

Folacin status is also unsatisfactory in many women, including those who are affluent.[4] This important B vitamin is low in many diets, is easily lost by bad cooking or processing practices, and is very commonly omitted from vitamin pills, so the frequency of folacin deficiency is perhaps not surprising. The incidence of folacin deficiency is high among women who use oral contraceptives, which may be due to an adverse effect of the drugs on absorption of the polyglutamate forms of food folacin.[5]

Obesity is common in young women, although less so than among older women. Being fat or being anxious about keeping slim leads to chronic self-imposed dieting that may further lower body stores of essential nutrients. Fat women are at least as likely to be poorly nourished as slender women. In the United States, this is especially true in poverty groups. A combination of being unemployed, without access to recreational sports, and on a limited food budget leads easily to consumption of too much cheap, filling food of poor nutritive value.

In all age and economic groups, dietary histories indicate unsatisfactory intakes of calcium, iron, and vitamin A, and often of B vitamins, vitamin C, and iodine.[6] It is likely that intake of the lesser known nutrients is also low, but this point has not been well studied.

Effect of Malnutrition on the Outcome of Pregnancy

An undernourished mother may still be able to produce a healthy child, though there is evidence that a larger percentage of babies in poor condition are born to groups of mothers who were in poor nutritive condition. Illustrative evidence that the nutritive condition of the mother during pregnancy frequently influences not only her own health but also the well-being of her child comes from investigations in Canada[7] and the United States,[8] among others.[1] In each case, pregnant women from low-income groups were studied during the later months of pregnancy, and for some time after birth of the children. At the Boston Lying-In Hospital, 216 women attending the prenatal clinic were classified according to whether their diets were considered good, fair, or poor. No attempt was made to influence the diet, and records were kept of condition of mother and baby at and after delivery. Mothers in the poorest diet group had more complications and difficult types of delivery, while all the stillborn babies and all but one of those who were premature or died soon after birth were born to mothers in this group. Conversely, a higher proportion of babies whose condition was rated at birth as superior or good were born to mothers who had had good or excellent diets during pregnancy (see Fig. 19–1). In the Toronto studies, the women in one group, whose diets were poor, received supplementary food. Those in another group had self-chosen diets but were trained in food selection. Those in the third group were given neither food nor instruction and served as controls. Those who received supplementary food had better health, both before and after delivery, fewer complications at delivery, also fewer miscarriages, stillbirths, or premature deliveries, than the mothers who ate poor diets during pregnancy. Beneficial effects of food supplements have also been reported from India.[9] These studies offer evidence of a direct relationship between quality of the prenatal diet and welfare of both mother and child.

Studies made in Europe following

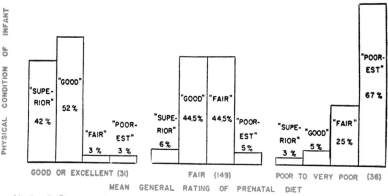

Figure 19–1. Influence of nutrition on condition of the infant during pregnancy, at birth and in the first two weeks of life. Note the high relative proportion of infants in superior or good physical condition born to mothers whose diet was rated as good or excellent, and the relatively large numbers of babies in fair or poorest condition in the group of mothers whose diet was rated as poor to very poor. (Courtesy of B. S. Burke and the *Journal of Nutrition.*)

severe food restrictions during the war years show disasters in reproduction—premature births, stillborn infants, infants below normal weight, and high neonatal death rate. In the Netherlands, food available to pregnant women provided on the average 1925 kcal and 61 gm of protein in 1944; by the spring of 1945, these allowances had fallen to 800 kcal and 35 gm of protein. About 50 percent of women became infertile, and there is an indication that the women who became pregnant were the better nourished. Birth weights of infants were decreased, but rose after relief feeding.[10] The situation was much worse during the siege of Leningrad, where the principal food available was rye bread of very poor quality. The total daily allowance for a working man was 300 to 350 gm of bread. At the height of the siege, the stillbirth rate rose to 56 percent and the incidence of prematurity was 40 percent. Birth weights were low and infant mortality was high.[11] These women were stressed in many ways, but poor nutrition is thought to have been a dominant factor in the poor outcomes of pregnancy. Ample supportive evidence is available from animal studies in which poor diets were fed during pregnancy.[1, 12] Not only do restricted laboratory and farm animals bear under-

sized young, but under severe conditions there is permanent stunting of growth and poor intellectual development.

Protein appears to be particularly important in both animal studies and human experience. In the United States, Dieckman[13] showed that there was an increased incidence of abortion when mothers were on a low-protein intake and, on the positive side, that the number of infants born in excellent condition increased steadily as the protein intake of the mothers was on a progressively higher level. Burke and her associates also found a positive relationship between maternal protein intake and infant weight, length, and physical well-being.[14] Adequate energy intake is also important, to guarantee that protein is well utilized.

Other investigators have failed to find a relationship between the nutrient content of self-selected diets and the quality of pregnancy.[15-17] In some studies the entire population appears to have been reasonably well-nourished, so differences due to minor variations in diet would not have been expected. The diet was poor in one Indian study, which has led to the totally unsupported suggestion that where diets have been poor for generations adaptive mechanisms may be developed that make for more efficient utilization of nutrients.[17]

In experimental animals, deficiency of specific nutrients at specific stages of fetal development causes malformation or loss of the fetus (see Chapters 5, 7, 9, and 12). Although there is no reason to believe that the same influences could not be manifest in the human fetus, such clear-cut effects have not been demonstrated in population studies. However, birth of deformed infants has occurred following the administration of folacin antagonists to pregnant women with cancer,[18] similar to the experience in laboratory animals (see Chap. 7). This evidence is sufficiently persuasive to emphasize that *pregnant women should adhere to a well balanced diet composed of a wide variety of foods.*

PREGNANCY

How the Child is Nourished

There is no direct connection, either nervous or circulatory, between the mother and the fetus, but interchange between the blood streams of mother and child takes place through the placenta (Fig. 19–2). This is a vascular organ on the inner surface of the uterus, in which the blood from the mother and the fetus are brought closely together so that interchange of constituents from one to the other is possible. Thus, the fetal blood takes up nutrients in the simple forms in which they are carried in the mother's blood and carries them to the fetus (through the umbilical cord), where they are built into the more complex substances needed to form the organs, muscles, and other tissues of the child.

Different Stages of Pregnancy

From the *first through the fourth months* of pregnancy, the need of materials for the growth of the fetus daily is so small as to be practically negligible. The mother should eat just what any woman should who wishes to preserve or build up her health and vitality. However, this is the period during which many women experience nausea or digestive disturbances. Nausea in early pregnancy is due usually to adjustments in establishing relationships between the fetus and the mother, not primarily due to misfunctioning of the digestive tract itself, and it should soon disappear. Food may be better tolerated in smaller meals at shorter intervals. Eating a few salted crackers before rising may help and certainly will do no harm. If vomiting is severe and prolonged, medical attention is advisable. In spite of optimistic claims, there is no clear evidence that administration of vitamins alleviates the nausea of early pregnancy in the well nourished patient. In fact, some vitamin-mineral supplements are not well tolerated, and *if prescribed*, these should be taken with, or immediately after, meals. By the beginning of the *second trimester of pregnancy*, the appetite and digestive abilities of the mother should be normal. The National Research Council recommends increased allowances for almost all the essential nutrients during pregnancy. These recommended allowances are found in Table 19–1, contrasted with those of a young, moderately active nonpregnant woman. Some of the extra nutrients allowed are for the building of tissues in the child, and some are intended for the protection of the mother's own tissues. In the early part of pregnancy the fetus gains hardly more than one gram of weight per day. Maternal tissues are growing during this time. The uterus and breasts enlarge, the placenta and amniotic fluid are formed, and the maternal blood volume expands. During the second trimester the mother stores a substantial amount of fat which provides a safety factor for the fetus against possible maternal food deprivation. By the sixth month the fetus is gaining

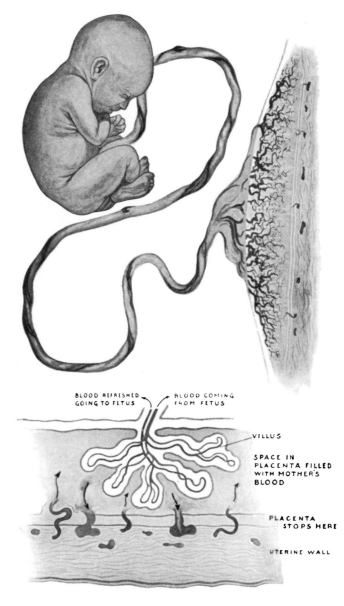

Figure 19–2. Diagram showing relations of maternal and fetal circulations. **Top,** The fetus is connected by the umbilical cord to the placenta, which in turn is attached to the wall of the uterus. **Bottom,** Detail of the fetal and maternal blood vessels in the placenta, with small vessels from and to the fetus immersed in a space filled with the mother's blood. (From Davis and Sheckler: *DeLee's Obstetrics for Nurses.*)

about 10 gm daily, but about half the total weight increase during gestation occurs in the last two months. Therefore, during the final months of pregnancy it is especially important that the diet be unusually rich in all the nutritive factors needed for the growing child. The extra energy needs should be met in the form of foods which also provide high-quality proteins, minerals, and vitamins.

The extra energy allowance suggested by the NRC is not large (200 kcal or 840 kJ per day). The energy value of new tissue laid down in pregnancy is about 50,000 kcal, of which a substantial portion is maternal fat. The basal metabolic rate is increased due to the energy requirement of fetal and supporting tissues and the added burden on the maternal heart and lungs. The total energy cost of a pregnancy is about

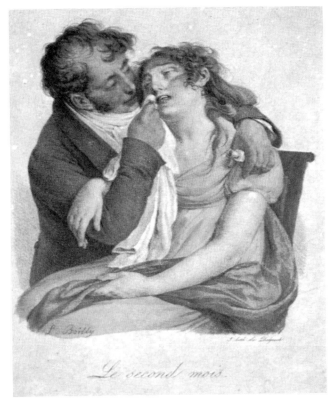

Figure 19–3. Old lithograph depicting the tribulations of the first weeks of pregnancy, some emotional, some physiological. Nausea and faintness disappear when maternal and placental circulatory systems are adjusted, and many women experience no difficulty whatsoever.

Le second mois.

Table 19–1. Dietary Allowances in Pregnancy and Lactation*

Nutritive Factors	Nonpregnant Woman, 18–35 years, 58 kg	During Pregnancy	During Lactation
Energy, kcal	2000	2200	3000
Protein, gm	55	65	75
Calcium, gm	0.8	1.2	1.3
Phosphorus, gm	0.8	1.2	1.3
Magnesium, mg	300	450	450
Iodine, μg	100	125	150
Iron, mg	18	18	18
Vitamin A, IU	5000	6000	8000
Thiamin, mg	1.0	1.1	1.5
Riboflavin, mg	1.5	1.8	2.0
Niacin (equiv.), mg	13	15	20
Folacin, mg	0.4	0.8	0.5
Vitamin B-6, mg	2.0	2.5	2.5
Vitamin B-12 μg	5	8	6
Vitamin C, mg	55	60	60
Vitamin D, IU	–	400	400
Vitamin E, IU	25	30	30

*National Research Council, recommendations of 1968.

80,000 kcal of metabolizable energy, or 285 kcal per day divided through the 280 days of gestation. The lower NRC allowance is based on the observation that women in the later months of pregnancy are often not very active physically. If the woman is active, and she should be to maintain fitness, her needs will be even greater than predicted because of the higher energy cost of moving a heavier, awkward body mass. Many women continue activity at home or at work much as before until very near term and their needs will be large. The additional energy allowance should be adjusted to the needs of the individual, so that the energy costs of building new tissues, of higher metabolic rate (in fetus), and of physical work load are met.

A normal and desirable weight gain during the 40 weeks of pregnancy is 24 to 28 pounds. Maternal complications are more frequently associated with marked over- or underweight at the time of conception and with wide deviation from normal *rate* of weight gain during pregnancy. Some studies have suggested an increased incidence of toxemia* in obese pregnant women but others have not. Large early weight gain has also been regarded as a bad omen of maternal complications. This fear has led to excessive concern with weight gain, especially in the obese woman. With family planning the obese woman can lose weight prior to pregnancy, but while she is pregnant she should *not* attempt to correct the pre-existing condition. If there is a tendency to excessive weight gain, it is far wiser to increase physical activity than to restrict food intake.

---

*Toxemia usually refers to a condition of blood poisoning as a result of microorganisms growing in the tissues or blood and/or the absorption of noxious materials from food and water. Toxemia of pregnancy differs and is a disorder of unidentified cause that is characterized by high blood pressure, protein in the urine, edema, headache, visual disturbances, and, in severe cases, convulsions and death.

Many slender women will need to gain more than the average 25 pounds. A study of 10,000 births showed that higher maternal weight gain was related to higher birth weight, a lower incidence of prematurity, and better growth and performance during the infant's first year of life.[19] The key consideration is that healthy tissue be laid down at a smooth progressive rate, irrespective of the total gain, and that the mother's health remain good. Some suggest that the weight gain may be spaced at about 4, 10, and 10 pounds in each of the three trimesters, but healthy women vary widely in this regard. Women carrying twins will gain about twice as much as those with singletons.

A Healthy Pregnancy

The nutritive needs during pregnancy are best met by a simple, wholesome diet, the basis of which is milk, eggs, meat, legumes, whole grains, fruits, and vegetables. If the diet taken before pregnancy was adequate, only simple modification is required to meet all additional nutrient allowances. Addition of two glasses of milk and one serving of dark green, leafy vegetables, with frequent substitution of fruit for rich dessert and organ meats for other meat, fish, or poultry, is sufficient. In general, the more fruits and vegetables taken the better, because these foods help to ensure the surplus of vitamins and minerals which is so very advantageous, without appreciably increasing caloric intake.

The daily diet during pregnancy should be built around the following foods, both as to types and amounts of foods daily:

Milk: 1 quart of whole or skimmed milk or yogurt.
Milk powder or canned milk may be substituted either as beverage or in cooking; 1 oz of Cheddar cheese may be substituted for one glass of milk.

Alternative sources of calcium are discussed in the preceding chapter.

Eggs: One, or at least five per week as such or used in cooking.

Meat: One large or two small servings of meat, fish, or poultry.

Frequent use of liver is desirable. Dry legumes (beans, peas, lentils) and nuts may be substituted with cautions as noted in the preceding chapter.

Vegetables and Fruits: Four or more large servings.

At least one serving should be a dark green leafy vegetable. One serving should be a vegetable or fruit high in vitamin C, such as green or red peppers, a citrus variety (orange, lemon, lime, grapefruit), papaya, melon, cabbage, or tomato.

Breads and cereals: Four slices of whole-grain bread.

Cereal, $1/2$ to $2/3$ c. ck., may be substituted for one slice of bread. Potatoes and whole-grain or enriched rice, corn meal, macaroni, spaghetti, barley, or wheat (bulgur) may also be used. Ready-to-eat cereal should be made from whole grain or have added bran or germ.

Fat: 2 tbsp of butter, margarine, or vegetable oil. If whole milk or milk products are used, 1 tbsp of vegetable oil may be sufficient, depending on energy needs.

Vitamin D: 400 IU from fortified milk or dietary supplement.

Fluid whole milk, canned evaporated milk, and some dry and skimmed milks are fortified with vitamin D at the level of 400 IU per quart. Some milk powder is not fortified, nor are cheese and ice cream. Package labels specify the addition of vitamin D.

Iodine: Iodized salt should be used in cooking and at the table.

One may supplement these foods to furnish calories sufficient for individual energy needs and desired weight gain, either by taking more of some foods just listed or other foods of one's choice. It should be remembered that the *energy needs vary* with weight and especially with degree of activity, so that the calorie allowance should be estimated individually, then increased in the second trimester of pregnancy by at least 200 kcal. A moderately active, 58 kg woman (as listed in first column of Table 19–1) who needs 2000 kcal normally should have 2200 kcal or more in the latter part of pregnancy. But an active woman whose ordinary daily energy need is about 2400 kcal requires at least 2600 kcal in late pregnancy. Also, a woman who begins pregnancy in an undernourished condition may need a more liberal energy allowance in order to gain some weight. Teenagers must add the pregnancy allowance to the higher energy values recommended for nonpregnant girls of the same maturity.

A woman who is overweight when she becomes pregnant will need to keep her physical activity level high, or increase it, in order not to add to her obesity. The diet should not be too restrictive, i.e., not below 36 kcal per kg ideal body weight. Foods containing sugar, starch, and fats should be the ones eliminated, rather than protein, minerals, and vitamin-bearing foods; skim milk may be substituted for whole milk.

Enough energy must be supplied so that there will be no need to burn protein merely as fuel. Obviously, all the essential amino acids are required for fetal growth, so it is advisable that at least half the protein in the diet should be from foods of animal origin (milk, meats, eggs).

Extra *calcium* for the mother during pregnancy (and lactation) goes far toward ensuring teeth of good quality and well calcified bones in the child. The teeth of the child are formed and in large part calcified during the latter half of fetal life and the first few months after birth. About 20 gm of calcium is present in the body of a full-term infant which means that the mother must supply 80 mg of *absorbed* calcium every day of pregnancy.

If the mother's diet is rich in *iron* during pregnancy, the child will be born with a liver well stored with iron, often a reserve sufficient to last through the months when it will be fed chiefly milk—a food of low iron content. The newly born infant has about 0.2 to 0.3 gm of iron in his body and another 0.5 gm is present in the placenta and extramaternal tissues. The average woman has about 0.3 gm of storage iron, and another 150 mg will be spared because she is not menstruating. This is only about half the amount needed even if maternal stores were to be totally depleted. Unless the diet is rich in iron, the baby will be born without a good iron reserve and the woman will become anemic. Supplementary iron is often prescribed, and a supplement of 15 mg per day should be ample. A folacin supplement may also be needed; 0.3 to 0.4 mg will meet the additional requirement for pregnancy.

Women are sometimes advised to restrict their salt intake when their weight gain is judged excessive and they are accumulating tissue fluid. Some gain in blood volume and other extracellular fluid is perfectly normal under the hormonal influences of pregnancy. Salt is a dietary essential, and neither maternal nor fetal tissues can be maintained satisfactorily without it.[20-22] The association of sodium, edema, and hypertension (Chapter 10) led to the practice of salt restriction as a medical measure in threatened toxemia, but a careful study by Robinson[22] of over 2000 women showed that there were fewer complications in the group instructed to take more salt than in the one told to restrict it.

If digestion is upset or there is difficulty in taking enough food, the regular meals may be reduced in size and extra nourishment given between meals in the form of easily tolerated foods, such as milk, eggnog, malted milk, cereal gruels, crackers, fruit, or fruit juice. If preferred, much of the milk may be taken in dishes, such as cream soups and custards. Meals may easily be made to fit into the family schedule, if foods for the family are wisely chosen—that

is, planned to be of high nutritive value and cooked simply.

The extra allowances of all the essential nutrients recommended for pregnancy are a protection for both mother and child. They provide an abundance of building materials for growth and development of the infant without any need to draw on the stores of these substances in the mother's body, and they help to build reserves in the baby of such nutrients as can be stored before birth.

LACTATION

Nutritive Requirements of Nursing Mother Higher Than for Pregnant Woman

During lactation, there is a very high need for energy, protein, minerals, and vitamins: (1) to cover the amounts secreted in the milk for nourishment of the infant, (2) to cover the "cost" of secreting the milk, and (3) to protect the mother's body. Energy requirement varies with the amount of milk produced, and intake must be regulated to the individual woman. A woman who is meeting all the needs of a 5 kg infant (11 pounds) must secrete about 800 ml of milk, providing about 600 kcal daily. The U.S. National Research Council recommends a supplement of 120 kcal for each 100 ml of milk produced. The energy value of the milk secreted accounts for about two-thirds of this allowance. The additional energy allowance was based on an assumption that conversion of dietary energy to secreted milk energy was in the order of 60 percent efficient. Later work in Scotland[23] has proved lactation to be over 90 percent efficient in energy conversion. This study compared women who were breast feeding their infants with those who gave bottle feedings, as to energy intake, physical activity level, and loss of body fat. Energy intakes of the two groups were 2716 and 2125 kcal, respectively; both were losing weight and the lactating women negligibly more. Energy available for milk formation was 618 kcal per day, and the calculated energy content of milk was 597 kcal.

A woman who has gained an adequate amount of weight during pregnancy should have a fat reserve that she can call on to meet lactational needs. This is a real benefit because during the first few weeks post partum a mother is often physically active and short on sleep and her food intake does not keep up with her needs. Body weight will be normalized without need for special effort at slimming, and the woman who carries through the whole of the reproductive cycle should not become fatter with each pregnancy. Although lactation performance is well maintained in spite of very inadequate intakes of energy,[24] the diet should be of good quality to prevent depletion of the maternal lean tissues and to guarantee adequate content of vitamins and trace minerals in the milk.

Human milk contains about 12 gm of protein per liter. In arriving at the recommended allowance of an additional 20 gm of protein per day during lactation, the National Research Council has assumed that the dietary protein is of lower quality than milk protein so that conversion is not 100 percent efficient and that milk production may exceed one liter per day. Successful lactation is achieved on lower protein intakes, but there is no clear evidence that this is not detrimental to the mother. The essential amino acids incorporated in milk proteins must be furnished liberally, so it is advisable to obtain the extra protein allowance from high-quality sources.

Because milk is so high in calcium and phosphorus, its secretion makes great demands for these mineral elements. If a mother increases her own milk intake by the amount she is providing to her child (an additional one pint to one quart daily), she will meet the high calcium needs, as well as the need for some other nutrients. Nursing mothers are often found to be in negative calcium and phosphorus balance. This causes a drain on the mother's

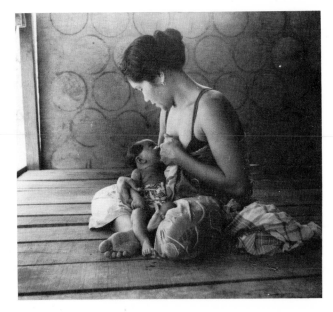

Figure 19–4. Breast feeding is the ideal method of providing nutrition for young infants. As evident in this picture of a Malaysian woman feeding her infant, the warm, close relationship is satisfying both to the mother and the child. (Courtesy of Dr. Christine Wilson, University of California.)

body, but it does not affect milk secretion. The vitamin content of human milk, especially the water-soluble vitamins, is largely dependent on the vitamin intake of the mother. Lactation, like pregnancy, is a period when borderline nutritional status may develop into frank deficiency. Allowances recommended for vitamins are about 50 percent more than those for nonpregnant women. Relatively little iron is secreted in milk (0.5 to 1.0 mg per day), and lactating women usually do not menstruate, so there is no added allowance for iron in lactation. Vitamin D (400 IU) in supplementary form is needed to ensure good utilization of calcium and phosphorus. The high allowances of various nutrients recommended during lactation may be seen by consulting Table 19–1.

Diet for Nursing Mothers

Recommendations for the diet in the nursing period are almost identical with those given for pregnancy, except that the need for almost all nutritive essentials is greater during lactation, especially as the infant grows and takes larger quantities of milk. The *quality* of the diet required remains essentially the same—a diet high in energy and containing liberal amounts of milk, eggs, fruits, and vegetables to furnish the extra protein, mineral salts, and vitamins needed.

Milk is the best food for protecting the mother's bones and teeth against any drain on calcium and phosphorus reserves to supply these elements in her milk. At least 1 quart of milk should be taken daily, or its equivalent in cheese or yogurt. It is a good thing to take supplementary nourishment just before nursing the baby in the middle of the morning and afternoon, and at bedtime. It is essential to have a plentiful intake of **fluids** (2 to 3 quarts from all sources) to provide the water in the milk secreted, in addition to that needed

by the mother. Fruit and vegetable juices are useful to give added fluids, as well as vitamins and minerals.

Many constituents other than nutrients are passed into milk. Excessive use of alcohol and artificially sweetened products is to be avoided during nursing periods for this reason. Drugs, including those sold without prescription, such as aspirin, laxatives, and sedatives, pass into the milk and should be taken only on the advice of a physician. Oral contraceptive agents are thought to affect lactation adversely,[25] but injected preparations have been used with no detected detriment.[26]

Technique of Breast Feeding

During the latter weeks of pregnancy, the mother should use extra care in cleansing the nipples, preferably without soap, and massage them as needed to assure protractility. The breasts should be mechanically supported by a well-fitting garment. Following delivery, the infant should be offered breast feeding as early and at as frequent intervals as possible, using both breasts. It is important that the infant receive the first flow (colostrum), as it contains much of the immune substances. The infant should not be given supplementary feedings because they decrease the appetite and vigor of sucking. If there is difficulty in the beginning, boiled water should be given from a spoon. When lactation is established, the baby should be suckled from alternate breasts at each feeding, or from both breasts if milk flow is light.

Advantages of Breast Feeding

In addition to the warmth, closeness and emotional satisfaction of breast feeding for both mother and child, there are clear superiorities of human milk for human infants.

Breast milk provides immune substances made by the mother that help the infant to resist infection during the early months of life, and use of breast milk favors the development of desirable strains of bacteria in the intestinal tract of the newborn. Furthermore, human milk is specially adapted for providing all nutrients needed in the right proportions for the rate of growth normal for infants and in forms easily handled by the baby's digestive tract. Cow s milk is designed for the calf, which should double its birth weight in about a third of the time that it takes an infant to do so. Therefore, cow's milk is more concentrated in certain building materials. The relative composition of human milk and cow's milk is shown in Table 19–2.

It can be seen that cow's milk contains about three times as much protein per 100 gm as human milk does and is much more concentrated in calcium and phosphorus, while human milk is higher in sugar content. When cow's milk is modified for infant feeding, the protein and inorganic substances are reduced by dilution and sugar (lactose, cane sugar, or corn syrup) is added to increase the energy value. Such modification makes it suitable for infant feeding but simultaneously dilutes its vitamin and trace mineral

Table 19–2. Nutrients in Human and Cow's Milk*

Nutrient	Human	Cow
	per 100 grams of milk	
Energy, kcal	77.0	65.0
Protein, gm	1.1	3.5
Fat, gm	4.0	3.5
Carbohydrate, gm	9.5	4.9
Calcium, mg	33.0	118.0
Phosphorus, mg	14.0	93.0
Iron, mg	0.1	Trace
Vitamin C, mg	5.0	1.0

*From Watt, B. K., and Merrill, A. L.: *Composition of Foods.* Agriculture Handbook No. 8, December, 1963, p. 39.

content and still does not provide various nutrients in the same relative proportions as in human milk. However, cow's milk formulas, as well as diets based on goat's or mare's milk, have been used successfully for infant feeding for years. When breast feeding is not feasible, pediatricians recommend formulas suited to the infant.

Human milk forms a much finer and more flocculent curd in the stomach than does cow s milk; moreover, cow's milk is liable to become contaminated with bacteria during its handling and storage. Even when boiled cow's milk is fed, great care is needed to have all utensils sterilzed and to store the bottles of formula in a cold place. All these difficulties are done away with when the baby is nursed by the mother. The milk is given direct from producer to consumer, and the child may take as much as desired with no chance of the formula not being readily handled by its digestive tract.

Most mothers can nurse their babies adequately and the advantages certainly warrant serious effort to do so, at least for the first three to six months.

To ensure good milk flow, dietary practices should be sound throughout pregnancy, as well as after the birth of the child. Successful nursing demands a quiet, contented life, in which food is intelligently chosen and sunshine, exercise, fresh air, and mental diversion are provided. Anxiety and fatigue react unfavorably on milk production. Breast feeding should be a happy and rewarding experience for both mother and child.

QUESTIONS AND PROBLEMS

1. Discuss the special problems and energy needs of the different periods of pregnancy. Do the needs for protein, mineral elements, and vitamins differ in early and late pregnancy, and if so, how?

2. By what selection of food groups could the higher energy need of the later months of pregnancy be satisfied and at the same time a diet rich in good quality protein, mineral elements and vitamins be provided? What food groups should be prominent in the diet during pregnancy?

3. How much weight should be gained in a singleton pregnancy? With twins? What tissues are laid down in pregnancy? Is a reserve of body fat advantageous or disadvantageous? Why?

4. Compare the allowances for each of the nutritive factors in late pregnancy with those for a woman who is nursing a baby (see Table 19–1). In what respects do the requirements in lactation differ from those in pregnancy, and why? Why are more calories, protein, calcium, phosphorus, and vitamins needed than are passed on to the baby in the mother's milk? Why do so many women become overweight when nursing a child? What factors in the diet, if taken in plentiful amounts, favor milk secretion? What environmental factors tend to suppress milk secretion?

5. Plan a day's meals for a woman in the last two months of pregnancy. Calculate the energy and protein in this diet, and compare with the allowances given in Table 19–1 to see if the diet is adequate in these respects. Can you make any suggestions as to how it might be altered to provide more liberal intake of mineral elements and vitamins? Does the woman need some vitamin D supplement, and why?

6. Plan a day's diet for a nursing mother and calculate the amount of calcium and vitamin A supplied to see if they are adequate. For meeting the calcium allowance, why are calcium pills not an adequate dietary supplement to use in place of milk? If the diet needs to be improved in these respects, what changes would you suggest?

REFERENCES

1. Committee on Maternal Nutrition, Food and Nutrition Board: Maternal nutrition and the course of pregnancy. Washington, D.C., NAS/NRC, 1970.

2. Hampton, M. C., Huenemann, R. L., Shapiro, L. R., and Mitchell, B. W.: Caloric and nutrient intakes of teenagers. J. Amer. Dietet. Assoc., *50*:385, 1967.

3. AMA Council on Foods and Nutrition: Iron deficiency in the United States. J. Amer. Med. Assoc., *203*:119, 1968.

4. Avery, B., and Ledger, W. J.: Folic acid metabolism in well-nourished pregnant women. Obstet. Gynec., *35*:616, 1970.

5. Streiff, R. R.: Folate deficiency and oral contraceptives. J. Amer. Med. Assoc., *214*:40, 1970.

6. Davis, T. R. A., Gershoff, S. N., and Gamble, D. F.: Review of studies of vitamin and mineral nutrition in the United States (1950–1968). J. Nutr. Ed., *1*:41, 1969.

7. Ebbs, J. H., Tisdall, F. F., and Scott, W. A.: The influence of prenatal diet on the mother and child. J. Nutr., *22*:515, 1941.

8. Burke, B. S., Beal, V. A., Kirkwood, S. B., and Stuart, H. C.: The influence of nutrition during pregnancy upon the condition of the infant at birth. J. Nutr., *25*: 569, 1943.

9. Devadas, R. P., Shenbagavalli, P. N., and Vijayalaskshmi, R.: The impact of an applied nutrition programme on the nutritional status of selected expectant women. Ind. J. Nutr. Dietet., *7*:293, 1970.

10. Smith, C. A.: The effect of wartime starvation in Holland upon pregnancy and its product. Amer. J. Obstet. Gynecol., *53*:599, 1947.

11. Antonov, A. N.: Children born during the siege of Leningrad in 1942. J. Pediat., *30*: 250, 1947.

12. Wigglesworth, J. S.: Pathological and experimental studies of intrauterine malnutrition. Proc. Nutr. Soc. (Gt. Brit.), *28*:31, 1969.

13. Dieckman, W. J., et al.: Observation on protein intake and the health of mother and baby. I. Clinical and laboratory findings. II. Food intake. J. Amer. Dietet. Assoc., *27*:1046, 1951.

14. Burke, B. S., Harding, V. V., and Stuart, H. C.: Nutrition studies during pregnancy. IV. Relation of protein content of mother's diet during pregnancy to birth length, birth weight, and condition of infant at birth. J. Pediat., *23*:506, 1943.

15. Thomson, A. M.: Diet in pregnancy. III. Diet in relation to course and outcome of pregnancy. Brit. J. Nutr., *13*:509, 1959.

16. McGanity, W. J., et al.: The Vanderbilt co-

operative study of maternal and infant nutrition. VI. Relationship of obstetric performance to nutrition. Amer. J. Obstet. Gynecol., *67*:501, 1954.

17. Bagchi, K., and Bose, A. K.: Effect of low nutrient intake during pregnancy on obstetrical performance and offspring. Amer. J. Clin. Nutr., *11*:586, 1962.

18. Thiersch, J. B.: Ciba Foundation Symposium on Congenital Malformations. London, 1960, pp. 152–154.

19. Singer, J. E., Westphal, M., and Niswander, K.: Relationship of weight gain during pregnancy to birth weight and infant growth and development in the first year of life. Obstet. Gynecol., *31*:417, 1968.

20. Kirksey, A., and Pike, R. L.: Some effects of high and low sodium intakes during pregnancy in the rat. I. Food consumption, weight gain, reproductive performance, electrolyte balances, plasma total protein and protein fractions in normal pregnancy. J. Nutr., 77:33, 1962.

21. Palomaki, J. F., and Lindheimer, M. D.: Sodium depletion simulating deterioration in a toxemic pregnancy. New Eng. J. Med., *282*:88, 1970.

22. Robinson, M.: Salt in pregnancy. Lancet, *1*:178, 1958.

23. Thomson, A. M., Hytten, F. E., and Billewicz, W. Z.: The energy cost of human lactation. Brit. J. Nutr., *24*:565, 1970.

24. Gopalan, C., and Belavady, B.: Nutrition and lactation. Fed. Proc., *20*:177, 1961.

25. Pincus, G.: *Control of Fertility.* New York, Academic Press, 1965.

26. Karim, M., et al.: Injected progestogen and lactation. Brit. Med. J., *1*:200, 1971.

SUPPLEMENTARY READING

Aitken, F. C., and Hytten, F. E.: Infant feeding: Comparison of breast and artificial feeding. Nutr. Abstr. Rev., *104*:341, 1960.

Bailey, P.: Vitamin K deficiency in early pregnancy. Brit. Med. J., *2*:1199, 1964.

Baumslag, N., Edelstein, T., and Metz, J.: Reduction of incidence of prematurity by folic acid supplementation in pregnancy. Brit. Med. J., *1*:16, 1970.

Beal, V. A.: Nutritional studies during pregnancy. J. Amer. Dietet. Assoc., *58*:312, 1971.

Bonnar, J., Goldberg, A., and Smith, J. A.: Do pregnant women take their iron? Lancet, *1*:457, 1969.

Brenner, W. E., and Hendricks, C. H.: Interdependence of blood pressure, weight gain, and fetal weight during normal human pregnancy. Health Services Rep., *87*:236, 1972.

Brin, M.: Abnormal tryptophan metabolism in pregnancy and with the oral contraceptive pill. II. Relative levels of vitamin B_6-vitamers in cord and maternal blood. Amer. J. Clin. Nutr., *24*:704, 1971.

Bruhn, C. M., and Pangborn, R. M.: Reported incidence of pica among migrant families. J. Amer. Dietet. Assoc., *58*:417, 1971.

Cantile, G. S. D., DeLeeuw, N. K. M., and Lowenstein, L.: Iron and folate nutrition in a group of private obstetrical patients. Amer. J. Clin. Nutr., *24*:637, 1971.

Cellier, K. M., and Hankin, M. E.: Studies of nutrition in pregnancy. Amer. J. Clin. Nutr., *13*:55, 1963.

Chanarin, I., and Rothman, D.: Further observations on the relation between iron and folate status in pregnancy. Brit. Med. J., 2:81, 1971.

Chopra, J. C., Camacho, R., Kevany, J., and Thompson, A. M.: Maternal nutrition and family planning. Amer. J. Clin. Nutr., *23*:1043, 1970.

Cooper, B. A., Cantile, G. S. D., and Brunton, L.: The case for folic acid supplements during pregnancy. Amer. J. Clin. Nutr., *23*:848, 1970.

Davies, P. A.: Feeding the newborn baby. Proc. Nutr. Soc. (Gt. Brit.), *28*:66, 1969.

Giroud, A.: *The Nutrition of the Embryo.* Springfield, Illinois, Charles C Thomas, 1970.

Gold, E. M.: Interconceptional nutrition. J. Amer. Dietet. Assoc., *55*:27, 1969.

György, P.: Orientation in infant feeding. Fed. Proc., *20*:169, 1961.

Hansen, A. E., et al.: Influence of diet on blood serum lipids in pregnant women and newborn infants. Amer. J. Clin. Nutr., *15*:11, 1964.

Hillman, R. W., et al.: Pyridoxine supplementation during pregnancy. Amer. J. Clin. Nutr., *12*:427, 1963.

Hytten, F. E., and Leitch, I.: *The Physiology of Human Pregnancy.* Oxford, Blackwell Publications, 1964.

Iyengar, L., and Apte, S. V.: Prophylaxis of anemia in pregnancy. Amer. J. Clin. Nutr., *23*:725, 1970.

Jeans, P. C.: Incidence of prematurity in relation to maternal nutrition. J. Amer. Dietet. Assoc., *31*:576, 1955.

Jelliffe, D. B., and Bennett, F. J.: Cultural and anthropological factors in infant and maternal nutrition. Fed. Proc., *20*:185, 1961.

Jelliffe, D. B., and Jelliffe, E. F. P., eds.: Symposium: The uniqueness of human milk. Amer. J. Clin. Nutr., *24*:968, 1971.

Lowenstein, L., et al.: Vitamin B_{12} in pregnancy and the puerperium. Amer. J. Clin. Nutr., *8*:265, 1960.

Macy, I. G.: *Physiological Adaptation and Nutritional Status During and After Pregnancy.* Detroit, Children's Fund of Michigan, 1954.

Metz, J.: Folate deficiency conditioned by lactation. Amer. J. Clin. Nutr., 23:843, 1970.

Moyer, E. C., et al.: *Nutritional Status of Mothers and Their Infants.* Detroit, Children's Fund of Michigan, 1954.

Oldham, H., and Sheft, B.: Effect of caloric intake on nitrogen utilization during pregnancy. J. Amer. Dietet. Assoc., 27:847, 1951.

Pike, R. L.: Sodium intake during pregnancy. J. Amer. Dietet. Assoc., 44:176, 1964.

Pike, R. L., and Gursky, D. S.: Further evidence of deleterious effects produced by sodium restriction during pregnancy. Amer. J. Clin. Nutr., 23:883, 1970.

Rose, D. P., and Braidman, I. P.: Excretion of tryptophan metabolites as affected by pregnancy, contraceptive steroids, and steroid hormones. Amer. J. Clin. Nutr., 24:673, 1971.

Seifrit, E.: Changes in beliefs and food practices in pregnancy. J. Amer. Dietet. Assoc., 39:455, 1961.

Southgate, D. A. T., and Barrett, I. M.: The intake and excretion of calorific constituents of milk by babies. Brit. J. Nutr., 20:363, 1966.

Thomson, A. M., and Billewitz, W. A.: Nutritional status. Maternal physique and reproductive efficiency. Proc. Nutr. Soc. (Gt. Brit.), 22:55, 1963.

Tracy, T., and Miller, G. L.: Obstetric problems of the massively obese. Obstet. Gynecol., 33:204, 1969.

Underwood, B. A., Hepner, R., and Abdullah, H.: Protein, lipid and fatty acids of human milk from Pakistani women during prolonged periods of lactation. Amer. J. Clin. Nutr., 23:400, 1970.

Widdowson, E. M.: How the foetus is fed. Proc. Nutr. Soc. (Gt. Brit.), 28:17, 1969.

Willoughby, M. L. N., and Jewell, F. G.: Folate status through pregnancy and in postpartum period. Brit. Med. J., 4:356, 1968.

World Health Organization: Nutrition in pregnancy and lactation. Geneva, WHO Tech. Rep. Ser. No. 302, 1965.

Nutrition Reviews

The effect of linoleic acid on reproduction in the hen. 24:122, 1966.

Pregnancy and pantothenic acid deficiency in the guinea pig. 24:169, 1966.

Zinc deficiency and congenital malformations in the rat. 25:157, 1967.

Folic acid and pregnancy I. 25:325, 1967.

Prenatal exposure to fluoride. 25:330, 1967.

Folic acid and pregnancy II. 26:5, 1968.

Present knowlege of nutrition in inborn errors of metabolism (by Craig, J. W.). 26:161, 1968.

Zinc and reproduction. 27:16, 1969.

Diet and mammary gland growth in the pregnant rat. 27:152, 1969.

Galactose toxicity and cellular growth of fetal brain. 28:55, 1970.

Plasma amino acids in maternal undernutrition. 28:91, 1970.

The efficiency of human milk production. 28:262, 1970.

Longitudinal studies of diet in pregnancy. 30:38, 1972.

To breast feed or not? 30:112, 1972.

twenty

Nutrition in Infancy and the Preschool Years

It is essential that infants and preschool children have good nutrition to insure that they grow and develop normally. Body tissues, including the cells of the brain, must have certain minimal levels of each nutrient so that the child's birthright—his full physical and intellectual potential—is reached. Indeed, this need begins at the moment of conception, continues throughout pregnancy (see Chap. 19), and is no less important after the baby is born.

From the time the brain is first formed, there is a crucial relationship between nutrition, brain growth, and final brain size, and there may also be a correlation between brain size and an individual's learning potential.[1]

Since nutritional needs begin before birth, it is evident that good feeding of the young child in itself will not necessarily guarantee totally optimal development. There are certain conditions in which the infant may have already received a poor start before birth with regard to nutrition (for example, because of a poorly functioning placenta or a severely malnourished mother). Yet evidence does exist that there can be a "catch-up" period in the first six to nine months of life, when nutritional deficiencies which occurred before birth may indeed be partially or, possibly, wholly corrected without permanent mental or physical damage to the child.

This chapter will center on the nutritional needs of a normal full term infant, from birth through the preschool years. In general, the discussion will also hold for premature and "small-for-gestational age" (tiny, but not premature) babies. However, in the first few weeks of life there are special considerations regarding the premature child's individual nutritional and physiologic needs, which will be mentioned briefly.

Ask a pediatrician about the most frequently voiced concerns by mothers of young infants, and he will probably tell you that infant feeding is one of them. Often he will find that parents lack the "basics" of this important subject; thus any reader contemplating being a parent at any time in the future may find this subject of personal and practical interest. In addition, with the current growth of day care centers, particularly for younger children, anyone — teachers, nurses, health workers — concerned with day-to-day care of children outside the home will need to be competent in the area of proper nutrition for the young growing child.

FEEDING OF THE INFANT, GENERAL CONSIDERATIONS

Growth

The healthy human infant needs food in order to (1) maintain minimal function (basal metabolism) of his body tissues; (2) generate activity, such as muscular movement in work and play; and (3) create new body cells and tissues, that is, to grow. Indeed, the normal infant's rate of growth in the first year is truly remarkable (see Fig. 20–1). He doubles in weight by age four to six months (while growing about 4 inches in length), and triples his birth weight by the age of one year (while increasing in length by about one-third). If this rate of weight gain continued, he would weigh about two and a half tons by his fifth birthday! On the average, he will gain about 6 ounces a week during the first year.

With this rapid rate of growth, it is easy to understand why the proper feeding of the young infant is critical to his present and future health and development.

The Newborn Infant

The healthy newborn infant is indeed a dependent creature, and of the few basic reflexes he is endowed with at birth, the natural sucking reflex for obtaining food is probably the most critical. Infants who are born prematurely may not have this sucking reflex developed fully and perfectly; they have been, in past years, "expected" to lose a certain amount of their already-low birth weight, partly because they were not immediately ready to feed successfully.

In recent years, fortunately, this "expected" weight loss of the premature has not been accepted as the norm, and pediatricians and nursery personnel have begun more energetic feeding practices in order to supply the important energy and nutritional needs of these high-risk babies. In fact, the premature and small babies' nutritional

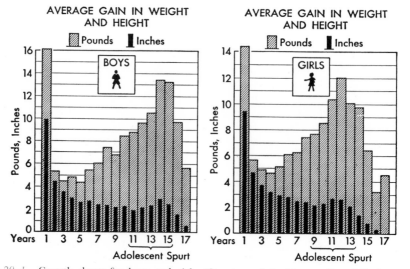

Figure 20–1. Growth charts for boys and girls. (Courtesy of the Metropolitan Life Insurance Co.)

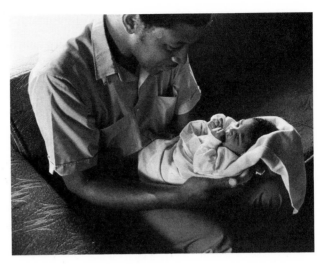

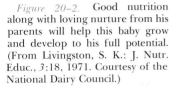

Figure 20–2. Good nutrition along with loving nurture from his parents will help this baby grow and develop to his full potential. (From Livingston, S. K.: J. Nutr. Educ., *3*:18, 1971. Courtesy of the National Dairy Council.)

needs are actually higher and more critical than the needs of the full term baby. For example, rather than waiting until the sucking reflex develops on its own, much-needed nutrients are now often given intravenously in the hospital nursery during the underweight infant's first hours of life. Thus, when given the calories and nutrients essential for their growth, the babies begin to grow and thrive at an earlier age than considered "normal" previously.[2]

Milk, the Infant's Primary Food

Breast and Bottle Feeding. Breast milk has been the most readily available and natural food for infants from the beginning of mankind; however, feeding bottles for infants have been found in archeological excavations of the Nile Basin.[3] This may be considered an indication of the agelessness of the controversy of "breast vs. bottle" in infant feeding. Historically, however, artificial feeding of infants (that is, with milk or concocted formula other than breast milk) has been fraught with appallingly poor results. It has been estimated that artificially fed babies in the period of the Industrial Revolution,

before any of the important bacteriological studies of Pasteur and Koch, had a mortality rate at least three times as high as breast-fed babies. At that time, the death rate already included two out of every three children before the age of five. The common practice of "wet-nursing" (breast feeding by a woman who was not the infant's mother and who very likely may have been nursing more than one child at a time) could not have been much more successful. Unfortunately, even today, in the less developed regions of the world, the increasing trend to the "higher status" practice of bottle feeding results in an increased infant sickness and death rate, because of (1) the lack of adequate sanitary preparation of bottles and milk substitutes and (2) the frequent inadequacy of nutritional content of these milk substitutes.

Presently in the United States, from 70 to 80 percent of all infants leaving hospital nurseries are bottle-fed.[4] Over the past 10 years, commercially prepared formulas have become more popular than evaporated milk formulas, as seen in Figure 20–3. This difference is due mainly to the ease and convenience of commercial formulas, since the standard evaporated milk formulas are more economical when properly

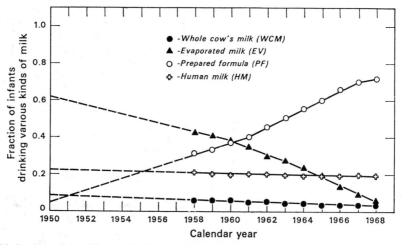

Figure 20–3. Use of the different kinds of milk from 1950 to 1968. Over the past two decades, the use of evaporated milk in infant feeding has declined while the use of prepared infant formulas has risen significantly. The incidence of breast feeding has remained stable at about 20 percent overall (although in selected populations, for example, students and university hospital clientele, the incidence of breast feeding at discharge from hospital may be as high as 70 to 80 percent). (From *Health Physics*, Vol. 19. Pergamon Press, 1970, p. 212.)

prepared under hygienic conditions and given with supplements.

Relative Merits, Breast vs. Bottle. Human milk is specifically adapted to the needs of human infants. The most common commercial formulas therefore are modified from cow's milk to approximate the known chemical composition of human breast milk (see Table 20–1). Thus each mother, according to her own personal feelings and preferences, can decide whether or not to breast feed with the full knowledge that either way the baby will receive an extremely nutritionally sound substance, a welcome advance over the questionable alternatives in past years. In fact, feeding by breast or by a properly prepared infant formula will in either case be a very satisfactory way to meet the baby's complete nutritional needs until the age of four to six months.

One advantage of breast feeding which has not been duplicated in any formula is the protective effect of human milk against infections, specifically, certain infantile diarrheas.[5] Babies fed

breast milk are also less likely to develop constipation and certain common infant allergies. A baby receiving bottle feedings who is held in a gentle and loving manner will be just as secure and happy as the breast-fed infant. Breast feeding, however, does make possible an exceptionally close and harmonious relationship that is pleasurable and satisfying to both infant and mother.

The total volume of milk required varies from infant to infant, with an average intake of about 3 ounces per pound (or, 175 to 200 ml per kg) of body weight in the first weeks of life (although a premature baby may need up to 4 to 5 ounces per pound), reduced to 1½ or 2 ounces per pound in the later months of infancy. Milk intake will vary with such factors as individual appetite, growth rate, body size, the amount of other liquids taken, and co-existent solid food intake. Most infants over a few weeks of age will consume in the general area of 1 quart of milk a day, with a standard deviation of intake of approximately 25 percent. An average of actual milk intakes per kilogram in a group of 95 healthy infants is presented in Figure 20–4.

The frequency of milk feeding begins at about seven to eight times a day and gradually decreases to five times a day at two months, by which time nearly all infants will be content to sleep throughout the night. There is no virtue in fixing rigid feeding times, nor in feeding completely haphazardly. If an infant (especially a breast-fed infant whose actual intake is not known) consistently demands food on less than a three-hour schedule, the possibility of a temporarily inadequate milk supply for that baby's needs should be con-

sidered. Healthy newborns will rapidly develop their own fairly regular feeding times.

Baby Foods; Starting on Solids

After the infant has been given only milk for a few weeks, many mothers begin to wonder about when to introduce solids. The general practice in the United States (as distinguished from certain underdeveloped areas of the world where, unfortunately, mother's milk may be all that is available for nourishment for the entire first year of life or even more) has been to intro-

Table 20–1. A Sample of the Variety of Milk Formulas

| | Human Milk | Cow's Milk, Fresh, Whole | Examples of: | | |
			MODIFIED INFANT FORMULA, BASED ON COW'S MILK*	SOY-BASED FORMULA	HYDROLYZED PROTEIN FORMULA
Calories/100 ml	67–72	67	67	67	67
Linoleic acid as percent of fatty acids	10.6	2.1	—	—	—
Gm/100 ml of:					
Protein	1.1–1.2	3.3	1.5	2.5	2.2
Carbohydrate	6.8–7.2	4.8	7.0	6.8	8.5
Fat	3.3–4.5	3.7	3.7	3.4	2.6
Water	87	87	87	87	87
Calcium: phosphorus ratio (mg/liter)	340:140	1250:960	550:430	800:630	1000:700
Vitamins/liter					
A, IU	1660–1898	1025–1425	1600	1500	1500
C, mg	51	11	50	50	50
D, IU	4–21	13–31†	400	400	400
B-1, mg	0.16–0.2	0.44	0.4	0.5	0.46
B-2, mg	0.36–0.4	1.75	0.6	1	1.8
B-6, mg	0.1	0.64	0.3	0.4	0.5
B-12, mcg	0.3	4	1.5	2	4.5
Pantothenic acid, mg	1.8	3.4	2	2.5	3.2
Niacin, mg	1.5	0.94	7	7	4
Folacin, mcg	25	27–100	50	170	50
K, mcg	15	60	35	80	18
E, IU	6.6	1.0	5	5	5
Iron, mg	0.3	—	1.4 (with iron— 8–12 mg)	8–10	12

*Adapted from Fomon[9] and manufacturers' data.
†400 IU when fortified.

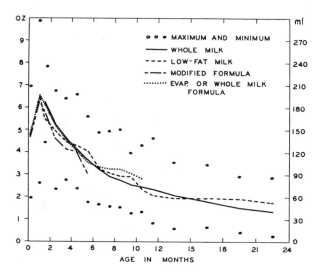

Figure 20-4. Volume intake per day of various types of formula or milk in the first two years of life per kilogram body weight (data from 95 infants in a longitudinal study). (From Beal, V. A.: J. Amer. Dietet. Assoc., 55:31, 1969.)

duce solid foods, that is, strained baby foods, at early ages. Approximately 90 percent of all infants will start solids at three months of age or less. Cereals and fruits are often introduced by one to two months of age, with yellow and green vegetables beginning in the second or third month, and meats in the fourth to fifth month. Many mothers, however, independently begin these foods earlier than the above commonly advised (although by no means absolutely standard) schedule. Although there is this tendency to feed solids, including meats, early, actually it is not until the baby reaches five or six months of age that nutritional need increases to a point not entirely met by milk alone. There is no evidence that early (that is, before one to two months) introduction of a reasonable amount of solid food is detrimental to the very adaptable human infant. However, the infant who is given solids early will simply cut down on his milk intake, thus resulting in no real increase of total food intake.

Recently there has been an effort to label containers of commercial baby foods more completely than has been done in the past so that the buyer can have full knowledge of what substances are included in the packaged or canned

foods which the infant will be eating. There have been questions regarding added ingredients in these foods, for example, concerning the use of monosodium glutamate, the sodium salt of glutamic acid, the addition of which was not necessary to any final food product itself but did serve to make the food taste better to mothers, at least. Wisely, the use of this substance has now been discontinued in most infant foods, because there has been a question raised regarding its safety.

The Diet of the Toddler and the Preschool Child

The infant is fed strained baby foods until the first teeth arrive at about five to ten months of age; then "junior foods," characterized by their soft chewable consistency, are begun. An alternative method is to skip the junior food stage entirely and begin puréed and semi-solid table foods when the infant's teeth appear. This is why a blender is a useful and practical addition to a household with a growing infant, for most fresh vegetables and fruits, as well as meats, may be prepared to the consistency enjoyed by the infant. For some families, this may be the preferred method of preparing all the baby's meals from early infancy on.

At around eight months to a year, the infant may be beginning to use a cup rather than the bottle or breast. By this time he should be taking, in addition to milk, a varied diet of cereal, green and yellow vegetables, meats, fruit juices, and fruit and custard desserts. He will also be chewing on bread and toast products.

During the second year of life the child should complete the transition to the cup. He should be drinking no less than three cups of milk a day and, again, eating a balanced diet with products from all four food groups (see Chap. 17). The mother will often complain about her child "losing appetite" during this year; but when the normal decline in the child's *rate* of growth after the first 12 months is understood, it will be clear that such decreased appetites indeed have a physiologic basis. In fact, this has been termed the "physiologic anorexia" (anorexia means loss of appetite) of the one-year-old, and mothers should be reassured that this is normal. Of course, the child should continue to be offered a balanced diet suitable for his age, with an emphasis on easily self-fed foods ("finger foods"), because this is a time that the child likes and requires a sense of independence, of doing things for himself. Some examples of protein-rich "finger foods" are peanut butter on crackers or bread strips, cheese squares, and hard-boiled eggs. These may also be offered as midmorning or midafternoon snacks, for the toddler and preschooler will often adapt more easily to smaller amounts of food offered five or six times a day than to a strict regimen of three large meals each day. A useful "rule of thumb" regarding minimal serving sizes for preschoolers is "one bite, or teaspoonful, for each year of age" of each separate food served. A common complaint about the child of this age is that "he won't eat vegetables." In this case, again one can attempt to encourage vegetables such as green beans and boiled carrots which can be easily picked up by the child. If all planning is to no avail, this may be the proper time for judicious use of supplemental vitamins so that parents do not find themselves forcing the food down the unwilling toddler.

In the preschool years the child continues to strive to assert his new feelings of self and independence, again resulting in possible "power struggles" at meal times. Firmness, consistency, and creativity on the part of the parents should continue to insure that the child receive the nutritional intake required for his activity and growth needs. For menu ideas and recommended servings, see Tables 20–2 and 20–3.

NUTRITIONAL REQUIREMENTS OF INFANTS AND PRESCHOOL CHILDREN

The last section introduced common problems and practices in infant and preschool feeding. The following section will focus on requirements and recommended daily intakes for specific nutrients needed in infants' and small children's diets, as well as practical guidelines which may help to insure that these requirements are met.

With regard to infants and children, needs for most types of nutrients are proportionately (per unit of size) higher than the needs of an adult. This applies to everything from the need for water (because of the child's relatively large surface area, and the thus proportionately larger evaporative water loss, as well as the relatively higher body water content of the child) to the need for protein, vitamins, and minerals. The relative requirement for energy is also greater in the child. For example, the newborn requires about 100 to 120 kcal per kg of body weight, while the average young adult needs 35 to 40 kcal per kg. See Table 20–4 for a sum-

Table 20 -2.   Foods Recommended for Children's Daily Diets,
Average Amounts for Different Age Groups*

Food	Preschool 2–5 yrs	Grade School 6–12 yrs.
Milk (or equivalent)	1–1½ pt (2–3 c.)	1–1½ pt (2–3 c.)
Meat, poultry, fish	2 oz (¼ c.)	2–4 oz
Second protein dish: sm. svg. meat, legumes, or nuts	3–4 tbsp	4–6 tbsp
Egg	1 whole egg	1 whole egg
Potatoes (or equiv. amt. rice, macaroni, spaghetti)	1 small or (3–4 tbsp)	1 med. to lg. or (4–5 tbsp)
Other cooked vegetables (green leafy† or deep yellow frequently)	3–4 tbsp at one or more meals	4–5 tbsp at one or more meals
Raw vegetables (carrots, lettuce, celery, etc.)	2 or more small pieces	¼ to ⅓ c.
Vitamin C food (citrus fruits, tomatoes, etc.)	1 med. orange or equiv.	1 med. orange or equiv.
Other fruits	⅓ c. at one or more meals	½ c. or more at one or more meals
Cereal, whole-grain, restored	½ c. or more	¾ c. or more
Bread, whole-grain	2 or more slices	2 or more slices
Butter or fortified margarine	1 tbsp	1 tbsp or more
Sweets	⅓ c. simple dessert at 1 or 2 meals	½ c. simple dessert at 1 or 2 meals
Vitamin D source	Enough to provide 400 U.S.P. units daily	

*Adapted from Krause, M. V.: *Food Nutrition and Diet Therapy.* 4th Ed. Philadelphia, W. B. Saunders Co., 1966.

†Green leafy vegetables are important every day because of their folic acid content; see text.

mary of the recommended dietary allowances for infants and children.

Protein

Protein allowances in this age group are in the range of 2 to 4 gm per kg per day. Breast milk gives approximately 2 gm per kg per day, and countless infants have thrived on this level of protein intake for the first five to six months. In many instances, however, the "requirement" has been published higher than this figure—for example, 3.5 to 4 gm per kg per day—causing some confusion. There has been evidence that premature babies, at least, will thrive on a formula allowing from 4 to 6 gm per kg per day of protein. Most popular commercial formulas have followed the general composition

of breast milk with a relatively lower protein (compared with cow's milk) content (see Table 20–1).

Carbohydrates

The usable carbohydrates in children's diets, as in adults', are sugars and starches (see Chap. 3). Also, as with adults, diets compatible with good health in children can contain varying quantities of carbohydrates, so there is not a definite allowance set. However, carbohydrates do make an essential contribution to meeting energy requirements of infants and children and in this way are extremely important. If insufficient carbohydrate is ingested to meet daily energy needs, the body must break down a certain portion of dietary and body protein to meet these needs.

Table 20–3. Practical Menu Suggestions for Children at Various Ages

1–2 Years	3–6 Years	7–12 Years
Breakfast	*Breakfast*	*Breakfast*
Orange juice	Orange juice	Banana
Oatmeal with milk	Bran flakes with milk	Farina with milk
Whole wheat toast	Whole wheat toast	Omelette – plain
Milk to drink	Milk to drink	Toast
		Milk to drink
Midmorning	*Midmorning*	
Juice	Raisins	
Lunch	*Lunch*	*Lunch*
Egg, soft poached	Egg salad sandwich with	Vegetable soup with rice
Mashed potato	lettuce	Peanut butter and jelly
Peas	Milk to drink	sandwich
Zwieback	Plain, crisp cookies (1–2)	Milk
Milk to drink	Custard pudding	Fresh peaches
Rice pudding		
Midafternoon	*Midafternoon*	*Midafternoon*
Milk	Juice	1–2 molasses cookies
Crackers with soft cheese	Apple and cheese wedges	Fruit juice or milk
spread		
Dinner	*Dinner*	*Dinner*
Fish sticks	Hamburger with tomato	Broiled chicken
Spinach or carrots	and lettuce	Baked potato
Bread and butter	Squash	Carrots and peas
Applesauce	Toast and butter	Shredded raw cabbage
Milk	Milk	salad
	Stewed prunes	Bread and butter
	Carrots and celery	Milk
		Apple tapioca pudding
		with thin custard sauce

A meal plan for a child for a day should be based on a knowledge of the "Basic 4" (Chap. 17). For example: *Breakfast:* milk group, 1; fruit-vegetable group, 1; bread-cereal group, 2. *Lunch:* meat-protein group, 1; bread-cereal group, 1; milk group, 1; vegetable-fruit group, 1. *Dinner:* meat-protein group, 1; milk group, 1; vegetable-fruit group, 2; bread-cereal group, 1. Additional servings may easily be added as midmorning or midafternoon snacks.

*Table 20–4. Recommended Daily Dietary Allowances for Infants and Children**

Age (Years)	Energy (kcal)	Protein (gm)	Vitamin A Activity (IU)	Vitamin D (IU)	Vitamin C (mg)	Folacin (mg)	Niacin (mg eq)	Riboflavin (mg)	Thiamin (mg)	Vitamin B-6 (mg)	Calcium (gm)	Iron (mg)
Infants												
0–1/6	kg × 120	kg × 2.2†	1500	400	35	0.05	5	0.4	0.2	0.2	0.4	6
1/6–1/2	kg × 110	kg × 2.0†	1500	400	35	0.05	7	0.5	0.4	0.3	0.5	10
1/2–1	kg × 100	kg × 1.8†	1500	400	35	0.1	8	0.6	0.5	0.4	0.6	15
Children												
1–2	1100	25	2000	400	40	0.1	8	0.6	0.6	0.5	0.7	15
2–3	1250	25	2000	400	40	0.2	8	0.7	0.6	0.6	0.8	15
3–4	1400	30	2500	400	40	0.2	9	0.8	0.7	0.7	0.8	10
4–6	1600	30	2500	400	40	0.2	11	0.9	0.8	0.9	0.8	10
6–8	2000	35	3500	400	40	0.2	13	1.1	1.0	1.0	0.9	10
8–10	2200	40	3500	400	40	0.3	15	1.2	1.1	1.2	1.0	10

*Not complete. For additional recommendations for vitamins E, B-12, phosphorus, iodine, and magnesium, see Table 1 of Appendix. (From Food and Nutrition Board: *Recommended Dietary Allowances.* 7th Ed. Washington, D.C., National Academy of Sciences, 1968.)
†Assumes protein equivalent to human milk. For proteins not 100 percent utilized, factors should be increased proportionately.

In the newborn, the most usual carbohydrates ingested are lactose, from milk, glucose, and sucrose. Nearly all infants (with a few exceptions; for example, those with a specific enzyme defect) can digest and absorb these sugars adequately, except if given in high concentrations, when diarrhea is likely to occur.

The infant is considered quite able to digest starches in the diet to glucose by the age of one month. The carbohydrate intake of the infant is important for both energy requirements and the maintenance of the plasma glucose level (important because of the need of brain cells to utilize glucose). The latter consideration is especially important in the case of the premature baby, because his liver glycogen stores at birth are incompletely formed and may be inadequate to maintain proper blood glucose levels for the first 24 to 48 hours of life unless glucose is given him.

During the first weeks of life, the caloric supply of certain milk formulas (specifically, evaporated milk and water formulas) may need to be supplemented with extra carbohydrate, commonly in the form of 2 to 4 gm (½ to 1 tsp) corn syrup per feeding, or possibly with early addition of cereal to the diet.

Fats

Fats contribute about half the energy requirement of the infant who is fed on milk alone. Infant formulas should provide at least 15 percent of the total calories as fat in order to meet the energy needs of infants within the relatively small quantity of food they can consume.

The essential fatty acid, linoleic acid, is important in promoting optimal health in infants. Without it, poor growth and a severe skin rash will result.[6] High quantities of linoleic acid are found in corn oil, cottonseed oil, soybean oil, and whole grain cereals, and one of these should be included in an infant's diet if he is being given primarily a skim milk formula. The minimal recommended level of linoleic acid is 3 percent of the total amount of calories. (Human milk contains 6 to 9 percent of calories as linoleic acid.)

Vitamins

Growing active children have a special need, relatively higher than adults, for a complete supply of the known vitamins. These vitamins can usually be supplied in a balanced, varied diet, but there are certain periods when supplements are advisable, especially in infancy when the baby's limited food intake sometimes makes an adult-type "balanced" diet impossible. Other possible periods when vitamin supplements may be indicated are (1) when the toddler is undergoing his stage of "physiologic anorexia," (2) in times of illness and other periods of possibly limited food intake, and (3) in specific disease entities requiring specific vitamins as part of the treatment.

Table 20–4 details the recommended daily allowances established for the vitamins. The *vitamin A* requirement is deduced from the fact that human milk apparently supplies an adequate amount of the vitamin for good health during the first year of life, and human milk contains 170 IU per 100 ml. (Thus, an infant ingesting 850 ml would ingest 1500 IU, which is then set as the RDA.)

In normal full term infants, intakes of as little as 100 IU a day of *vitamin D* have prevented rickets. With inadequate vitamin D intake, premature infants are more prone to develop rickets because of their rapid growth rate. Assuming good intakes of calcium and phosphate, 100 to 200 IU of vitamin D per day will prevent this occurrence of rickets. (Formulas supplemented with the usual amount of vitamin D cannot be depended on as the tiny infant's total supply of this vitamin, because of the small amount of total formula ingested per day.[7]) The recommended level of 400 IU is intended to prevent rachitic symptoms in all babies, small or of normal size. This is also the level recommended for growing children and adults. Sunlight (certain ultraviolet wavelengths) is an alternative way to meet the need for vitamin D, through conversion of 7-dehydrocholesterol in the skin to vitamin D_3. An infant wearing the normal amount of clothes would probably receive an antirachitic dose of sunlight in approximately a 30 to 60 minute exposure per day, but because this is not often feasible in infants, this vitamin is usually included as a supplement. Vitamin D in the mother's diet does not pass to breast milk to a significant extent (which is also the case with cow's milk, and is the reason that commercial cow's milk is supplemented with this vitamin), and thus breast-fed infants should receive supplemental vitamin D. This vitamin is now included as a routine supplement in all commercial infant formulas, including evaporated milk.

The adverse effects of excess quantities of the aforementioned two vitamins, especially vitamin D, cannot be overemphasized. An infant who repeatedly receives more than 1800 to 3000 IU of vitamin D per day is in danger of manifesting toxic signs of overuse which may lead to hypercalcemia and other complications. Thus the RDA of 400 IU should not be consistently or significantly exceeded. This is sometimes a difficult task, because of the multiplicity of vitamin D fortified foods. Vitamin A may also be toxic if an infant is given dosages as low as 18,500 IU per day for one to three months.

Human milk is rich in *vitamin E*, and will meet the infant's requirement, while cow's milk is relatively low (about one-half to one-tenth of the amount in breast milk). Supplementation with this vitamin has been particularly advised for premature infants because of negligible placental transfer of this vitamin. A syndrome of megaloblastic anemia, rash, and other lesser signs, which is correlated with low vitamin E levels, and which disappears with the administration of supplemental vitamin E, has been described in six- to eight-week-old premature babies.[8] Good natural sources of vitamin E include salad oils, shortening and margarine. A toxicity syndrome has not been described.

Because of low values of plasmaclotting factors, the newborn infant has a chance of abnormal bleeding in the first few days of life. Thus *vitamin K*, important in attaining the normal levels of prothrombin and other clotting factors, is usually given in injection form to newborns (0.5 mg of an aqueous preparation). Adding vitamin K supplements to expectant mothers' diets during the last month to help raise the newborn's level of vitamin K has also been recommended as a possible prenatal preventive measure.[9]

The recommended daily allowance of *vitamin C*, 35 mg, is found in 850 ml of breast milk of generally well-nourished mothers, an average daily milk intake for a three-month-old. The vitamin C content of cow's milk is about one-fifth this amount, and, in addition, treatment of cow's milk for infant use (for example, boiling, evaporation, drying, etc.) contributes to the destruction of this relatively unstable vitamin, destroying what little is present. Thus, most infant formulas must be and are fortified because of the importance of vitamin C in the infant's diet.

Often, pediatricians will recommend that the infant avoid citrus fruits and juices up to the age of a year or so in order to prevent the development of possible allergic reactions to these foods. In these cases supplemental vitamin C should be given in the form of vitamin drops when the infant is taken off prepared formulas or breast milk and started on regular milk.

The *B vitamins*—folacin, niacin, pantothenic acid, riboflavin, thiamin, vitamins B-6, B-12, biotin, and choline—are discussed in detail in Chapter 7.

All the B complex vitamins are present in milk (both cow's milk and breast milk from generally well-nourished mothers) in sufficient amounts to meet the recommended daily allowances for infants who are on a normal milk intake. A diet with B complex vitamins in excess of the requirements is not considered hazardous, because the unneeded amounts will be excreted in the urine (as is also the case with ascorbic acid).

Generally, B complex vitamin deficiency states in infants and children are rare in the United States. However, there are certain specific points to be made about vitamin B-12 and folic acid. *Vitamin B-12* is not found in any plant source, unlike the rest of the B complex vitamins. Therefore, a pregnant woman who is on a strict "macrobiotic" or vegetarian diet and who does not have a large intake of milk or eggs (which are, along with meat and fish, the only food sources of this vitamin) may give birth to an infant with a low vitamin B-12 level who is at high risk for developing a deficiency state which includes megaloblastic anemia. Thus, pregnant mothers on this type of diet should receive ample information and education as to the possible harm it will cause to the health of the unborn child.

Folacin is found both in meats and in green leafy vegetables as well as in most milk. However, it is present only in insignificant amounts in goat's milk, which is occasionally used as the primary milk in an allergy-prone infant or child (although commercially prepared, fortified, nonallergenic formulas are replacing it in most cases). Thus any infant on goat's milk as a primary food should receive folacin supplementation at the recommended level of 50 mcg per day to prevent the deficiency state characterized by megaloblastic anemia. One further word concerning premature infants: as with several other nutrients, their stores of folacin may be quite low, and they may need slightly higher levels of this vitamin than are found in cow's

milk and most infant formulas.* Also with regard to folacin, it has been shown that strained baby foods which have been commercially prepared contain significantly lower amounts of this vitamin than do the fresh vegetables.

Minerals

The infant's diet must include all the elements and the inorganic radicals essential for normal metabolism and growth. The major minerals needed by the infant occur in generous amounts in human milk, cow's milk and many other foods common in the infant's diet. (For a review of each mineral and its specific role, see Chaps. 11 and 12.) However, iron and fluorine are low in both human and cow's milk. Calcium and phosphorus are particularly important for skeletal growth, as well as for normal body physiology. The requirements for sodium, potassium, and chloride are particularly important to consider in the care and management of sick infants; this is a specialized topic and is not covered here.

Calcium and Phosphorus

Calcium makes up 1.5 to 2 percent of the adult's body weight, with 99 percent being present in bones and teeth; thus it is extremely important in the growth and development of these structures in children. During increased periods of growth, such as in infancy, the calcium absorption rate is higher than when the growth rate slows. Vitamin D, of course, is necessary for this absorption. The advisable intake for calcium is set at twice the calculated requirement of a breast-fed baby, because calcium absorption may be different in infants fed other than human milk.

Usually, the allowance for calcium

---

*A quantitative analysis of all vitamins found in the different types of infant formulas are found in Fomon.[9]

approximately equals the phosphate allowance, except in the young infant, in whom an overliberal phosphate intake may contribute to hypocalcemic tetany. (Human milk contains approximately twice as much calcium as phosphorus.) In older infants, the phosphate allowance may be increased to 80 percent of the calcium allowance, as is found in cow's milk.

A child who is not receiving his required intake of calcium and phosphorus (found primarily in milk and milk products) will still continue to grow, but the mineralization of bones and teeth will not be optimal (see also Chap. 11).

Iron

The importance of this mineral in the diet of infants and children has long been recognized. Recently, definite recommendations have been put forth to insure that youngsters will be protected from the anemia which results from lack of iron in the diet.

The usual age at which the anemia of iron deficiency begins to appear, if present, is six to 12 months. Up to six months of age, the term infant's iron stores, which were deposited in fetal life, are generally adequate for body needs (e.g., for the production of hemoglobin). After that age, body stores must be resupplied by diet to insure proper blood formation.

The usual hemoglobin level at birth is high, at 16 to 18 gm, and falls normally to a level of 10 to 11 gm at three to four months. The level of hemoglobin should be maintained at least at this level throughout the first year (and later), and additional dietary iron is now recommended during even the early months of infancy so that iron supplies will not be depleted at six months.

Regarding the recommended daily dose, it has been calculated that the infant can be expected to need a total of about 2000 mg of iron during the first year of life, and this results in a

daily need, according to Fomon,[9] of at least 6 mg a day (beginning at birth), or 8 mg a day (if supplements are begun at three months of age). This requirement can best be met in the very young infant by (1) an iron-supplemented formula, costing no more than regular formula, (2) iron drops, or (3) about four to six tablespoons of a packaged iron-fortified infant cereal. Iron requirements in infancy have also been calculated by weight, but the above method of calculating recommendations is probably more rational and easily understood. The recommended intakes by weight are 1 mg per kg per day for term infants and 2 mg per kg per day for low birth weight infants. During the preschool years, through age three, the allowance is 15 mg a day. For other more detailed remarks on iron requirements, functions, absorption, and metabolism, see Chapter 12.

Fluorine

This element is particularly important in early infancy and childhood because of its well-known effect in the prevention of dental caries. It may be given from early infancy on.

If there is fluoridation of the water supply at approximately 1 ppm, the baby whose powdered formula is made with that water will receive his recommended fluoride intake per day, and the infant receiving equal parts water and formula will also receive his recommended fluorine. However, if the infant is on "ready to serve" formula, or is breast fed,* fluoridated water is of no help and he will need other sources of fluoride, just as will the infant living in a community without fluoridation of water supplies. (The young infant will not take in sufficient quantities of supplemental water to give enough fluoride

---

*Breast milk contains less than 0.03 ppm of fluoride, regardless of the mother's fluoride intake. Cow's milk contains slightly more, but still not nearly enough to meet the infant's requirement.[10]

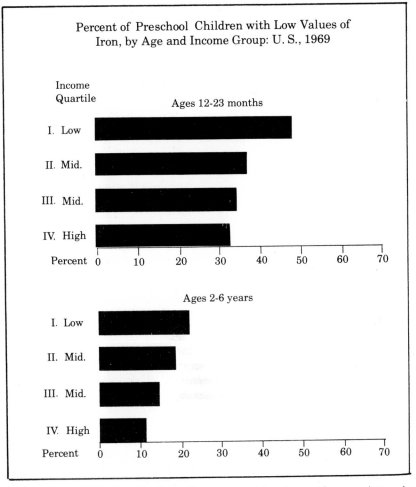

Figure 20–5. An example of the findings of poorer nutrition, here with serum iron values as an indicator, of preschool children in low income families when compared with children of the same age in families with higher incomes. (From *Profiles of Children: 1970 White House Conference on Children,* p. 66. Washington, D.C., U.S. Government Printing Office.)

to be of maximal protection.) Supplemental fluoride preparations are available only on prescription.

To review, then, the role of supplemental vitamins and minerals in infant feeding is summarized as follows:

Period Before Introduction
of Solid Foods

VITAMINS. 1. When an infant is on a popular commercially prepared in-

fant formula, he will generally receive the required dosages of all vitamins by taking a quart or nearly a quart of milk a day. (For a small infant then, or a baby who is a "slow starter" to milk feedings, supplemental vitamins are in order until a sufficient intake of milk is reached.)

2. When an infant is on an evaporated milk and water formula (only), he should receive a vitamin C supplementation daily.

3. The successfully nursing baby should receive vitamin D supplementa-

tion (400 IU) at least until that time when the mother and the doctor feel he is ready to "sun" for a period of one-half to one hour a day.

MINERALS. The iron requirement, 6 to 8 mg a day from the first to third month to the sixth month, may be met most easily by an iron-fortified formula, or by iron drops for the breast-fed baby.

*The Period After Introduction
of Solid Foods*

VITAMINS. If a balanced and varied diet (including cereals and bread products; citrus fruits and juices; green and yellow vegetables; and meat, eggs, and milk products) is taken well by the infant or child, supplements will not usually be necessary, and indeed an excess of vitamins A and D is known to be harmful. However, if the child (commonly the one- or two-year-old) refuses for days to eat foods from certain food groups (vegetables, for example!), a limited period of "educated" supplementation (for the vitamins present in that food group) is acceptable.

MINERALS. 1. The iron requirement may now be met by a balanced diet; however, in some cases supplementation of 6 to 8 mg until the end of the first year will be recommended by the pediatrician.

2. Fluoride supplementation (0.5 to 1 mg) should be added (with the approval of a physician) if the community water supply contains less than recommended amounts of fluorine, if the child is not receiving a liberal intake of the supplemented water, or if the infant is breast fed.

SPECIAL CONCERNS IN INFANT AND CHILDHOOD FEEDING

Food Allergies

Food allergies are often a subject of concern to parents attempting to give their children a complete and balanced diet. There are different types of food allergies.

MILK ALLERGY. This has also been termed milk sensitivity, or milk intolerance. This last phrase should probably be specifically reserved for the intolerance to milk that results from the very rare congenital absence or decreased supply of lactase, the enzyme which digests the milk sugar lactose. It is not a true allergy (see Chap. 13).

Estimates of the incidence of true cow's milk allergy in a total population range from 0.1 to 3 percent. It tends to run in families, and an infant who has an allergy to milk may also be allergic to other common food allergens, such as citrus fruits or egg whites.

Cow's milk allergy in susceptible infants is commonly manifested by frequent loose stools, frequent respiratory infections, and/or allergic skin reactions, usually eczema. More serious problems, such as shock (cardiovascular collapse), may rarely occur. The symptoms may occur as early as two to four weeks of age, or later during the preschool years. Symptoms will begin in a susceptible breast-fed child soon after the first cow's milk feedings are given.

Thus, it may sometimes be necessary, for a certain child with specific symptoms, to eliminate cow's milk and milk products from the diet. In these cases, there are excellent cow's milk substitutes that have been developed which provide essentially all nutrients normally found in milk. They also have usually added vitamin and mineral supplementation. It has been shown that infants' growth curves, when given these milk substitutes, are no different from the curves of infants given breast milk. However, in the older child, the milk substitutes may be refused, and in these cases care must be taken that these children do, in fact, receive a proper diet. For example, supplemental calcium may be warranted in these cases. One further optimistic note about true milk allergy is that most children affected in infancy may be able to tolerate cows milk by the age of two to three years.

OTHER FOOD ALLERGIES.   Mothers of small infants are usually advised by their pediatricians to avoid, at least in the first few months, certain foods which are thought to be commonly allergenic at early ages. The classic examples of these foods would include wheat, citrus fruits, egg whites, nuts, and chocolate. (A child whose parent[s] had a true milk allergy would also often be advised to use a cow's milk substitute from birth.)

Allergies caused by foods are not as common as inhalant (pollen, etc.) allergies; however, they do occur more frequently in infants and young children than in adults, and this is why a preventive approach to the common food allergies is usually taken. Often a child will have an allergy to more than one food. The young child has a greater tendency to absorb unaltered protein and thus to have a greater potential for setting up antigen-antibody reactions which comprise the allergic response.

There are two types of allergic reactions to foods. One is immediate, with the rapid occurrence of symptoms, and often may appear after the ingestion of fish, other seafood, berries and nuts. The other type is a delayed response which may occur hours or days after the allergenic food (commonly wheat, milk, eggs, oranges, or chocolate) is eaten.

A child who is suspected of having a food allergy should be on a trial period of elimination of the food for about six weeks to see if symptoms will clear. Again, a child with a known food allergy will require special menu planning to allow for a balanced, palatable, and enjoyable diet.

Failure to Thrive

This is a general term used by pediatricians and others to describe any infant who fails to attain his minimal expected gains in growth and development. It is a problem that requires expert diagnostic study and therapeutic steps. The most common cause is some form of failure to receive adequate nurture and nutrition to meet bodily needs, a process which may even start, as mentioned previously, before birth.

The failure may be at the level of food intake or there may be a problem in digestion, assimilation, metabolism, or utilization of food.

Certain specific examples of known illnesses in which an infant may fail to thrive are the celiac syndrome (intestinal mucosal hypersensitivity to wheat protein), cystic fibrosis (a complex disease which includes a malabsorption state), galactosemia, and disaccharide deficiency. There are innumerable other etiologies, but the common cause of inadequate food should not be overlooked. Proper nutritional therapy and rehabilitation in these particular cases is of prime importance.

Overnutrition in Infancy

The "chubby" baby—is he headed for an unhappy teenage and adult bout with obesity? Evidence is beginning to accumulate that the overweight baby does indeed have a higher chance for obesity in later life.

In the average six-month-old infant, 50 percent of the body weight is normally fat. In the first six months of life, the normal baby will gain 38 percent of his total weight gain from fat, while from six to 12 months, 11 percent of the gain will be from fat. However, an increase over this "normal" amount is thought to lead to the formation of a permanently increased number of fat cells in the body. Later, decreasing the amount of calories taken in will decrease the amount of fat contained in the cells but cannot "subtract" from the actual number of cells present. This may have implications for later ease or difficulty of weight loss.

It has also been shown that babies who gain weight rapidly in infancy obtain a greater height and weight at the age of six to eight years. Also, there is an increased chance of obesity in later childhood if there was an excessive weight gain in infancy.[11]

Overweight babies are usually found to be less active and energetic than their slimmer companions. Thus, overfeeding of food such as milk and/or solids may not be the only culprit causing later obesity; there may also be an inherent predisposition in certain infants, for reasons not fully understood.

Pica and Lead Poisoning

"Pica" is a term used to designate the tendency of certain people to eat substances (paper, plaster, paint, laundry starch, dirt) which usually are considered inedible. There are two types of pica: (1) "malignant, cachectic" pica, a rare form which is associated with a grossly inadequate diet; and (2) "benign" pica, the more common form, which has never been satisfactorily proved to be associated with malnutrition. This is practiced by the child who eats, for example, the peeling paint of windowsills, or the pregnant woman who eats clay or laundry starch. However, in the case of children, this latter form should not be termed "benign," because there can be at least one specific serious complication associated with it. If the substances ingested (paint, plaster, etc.) contain _lead_, lead poisoning may result. Thus it is often not a totally "benign" habit.

Infant Feeding in Special Conditions

As important as proper feeding is to children who are well, it becomes critically important in times of special needs such as illness, as well as during rapid growth periods.

The importance of prenatal nutrition has already been discussed. The topic of the feeding of premature infants has also been mentioned, and this entire area of the care of premature, low birth weight, and sick newborns is truly a subspecialty of its own.

Disease treatments which call for specialized nutritional knowledge include those for illnesses in which the body lacks certain enzymes required for proper digestion and metabolism of ingested foods. Foods must be carefully selected in these cases to avoid the illness symptoms which arise often only when the unacceptable food is eaten. Examples of disease states in children for which special nutritional expertise is needed include phenylketonuria (PKU), galactosemia, hyperlipidemia, food allergies (see p. 472), lactose intolerance, disaccharidase deficiencies and chronic diarrheas. Individuals with these conditions should be under supervision of their physicians whenever possible.

Vegetarian Diets for Children

Can a child be fed successfully on a vegetarian diet? The answer is a qualified yes. It is true that a diet excluding meat protein will allow for adequate growth and development of a child, _provided_ it is based on sound nutritional knowledge. There are different "levels" of vegetarian diets used by their advocates—ranging from diets that allow eggs and milk as well as fruits, cereal products, varied vegetables, legumes and nuts, to diets that include primarily cereals and water. The first type mentioned (the lacto-ovo-vegetarian type) would be expected to provide for complete nutritional needs _if_ the following criteria are met: (1) the protein sources must be varied (that is, come from different legumes, grains, and vegetables) in order to supply the essential amino acids, _all_ of which are not found in any _one_ vegetarian food; (2) there is an adequate supply of folacin and vitamin C (sometimes low in these diets); (3) there is a form of iodized salt used;

and (4) the diet does in fact include plentiful allowances of milk, cheese, and eggs. The latter foods are important because they would be the sole source of vitamin B-12 in this meatless diet, and they also help supply important amino acids, minerals such as calcium and iron, and other vitamins such as vitamin A. Vegetarian diets other than this varied lacto-ovo-vegetarian type would not generally be satisfactory for children. It should be obvious by now that to try to raise infants and children without some form of milk or its complete equivalent is very difficult and nutritionally unwise.

Infant and Child Nutrition in Developing Countries

The discussion has focused so far on the nutritional needs and practices of children of the United States and countries of a similar economic level. Countries, however, with a serious discrepancy between population (too many people) and food (too little) have problems of infant feeding not even touched upon here. Their infant and childhood mortality rates are very high—to a large part, as a result of the combined effects of malnutrition, infection, poor economic conditions, and lack of good information about nutrition and health.

Special areas of concern are (1) the infant who remains breast-fed without other adequate food intake up to two or three years of age, and (2) often even worse, the toddler who is suddenly weaned from the breast at the arrival of a new baby who demands all the mother's breast milk. This toddler is then deprived of even this minimal supply of his only high nutrient food, other portions of his typical weaning diet

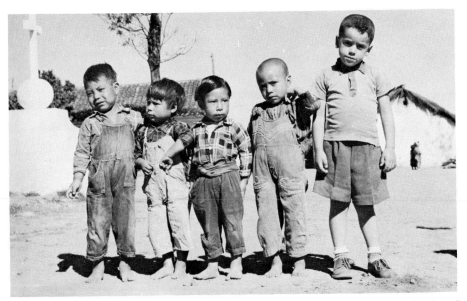

Figure 20–6. Marked difference in growth and general nutritive condition of Guatemalan boys four to five years of age, contrasting village children reared on the native diet (corn and beans as chief food staples) with a boy of same age group from a professional man's family, in which the diet was superior. The latter boy (at right) is of normal height and weight for this age group; the others show stunted growth and other evidences of poor nutrition. Supplementing the poor diets to meet nutritive needs results in better growth and condition, but tissue damages caused by early deprivation may persist into later life. (Courtesy of Dr. Miguel A. Guzman, Institute of Nutrition for Central American and Panama.)

being mainly carbohydrate. Custom usually demands that the few high nutrient foods will go first (and often, only) to the adult males of the tribe and family. In some areas, there are also cultural food taboos which effectively deny certain protein-rich foods, such as eggs, to pregnant women and young children.

The increasing practice of bottle feeding (often with the misguided attempt to gain "status" in the eyes of neighbors), even in the most underdeveloped areas, is also a subject of concern. The advantages of breast feeding in these areas are *very* high, since the facilities for safe, sterile preparation and storage of bottle feedings are limited. (In fact, the infant is lucky if he actually receives *milk* in the bottle — in one location, rice water was given because it "looked like" the European pictures of bottled milk formulas!)

Thus, it is clear that childhood nutrition is a very real and high-priority concern in many parts of the world. Childhood undernutrition is not, unfortunately, completely unknown even in the generally more advantaged United States. This is particularly true in economically deprived areas.

Unanswered Questions

Areas in the field of infant and childhood nutrition which are under study and are as yet not completely resolved include the following:

1. The final relation between fetal undernutrition and later intellectual development.
2. The possible role that the overconsumption of salt in infancy may play in later high blood pressure conditions.
3. The role of cholesterol in the diet of childhood and in the later onset of atherosclerotic heart disease.
4. The possible relation between short periods of undernutrition and

longer life spans. For example, undernutrition in certain laboratory animals at weaning results in their living longer than similar well-fed animals.
5. The final implications of any long-term effects of early obesity and over-nutrition.

More study, research, and experience will be required before we know the final answers to these questions and to problems in other areas of infant and childhood nutrition. Above all, there is a real need for *application* of nutritional knowledge already gathered to help insure optimal health and development for all the world's infants and children — from children in your own neighborhood to those in the farthest lands.

QUESTIONS AND PROBLEMS

1. By what age will the newborn infant normally double his birth weight? Triple it?
2. List three major differences between breast milk and undiluted, unmodified cow's milk.
3. What is an average daily milk intake for a six-month-old child weighing 15 pounds (7 kg)?
4. By what age should the infant be on a diet which includes meats and other solids?
5. What are advisable dietary supplements for a three-month-old infant in a rural community (no community water supply, no natural fluoridation of local water) fed on an evaporated milk formula?
6. Name three foods which might be suspected if a nine-month-old infant begins to develop signs of allergy.
7. What would you advise a vegetarian mother who asks you about the adequacy of the "vegetarian" diet which she feeds her two-year-old?
8. Prepare a day's sample menu (including snacks) for a day care center taking care of three- to five-year-olds, open from 7 a.m. to 6 p.m.

REFERENCES

1. Winick, M.: Pediatrics, *47*:969, 1971.
2. Babson, S. G.: J. Pediat., *79*:694, 1971; Davidson, M.: Pediat. Clin. N. Amer., *17*: 913, 1970.
3. Wood, A. L.: J. Amer. Dietet. Assoc., *31*:474, 1955.
4. Rivera, J.: Amer. J. Pub. Health, *61*:277, 1971.
5. Bullen, C., and Willis, A. T.: Brit. Med. J., *3*:338, 1971; South, M. A.: J. Pediat., *79*:1, 1971.
6. Hansen, A. E., et al.: Pediatrics, *31*(Part II): 171, 1963.
7. Lewin, P. K., et al.: J. Pediat., *78*:207, 1971.
8. Ritchie, J. H., Fish, M. B., McMasters, V., and Grossman, M.: New Eng. J. Med., *279*: 1185, 1968.
9. Fomon, S.: *Infant Nutrition.* Philadelphia, W. B. Saunders Co., 1967.
10. Ericsson, Y., and Ribelius, U.: Acta Paediat. Scand., *59*:424, 1970.
11. Eid, E. E.: Brit. Med. J., *2*:74, 1970.

SUPPLEMENTARY READING

General, History, and Reviews

Anderson, T. A., and Fomon, S. J.: Commercially prepared strained and junior foods for infants. J. Amer. Dietet. Assoc., *58*:520, 1971.

Committee on Nutrition: Factors affecting food intake. Pediatrics, *33*:135, 1964; On the feeding of solid foods to infants. Pediatrics, *21*:685, 1958.

Filer, L. J., and Martinez, G. A.: Intake of selected nutrients by infants in the United States: An evaluation of 4,000 representative six-month-olds. Clin. Pediat., *3*:633, 1964.

Fomon, S. J.: A pediatrician looks at early nutrition. Bull. N. Y. Acad. Med., *47*:569, 1971.

Fomon, S. J., Thomas, L. N., and Filer, L. J., Jr.: Acceptance of unsalted strained foods by normal infants. J. Pediat., *76*:242, 1970.

Harris, L. E., and Chan, J. C. M.: Infant feeding practices. Amer. J. Dis. Child., *117*:483, 1969.

Heseltine, M. M., and Pitts, J. L.: Economy in nutrition and feeding of infants. Amer. J. Pub. Health, *56*:1756, 1966.

Hill, L. F.: Infant feeding: Historical and current. Ped. Clin. N. Amer., *14*:255, 1967.

Jackson, R. L., Hanna, F. M., and Flynn, M. A.: Nutritional requirements of infants and children. Ped. Clin. N. Amer., *9*:879, 1962.

Juhas, L.: Day-care for children—recent developments and their implications for dietitians. J. Amer. Dietet. Assoc., *57*:139, 1970.

Kekomäki, M.: Food requirements in normal children. Acta Anaesth. Scand., *14*:18, 1970.

Martin, E. A.: *Roberts' Nutrition Work with Children.* Chicago, University of Chicago Press, 1954.

McWilliams, M.: *Nutrition for the Growing Years.* New York, John Wiley & Sons, 1967.

O'Grady, R. S.: Feeding behavior in infants. Amer. J. Nurs., *71*:736, 1971.

Willis, N. H.: *Basic Infant Nutrition: Birth to Six Months: A Syllabus.* Philadelphia, J. B. Lippincott, 1964.

Wood, A. L.: The history of artificial feeding of infants. J. Amer. Dietet. Assoc., *31*:474, 1955.

Ziegler, E. E., and Fomon, S. J.: Fluid intake, renal solute load, and water balance in infancy. J. Pediat., *78*:561, 1971.

Nutrition Reviews

Protection of the infant diet: Government and industry. *24*:195, 1966.

Early feeding of the premature infant. *24*:295, 1966.

Salt in the infant's diet. *25*:82, 1967.

Dietary solute load and the premature infant. *25*:143, 1967.

Absorption of milk protein by infants. *25*:223, 1967.

Solid foods in the nutrition of young infants. *25*:233, 1967.

Some economic and social aspects of infant feeding. *25*:255, 1967.

Nutrients and genes: Interactions in development (by Hurley, L. S.). *27*:3, 1969.

Salt in infant foods (by Filer, L. J., Jr.). *29*:27, 1971.

Modified food starches for use in infant foods (by Filer, L. J., Jr.). *29*:55, 1971.

Prenatal nutrition and the human fetus. *29*:197, 1971.

Growth and Mental Development

Cheek, D. B., Graystone, J. E., and Read, M. S.: Cellular growth, nutrition and development. Pediatrics, *45*:315, 1970.

Dugdale, A. E., Chen, S. T., and Hewitt, G.: Patterns of growth and nutrition in childhood. Amer. J. Clin. Nutr., *23*:1280, 1970.

Giok, L. T., Rose, C. S., and György, P.: Influence of early malnutrition on some aspects of the health of school-age children. Amer. J. Clin. Nutr., *20*:1280, 1967.

Graham, G. G.: Effect of infantile malnutrition on growth. Fed. Proc., *26*:139, 1967.

Hansen, J. D. L., Freesemann, C., Moodie, A. D., and Evans, D. E.: What does nutritional growth retardation imply? Pediatrics, *47*: 299, 1971.

Holliday, M. A.: Metabolic rate and organ size during growth from infancy to maturity and during late gestation and early infancy. Pediatrics, *47*:169, 1971.

Latham, M. C., and Cobos, F.: The effects of malnutrition on intellectual development and learning. Amer. J. Pub. Health, *61*: 1307, 1971.

Osofsky, H. J.: Antenatal malnutrition: Its relationship to subsequent infant and child development. Amer. J. Obstet. Gynecol., *105*:1150, 1969.

Rueda-Williamson, R., and Rose, H. E.: Growth and nutrition of infants: The influence of diet and other factors on growth. Pediatrics, *30*:639, 1962.

Scrimshaw, N. S., and Gorden, J. E. (eds.): *Malnutrition, Learning and Behavior.* Cambridge, Mass., MIT Press, 1968.

Wingerd, J., Schoen, E. J., and Solomon, I. L.: Growth standards in the first two years of life based on measurements of white and black children in a prepaid health care program. Pediatrics, *47*:818, 1971.

Winick, M.: Cellular growth during early malnutrition. Pediatrics, *47*:969, 1971.

Woodruff, C.: Nutritional aspects of metabolism of growth and development. J. Amer. Med. Assoc., *196*:214, 1966.

Nutrition Reviews

Response of young infants to growth hormone. *24*:134, 1966.

Subsequent growth of children treated for malnutrition. *24*:267, 1966.

Iron deficiency and growth. *24*:330, 1966.

Nutrition and learning behavior. *25*:20, 1967.

Underfeeding and brain development. *25*:334, 1967.

Undernutrition in children and subsequent brain growth and intellectual development. *26*: 197, 1968.

The infant brain following severe malnutrition. *27*:251, 1969.

Environment and growth. *27*:282, 1969.

Emotional deprivation and growth failure. *28*:36, 1970.

Malnutrition and physical and mental development. *28*:176, 1970.

Cellular growth in infantile malnutrition. *29*:6, 1971.

Breast and Bottle Feeding

Applebaum, R. M.: The modern management of successful breast feeding. Pediat. Clin. N. Amer., *17*:203, 1970.

Arena, J. M.: Contamination of the ideal food. Nutr. Today, *5*:2, Winter 1970.

Beal, V. A.: Breast- and formula-feeding of infants. J. Amer. Dietet. Assoc., *55*:31, 1969.

Berenberg, W., Mandell, F., and Fellers, F. X.: Hazards of skimmed milk, unboiled and boiled. Pediatrics, *44*:734, 1969.

Catz, C. S., and Giacoia, G. P.: Drugs and breast milk. Pediat. Clin., *19*:151, 1972.

Jelliffe, D. B., and Jelliffe, E. F. P. (eds.): Symposium: The uniqueness of human milk. Amer. J. Clin. Nutr., *24*:968, 1971.

Ordway, N. K.: Formula feeding of infants in the first months. Postgrad. Med., *48*:167, 1970.

Owen, G. M.: Modification of cow's milk for infant formulas: Current practices. Amer. J. Clin. Nutr., *22*:1150, 1969.

Rivera, J.: The frequency of use of various kinds of milk during infancy in middle and lower-income families. Amer. J. Pub. Health, *61*:277, 1971.

Sellars, W. A., et al.: New growth charts: Soy, cow, and breast milk comparison. Ann. Allergy, *29*:126, 1971.

Straub, C. P.: Nutritional intake of infants. II. Effect of milk or milk formula. J. Amer. Dietet. Assoc., *54*:387, 1969.

Williams, H. H.: Differences between cow's and human milk. J. Amer. Med. Assoc., *175*: 104, 1961.

Nutrition Reviews

Hypocalcemia in newborn infants fed cows' milk. *26*:299, 1968.

Gastrointestinal milk allergy in infants. *27*:7, 1969.

Preschool Nutrition

Blix, G. (ed.): *Symposia of the Swedish Nutrition Foundation. VII. Nutrition in Preschool and School Age.* Uppsala, Almqvist & Wiksells, 1969.

Dwyer, F. M., Dwyer, J. T., and Mayer, J.: Feeding the preschool child. Postgrad. Med., *47*:267, 1970.

Food and Nutrition Board: Pre-school child malnutrition: Primary deterrent to human progress. Summary of international conference on Prevention of Malnutrition in the Pre-School Child. Washington, D.C., National Academy of Sciences–National Research Council, 1964.

Jelliffe, D. B., and Jelliffe, E. F. P.: A bookshelf of nutrition programs for pre-school children—a recent selected bibliography. Amer. J. Pub. Health, *62*:469, 1972.

Nutrition Reviews

Nutrition evaluation of preschool children. *30*: 34, 1972.

Nutritional status and the "hydroxyproline index" in Mississippi preschool children. *30*:87, 1972.

Nutritional Requirements

Carbohydrates, Proteins, Fat

Cox, W. M., Jr., and Filer, L. J., Jr.: Protein intake for low-birth-weight infants. J. Pediat., *74*:1016, 1969.

Hanna, F. M., Navarrete, D. A., and Hsu, F. A.: Calcium–fatty acid absorption in term infants fed human milk and prepared formulas simulating human milk. Pediatrics, *45*:216, 1970.

Vitamins

Committee on Drugs and Nutrition: Use and abuse of vitamin A. Pediatrics, *48*:655, 1971.

Committee on Nutrition: The prophylactic requirement and the toxicity of vitamin D. Pediatrics, *31*:512, 1963; Vitamin K supplementation for infants receiving milk substitute infant formulas and for those with fat malabsorption. Pediatrics, *48*:483, 1971.

Hoppner, K.: Free and total folate activity in strained baby foods. J. Inst. Can. Technol. Aliment., *4*:51, 1971.

Jusko, W. J., et al.: Riboflavin absorption and excretion in the neonate. Pediatrics, *45*:945, 1970.

Lampkin, B. C., and Saunders, E. F.: Nutritional vitamin B_{12} deficiency in an infant. J. Pediat., *75*:1053, 1969.

Roberts, P. M., Arrowsmith, D. E., Rau, S. M., and Monk-Jones, M. E.: Folate state of premature infants. Arch. Dis. Child., *44*: 637, 1969.

Seelig, M. S.: Vitamin D and cardiovascular, renal, and brain damage in infancy and childhood. Ann. N. Y. Acad. Sci., *147*: 537, 1969.

Minerals

Al-Rashid, R, and Spangler, J.: Neonatal copper deficiency. New Eng. J. Med., *285*:841, 1971.

Anonymous: Iron-deficiency anemia in infants and preschool children. Dairy Council Digest, *43*:1, 1972.

Barltrop, D., and Oppé, T. E.: Dietary factors in neonatal calcium homoeostasis. Lancet, *2*:1333, 1970.

Caddell, J. L.: A review of magnesium deficiency in children. Pediat. Digest, *12*:30, 1970.

Committee on Nutrition: Iron balance and requirements in infancy. Pediatrics, *43*:134, 1969; Iron-fortified formulas. Pediatrics, *47*:786, 1971.

Cordano, A., Baerti, J. M., and Graham, G. G.: Copper deficiency in infancy. Pediatrics, *34*:324, 1964.

Coussons, H.: Magnesium metabolism in infants and children. Postgrad. Med., *46*:135, 1969.

Eminians, J., Ziai, M., and Reinhold, J. G.: Zinc metabolism: The possible roles played by zinc deficiency in malnutrition of children. Clin. Pediat., *6*:603, 1967.

Harris, I., and Wilkinson, A. W.: Magnesium depletion in children. Lancet, *2*:735, 1971.

Murthy, G. K., and Rhea, U. S.: Cadmium, copper, iron, lead, manganese, and zinc in evaporated milk, infant products, and human milk, J. Dairy Sci., *54*:1001, 1971.

Oberleas, D., and Prasad, A. S.: Adequacy of trace minerals in bovine milk for human consumption. Amer. J. Clin. Nutr., *22*:196, 1969.

Oppé, T. E., and Redstone, D.: Calcium and phosphorus levels in healthy newborn infants given various types of milk. Lancet, *1*:1045, 1968.

Oski, F. A.: Iron-fortified formulas in infancy: Best form of iron supplementation? J. Pediat., *80*:524, 1972.

Say, B., Özsoylu, S., and Berkel, I.: Geophagia associated with iron-deficiency anemia, hepatosplenomegaly, hypogonadism, and dwarfism: A syndrome probably associated with zinc deficiency. Clin. Pediat., *8*:661, 1969.

Seely, J. et al.: Copper deficiency in a premature infant fed an iron fortified formula. New Eng. J. Med., *286*:109, 1972.

Williams, M. L., et al.: Calcium and fat absorption in neonatal period. Amer. J. Clin. Nutr., *23*:1322, 1970.

Nutrition Reviews

Safe levels of vitamin D intake for infants. *24*: 230, 1966.

Chromium and carbohydrate metabolism in infantile malnutrition. *26*:235, 1968.

Calories and activity in infants. *26*:239, 1968.

Calcium, phosphorus, and strontium metabolism in infants. *27*:254, 1969.

Special Topics

Aykroyd, W. R.: Nutrition and mortality in infancy and early childhood: Past and present relationships. Amer. J. Clin. Nutr., *24*:480, 1971.

Eid, E. E.: Follow-up of physical growth of children who had excessive weight gain in the first six months of life. Brit. Med. J., *2*:74, 1970.

Erhard, D.: Nutrition education for the 'now' generation. J. Nutr. Ed., *2*:135, 1971.

Feeney, M. C.: Nutritional and dietary management of food allergy in children. Amer. J. Clin. Nutr., *22*:103, 1969.

Fredrickson, D. S., ed.: Symposium: Factors in childhood that influence the development of atherosclerosis and hypertension. Amer. J. Clin. Nutr., *25*:222, 1972.

Freier, S., and Kletter, B.: Milk allergy in infants and young children. Clin. Pediat., *9*:449, 1970.

Gokulanathan, K. S., and Verghese, K. P.: Sociocultural malnutrition: Syndrome of nutritional imbalance, growth disturbances and chronic infection. Clin. Pediat., *9*:439, 1970.

Guthrie, H. A.: Infant feeding practices—a predisposing factor in hypertension? Amer. J. Clin. Nutr., *21*:863, 1968.

György, P.: Prevention of malnutrition as a problem of ecology. Pediat. Res., *2*:389, 1968.

Jelliffe, D. B., and Jelliffe, E. F. P.: The urban avalanche and child nutrition. II. Special problems in developing countries. J. Amer. Dietet. Assoc., *57*:114, 1970.

Johnstone, D. E., and Dutton, A. M.: Dietary prophylaxis of allergic disease in children. New Eng. J. Med., *274*:715, 1966.

Kildeberg, P., and Winters, R.: Infant feeding and blood acid-base status. Pediatrics, *49*: 801, 1972.

Kohler, E. E., and Good, T. A.: The infant who fails to thrive. Hosp. Prac., *4*:54, 1969.

Sanjur, D. M., Cravioto, J., Rosales, L., and van Veen, A.: *Infant Feeding and Weaning Practices in a Rural Preindustrial Setting: A Sociocultural Approach.* Uppsala, Almqvist & Wiksells, 1970.

Smith, C. A., and Berenberg, W.: The concept of failure to thrive. Pediatrics, *46*:661, 1970.

Swaminathan, M.: The nutrition and feeding of infants and preschool children in the developing countries. World Rev. Nutr. Dietet., *9*:85, 1968.

Taitz, L. S.: Infantile overnutrition among artificially fed infants in the Sheffield region. Brit. Med. J., *1*:315, 1971.

Nutrition Reviews

Gastrectomy in children. *24*:8, 1966.

Hypermetabolism and undernutrition. *24*:68, 1966.

Long-term effects of severe infantile malnutrition. *25*:261, 1967.

Prognosis for malnourished infants. *25*:332, 1967.

Renal function in infantile malnutrition. *25*:350, 1967.

Magnesium toxicity in the newborn. *26*:139, 1968.

Measles and malnutrition. *26*:323, 1968.

Recovery rates of children following protein-calorie malnutrition. *28*:118, 1970.

twenty-one

Nutrition and Physical Work Performance

Sound nutrition and a sensible program of physical activity are two of the chief requirements for health. Most people are aware of the need for a good diet, whether or not they take one, but few people seem to realize how important exercise is to their general well-being. Exercise is a dominant variable in energy balance (total energy expenditure). Energy intake is not adequately regulated to prevent obesity unless enough physical work is done (Chapter 15).

Even a modest but diligently followed program of training has been shown to alter the body composition of sedentary middle-aged men. In one study the men were required to walk only 40 minutes at a speed of 4 to 5 miles per hour four times a week, and yet their weight and body fat were somewhat reduced and their cardiovascular fitness was significantly improved.[1] Measurements of old men showed that among those in the eighth decade of life the ones who were most active had the highest amount of lean body tissue and their muscle strength was equal to that of inactive men who were ten years

younger.[2] Physical activity (defined as any amount of habitual running) was also shown to be equivalent to a difference of ten years of age as regards parameters of physical fitness in middle-aged men.[3] Fitness is also related in a desirable way to a number of factors associated with risk of heart disease. Inactivity is associated with loss of bone substance (osteoporosis), and the epidemiology of hip fracture suggests that hard physical work throughout life protects against it.[4]

It has been suggested that lack of physical activity and sports in childhood leads to underdeveloped abdominal muscles and weak connective tissue sheaths that then contribute to chronic low back pain in women after pregnancy.[5] Women often restrict physical activity due to the old-fashioned notion that menses are made difficult by vigorous movement. In most women fitness is slightly reduced two to six days before the onset of menstruation,[6] yet women athletes perform superbly throughout the menstrual cycle. The last months of pregnancy place a great burden on the maternal circulation.

When the mother does physical work, her muscles compete with the placenta for blood and if her heart is small it may not adequately cope with the double burden. Pregnant women with small hearts have an increased risk of premature delivery.[6] One way to assure good development of the musculature and the cardiovascular system is by a program of regular physical exercise throughout life, for women as well as for men.

Psychologists also point out beneficial effects of physical activity. Exercise is said to be an outlet for unconsumed accumulated energy and so reduces "free floating tension" and channels aggression outward. Fretfulness, restlessness and insomnia are outcomes ascribed to failure to relieve tension by physical activity.[7]

Neither adults nor teenagers are very active in typical Western cultures. Although American teenagers were found to spend a bit more time in moderate and strenuous activity than adults of the same sex, girls spent 95 percent of their time asleep and in activities classed as very light (2.5 kcal per minute or less) or light (2.5 to 4.9 kcal per minute), and boys spent over 90 percent of their time in like activities.[8] Australian youth spent 78 to 80 percent of their time lying or sitting, 14 to 20 percent in very light activity, and only 1.5 to 4.4 percent in any activity that involved greater energy expenditure than walking.[9]

Work Capacity

The ability to perform work is dependent on energy-yielding processes in muscle cells. For muscle cells to work they must have oxygen which comes from the lungs via the blood and is taken up by the muscle cell. The ability to work can be limited by failure of any one of these processes: inadequate lung capacity, inadequate capability of the heart to pump blood, inadequate oxygen-carrying power of the blood, or failure of the peripheral circulation to supply enough blood to the working muscle. In some disease conditions or in very heavy smokers lung power may be limiting, but generally it is cardiovascular factors that limit work. During exercise blood is diverted from the organs to the maximum extent feasible to supply the working muscles and the heart. As illustrated in Figure 21–1, the combined effect of diversion of blood circulation and increased heart pumping action augments the blood supply to the muscles by thirty-fold.[10] Anemia is one condition in which oxygen transport is limited. Low blood hemoglobin levels in anemic patients and the sharp drop in hemoglobin occasioned by blood donation in healthy women reduce blood buffering power and capacity to transport oxygen and have a detrimental effect on work performance.[11] In sedentary but normal persons, limitation is usually due to poor cardiovascular fitness, and the heart then has to work very hard to pump blood at levels of work that are well tolerated by persons who are more fit.

Since work requires energy expenditure and that involves oxygen, higher work levels are always associated with higher tissue uptake of oxygen and more oxygen removal in respiration. *Maximal oxygen uptake* is the greatest amount of oxygen a person can take in during exercise and so reflects his ability to transport oxygen to his tissues (Fig. 21–2). Thus, maximal oxygen uptake is one index of fitness. For average middle-aged men the maximal oxygen uptake is 35 to 40 ml per kg of body weight per minute, or about 2.5 liters of oxygen per minute. In well-trained young athletes, maximal oxygen uptake is about 70 ml per kg per minute.

When people work at very high rates, oxygen supplied to the tissues is not sufficient to oxidize muscle glycogen completely and an intermediate compound, lactic acid, accumulates. (See

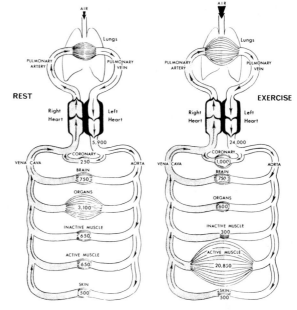

Figure 21–1. Schematic representation of the blood circulation of a sedentary man during standing rest and during exercise at the maximal oxygen uptake. Organs include kidneys, liver, gastrointestinal tract, and others. Blood flow is given in milliliters per minute. (Courtesy of Drs. Mitchell and Blomqvist and the New England Journal of Medicine.[10])

section on glycolysis, Chapter 14.) After the work is completed, the person continues to breathe heavily and takes up additional oxygen until the lactic acid is completely metabolized and tissue stores are repleted. This is referred to as an *anaerobic work* situation, and the person is said to accumulate an oxygen debt. Man can accumulate a debt equal to 2 to 5 liters of oxygen.

Work at lower intensity that is performed without building up lactic acid in the tissues is called *aerobic work*. For most healthy people, the limit of aerobic work capacity approximates the energy expenditure of a brisk walk and corresponds to use of just over 1 liter of oxygen or 5 kcal per minute.[2] This is about four to five times the resting metabolic rate (Chapter 2). Work at or below the aerobic capacity is called steady state work because it can be continued steadily for long periods without fatigue.

How long a person can work at a time without a break obviously varies according to the work rate. This is an important consideration in industry where rest periods must be established and in endurance sports events where the work must be paced. If the work task is at or below the aerobic capacity, rest periods are not needed. Durnin and Passmore suggest that rest periods can be calculated simply according to multiples of the aerobic capacity.[12] If the work task requires 7.5 kcal per minute and the aerobic capacity is 5 kcal, then 30 minutes of rest will be needed for every hour worked; if the task is one requiring 10 kcal per minute, then the rest periods will have to be the same length as the work periods. For maximum work output it is best to work and rest for short periods — ten minutes of work and five minutes of rest in a hillclimb, for instance. Otherwise, the work pace must be slowed so that expenditure rate does not exceed the aerobic capacity of the workers. The value of 5 kcal per minute suggests a maximum work output of 2400 kcal per eight-hour work-shift and coincides well with actual observations of sustained hard industrial work, such as coal mining and nonmechanized agriculture.[12] The trained athlete is capable of sustained work at about ten times his resting rate,

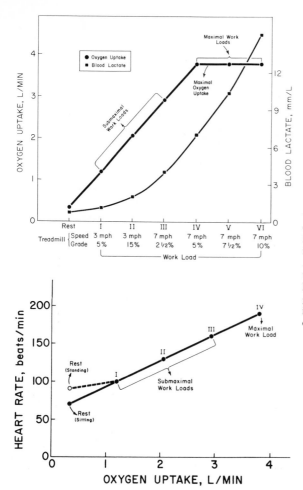

Figure 21–2. **A,** Maximal oxygen uptake determined by means of a motor-driven treadmill. The man does increasingly harder work until the capacity to take in oxygen reaches its limit. After this point, lactic acid rises because there is not enough oxygen to metabolize glycogen completely. **B,** With progressively increasing exercise loads there is a linear relation between heart rate and oxygen uptake.
(Courtesy of Drs. Mitchell and Blomqvist and the New England Journal of Medicine.[10])

but he does become fatigued and does accumulate an oxygen debt during this load of work.

In a study of the energy needs of college football players,[13] food eaten at the training table and between meal snacks amounted to 5600 kcal per day during playing season and the men were not gaining weight. The men averaged 80 kg (small, perhaps, but it was the Harvard team), which would indicate an expected energy requirement in the order of 3200 kcal per day if the men had pursued a usual collegiate pattern of moderate activity rather than sports. The difference between ordinary needs and those of the team, 2400 kcal, should be ascribable in some way to football practice and competition. This activity occupied only two hours a day, indicating an energy expenditure rate of 1200 kcal per hour, nearly 20 times the basal metabolic rate, which is above a level that is usually sustainable for an extended period. The extra energy need of the team probably reflects in part a continued high rate of metabolism after the exercise was concluded. Benedict's classic research on energy metabolism in the early 1900's included an observation that metabolism during sleep was 25 percent higher when very severe work had been performed one hour earlier than when the sleep followed a day of rest; sleeping metabolic rate was still 10 to 15 percent higher as long as seven hours after severe work. This continued effect of exercise on resting metabolism was mentioned in Chapter 2 and is repeated here as a reminder that calculations of total energy need based on activity categories are only rough approximations. The only satisfactory basis for judging energy need is by maintenance of ideal body weight, because physical work affects the body in ways which have not yet been adequately explained.

Mechanical Work Efficiency

The efficiency with which work is performed can be calculated from the amount of energy metabolized if the amount of mechanical work performed can be measured. In the laboratory this can be accomplished by having the person pedal a stationary bicycle at a stipulated speed against a set resistance, or walk at a given rate and incline on a motor-driven treadmill. *Gross efficiency is the ratio of mechanical work performed to the total energy expended. Net efficiency* is the ratio of mechanical work to the increment of the work energy expenditure *above the resting metabolic rate.*

Mechanical work efficiency varies considerably. It is influenced by the type of work performed, previous training or practice, fatigue, the amount of the load, and the speed and conditions under which the work is done. A healthy person performs usual work tasks with about 25 percent net efficiency, which means that he consumes four times as much energy as is represented in the work actually performed. When the person is fit and accustomed to the task (e.g., in trained bicycle riders), efficiencies as high as 33 percent

have been obtained. Under unfavorable conditions, such as an unaccustomed task, too heavy a load, too high a rate of speed, inconvenient posture for the task, or fatigue, net mechanical efficiency may fall as low as 10 percent. Low mechanical efficiency means that work is accomplished at a greater cost—that is, more energy and oxygen are needed to produce a given amount of external work, a larger proportion of the energy appearing as heat under these conditions.

Fuel for Muscular Work and Performance Capacity

The source of energy for muscular work is ATP generated from the common metabolic pathways (Chapter 14) or, in the short term, from creatine phosphate stored in the muscle. Creatine is a nitrogen-containing compound synthesized in the body from amino acids. It combines with phosphate from ATP in a high-energy linkage, forming creatine phosphate and ADP. When ATP is needed for the initial stages of muscular work, the reverse reaction of creatine phosphate with ADP yields ATP for muscle contraction, and creatine. The latter is again regenerated to creatine phosphate when ATP is abundant.

The nature of the substance undergoing metabolism can be determined by measuring the amount of oxygen used and the amount of carbon dioxide formed during metabolism. If carbohydrate is being metabolized, one molecule of carbon dioxide is formed for every molecule of oxygen used, according to the following equation for glucose:

$$C_6H_{12}O_6 + 6\ O_2 \rightarrow 6\ CO_2 + 6\ H_2O$$

The ratio of carbon dioxide produced to oxygen used is called the *respiratory quotient*, which is abbreviated to RQ. In the glucose example, $6\ CO_2/6\ O_2$ equals an RQ of 1.0. For complete metabolism of fat, the RQ is about 0.7 as illustrated for stearic acid:

$$C_{18}H_{36}O_2 + 26\ O_2 \rightarrow 18\ CO_2 + 18\ H_2O$$

and $18\ CO_2/26\ O_2$ equals 0.7. If the volume and composition of air inhaled and exhaled during work are known, both the energy expended and the composition of the source of energy can be ascertained.

Formerly carbohydrate was thought to be the only energy source for physical work, but present information indicates that carbohydrate plays a dominant role only in heavy exercise when oxygen supply to the muscle becomes limiting. During steady state work, fat provides about half of the energy. The fat utilized comes from lipid pools in the muscle tissue and fatty acids mobilized from adipose tissue and transported to the working muscle by the blood. Protein is not used for work energy to any great extent.

To determine if the metabolic mixture utilized during work does affect work performance, two types of studies have been made. In one, persons were fed a normal diet or one very high in either of the work-energy sources (fat or carbohydrate) for some period of time to foster preferential use of that source during work. Other studies emphasized the composition of meals taken just prior to an event. Carbohydrate has more oxygen in its composition than does fat, and about 10 percent less oxygen is needed per unit of energy when carbohydrate is metabolized, so theoretically preferential utilization of carbohydrate should be beneficial when oxygen limits work.

Diets containing little or no carbohydrate have adverse effects on performance in every study. One experiment compared a diet containing less than 5 percent with one supplying over 90 percent of energy as carbohydrate. Capacity for hard physical work was reduced by one-half with the high-fat diet and increased by one-fourth with the high-carbohydrate regimen, as compared with performance during normal diet periods. Other studies confirm these findings and indicate that one factor involved is the amount of glycogen present in the muscle. Swedish investigators measured performance capacity (work to exhaustion in a standard bicycle test) and obtained samples of muscle by needle biopsy from a group of men fed three diets. Time to exhaustion was 114 minutes with a normal diet, 57 minutes when the diet was made up exclusively of high-protein and high-fat foods, and 167 minutes when the diet was high in carbohydrate. After the normal mixed diet, glycogen content was found to be 1.75 gm per 100 gm wet muscle before exercise; after three days of carbohydrate-free diet it was 0.63 gm, and after the same period of high-carbohydrate feeding, 3.51 gm.[14]

When men fed a normal mixed diet worked at a rate of about 75 percent of their maximum oxygen uptake, glycogen content of muscle was almost completely depleted in 90 minutes, but blood sugar was satisfactorily maintained. Past this point, evidence indicates that blood sugar falls and constitutes a final limit to performance. Administration of glucose at the point of exhaustion allows work to proceed for an additional period of time.[14]

Diets based on the principle of improving the fuel for muscular work have been developed and enthusiastically adopted in Europe. It is difficult to say if this has a significant effect on the outcome of athletic competition, because there are uncontrollable differences in skills and training between competitors and in environmental factors between events. Also, strength of belief in the efficacy of a treatment may be sufficient to make the treatment effective, a point that is difficult to rule out even in laboratory studies involving subjective acknowledgment of "fatigue." However, this treatment does have a sound basis in theory and a reasonable body of experimental evidence in support of it.

The preparation recommended by Åstrand[14] for competition in endurance events exceeding 30 to 60 minutes' duration is as follows:

1. One week before the competition, exercise to exhaustion the same muscles that will be used in the event. This is done to exhaust the glycogen stores.

2. For the next three days eat a diet made up almost exclusively of foods high in protein and fat (In our opinion it should contain a minimum of 80 gm of carbohydrate.) (See Table 21–1). This is to keep the glycogen content low.

3. As the competition nears, add large quantities of carbohydrate to the diet. Åstrand emphasizes that the carbohydrate should be *added* while maintaining the intake of protein and fat.

Åstrand's tests show that muscle glycogen can exceed 4 gm per 100 gm of muscle with this regimen and that total muscle glycogen stores could be as high as 700 gm. This would represent a reserve of about 2800 kcal if completely metabolized or half that if lactic acid were the end-product due to anaerobic work metabolism. This is approximately double the usual reserve capacity in trained athletes.

Studies of the composition of meals taken just before competition do not indicate any special benefit of one mixture of energy sources over another. Glucose has been compared with sucrose, and although there was a small difference in RQ, physical efficiency was the same with the two sugars.[15] Åstrand's practical advice in this connection is that before a competition an athlete should eat according to his own wishes based on the advice of his coach and experience of his own reactions in

Table 21–1. *Diets for Use in the Åstrand Regimen for Enhanced Muscle Glycogen Storage*

Days 4–6 Before an Event	*Days 1–3 Before an Event*
HIGH ENERGY-LOW CARBOHYDRATE DIET	VERY HIGH ENERGY-HIGH CARBOHYDRATE DIET
Breakfast	
½ grapefruit or ½ c. grapefruit juice or berries	1 c. orange or pineapple juice
2 eggs	Hot cereal as desired
Generous serving bacon, ham or sausage	Eggs and/or hot cakes
Butter or margarine as desired	Generous serving bacon, ham or sausage
1 thin slice whole wheat bread	Butter or margarine as desired
1 c. whole milk or half and half	2–4 slices whole grain bread
	Chocolate or cocoa as desired
Luncheon and Dinner	
Clear bouillon or ½ c. tomato juice	Cream or legume soup or chowder
Large serving fish, poultry or liver (> 6 oz)	Large serving fish, poultry or liver (> 6 oz)
Mixed green (only) salad or 1 c. cooked green vegetable	Added beans or fruits
Salad dressing, butter or margarine as desired	Salad dressing, butter or margarine as desired
1 c. whole milk or half and half	1 c. whole milk, half and half, or milkshake
Artificially sweetened gelatin with whipped cream (no sugar)	2–4 slices whole grain bread or rolls or potato
	Pie, cake, pudding or ice cream
Snacks	
Cheddar cheese	Fruits, especially dates, raisins, apples, bananas
Nuts	More milk or milkshakes
1 slice whole grain bread	Cookies or candy
Artificially sweetened lemonade	

sports competition. Some additional suggestions are given in the later section on feeding just before work (p. 490).

*Nutritional Deficiency
and Performance*

Among factors known to be detrimental to performance, two are outstanding: *dehydration* and *food deprivation*. Evidence on these points comes from careful laboratory studies and abundant field experience. Of the two, dehydration is the more immediate and serious risk. Normally, voluntary drinking is stimulated when the body water content drops by 1 percent, but during exercise voluntary intake is inhibited and water balance may not be attained until hours or days after a severe bout of work with high rates of water loss as sweat. In a comfortable environment water loss due to sweating during moderate exercise will be about 1 liter per hour; at higher work output or in the heat, loss may be two to four times that rate (Chapter 10). Physical performance begins to deteriorate when the water deficit exceeds 3 percent of body weight.

In spite of this evidence, extremely ill-advised practices are used to meet weight ranges in competitive sports such as wrestling — practices that include withholding water, wearing rubberized apparel and inducing vomiting. The American Medical Association's Committee on Medical Aspects of Sports has this to say about indiscriminate weight control practices: "If weight loss is excessive, the boy's competitive abilities are impaired. If his weight loss is contrived to circumvent a regulation, his ethics have been compromised. If he has an unsuspected metabolic problem or if the weight reduction scheme is extreme, health could be seriously affected."[16]

There is a serious question as to how much weight (other than water) an athlete can safely lose without impairing

his performance. Any amount of *excess* fat can be trimmed off to advantage, and reducing weight to the desirable level for height and age is a logical and defensible point. In the famous Minnesota studies of conscientious objectors on a semistarvation regimen, loss of 25 percent of body weight over a six-month period resulted in diminished work performance, endurance, and strength of the large muscles. Later studies in the same laboratory tested more severely restricted diets of 580 and 1010 kcal per day. The 580 kcal diet was inadequate to maintain blood sugar levels for work and can be dismissed from further consideration. With the higher energy intake, loss of hand strength and lowering of maximal oxygen uptake occurred when the men lost 10 percent or more of body weight. Low work loads can be accomplished for a few days in an emergency, especially if at least 100 gm of carbohydrate, a few grams of salt (such as bouillon cubes), and adequate water are consumed, but this is not compatible with top performance capability.

A sensible plan of weight control, suggested by the AMA Committee, is to undertake ". . . an intensive conditioning program related to the demands of [the sport] for at least four weeks, preferably six, without emphasis on [body] weight. . . . At the end of this period and without altering the daily training routine, [record] weight in a pre-breakfast, post-micturition state. Consider this weight the minimal effective weight for competition as well as certification purposes."[16] A program of this kind that includes sound nutrition education is ideal and is especially important for young people who participate in more than one sport according to the season and for which weight advantages differ, such as football and wrestling. Alternating attempts to gain and lose weight cannot help but be detrimental.

Vitamin deficiencies of all kinds are damaging to work performance.[15] How long performance can be maintained when one or more vitamins are omitted from the diet will vary with the amount of tissue reserves of the nutrient the individual has and the role that the specific nutrient plays in work metabolism. On the basis of their participation in the metabolic pathways, lack of the B vitamins would be expected to have the most immediate effects, and this is borne out by investigations of the subject. Lack of thiamin is evident in a few days or weeks, and the symptoms of deficiency appear earlier in men fed a deficient diet who are actively working than in those who are sedentary. This early damage to performance is probably true of most of the B complex vitamins, but effects of lack of vitamin A do not appear for months in previously well-nourished subjects.

Deficiencies of minerals other than sodium (Chapter 10) have not been well-studied, but because of their important role in neuromuscular transmission and as enzyme cofactors, detrimental effects would certainly be expected. The skeleton provides an essential reserve of calcium which is withdrawn to maintain blood levels of ionized calcium and the liver holds some stores of the trace minerals, but these are variable according to the quality of the usual diet. When effects of mineral deficiencies other than the electrolytes are examined, one would expect them to appear only after periods of weeks or months, or when there are abnormal losses due to diarrhea or vomiting.

Total deprivation of protein with adequate energy intake for two weeks has not been shown to alter performance of fixed work tasks in a laboratory nor to reduce muscular strength. The men do complain of feeling less "fit" subjectively and the blood volume is reduced somewhat, which would be disadvantageous in high-performance work situations and competitive sports. However, lower levels of protein intake, 50 to 60 gm a day, which are much be-

low intakes for athletes and men engaged in hard physical labor, have not been shown to affect adversely the performance of persons who are *already trained.*[15]

Diets During Physical Training

Nutrition is an important feature of any training program. Education of coaches and athletes is needed as to both nutritional needs and the role of different foods in the diet. A study of Australian Olympic athletes showed great variability in their diets and in their nutrition knowledge. Intakes of some nutrients were much higher than is required, particularly protein, calcium, and vitamin C, and although these are usually harmless, the diets would be uneconomic. Some diets were below recommended levels of thiamin if the large energy need of the athletes is taken into account. Records in the competition showed that those whose thiamin intake was adequate placed better, some winning medals, in comparison with the ones whose diets were suboptimal in thiamin content.[17]

During training there is an increased need for protein, in the order of 2 gm per kilogram of body weight. Muscle tissue must be built, and there is an increase of plasma protein and of iron-containing muscle and blood proteins. During very strenuous, stressful physical work the red blood cells become fragile and there is a transient anemia that is corrected after about two weeks of training[18] if the diet is adequate in protein and iron reserves are normal.

The higher energy needs of physical activity must be met, but there is often some loss of body weight and a shift in body composition toward more lean and less fat. This is seen in both military recruits and athletes in training. On the other hand, body weight is apt to increase in persons who are below average weight at the time training begins. Along with increased energy requirements there are increased needs for the B vitamins (see Chapter 7 and Appendix).

The diet must be adequate in all essential nutrients, but there is no evidence that supernormal intakes of nutrients (except as cited above) will do anything to improve work capacity.[15] There have been hopeful claims for exotic foods such as royal jelly, mysterious benefits have been ascribed to wheat germ oil and lecithin, and a number of "ergogenic" substances have been tested with a view toward expanding the creatine phosphate pool (glycine, gelatin [which is one-fourth glycine] and creatine *per se*). Salts of the nonessential amino acid, aspartic acid, have also been suggested as improving neuromuscular excitability. None of these has proved to be of benefit in carefully controlled studies. A good diet—one based on meat, milk, fish, poultry and eggs, whole grain cereals, legumes and nuts, leafy green vegetables, and other vegetables and fruits—will meet all the nutritional requirements of athletes and persons engaged in hard physical labor. Vitamin pills and special supplements are not needed and should not be relied upon because they may lull the individual into thinking he has met his nutritional needs when in reality he may still be lacking in protein and minerals.

Feeding Just Before and During Work

Industrial experience indicates that frequent feeding is beneficial to work output, which may be due either to meal spacing or to the physical and psychological benefit of rest periods. In any case, more frequent intake of smaller amounts of food may be desirable (Chapter 18). Omission of breakfast does lead to poorer work performance, and blood sugar falls to undesirably low levels with continued deprivation of food.

Eating before athletic competitions

has been a subject of lively controversy. Small balanced meals of 500 to 800 kcal have not been shown to have any adverse effect on a variety of athletic performances conducted in a test situation. The tension and stress of game competition may be another matter, and the experience of seasoned coaches and athletes is a good practical guide. There is general agreement that high protein meals are undesirable just before competition. The usual recommendation is to eat a light balanced meal high in carbohydrate, which seems a sensible approach.

The American Association for Health, Physical Education and Recreation offers the following suggestions for a meal to be eaten three to four hours before competition:[19] one serving of roasted or broiled meat or poultry; one serving of mashed potatoes or a baked potato or one-half cup of macaroni, rice, etc.; one serving of vegetables; one cup of skim milk; one teaspoon of fat spread; two teaspoons of jelly or other sweet; one serving of fruit or juice; one serving of sugar cookies or plain cake. Take one or two cups of extra beverages and salt the food well.

This group also suggests that a commercial or home-prepared formula may be substituted for a normal meal and is preferred by some athletes. However, these formulas are usually based on milk plus added milk solids, and so are high in lactose content, which sugar is not well tolerated by many Oriental and African populations and some others (Chapter 13).

Coffee and tea are best omitted except by people who are thoroughly habituated to their use. Alcohol is quite deleterious to coordination and judgment.

During competition that involves much sweating, it is essential that water losses be replaced. Sweat is less concentrated in minerals than is plasma, and the fluid used to replace it should be also (Chapter 10). In short-term sports, salt is not a problem, and the fluid given could be water or sweetened lemonade. However, for continued high work output or in severe heat, salt will be needed. Since salt absorption is improved if glucose is present for absorption at the same time, workers and athletes in endurance events should take some carbohydrate as well as salt and water. For this purpose a 0.2 percent salt solution can be drunk or used as the base of a flavored, sweetened beverage, or carbohydrate may be taken in the form of hard candy or fruit jellies along with the salt solution. Workers and climbers may prefer a snack of dried fruits and salted crackers or chips with water or an accustomed beverage. The important consideration is replacement of water and salt, not the form in which these are given.

QUESTIONS AND PROBLEMS

1. What are the advantages of exercise? How does exercise affect body weight? Food intake? Fitness?

2. What factors affect work capacity? What is meant by maximal oxygen uptake? Distinguish between aerobic and anaerobic work. How should work and rest cycles be spaced?

3. How much additional energy intake will be required by an athlete? A worker in heavy industry? (Consult the tables in Chapter 2.) Do all sports have high energy demands? Make a list of high- and low-energy cost recreations. How much of your time is spent in activities requiring more energy than in walking?

4. What is the fuel for muscular work? How is this determined? Define RQ and tell how it is measured. How much glycogen is present in muscle and what affects this amount? Of what importance is muscle glycogen? Liver glycogen?

5. What effect does nutritional deficiency have on work performance? On fitness and training? Why does dehydration have serious effects on per-formance? How is dehydration prevented?

6. Make up a menu for a meal to be eaten three to four hours before a sports event. Devise a liquid formula from inexpensive ingredients that would provide about the same nutrients.

REFERENCES

1. Pollock, M. L., et al.: Effects of walking on body composition and cardiovascular function of middle-aged men. J. Appl. Physiol., *30*:126, 1971.
2. Kuta, I., Parizkova, J., and Dycka, J.: Muscle strength and lean body mass in old men. J. Appl. Physiol., 29:168, 1970.
3. McDonough, J. R., Kusumi, F., and Bruce, R. A.: Variations in maximal oxygen with physical activity in middle-aged men. Circulation, *41*:743, 1970.
4. Chalmers, J., and Ho, K. C.: Geographical variations in senile osteoporosis. The association with physical activity. J. Bone, Joint Surg., 52:667, 1970.
5. Gendel, E. S.: Pregnancy, fitness and sports. J. Amer. Med. Assoc., *201*:751, 1967.
6. Karvonen, M. J.: Women and men at work. World Health, p. 3, January, 1971.
7. Kreitler, H., and Kreitler, S.: Movement and aging: A psychological approach. Med. and Sport, *4*:302, 1970.
8. Huenemann, R. L., et al.: Teen-agers; activities and attitudes towards activity. J. Amer. Dietet. Assoc., *51*:433, 1967.
9. McNaughton, J. W., and Cahn, A. J.: A study of the food intake and activity of a group of urban adolescents. Brit. J. Nutr., *24*:331, 1970.
10. Mitchell, J. H., and Blomqvist, G.: Maximal oxygen uptake. New Eng. J. Med., *284*:1018, 1971.
11. Anderson, H. T., and Barkue, H.: Iron deficiency and muscular work performance. Scand. J. Lab. Clin. Invest., 25:supp 114, 1970.
12. Durnin, J. V. G. A., and Passmore, R.: *Energy, Work and Leisure.* London, Heinemann Educ. Books, Ltd., 1967.
13. Edwards, H. T., Thorndike, A., Jr., and Dill, D. B.: The energy requirement in strenuous muscular exercise. New Eng. J. Med., *213*:532, 1935.
14. Åstrand, P. O.: Diet and athletic performance. Fed. Proc., *26*:1772, 1967, and Nutr. Today, *3*(2):9, 1968.
15. Mayer, J., and Bullen, B.: Nutrition and athletic performance. Physiol. Rev., *40*:369, 1960.
16. Slocum, D. B., et al.: Wrestling and weight

control. J. Amer. Med. Assoc., *201*:541, 1967.

17. Steel, J. E.: A nutritional study of Australian olympic athletes. Med. J. Australia, *2*:119, 1970.

18. Yoshimura, H.: Anemia during physical training (sports anemia). Nutr. Rev., *28*: 251, 1970.

19. American Assoc. Health, Physical Education and Recreation: *Nutrition for Athletes: A Handbook for Coaches.* Washington, D.C., 1971.

SUPPLEMENTARY READING

Ahrens, R. A., Bishop, C. L., and Berdanier, C. D.: Effect of age and dietary carbohydrate source on the responses of rats to forced exercise. J. Nutr., *102*:241, 1972.

Asprey, G. M., Alley, L. E., and Tuttle, W. W.: Effect of eating at various times on subsequent performances in the one-mile freestyle swim. Res. Quart., *39*:231, 1968.

Bailey, D. A., et al.: Vitamin C supplementation related to physiological response to exercise in smoking and nonsmoking subjects. Amer. J. Clin. Nutr., *23*:905, 1970.

Celejowa, I., and Homa, M.: Food intake, nitrogen, and energy balance in Polish weight lifters, during a training camp. Nutr. Metab., *12*:259, 1970.

Chávez, A., Martinez, C., and Bourges, H.: Nutrition and development of infants from poor rural areas. 2. Nutritional level and physical activity. Nutr. Rep. Int'l., *5*:139, 1972.

Consolazio, C. F., and Johnson, H. L.: Dietary carbohydrate and work capacity. Amer. J. Clin. Nutr., *25*:85, 1972.

Covell, B., Eldin, N., and Passmore, R.: Energy expenditure of young men during the weekend. Lancet, *1*:727, 1965.

Issekutz, B., Jr.: Interrelationships of free fatty acids, lactic acid, and glucose in muscle metabolism. In Briskey, E. J., Cassena, R. G., and Marsh, B. B. (eds.): *The Physiology and Biochemistry of Muscle as a Food,* Vol. 2. Madison, University of Wisconsin Press, 1970.

Mayer, J.: Nutrition, exercise and cardiovascular disease. Fed. Proc., *26*:1768, 1967; What are champions made of? Family Health, *4*:24, 1972.

Mitchell, J. W., Nadel, E. R., and Stolwijk, J. A. J.: Respiratory weight losses during exercise. J. Appl. Physiol., *32*:474, 1972.

Osnes, J., and Hermansen, L.: Acid-base balance after maximal exercise of short duration. J. Appl. Physiol., *32*:59, 1972.

Skubic, V., and Kodgkins, J.: Energy expenditure of women participants in selected individual sports. J. Appl. Physiol., *21*:133, 1966.

Westerman, R.: Fluid and electrolyte replacement in sweating athletes. J. Amer. Med. Assoc., *212*:1713, 1970.

Nutrition Reviews

Alcohol metabolism during rest and exercise. *24*:239, 1966.

The effect of exercise on serum lipids. *25*:197, 1967.

Dietary influence on physical and behavioral development of rats. *25*:280, 1967.

Exercise and gastrointestinal absorption in human beings. *26*:167, 1968.

Calories and activity in infants. *26*:239, 1968.

Physical training and cardiovascular status. *27*: 103, 1969.

Exercise and cholesterol catabolism. *28*:211, 1970.

Responses of rat heart muscle to exercise. *29*:116, 1971.

Diet, exercise, and endurance. *30*:86, 1972.

twenty-two

Dental Health, Nutrition, and Diet

Dental ill health is one of the most widespread and costly diseases with a nutrition component in this country. Besides untold suffering from toothaches and embarrassment from missing front teeth, the total dental bill in the United States since 1970 has been over four billion dollars a year.

Understanding of the complex issues of the two most important causes of dental disease, dental decay and periodontal (gum) disease, has greatly progressed in the past few decades. Awareness of the factors involved in dental ill-health is an important step toward appreciation and maintenance of healthy teeth and gums. There is a double relationship between oral health and nutrition in that, first, good nutrition is important for developing and maintaining healthy and sound teeth and gum structures and, in turn, healthy dental structures are needed so that an adequate diet may be consumed at all ages (see Fig. 22–1).

What exactly is dental disease? Why are "permanent" teeth lost? How can tooth loss and cavities be prevented, and how does diet play a role in this? In order to answer these questions, this chapter reviews the current concepts regarding the causes of dental decay and periodontal disease, with special emphasis on the role of dietary factors.

A look at the enormity of the dental disease problem in the United States is important here. Of similar concern is the problem of availability of adequate acute and preventive dental care services for all segments of the population. This is reflected in the many statistics which point out that dental problems are most prevalent and severe in the lower socio-economic groups.

Evidence of the spread of both dental decay and periodontal disease and their secondary result, loss of natural teeth, is documented in statistics such as the following:

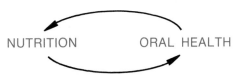

Figure 22–1. Good nutrition is necessary for oral health, and oral health is necessary for good nutrition.

1. Over 20 million Americans have lost all their teeth.

2. According to present rates, one out of every five Americans by the age of 45 will need dentures.

3. At least half of those who are 65 or older have *no* natural teeth left.

4. People with low family income and minimal education tend to lose teeth earlier and more frequently than people with higher earnings and levels of education.

5. There is an estimated number of one billion unfilled cavities in the American population today (an average of nearly six per person with teeth).

6. The cost of treatment for dental disease (seven billion dollars a year) requires one-ninth of the family health dollar.

7. Half the children under 15 in the United States have never been to a dentist (up to 80 percent of this group living in poverty areas).

8. One-third of the entire population receive no dental care except, possibly, emergency procedures for relief from pain.

9. In children under the age of five, one out of ten has eight or more unfilled cavities. The incidence of decayed, missing, or filled teeth ("DMF") then rises rapidly in the ages six to nine, slightly less rapidly to age 15, and again is high during the teen years.

Thus there appears to be a pattern of neglect (including nutrition neglect) surrounding oral health, leading to painful teeth and unhealthy gums. These in turn result in tooth loss and need for artificial replacements for normal tooth functions.

DEVELOPMENTAL ANATOMY OF THE TOOTH, AND ROLE OF NUTRITION

Nutrition plays an important part in future tooth development even prior to birth. The genetic make-up of the individual provides the pattern for the tooth and other oral development, but this is only a pattern. Unless the environment supplies adequate nutrients, the genetic potential is not realized. Thus the pregnant mother must receive generous supplies of calcium, protein, iron, and vitamins, especially A, C, and D, for good oral development (see other sections on these subjects). Examples of how specific nutrients are related to tooth development are the following:

1. Vitamin D aids in absorption and utilization of calcium, promoting the deposition of both calcium and phosphorus in teeth. Excessive vitamin D in pregnant animals leads to badly shaped jaws in the offspring, with resultant faulty bite or malocclusion.

2. Vitamins C and A affect the functional activities of the formative cells. Vitamin C is important for calcification of *dentin* (the inner tooth structure), and vitamin A is necessary for optimal calcification and development of *enamel* (the outer coat of the tooth).

3. In animal studies, specific nutritional deficiencies, or vitamin excesses in some cases, cause defective development of oral structures—for example, cleft palate seen in offspring when maternal diets are deficient in vitamin E, vitamin A, a number of the B vitamins, and many minerals.

4. Low protein and correspondingly high carbohydrate in the diet of pregnant rats has been shown to be associated with reduction in the size of molars, delay in the eruption of certain teeth, and increased susceptibility to carious lesions.

Thus in experimental animals, there are demonstrated relationships between nutritional factors and microscopic structure, chemical composition, tooth shape and size, eruption time, and susceptibility to caries, as well as to jaw malformations.

Although specific oral and dental malformations as a result of specific nutritional deficiencies have not been experimentally demonstrated in humans, optimal development and size and shape of the teeth are undoubtedly related to the intake of a balanced and adequate diet. The very important role of a specific nutrient, fluoride, in tooth development will be discussed later in the chapter (see also Chap. 12).

The basic structure of the tooth and adjacent gum area is shown in Figure 22–2. The tooth is composed of four separate tissues:

Enamel, the outer layer, is the most durable of all body tissues. It is primarily (95 percent) inorganic in nature, with its major constituents being calcium, phosphorus, magnesium, and carbonate. It can function as a semipermeable membrane.

Dentin (the major part of core of the hard portion of the tooth) is 80 percent inorganic, composed mainly of calcium and phosphorus. It extends almost the entire length of the tooth, and is covered by enamel on the crown, and by cementum on the roots. Unlike enamel, it is a very sensitive portion of the tooth.

Cementum is also a calcified tissue which is presumed to be similar in composition to bone and dentin. It acts as a surface for the attachment of the fibers (periodontal ligaments) that hold the tooth to the surrounding tissues.

Pulp, the soft part in the tooth's center, is a vital tissue containing nerves, lymph, blood vessels, and fibrous tissue. It extends for about four-fifths of the length of the tooth, with communication to the general nutritional and nervous systems through the root.

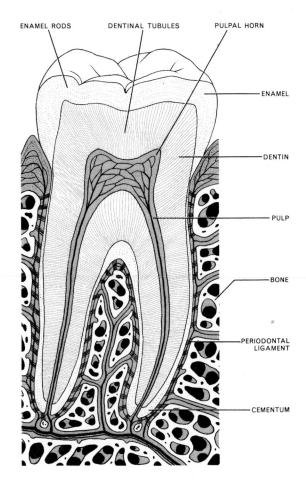

Figure 22–2. The anatomy of the tooth and surrounding structures. (From Morrey, L. W., and Nelsen, R. J.: *Dental Science Handbook.* Washington, D.C., Superintendent of Documents, 1970. Copyright by the American Dental Association. Reprinted by permission.)

ENAMEL RODS   DENTINAL TUBULES   PULPAL HORN

ENAMEL

DENTIN

PULP

BONE

PERIODONTAL LIGAMENT

CEMENTUM

The *periodontal tissues* make up the gums and the tissues which hold the teeth in place. They contain much connective tissue.

Not only *permanent* teeth, but also the *deciduous* or "baby" teeth, the teeth which are lost before the permanent teeth erupt, are important. If these primary teeth are lost too early through neglect or any other reason, the spacing of the permanent teeth may be affected, and there may be irregularities in their proper positioning. A diagram of the permanent teeth is seen in Figure 22–3.

DENTAL CARIES

The two major causes of the all-too-common problems of dental ill health

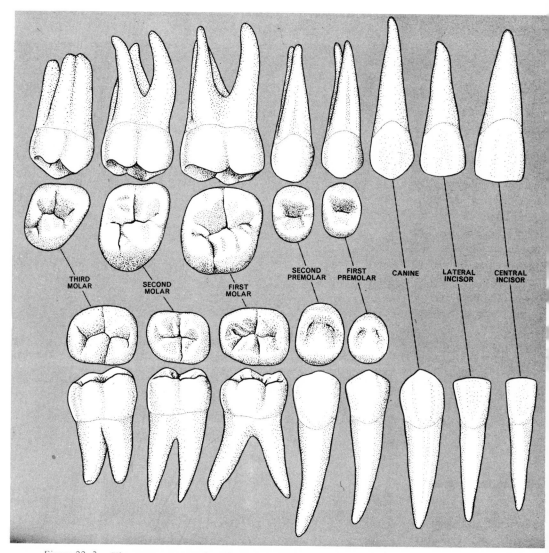

Figure 22–3. The permanent teeth. The incisors are for cutting; the premolars and molars are for grinding food. The canine teeth are used primarily to tear or shred food. (From Morrey, L. W., and Nelsen, R. J.: *Dental Science Handbook.* Washington, D. C., Superintendent of Documents, 1970. Copyright by the American Dental Association. Reprinted by permission.)

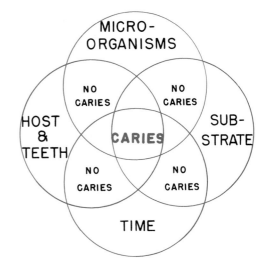

Figure 22–4. The four circles represent the factors involved in the formation of dental caries. All four factors must be acting together (overlapping of the circles) for caries to occur. (From Newbrun, E.: *Etiology of Dental Caries.* San Francisco, University of California, 1971.)

and subsequent tooth loss are *dental caries* (from the Greek word for "rottenness") or "cavities" as they are generally known, and *periodontal disease* (disease of the gums and jaw structures which hold the teeth), the first stage of which is *gingivitis* or gum inflammation. A severe form of gum disease is commonly known as "pyorrhea."

This section will summarize what is presently known about the mechanisms of these problems as they relate to the role of diet and nutrition.

Tooth loss prior to age 35 is primarily due to dental caries. The cause of dental caries is related to the combined role of four major factors—characteristics of the *host* where the teeth are present, actions of specific *bacteria* in the mouth, the presence of certain *substrates* in the diet which are needed for the bacterial actions, and the passage of *time* necessary for the development of caries.

Dental caries has been termed one of the oldest diseases of man: wall paintings depicting dental problems of Cro-Magnon man (22,000 years ago) have been found. Early theories on the cause of dental decay ranged from invasion by worms, to "gangrene" beginning in the inside of the tooth, to an imbalance of the four bodily "humours." Aristotle noticed that soft

sweet figs adhered to teeth, putrefied, and produced damage.

In 1600 an English writer[1] noted a relationship between carbohydrate intake and poor teeth, with the following observation, "overuse of most confections and sugar plummes . . . rotteth the teeth and maketh them look black." In the early nineteenth century, a chemical theory on the origin of dental caries was postulated. It related carious teeth to "a chemical agent" (acid) produced when food putrefied on tooth enamel. Then in the mid-nineteenth century, with the early use of the microscope, bacteria were seen on teeth, and the ground was laid for the presently accepted cause of dental caries (see Fig. 22–5). Ever since Miller in 1890 first demonstrated that the action of salivary bacteria on carbohydrates caused decalcification of enamel, this fact of acid formation from bacterial action on ingested carbohydrates has seldom been questioned. An example of a study which provided proof of the effect of food is one made in 1938 which showed a significant difference in the number of dental caries between two groups of children—one group who had a balanced diet with no in-between-meal sweets, and who had no caries; and the second group with a poor diet

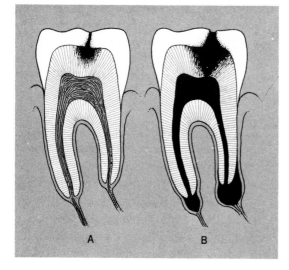

Figure 22-5. The progress of decay: **A,** The bacteria have penetrated the enamel and attacked the softer dentin. **B,** The bacteria have penetrated the dentin and killed the pulp, and infection has spread to the root. At this point the tooth may have to be removed. (From Morrey, L. W., and Nelsen, R. J.: *Dental Science Handbook.* Washington, D.C., Superintendent of Documents, 1970. Copyright by the American Dental Association. Reprinted by permission.)

(specifically low in vegetables, fruits, and vitamin D) and large amounts of sweets daily, who had an extremely high incidence of caries.[2] This study is one of the many that have associated dietary factors—such as type of food, clearance rate of food, frequency of eating, and "detergent" (leading to reduction in oral debris) effects of foods— with caries and documented the diet's specific effects on caries. Many more could be cited. We will study each of the factors known to cause dental caries.

The Effect of Physical Properties of Foods

Physical properties of foods, such as adhesiveness, solubility, and viscosity, may modify the caries-producing potential of foods. However, few good studies on humans have been done concerning this subject. A summary of certain physical and chemical factors which are thought to influence caries development is presented in Table 22–1. The "cariogenic factors" in foods mentioned in the table are of major importance and will be explained in detail.

The Effect of Food on the Microbiology of the Oral Cavity

Plaque is an important term in discussing dental caries. It is the layer of foreign material which accumulates over a period of weeks on even a cleaned tooth surface, to which it develops a tenacious attachment. It is composed primarily of bacteria and their by-products (see Fig. 22–6). Sugars diffuse easily into the plaque. The plaque is colonized by several types of bacteria, both *cariogenic* (those which cause caries and which live mainly on sucrose and other carbohydrates from food) and not. The most important cariogenic bacteria are streptococcal types. These bacteria ferment dietary carbohydrates to form, principally, lactic acid (see Fig. 22–6) which, at susceptible sites, initiates the carious lesion by demineralizing the enamel surface.

Caries do not develop in germ-free animals. Antibiotics when fed to animals are effective in reducing the incidence and severity of caries. In addition, children receiving ongoing antibiotic therapy effective against streptococcal bacteria (for example, in certain heart conditions) are known to have fewer

*Table 22-1. Interplay of Physical and Chemical Factors in Food Cariogenicity**

Highly retentive

Slowly soluble

High in cariogenic factors

Low in caries inhibitory factors

Maximal cariogenicity

Nonretentive

Rapidly soluble

Low in cariogenic factors

High in caries inhibitory factors

Minimal cariogenicity

*From Caldwell, R. C.: J. Dent. Res., *49*:1293, 1970.

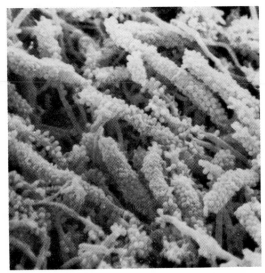

Figure 22–6. Dental plaque, shown here in a scanning electron micrograph, is composed of countless bacteria and contributes to the tooth decay process. (From Jones, S. J.: Dent. Abst., *17*:8, 1972.)

caries in their teeth than children not receiving such antibiotics.

Further evidence to implicate the role of bacteria in caries is that specific bacteria have been isolated and cultivated from carious lesions. By inoculating them in germ-free animals, caries have developed. *Streptococcus mutans* and *Streptococcus sanguis* are examples of two common caries-causing bacteria. For many years Lactobacillus strains were thought to be the culprits in caries. However, it has since been shown that (1) they account for only 1/10,000 of all dental flora and (2) they are found in carious lesions more as a result than as a cause of the lesions.

Thus dental caries is basically a local disease of the teeth subject to the influence of those dietary components which provide the caries-causing bacteria with their necessary growth material, including a dietary source of essential amino acids, vitamins, and minerals in addition to carbohydrate. Caries is indeed a type of bacterial infection.

The caries-producing strains also have the ability to convert sucrose (or its components glucose or fructose) into the extracellular polysaccharide, *dextran* (a complex carbohydrate), and others into an intracellular polysaccharide, *amylopectin*. The dextran so produced is a sticky, insoluble, relatively inert substance that causes plaque to adhere to the teeth and appears to serve as a barrier to buffer systems in the saliva which might otherwise neutralize the acids formed by the bacteria in the plaque. During periods in which the diet is sugar-free, the *intra*cellular polysaccharide of the plaque is available for fermentation and maintenance of acid production. This production of polysaccharides by specific bacteria has been shown to be correlated with caries incidence. In fact, organisms which have lost their property to make the insoluble extracellular polysaccharides are no longer caries-producing.[3]

The Role of Fermentable Carbohydrates in Dental Caries, with Emphasis on Sucrose

The association of food and caries has been made ever since it was observed that caries occur almost exclusively on tooth surfaces where self-cleansing mechanisms are least effective. Food is a necessary factor in allowing the cariogenic, dextran-producing plaque bacteria to actually begin causing caries. Dietary sucrose, specifically, is used by the plaque bacteria to produce and support caries development.

With the aid of carbohydrates to ferment, the plaque bacteria will produce an acid medium (of about a pH of 4.5 to 5.5) by the formation of lactic acid, and to a lesser extent, acetic, propionic, and butyric acid. The drop in plaque pH may remain for up to two hours after sucrose ingestion. Lactic

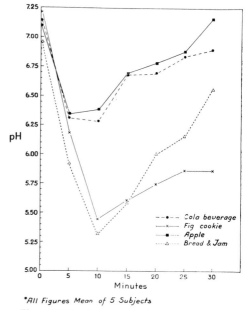

Plaque pH After Eating Different Foods

*All Figures Mean of 5 Subjects

Figure 22–7. Some examples of the changes in plaque pH following eating of different foods. (From Ludwig, T. G., and Bibby, B. G.: J. Dent. Res., *36*:56, 1957.)

acid is a much stronger acid than acetic or proprionic acid, and therefore probably more effective in enamel demineralization. An example of pH change observed in plaque after the ingestion of various foods is seen in Figure 22–7.

The important role of sucrose in the etiology of dental decay has been elucidated by epidemiological and chemical studies as well as controlled studies on animals and humans. For example:

1. During World War II, sugar consumption in Europe was severely restricted, and caries dropped significantly two years thereafter. When the sugar intake increased again, caries recurred at previous levels.

2. Rampant caries (especially in the front teeth, a rare location) have been observed with frequency in children who fall asleep either sucking on a pacifier soaked with sugar solution, or on a bottle of apple juice or milk with sugar (see Fig. 22–8).

3. A Scandinavian study (the Vipeholm study) is a classic which compared cariogenicity of various foods in humans.[4] For example, subjects who ate sticky toffee several times a day had 12 times as much caries development as controls without this sugar intake. A sugar solution, however, produced only twice as many carious surfaces as in controls, demonstrating the importance of clearance factors (how long the food stays in the mouth).

4. In one *in vitro* study, sucrose was reported to be the only sugar that would support plaque formation by caries-conducive *streptococci*.

5. People with a genetic defect known as hereditary fructose intolerance will avoid all sucrose- and fructose-containing foods because eating such foods gives unpleasant symptoms (nausea, vomiting, etc.). Their dental health is excellent, and their teeth often show total absence of dental caries.[5]

6. In one small South Atlantic island, dental decay was virtually nonexistent before the advent of Westernized foods and sweets. Twenty years later, after

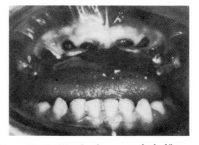

Figure 22–8. Teeth of a two and a half-year-old child who frequently received apple juice in a baby bottle. Note the nearly complete destruction of upper teeth by caries. (Lower teeth are thought to have been protected because of the position of the tongue and lower lip during sucking.) (From Kaplan, H., and Rabbach, V. P.: Apple Juice and Dental Caries. Bambino. Children's Hospital Medical Center, Oakland, California, Winter 1971.)

the inhabitants began consuming an average of 0.5 kg of sugar a week, one-half of permanent molars were carious in those 20 years old and under.

7. England has had documented increase in consumption of sugar of from 20 pounds to 110 pounds per person over the last 100 years, and there has been a nearly parallel rise in caries prevalence.

8. Widely different cavity counts were found in eight countries, and sugar consumption followed the same pattern (with highest caries incidence and sugar intake found in the United States and Central and South America).[6]

9. Hopewood House, a children's home in Australia, gave a diet completely free of sugar and other refined carbohydrates, and the children there had a caries prevalence of about 10 percent that of the general population of that age group in Australia.

10. Sucrose supports the most rapidly progressive caries in the hamster and rat in multiple studies. Fructose, lactose, and, lastly, glucose, also result in caries formation, but with more time than is necessary for sucrose.

11. Maltose, lactose, fructose, and glucose can be used by the plaque bacteria for synthesis of cell wall, capsular,

and intracellular polysaccharides, as well as in forming organic acids; but, unlike sucrose, they *cannot* be utilized in the creation of *extra*cellular polysaccharides. Starches probably cannot diffuse into plaque because of the relatively large size of the molecules. See Figure 22–9 for a diagrammatic summary of the metabolism of ingested carbohydrates.

Thus, the integral role of sucrose in caries is documented. Other foods have also been studied as to their relative potential to produce caries. For example, any fruit has been classed as potentially harmful if it has a pH under 4.5. Of course, certain low-acid fruits, apples, for example, also have a "detergent" effect, a positive effect shared by such foods as raw carrots and celery, and this is thought by some dentists to be helpful in the prevention of caries by "scraping away" some of the plaque accumulation on the teeth.

Different grains in (unsweetened) cereal products have also been studied. Corn was found to result in the largest

amount of enamel dissolution by plaque bacteria, and wheat and oat cereals were found to cause the least.

One further observation pertaining to the relationship of nutrition and dental health has been that in extremely poorly nourished populations, for example, overpopulated countries, the incidence of caries has been low. This observation has sometimes been interpreted as evidence for the *lack* of necessary association between a good diet and good teeth. However, these populations had *negligible*, if any, sucrose in their diet. The lack of this substance permitted their teeth, although probably less than optimally developed and shaped with a lifelong history of malnutrition, to remain free of the effects of the cariogenic plaque bacteria dependent on sucrose, and thus, free of caries.

The Role of the Time Factor and the Frequency of Eating

The time factor is included in Figure 22–4, which depicts the multifactorial

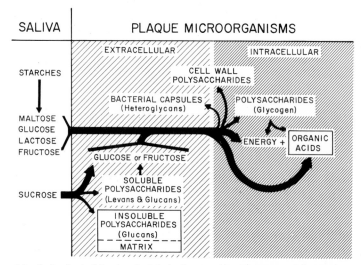

Figure 22–9. Metabolic fate of ingested carbohydrates, showing both extracellular and intracellular end products. Heavy arrows represent major pathways, and end products which are particularly harmful to the teeth are shown in the boxes. (From Newbrun, E.: *Etiology of Dental Caries.* San Francisco, University of California, 1971.)

etiology of dental caries, for three basic reasons:

1. A beginning small eroded spot (just barely detectable) will progress to clinical caries on an average of anywhere from one to two years, under normal conditions. If an early eroded spot, decalcified enamel, for example, starts, and then careful preventive measures are undertaken (dietary and oral hygiene measures: see later section), the development of the caries may be halted but the eroded spot can never revert to normal.

2. The "age" of the tooth plays a part in caries susceptibility. A tooth is most likely to develop caries from two to four years after eruption. This may have to do with the fact that complete enamel "maturation" takes this long, and when the enamel is fully matured it is more resistant to caries formation. This helps to explain why young children and teenagers (with fairly new deciduous and permanent teeth, respectively) have higher caries rates than other ages.

3. A primary factor in the onset of caries is the frequent between-meal eating of sweets, rather than the total sugar intake. The *more often* the sweets are in contact with the teeth, the *longer* the exposure to acid decalcification, and the *worse* the caries incidence will be (see Fig. 22–10).

This overriding importance of the frequency of exposure to sweets was first documented by the Vipeholm study,[4] where the outstanding difference between groups was in the frequency of eating. That is, the groups that ate between meals had more caries than the control groups who ate only at mealtimes, *regardless* of the *total* amount of sugar intake per day. This applies to sticky sweets and candy and to the more rapidly cleared sucrose solutions (such as soft drinks). For example, caries have been produced in humans in *three weeks* after mouth rinses with a sucrose solution nine times a day.

Many researchers are in the process

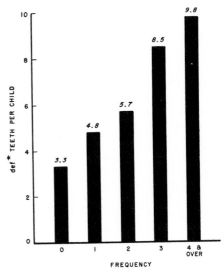

* Includes extracted primary molars.

Figure 22–10. The effect of between-meal eating on caries activity in children. This shows that the more snacks children ate, the higher was the incidence of decay. (From Weiss, R. L., and Trithart, A. H.: Amer. J. Public Health, *50*:1097, 1960.)

of looking for safe and acceptable sugar substitutes which will *not* be a culprit in dental caries and which might be used in snacks and desserts in place of sucrose.

Starches are not totally immune from suspicion as caries producers. They may be metabolized by certain (non-streptococcal) oral bacteria, to polysaccharides, which then may become part of the plaque matrix, undergo breakdown by caries-causing bacteria, and thus institute the decay process.

And, finally, if sucrose itself cannot be avoided in the diet, it should be removed from the teeth as quickly as possible by prompt oral hygiene measures. This is because as long as it is present in the plaque the bacterial enzymes will continue to utilize it to form plaque matrix material (insoluble polysaccharide) and fructose, the latter being then fermented by the plaque to form organic acids. These reactions occur most rapidly in the first few hours after sucrose ingestion.

The Role of Fluoride

Fluoride is the only dietary trace element so far proved to be effective in producing decay-resistant teeth in humans. The beneficial effects of fluoride on teeth have been known for over 70 years, and there have been over 10,000 articles on fluoride and dental health printed in the world's scientific journals. At present, fluoridation programs reach over 150 million people throughout the world.

The incidence of dental caries in both the deciduous and the permanent teeth is reduced about *60 percent* in children who drink water containing about one part per million (1 mg per

liter) of fluorine throughout the period of tooth development. See Figure 22–11 for the results of one important study documenting the results of fluoridation in a community. The caries decrement is smaller when fluoridated water consumption (or dietary fluoride supplementation) is started at a later age. There are also indications that caries inhibition attributable to fluoridated water is not merely temporary but continues throughout adult life. Most foods contain only trace amounts of fluorides, with the average American diet, exclusive of water, containing 0.2 to 0.5 mg of fluoride. Inclusion of water containing 1 ppm of fluoride thus raises the intake to an estimated 1.5 to 2.0 mg of fluoride per day. The safety of fluoridation has been well documented by the World Health Organization. Mottling of teeth does occur with overuse of fluoride, but only in the years from one to six. (See also Chap. 12.) Fluoride is cleared very rapidly by the kidneys; thus small amounts do not accumulate in the body in sufficient quantities to produce any health hazard.

The mode of action of fluorides in preventing dental caries is unique, and is related to its accumulation in enamel. It renders the structure of the enamel of the tooth more stable and less soluble to acid. It may also act as an enzyme inhibitor on the bacteria of the plaque.[7] There appears to be a lesser protective effect on permanent teeth posteruptively than pre-eruptively, with the teeth most recently erupted (still not totally "matured") being benefited most. No posteruptive effect on baby teeth has been yet documented. Thus in order to protect the *deciduous* teeth, fluoride must be ingested during the *first year* of life.

The use of fluorine tablets does not appear to be quite as efficacious as fluoridation of water, perhaps primarily because they rely on daily cooperation of parent and child. In one study, only 50 percent of families continued giving the pills for the recommended number

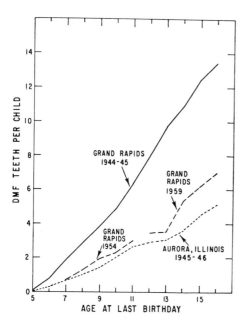

Figure 22–11. This diagram shows the beneficial results of a 15-year period of fluoridation in Grand Rapids, Michigan. It presents the dental caries experience in terms of decayed, missing, and filled teeth ("DMF") per child for Grand Rapids, both before and 15 years after fluoridation, and includes caries data from Aurora, Illinois, a community with natural water fluoridation, for comparison. (From Arnold, F. A., Jr., et al.: J. Amer. Dent. Assoc., *65*:780, 1962.)

of years, and this is probably a generous estimate. Fluoride tablets, which require a doctor's prescription, are more costly than community water fluoridation, which costs only five to 15 cents per person per year.

The use of fluorides applied topically to the teeth is possible in a practical way by using fluorine-containing toothpastes. They have a significant, although low, preventive value (giving about 20 percent reduction in incidence of new carious surfaces). Fluoride applications to the teeth are known to be of preventive value but require a dental assist.

Studies have shown that there are definite reductions in family dental bills after water fluoridation programs at the United States Public Health Service recommended level have begun. For example, the cost of initial dental care of a typical child dropped from $32 to $14 after fluoridation was instituted in one community, and the yearly

maintenance cost fell from $11 to $6.[8] Similarly, the Head Start Program has found that it must pay from three to ten times as much for dental services for an enrolled child from a nonfluoridated area as it does for such services for a child from a community with fluoridation.

With so much evidence as to the usefulness and safety of fluoridation, and its unanimous recommendation by scientific bodies,* to what extent is it in use in the United States? Unfortunately, not at anywhere near 100 percent. The varying use of fluoridation in the different states in 1967 is shown in Figure 22–12. The Public Health

---

*The United States Public Health Service was the first to endorse fluoridation, in 1945. Since then it has been endorsed by the American Dental Association, the American Medical Association, the World Health Organization, the American Public Health Association, the American Institute of Nutrition, and the Food and Nutrition Board, among others.

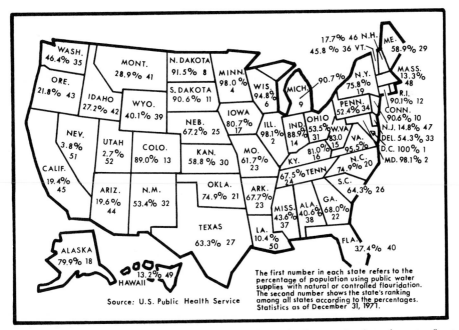

Figure 22–12.   How does your state stand on fluoridation? The first number in each state refers to the percentage of its population on public water supplies with natural or controlled fluoridation. The second number shows the state's position in a ranking of all states according to percentages. Statistics as of December 31, 1971

Service estimates that at the end of 1970, a total of 92 million Americans (out of about 206 million) were receiving fluoridated water. Eight million of that total were receiving water with fluoride found in it naturally. (It was on this type of population that initial observations noting the beneficial effects of fluoride were made.) Regarding the varying pattern of fluoridation, it was noted that in 1960–69, the prevalence of caries-free recruits in the military correlated highly with the availability of fluoride in the water supply of their community.

Further considerations regarding the practicalities of fluoridation include the following:

1. It has been estimated that about 40 percent of Americans do not have access to a community water supply. In these areas, fluoridation of school water is feasible and should be recommended, as well as dietary fluoride supplementation in the preschool years.

2. There is variability in exact water consumption of children. In one study, the mean intake of water was 470 ml at one to three years, which gradually increased to 990 ml at 10 to 12 years. Yet, in another study, an average of 300 ml of water was consumed at one year old and about 400 ml at five years old. In other words, the average intake of fluoride from water averages 0.3 to 0.4 mg a day for these children when water is fluoridated at 1 ppm. The actual fluoride intake recommended by the American Dental Association (1958) is as follows: 1 mg per day from birth to two years; 1 mg every other day from two to three years; and 1 mg a day from three years on. Thus it is seen that at most ages, even with water fluoridation, there is a case for individualized use of fluoride supplements in liquid or tablet form.

3. In hot climates, where there is a high intake of water, fluoridation concentration should be less than in colder climates.

4. The legal validity of fluoridation has been thoroughly tested in the United States in the last decades, and has been invariably confirmed. It is thus not considered a "compulsory medication," as opponents charge, but as a rightful preventive measure. At least four states (Connecticut, Minnesota, Illinois, and Delaware) have now passed legislation to require fluoridation in all community water supplies.

Countries in addition to the United States which have fluoridation in a good number of communities are Australia, Brazil, Canada, Chile, Czechoslovakia, Ireland, the Netherlands, New Zealand, and the U.S.S.R. The further use of added fluoride for drinking water will probably be rapidly increasing throughout the world.

Role of Other Nutrient Factors

It should be added that other nutrients, such as molybdenum and vanadium (as well as vitamin B-6) have been reported to help protect against caries development in the experimental animal. A variety of studies suggest but do not conclusively prove that there are relationships between caries prevalence and a wide variety of trace elements other than fluorine in either man or experimental animals. More research is needed regarding these possible relationships. The mechanisms for the role of these minerals may have to do with increasing the resistance of enamel or with changing the properties of saliva or plaque.

In animals, phosphate supplementation of food helps to decrease caries susceptibility by lowering the solubility rate of enamel, but this has not been proved in humans. There is no evidence for any direct role of calcium in decreasing caries after the tooth is formed.

Highly acid foods, such as undiluted lemon juice or soft drinks with a high phosphoric acid content, are known to be able to dissolve or etch tooth enamel after long-time contact periods. The usual short-time exposure, along with the buffering effect of saliva, probably results in little or no damage.

PERIODONTAL DISEASE AND NUTRITION

*Periodontal disease** (disease of the gums and other tissues surrounding the teeth), like caries, is an ancient malady of mankind and one still prevalent throughout the world. Tooth loss after the age of 35 in this country is usually due to the effects of periodontal disease, because it results in the loss of healthy supporting tissues for viable teeth. Periodontal disease and its effects thus worsen with increasing age, but the potential for advanced disease may start at an early age.

What are the factors which cause poor periodontal health? Local factors in the mouth, such as the state of oral cleanliness and hygiene, and, again, the effect of foods which either encourage or discourage bacterial growth at gingival (gum) margins are all-important. Rates of periodontal disease incidence are highest in populations with the poorest states of oral hygiene (for example, in countries with very few dentists, as well as in segments of the American population with limited access to dental care, as is common in low socio-economic groups). No specific environmental factors (such as sugar, as in the case of caries) have been identified as the key factors in periodontal disease, other than the state of oral cleanliness.

There have been no consistent correlations between specific nutrient intake and periodontal disease. Vitamin A and vitamin E have shown some positive correlations, but firm evidence is lacking. Certain acute periodontal problems— for example, scurvy with its bleeding gums and diseased gums often found in niacin deficiency—do stem from a lack of nutrients in the diet, but these

---

*From the two Greek words, "peri" and "odont," meaning "around tooth."

are not examples of classic periodontal disease.

Experimental studies have shown that protein starvation and magnesium deficiency may adversely affect the periodontium in man. An advanced stage of bone and periodontal destruction has been seen with protein deficiency. In addition to contributing to tissue growth and resistance, proteins are also important in endocrine function, whose hormones help in proper maintenance of periodontal tissue. Experimental magnesium lack in animals can cause imperfect development of the alveolar bone, widening of the periodontal membrane, gingival enlargement, and loosening of the teeth. In humans, iron deficiency has been shown to be related to unhealthy gingival tissues, especially in females. Other studies have suggested that fluoride has a mild but definite beneficial effect on periodontal health.[9]

In theory, calcium and phosphorus deficiency, if severe enough, could also affect the bone which helps support the tooth.

Bacterial masses, or plaque, are again key culprits in periodontal disease. The bacteria accumulations on the tooth surfaces closest to the gingival margins are implicated in this case. In addition, the subsequent accumulation of *calculus* (a mixture of minerals) occurs on the teeth and under loosened gingival margins. These factors lead to inflammation and infection of the periodontal tissues, known as *gingivitis*. This gingivitis, if untreated, is followed by loosening and destruction of the periodontal fibers or ligaments (see Fig. 22–2).

The last stage of periodontal disease is gradual resorption of the alveolar bone which supports the tooth, with consequent tooth loosening and finally, tooth loss. From this description of the less-than-welcome effects of periodontal disease, it is easy to see the effect that advanced disease will have on the diet. An affected individual will choose foods which are easy to chew but which, unfortunately, are often soft carbohydrates.

Good nutrition, then, is important in the control of gingival and periodontal disease in a preventive sense, that is, in maintaining optimally healthy tissues, resistant to disease. However, only when there is clear evidence of an acute systemic nutritional problem can it be said that nutrition has a direct effect.

Dietary control of sugars is also important here because of the incrimination of the role of bacterial plaque in the process of this problem. In addition, certain foods can be of some physical help to those affected with periodontal disease. Firm, fibrous foods may help to promote natural cleansing.

PREVENTION OF DENTAL DISEASE

Prevention must be the key to the problem of dental disease. Nutrition has been discussed as a general and specific factor. In addition, with the use of continual careful oral hygiene methods to control and to remove plaque and local irritants, most dental disease could be prevented.

Oral hygiene measures include proper tooth brushing supplemented by other cleansing aids such as dental floss, intradental cleansers, and water irrigation under pressure. If plaque is thus broken up every 24 hours, the activity of the plaque bacteria will be stopped before the underlying enamel begins to decalcify. Tooth brushing is particularly important prior to sleep, for in sleep salivary production decreases and thus there is a decrease in the natural salivary buffers which help to partially counteract the effects of the acid-producing bacteria.

The role of diet, and especially of sugars, has been discussed in detail. Control measures relating to their role include the following:

Table 22–2. "Caries-Potentiality" of Representative Foods*

Food	Total Sugar Content (Percent)	"Caries Potentiality"
Caramel	64.0	27
Honey + bread + butter	19.0	24
Honey	72.8	18
Sweet cookies (biscuits)	9.0	18
Marmalade	65.3	10
Marmalade + bread + butter	16.3	9
Ice cream	2.4	9
Potatoes (boiled)	0.8	7
Potatoes (fried)	3.9	7
White bread + butter	1.5	7
Coarse rye bread + butter	2.3	7
Milk	3.8	6
Apple	7.5	5
Orange	6.5	3
Lemonade	9.3	2
Carrot (boiled)	2.4	1

*Adapted from Dunning, J. M.: *Principles of Dental Public Health.* Cambridge, Harvard University Press, 1970. Calculated from sugar concentrations in saliva and how long they remained high after eating each specific food. In general, those with the lowest scores should be used instead of those with highest scores if optimal dental health is desired.

1. Avoid foods with the highest caries potentials (Table 22–2).
2. Use cheese, nuts, and raw vegetables and fruits instead of candy and cookies for snacks.
3. Avoid sticky candy and such candy as "all day suckers," as well as frequent soft drinks or fruit juices.
4. Consume carbohydrates mainly at meals.
5. Use a diet that provides good general nutrition, especially in children, for optimal developmental protection of the teeth.
6. Insure for all an adequate intake of fluoride either in water or supplement form.

Dental disease has been shown to be caused by factors that are accessible, controllable, and correctable, and improvement of individual dental health is within the reach of everyone, with the aid of his dentist. The amount of decay and gingival disease found is really an index of inadequate application of preventive procedures.

SUMMARY

The most important factors in individual and community dental health and the role of nutrition are summarized as follows:

1. Sucrose plays an integral role in the formation and activity of bacterial plaque, the precursor of dental disease. Decreasing the amount and frequency of sugar intake is thus a key preventive measure.

2. Fluoridation is the easiest and most effective method of caries resistance and prevention, with a decrease of up to 66 percent of caries in communities with a fluoridated water supply.

3. Increased application of oral hygiene measures to decrease accumulation and activity of plaque is important in both caries and periodontal disease control.

4. A balanced and varied general diet from infancy on (including fluoride supplements if fluoride is not in the water supply) will give the basis for tissue health and optimal resistance to dental disease.

With all these identifiable relationships between good diets, good oral cleanliness, and good teeth, it is no wonder that dentists very often take much interest in the subject of nutrition.

QUESTIONS AND PROBLEMS

1. Name the dental structures. What nutrients are found in these structures? Which other nutrients are necessary for formation of these structures?

2. Which foods are associated with a high incidence of dental caries? Which foods are helpful in preventing decay? Why?

3. Plan a lunch that may be carried from home, that provides one-third of the daily nutrient needs of an eight-year-old child and that will not foster dental caries.

4. How does fluoride aid in prevention of caries? How may fluoride be administered? Which method is most practical? What is the fluoride level of the water in your community?

REFERENCES

1. Hardwick, J. L.: Brit. Dent. J., *108*:9, 1960.
2. Read, T., and Knowles, E.: Brit. Dent. J., *64*: 185, 1938.
3. de Stoppelaar, J. D., et al.: Arch. Oral Biol., *16*:971, 1971.
4. Gustafsson, B. E., et al.: Acta Odont. Scand., *11*:232, 1954.
5. Newbrun, E.: Odont. Revy, *18*:373, 1967.
6. Dunning, J. M.: *Principles of Dental Public Health.* Cambridge, Harvard University Press, 1970.
7. Jenkins, G. N.: Internat. Dent. J., *17*:552, 1967.
8. Ast, D. B., Cons, N. C., Carlos, J. P., and Maiwald, A.: Amer. J. Pub. Health, 55:811, 1965.
9. Englander, H. R., Kesel, R. G., and Gupta, O. P.: Internat. Assoc. Dental Res. Abs., 40th general meeting, 1962.

SUPPLEMENTARY READING

General, History, and Reviews

Berman, D. S.: Dental caries — a review. Nutrition, 25:154, 1971.
Dunning, J. M.: *Principles of Dental Public Health.* Cambridge, Harvard University Press, 1970.
Morrey, L. W., and Nelsen, R. J. (eds.): *Dental Science Handbook.* Washington, D.C., Superintendent of Documents, 1970.
Newbrun, E.: *Etiology of Dental Caries.* San Francisco, University of California, 1971.
Nizel, A. E.: *The Science of Nutrition and Its Application in Clinical Dentistry.* Philadelphia, W. B. Saunders, 1967; *Nutrition in Preventive Dentistry: Science and Practice.* Philadelphia, W. B. Saunders, 1972.
Proceedings of Workshop Conference, Eastman Dental Center: Role of human foodstuffs in caries (symposium). J. Dent. Res., *49*: 1191, 1970.
Sumnicht, R. W.: Research in preventive dentistry. J. Amer. Dent. Assoc., *79*:1193, 1969.

Fluoridation

Babeaux, W. L., and Zipkin, I.: Dental aspects of the prenatal administration of fluoride. J. Oral Therap. Pharmacol., *3*:124, 1966.
Hadjimarkos, D. M.: Fluoride content of sea salt in dental caries prevention. Amer. J. Clin. Nutr., *25*:123, 1972.
Hodge, H. C., and Smith, F. A.: Effects of fluorides on bones and teeth. In Simons, J. H. (ed.): *Fluorine Chemistry IV.* New York, Academic Press, 1965.
Horowitz, H. S.: School water fluoridation. Amer. Family Physician, *1*:85, 1970; Effect of school water fluoridation on dental caries: Final results in Elk Lake, Pennsylvania

after 12 years. J. Amer. Dental Assoc., *84*:
832, 1972.

Knutson, J. W.: Water fluoridation after 25 years.
J. Amer. Dent. Assoc., *80*:765, 1970.

McClure, F. J.: *Water Fluoridation: The Search and
the Victory.* Bethesda, Maryland, National
Institutes of Health, 1970.

Sapolsky, H. M.: Science, voters, and the fluoridation controversy. Science, *162*:427, 1968.

U.S. Department of Health, Education, and Welfare: A Guide to Reading on Fluoridation.
Public Health Service Publication No.
1680. Bethesda, Maryland, 1967.

World Health Organization: *Fluorides and Human
Health.* Geneva, WHO Monograph No. 59,
1970.

of plaque polysaccharides to growth of
cariogenic microorganisms. Arch. Oral
Biol., *16*:855, 1971.

Scherp, H. W.: Dental caries: Prospects for prevention. Science, *173*:1199, 1971.

Stahl, S. S.: Nutritional influences on periodontal
disease. World Rev. Nutr. Dietet., *13*:277,
1971.

Stephan, R. M.: Effects of different types of human foods on dental health in experimental animals. J. Dent. Res., *45*:1551,
1966.

Zengo, A. N., and Mandel, I. D.: Sucrose tasting
and dental caries in man. Arch. Oral Biol.,
17:605, 1972.

Other References

Anonymous: Nutrition in oral health: Research
and practice. Dairy Council Digest, *40*:31,
1969.

Dreizen, S.: Diet and dental decay. Postgrad.
Med., *43*:233, 1968.

Glickman, I.: Periodontal disease. New Eng. J.
Med., *284*:1071, 1971.

Gordon, R. H.: Meeting dental health needs of
the aged. Amer. J. Pub. Health, *62*:385,
1972.

Parker, R. B., and Creamer, H. R.: Contribution

Nutrition Reviews

Rampant caries in the pre-school child. *24*:297,
1966.

The effect of phosphates in breakfast cereals on
dental caries. *25*:263, 1967.

Fluoride concentration in enamel and bone. *26*:
75, 1968.

Phosphates and dental caries. *26*:81, 1968.

Interactions of diet and microflora in experimental dental caries. *26*:119, 1968.

Effect of synthetic amino acid diets upon tooth
decay. *26*:145, 1968.

twenty-three

Overweight and Underweight

OVERWEIGHT

Obesity is one of our most pressing health problems. Many people accept as normal the gradual accumulation of weight which so often comes in the later years of life, disregarding the health risks that it brings with it. Some persuade themselves that they are not *much* overweight, just enough to be "pleasingly plump" and it is better to be happy than to diet. Others are embarrassed by a mountain of flesh and find it hard to get about, but seem to regard the matter as something determined by fate rather than by themselves. Not all the overweights are middle-aged or over. We have overweight young people, children, and even overweight babies.

Disadvantages and Dangers of Excess Weight

Obesity carries with it increased risk of illness and death from a number of diseases: heart disease, high blood pressure, stroke, kidney disease, gallstones, cirrhosis of the liver and, especially, diabetes. Fat people have difficulties with their feet and back because of the added burden of weight on the skeleton. They suffer from shortness of breath, especially on exertion, and have increased surgical risk. Our culture favors a lean look, so the obese are handicapped socially, in employment, and in school admission.

The health hazards that accompany overweight — increased prevalence of heart and circulatory diseases, and diabetes — are naturally increased with a larger excess of weight and with advancing years. For instance, in the 40- to 44-year-old age bracket 20 percent excess over normal weight carries with it a 30 to 40 percent increase in mortality above the expected rate, while a 40 percent excess of weight involves an 80 to 100 percent increase in mortality. Put another way, a 50-year-old man who is 50 pounds overweight has about half the life expectancy of one of the same age who is of normal weight.

Everyone should check his weight occasionally with some tables that show the normal weight for his height.

511

Tables based on the actual *average* weights of the population at various ages are not good for this purpose, because so many otherwise normal people show some degree of overweight after 40 that these figures are too high to represent the *optimum* weight so far as health is concerned. Physicians and life insurance companies now feel that, for the sake of health and longevity, it is best to weigh no more in the years after 25 or 30 than is normal for height and body build at that age. Table 23–1 gives desirable weights that men and women should maintain at 25 years of age and in later life. An individual who weighs 15 percent more than the theoretical normal for his height must be classed as mildly obese while one who is 25 percent or more overweight is grossly *obese.*

Obesity in children is common and presents special problems. It handicaps a child socially and in games or sports that involve moving mass in running or jumping. Although overweight in childhood may not carry the same predisposition to functional diseases that it does with adults, if it is not corrected and the child trained to dietary habits

that will keep weight down to normal for his height, he will very likely go on to become an obese adult. A reducing regimen for a child must be carefully planned to decrease energy intake but to furnish liberally all nutrients needed for growth — proteins, minerals, and vitamins. Although dietary restriction cannot be as drastic or weight readjustment as rapid for children as for adults, the retraining in food habits is especially important.

*Measurement and Form
of Body Fat*

Weight tables provide a convenient guide to desirable body weight, but what we are really concerned with is the amount of body fat an individual carries. A football player may be distinctly overweight for height, yet he may be not in the least obese in terms of having excess adipose tissue. Others who are underweight for height may have a larger percentage of adipose tissue than heavier people who are more physically fit. The goal of any reducing program is not to normalize

Table 23–1. Suggested Weights for Heights*

Height		Median Weight			
		Men		Women	
IN	CM	LB	KG	LB	KG
60	152			109 ± 9	49.5 ± 4
62	158			115 ± 9	52.2 ± 4
64	163	133 ± 11	60.5 ± 5	122 ± 10	55.5 ± 5
66	168	142 ± 11	64.5 ± 5	129 ± 10	58.6 ± 5
68	173	151 ± 14	68.6 ± 6	136 ± 10	61.8 ± 5
70	178	159 ± 14	72.3 ± 6	144 ± 11	65.5 ± 5
72	183	167 ± 15	75.9 ± 7	152 ± 12	69.0 ± 5
74	188	175 ± 15	79.5 ± 7		
76	193	182 ± 16	82.7 ± 7		

*From Food and Nutrition Board: *Recommended Dietary Allowances.* 7th Ed. Washington, D.C., National Academy of Sciences, 1968. Modified from Table 80, Hathaway and Ford, 1960, "Heights and Weights of Adults in the U.S.," *Home Economics Research Report No. 10,* ARS, USDA. Weights were based on those of college men and women. Measurements were made without shoes or other clothing. ± refers to the weight range between the 25th and 75th percentile of each height category.

body weight arbitrarily but to reduce to normal the amount of stored fat in the body.

A number of ways have been worked out to measure body fatness. Many of these are complex, involving use of radioisotopes or elaborate equipment, but others are relatively simple and ingenious. Fat has a lower specific gravity than water; hence, excess tissue fat tends to buoy up the body when immersed in water. Behnke[1] has utilized this principle in order to determine the ratio of lean to fatty tissues in the body. The body weight, taken when immersed in water and divided by the weight of the water displaced, is a true index of the relative amount of body fat. Obviously, a low specific gravity of the body indicates a relatively large proportion of body fat, and vice versa.

Estimates of the amount of subcutaneous fat in various parts of the body may also be made from the thickness of folds of skin and fat pinched up in several places (the upper back, abdomen, chest, arms or legs), as measured accurately by calipers.[2] By mathematical equations, body fat may be estimated from skinfold measurements. The "educated pinch" has even been suggested for the ordinary layman as a general guide in judging overfatness (obesity). If such a skinfold proves to be over an inch (25 mm) in thickness, it is an indication to reduce weight.

Body fatness may also be calculated from "envelope measurements" of the body (torso, legs, and arms, especially circumference of thigh and buttocks). Young and Blondin[3] found that constants derived from such measurements on individual young women formed a fairly accurate basis for estimating body weight and relative fatness. Brožek has published a review of methods for determining the relative amounts of fat, lean tissues, and water in the body.[4]

Body fat is stored mainly in the specialized cells of *adipose tissue*. When filled with fat, adipose tissue has about 85 to 90 percent fat, 2 percent protein and 10 percent water. This fat is formed in the cells from precursors brought in the blood and fatty acids are released from the cells when there is a demand for energy. Excess fat may be stored in adipose tissue cells that are not yet filled or new cells will be made if necessary. Insulin is required to store fat, and adrenal and pituitary hormones are involved in mobilizing it in response to need. The energy value of adipose tissue is about 8 kcal per gram or 3600 kcal per pound (33.5 MJ per kg.)*

Causes of Obesity

The chief causes of obesity are overeating and inactivity, usually in combination. People seem not to recognize that they are overeating, yet it is an easy thing to do, especially as one grows older and less inclined to physical exertion. Most Americans exercise little. We tend toward spectator sports, riding in cars, and sitting while we work. Also, we tend to adjust the temperature of our homes and places of work and entertainment and to dress in a way that minimizes the amount of energy used in body temperature regulation. If appetite and former food habits encourage one to take more food than needed, the fat accumulates. Only a relatively small excess daily may in time add considerable weight. Too large portions of food or fat and sugar added to foods may give a *surplus* of energy intake over output that will cause several pounds to be added in a few months, or 20 to 30 pounds extra weight in a few years time. For instance, the addition of one martini or one ounce of milk chocolate a day in three weeks adds the energy equivalent of one pound of adipose tissue.

Studies of obese children and adults have revealed that most of them ate about as much as individuals of normal

---

*1 kcal = 4.184 kJ = 0.004 MJ (MegaJoules). See Chapter 2 and Table 5 in the Appendix.

weight but that they were much less active physically. Thus, they were over-eating, but only relative to their needs. Inactivity is not accompanied by a commensurate decrease in appetite at very low levels of work output in animals or people (Fig. 23–1). Rats become obese if confined to small cages where their movement is restricted, and the standard way for a farmer to finish a steer, or fatten a goose for pâté de foie gras, is to limit exercise by penning and provide plenty of food. These same animals—rats, cattle, and fowl—better adjust intake to output when they are free to range and must forage for food. Control of activity alone, by forcing a rat to run in an activity wheel, allows the animal to remain lean while eating to appetite from freely available food. This indicates that of the two factors—food and exercise—exercise is probably

the more important.[5] Again the difference need not be large: 30 minutes of walking each day in three weeks adds up to one pound of adipose tissue.

People often fail to perceive underactivity and overconsumption as the cause of their weight gain. Instead they offer such comments as: "it is in the family to be stout," or "something must be the matter with my glands," or "no matter how little I eat, I don't lose weight." In most cases, a family tendency to stoutness has no more mysterious causes than an inactive temperament, combined with contributory food habits such as a preference for sweets and fatty foods. A few people do have an inherited tendency to put on weight more readily than most people do, just as some strains of animals have slimmer of fatter body conformation (lard hogs versus bacon hogs). Studies of identical

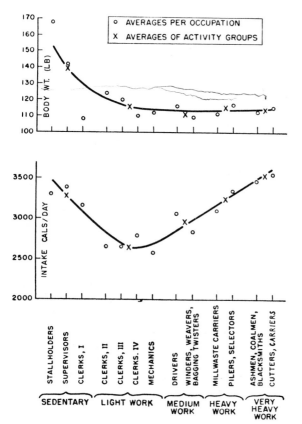

Figure 23–1. Body weight and energy intake as a function of physical activity. (Courtesy of Mayer and Bullen; reprinted from Physiological Reviews.)

twins raised in different environments show that some genetic influence exists in man but, at the same time, show a dominant effect of environmental factors, the life style.[5] Inbreeding has produced strains of mice that are obese from birth, and these have provided many useful clues in research concerning obesity. Fortunately, man limits the development of the genetic characteristic by his taboos on familial marriages.

In some cases, obesity is conditioned by inactivity of some one or more of the endocrine glands (thyroid, pituitary, or sex glands), but these people are distinctly in the minority. Studies on groups of obese people show that, in most cases, their basal metabolism is about the same per unit of surface area, as that in individuals of normal weight. However, they may exercise very little, and in contrast to their lower fuel needs, their intake of energy-bearing foods is in excess of their body needs, even though their total food intake may be below that of their leaner, more active friends.

Since psychology has come to be recognized, physicians have concluded that some persons may overeat to compensate for emotional insecurity or frustration. Such people need to have the cause of their unusual craving for food (bulemia) resolved and to be made aware of the disadvantages of their behavior. Persons must see advantages to be gained from changing food habits, before they are willing to do so.

Experimental Work on Obesity

The primary causes of obesity in man are, as we have noted, too much food, too little exercise, or both. These are really all one fundamental cause, an error in regulating the amount of energy eaten in proportion to need. This type of obesity is called *regulatory obesity*. Physiological control of hunger and appetite was considered in Chapter 15. Interesting studies by psychologists have shed new light on this complex problem, and indicate that for some as yet unexplained reason, obese people fail to respond to the internal cues that tell a body when food is needed and when it has had enough. What they do respond to is external stimuli, the presence or sight of food. One study showed that fat college students would eat more of three sandwiches put before them in a test situation than would normal-weight or thin students. However, if the subjects had to go to a refrigerator to obtain the sandwiches, the fat ones ate less than did those of normal weight.[6] This suggests that the fat students did not recognize biologically if or how hungry they were. Palatability is another factor. VanItallie and Hashim made freely available a bland and not distasteful formula diet to adults of normal weight and to fat ones; the normals soon learned to take enough to maintain their body weight constant, but the fat ones did not meet their needs and lost weight.[7]

Mayer and his colleagues[5] have described other types of obesity broadly categorized as *metabolic obesity*, in which the rate of fat synthesis is greater than normal or the rate of mobilization of fat from adipose tissue is depressed. One of these is seen in genetically obese-hyperglycemic mice, so called because they are fat and have elevated levels of sugar in the blood. The adipose tissue of these mice differs from normal in having high coenzyme A activity and an increased rate of fat synthesis from acetate precursors (refer to Chapter 14); diminished responsiveness to hormonal triggering of fat release; and an excess amount of a fat-forming enzyme. Mice that have this genetic makeup can be reduced in body weight by food restriction, but they continue to have a higher percentage of body fat than do normal mice of the same body weight.

Yet another theory of obesity may have important implications as to the problem that obese people have in staying lean once they have reduced and to the need for a preventive approach to obesity. Studies of adipose tissue of normal, fat, and formerly fat people show that the tissue of the obese has more cells than normal.[8] It is thought that these cells when lacking in fat send chemical messages that elicit eating behavior. Thus, if fewer cells were formed, if children were not allowed to become fat by overfeeding in infancy and the early years of childhood, they would not have a reservoir of demanding adipose cells.

Other lines of research raise questions as to whether it is possible to express the energy required for weight maintenance with the degree of mathematical accuracy formerly assumed. It may be that the total amount of energy needed depends to some extent on the relative proportions of the three classes of energy nutrients provided in the diet and to adaptive body mechanisms. Miller and Payne, working with animals, found the energy intakes required to keep body weight constant varied with individuals over a wide range, which led them to explore the problem in greater depth.[9] Particularly spectacular was an experiment with two pigs, one of which required almost five times the amount of energy for weight maintenance as did the other. This could not be accounted for by differences in digestibility, loss in urine, storage of fat, or physical activity. The pig which required the high energy intake for weight maintenance had a diet containing only half as much protein as did the other. After 40 days, the diets were reversed and the pig which formerly required high energy adjusted to maintain weight at the lower intake level, and vice versa, showing that the difference was due to the diet rather than to individual differences in the pigs.

Miller and Mumford have briefly reported similar experience in two human subjects in whom body weight was maintained constant, first during a period of seven weeks in which they consumed about 2400 to 2500 kcal per day (9 and 12 percent of the energy from protein), and then during six weeks of ingestion of diets providing 500 and 900 kcal *more* per day (2.5 percent of total energy from protein).[10] The excess energy consumed was enough to add 4.3 kg body weight in one case and 2.6 kg in the other, and yet no weight was gained. The authors do not offer full explanation, but they suggest that some of the food energy may be converted directly into heat and thus be unavailable for the internal and external work needs of the body.

Cohn has shown that the frequency of eating also affects nutrient utilization in experimental animals,[11] and similar responses have been inferred from observations of weight changes in man.[12] Administration of large meals at infrequent intervals is associated with decreased energy need for weight maintenance, increased deposition of body fat, and decreased deposition of body protein, as compared with a "nibbling" pattern of food intake (frequent small meals). It is known that the body adapts to long-term (days) food deprivation in such a way that a second period of fasting causes less loss of weight and acidosis than did the first fasting experience. It may be that the altered nutrient utilization of meal-fed animals represents comparable adaptation to short-term food deprivation (hours).

In conclusion, modern research suggests that obesity may not be a single entity, but one symptom which has many causes. Knowledge of these may one day yield effective methods of therapy. Whatever the contributing causes, the final one is always the same: the food intake of that individual is greater than his need. Prevention shows more promise than therapy in dealing with the problem.

Disorders Related to Obesity

Several of the diseases that are common in adults are associated with obesity as noted earlier, and these diseases are related to one another. A particular kind of circulatory disorder, atherosclerosis, is common in diabetics; people with atherosclerotic heart disease often have high blood pressure (hypertension); and in both cases they are likely to be obese. However, not all people who have these disorders are obese, and not all people who are obese will inevitably develop these diseases.

ATHEROSCLEROSIS AND CORONARY HEART DISEASE. Atherosclerosis is a kind of hardening of the arteries, a degenerative condition in which cholesterol and large lipoproteins are deposited on the interior wall of arteries. When this occurs the space in the blood vessel is narrowed. A blood clot (thrombus) may form in the narrowed vessel, closing off the supply of blood with its oxygen and nutrients to the organ or tissue served by the blood vessel. If a clot is formed in one of the small arteries that nourishes the heart muscle (a coronary vessel), a portion of the muscle will die. If the damage is extensive, the heart may be unable to function and the patient dies. If the damage is small or if the person has a well-developed circulatory system due to regular hard exercise, the heart may be able to continue to pump blood and the muscle will heal. The risk of coronary thrombosis becomes high at about middle age in men and after menopause in women and is increased in persons who have the following characteristics: high levels of blood cholesterol and/or neutral fat (triglycerides), high blood pressure, family history of heart disease, obesity, sedentary occupation, and cigarette-smoking.

Literally thousands of papers on this subject have been published since 1914 when atherosclerosis was first experimentally induced by feeding rabbits large amounts of cholesterol, a substance foreign to the metabolism of these animals which normally eat only plant foods. Then followed surveys on the fat content of the diet, the blood cholesterol levels, and the incidence of coronary heart disease among peoples in various parts of the world. These surveys indicated that levels of blood cholesterol tended to be higher and heart disease more common in the more prosperous nations, where more fats and especially more animal fats are eaten. However, because two facts occur coincidentally is not proof that one is the *cause* of the other, and *many factors other than dietary fat and cholesterol* are known to be associated with heart disease.

Considerable variation is observed in the blood cholesterol level among normal individuals, irrespective of their diet. There is a familial tendency toward higher levels of cholesterol, and blood cholesterol may also show sudden variations due to emotional or environmental factors. For example, a man may have high blood cholesterol when under tension on his job and two weeks later, when relaxed on vacation, have a normal level of this substance in the blood, with no significant change in diet. Factors such as lack of exercise, overeating, and stress and strain of life decidedly affect the incidence of high blood pressure and heart disease. This was strikingly shown in a joint study by investigations at Harvard University and at Trinity College, Dublin. They collected data on Irish-born men who had emigrated to the Boston area and their brothers who had remained in Ireland, chiefly engaged in agriculture. Although the study will continue for some years, a progress report was issued in 1964, and included data on 174 pairs of brothers (one in Ireland, one in Boston).[13] Although the diet of those in Ireland was higher in total energy, starchy foods, and animal fats (almost twice as much butter), the incidence of heart disease was considerably higher among the urbanized, sedentary American residents than among their paired brothers, who had been living a more active life. Several other studies involving comparisons of occupational groups within a country emphasize the importance of physical activity and energy balance: San Francisco longshoremen have a lower incidence of heart disease than do warehouse workers,[14] London bus conductors than drivers, and British postmen than bank clerks.[15]

There is ample evidence to show that ingestion of considerable amounts of saturated fatty acids, or of animal fats which have a high proportion of saturated (S) to polyunsaturated (P) fatty acids, tends to increase levels of total lipids and of cholesterol in the blood. Conversely, inclusion in the diet of a higher proportion of vegetable fats, rich in polyunsaturated fatty acids (a high P/S ratio), tends to lower the content of lipids and cholesterol in the blood. However, there are conflicting reports as to the effect of these dietary factors on the *occurrence of heart attacks per se*. Some studies show moderate success in terms of frequency and severity of coronary episodes among men whose diet is modified to provide a higher P/S ratio and, inevitably, less cholesterol (since cholesterol is found only in animal tissues and animal fat is restricted in these diets). Others have failed to prove a beneficial effect of such changes. This is not surprising, because the disease process is known to begin early in life, in childhood, and such studies have involved middle-aged or older men in whom the disease might already be well advanced. Also, we know that there are several different types of disorders in which blood lipids are elevated and that these respond to different dietary treatments.[16] Some types require rigid restriction of the amount of carbohydrate in the diet, and the fat level may be indifferent. Not all carbohydrates even behave the same: sucrose and fructose are more likely to elevate blood lipids than is starch.[17] Other types of blood lipid disorders do need to have less total fat in the diet, some profit by limitation of cholesterol intake, and some need a high ratio of P/S fatty acids. Some must have alcohol reduced or eliminated. Proper treatment can only be chosen after diagnosis based on complete analysis of the blood lipid patterns.

Considering the frequency of the various types of blood lipid disorders and based on epidemiologic evidence, the consensus of medical opinion is that people would do well to prevent or correct obesity, take more exercise, and reduce their total fat intake while substituting *moderate* amounts of vegetable fats with high P/S ratios for meat and milk fats. It is equally wise, on nutritional grounds as well as health ones, to reduce the amount of sucrose in the diet. This does not mean that diets should be so distorted that they constitute a bar to the needed intake of animal foods nor that all gustatory pleasure should be denied—only that moderation should be practiced in the use of animal fats and sweets. Although it is outside the province of this book, elimination of smoking is a very important preventive measure.

HYPERTENSION. High blood pressure is thought to have several causes, mainly renal and endocrine in origin. Some hypertensive patients are thin, but the incidence is markedly increased in persons who are obese, for reasons that are obscure. The trait is familial, and environmental factors probably play a role in permitting the potential tendency to become manifest. Epidemiologic evidence linking salt and high blood pressure was discussed in Chapter 10, but sodium is only one of a number of possible contributing factors. Recent research implicates a toxic trace mineral, cadmium.[18] The presence or absence of mineral elements in water is also associated with atherosclerosis and coronary heart disease; it has been observed that incidence is lower in regions that have hard water.[19] Again, there is no explanation for this finding.

DIABETES. When the word "diabetes" is used alone, it refers to a metabolic disease involving inadequate insulin function. The proper name is diabetes mellitus, a combination of the Greek word for "siphon" and the Latin word for "honey," referring to the fact that a dominant symptom of diabetes is excretion of large amounts of urine containing sugar. Diabetes is inheritable, and both members of a pair of identical twins will develop the disease. The severe disorder, as it occurs in young people, is quite different from the variety that develops at or past middle age, most commonly in obese people.

The reason obesity causes or accompanies maturity-onset diabetes in genetically predisposed individuals is uncertain. It is known that the disorder is less likely to occur in people who remain lean, and the mild form may be controlled simply by reducing weight to normal and increasing the amount of physical exercise. There is no clear evidence that dietary carbohydrate in general or sucrose in particular are causally related to diabetes, although this has been suggested,[20] but restriction of dietary sugar is an important aspect of dietary treatment. Attention is now being given to a possible association of various mineral deficiencies and diabetes, because of their role in the formation and utilization of insulin (zinc, magnesium, chromium, potassium),[21] but there is as yet no evidence that lack of these is a factor in the disease as it commonly occurs.

UNDERWEIGHT

Malnutrition Versus Underweight

The terms *malnutrition* and *underweight* are not synonymous, though the two conditions often occur together. Underweight results from an intake of energy insufficient to meet the body's needs, just as overweight results from a surplus energy intake. Malnutrition is a broader term: it means, literally, *bad* (from *mal*) *nutrition*, whether due to deficiency or excess of one or more nutrients in relation to the tissue needs.

The obese person is badly overnourished with respect to energy foods; the emaciated person is underweight due to supplies of food energy insufficient to meet body needs. Either may also be malnourished relative to other nutrients.

Undernutrition may be brought about in many different ways. The food may be inadequate either as to *quantity* or *quality*. Or the food supply may be all right, but *digestion* and *absorption* may be so poor that the food materials are not taken into the blood stream. *Living habits* or *environment*, which react on the individual so as to bring about poor appetite, aversion to particular foods, or refusal to take food are naturally unfavorable to nutrition, as are also absorbed toxins from various *infections* in the body. In short, anything which tends to interfere with the intake of some essential material or make the total amount of intake low, and anything which interferes with the normal processes by which food is utilized in the body, tends to bring about a condition of undernourishment, which will be more or less severe depending on the extent of the deficiency thus brought about.

Overweight malnourished persons, either children or adults, usually have enough subcutaneous fat so that they may look well nourished to the superficial observer. This combination of fatness and poor vitamin-mineral status may be found among the poor, whose low income forces them to fill up on the cheaper high-energy foods (starchy foods, cheaper fats, and sweets) and does not allow them to buy enough of the body-building foods (meat, milk, fruits, and vegetables). Such malnourished individuals are also found among the well-to-do who simply prefer to eat the wrong types of food. Their color is usually poor, their flesh flabby, and their bones and teeth of poor quality. They are often *anemic* and *listless*, tire quickly, and when seriously ill, are more apt to succumb than persons who have better nourished tissues and greater vitality. It is in these ways that their malnourished condition shows.

Underweight and Health Status

Underweight without lack of minerals and vitamins may or may not be serious, depending on the degree of underweight and the age at which it occurs. The average weights (found in tables) are not necessarily the normal or the best for every individual. There are times when it is advantageous to be somewhat under the average weight for height. This is true of middle-aged or older persons, especially if they have any tendencies to diabetes, high blood pressure, or heart or kidney ailments. Life insurance companies tell us that for older adults a slight degree of underweight increases health and life expectancy. This does not mean underweight to the point of malnutrition. Some older people, especially those of

small means, live on such abstemious diets as to lead to serious malnutrition. However, it is with *children* and *young adults* that severe underweight is almost sure to be a disadvantage. In general, we may say that to be more than 7 to 10 percent below the average weight for one's height and type of body build* usually means lowered vigor.

Normally the body profits from having some stores of fatty tissue, as well as reserves of the other nutrients to draw on in times of extra stress. The fatty tissues not only serve as reserve energy but as padding about the nerve plexuses and the abdominal organs. The very thin person has a scrawny ap-

---

*The average weight and height of boys and girls at given ages are found in the Appendix. Adult weights are given on page 512 (and Tables 10 and 11 of the Appendix). If underweight, deduct the present weight from the average or desirable one and calculate what percent this deficiency in pounds is of the proper or ideal weight. For example, a young woman finds that she is supposed to weigh 120 lb, but weighs only 108 lb; she is 12 lb, or 10 percent, underweight.

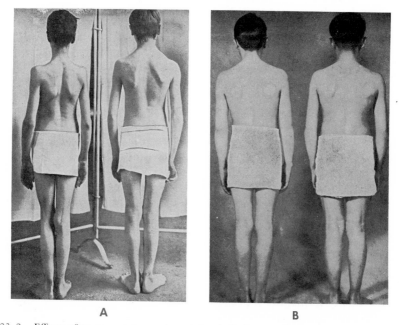

      A   **B**

Figure 23–2. Effects of treatment for underweight. **A,** Before, and **B,** After treatment at a rehabilitation camp. Notice that the boys have well-developed bodies but were simply thin. (From Emerson: *Nutrition and Growth in Children,* D. Appleton and Co.)

pearance and a tendency to chill easily owing to lack of a normal layer of subcutaneous fat (Fig. 23–2). Such persons readily experience physical fatigue and are more susceptible to the effects of infections. Their basal metabolism may be lowered and they are disinclined to any physical exertion, for their bodies are conserving energy. This is what we call living on a lower nutritional level.

Chronic Energy Shortage and Starvation

The disadvantages of becoming accustomed to living on a low level of energy intake were evident in experiments on otherwise healthy people. Benedict studied the effect of sharply reduced energy intake on healthy young men in the early 1900's and this type of study was repeated during World War II on a group of conscientious objectors at the University of Minnesota by Keys and associates. In both cases, the young men, who had previously taken well over 3000 kcal daily, submitted to a drastic reduction of energy intake until they had lost body weight on an average of 12 percent in the earlier set of experiments and 24 percent in the later ones. Their weight was then kept stable on a somewhat higher but still restricted energy level (1950 kcal in Benedict's group, 1550 kcal in Keys' experiments). At this lower nutritional level the men reported that they felt well but had less energy and had to drive themselves to do their accustomed tasks, and they tired sooner in various gymnasium tests. Keys' subjects subsisted on the low level of intake for six months and developed some more serious symptoms — depression, anemia, edema, slowing of heart beat, and others. They showed marked lack of endurance, tired easily, and reduced unnecessary movements to a minimum. When returned to their former level of energy consumption, they recovered their vitality, but it took considerable time to restore them to buoyant health.[22]

Severe undernutrition, to the point of starvation, comes about when there is famine due to crop failure or war, or it may result from serious diseases of the gastrointestinal tract that impair digestion or absorption of food. In some cases it is due to a psychiatric disorder (anorexia nervosa). Loss of about 25 percent of body weight is without serious permanent damage in healthy adults of normal weight, but losses in the order of 50 percent are not compatible with recovery. In Europe, during and after the long period of underfeeding in World War II, there was an increase of stillbirths and of babies who died soon after birth (Chapter 19). Wastage of muscle, edema due to lack of plasma protein, and lessened digestive capacity were seen in the severe cases. Tuberculosis and other infectious diseases flared up among both young mothers and children during the postwar years. Even today, among the poor in the teeming populations of Asia, the Middle East, Africa, southern Italy, and South America, there are millions who exist on a very low nutritional level because of insufficiency of energy (complicated by shortage of other nutrients), and we see the results in general misery and disease. The grave consequences of protein-energy malnutrition in children have been described in Chapter 5.

Total fasting* has been used as a therapeutic measure for grossly obese patients, but it is not to be recommended. Even with large energy reserves available in the body, total lack of food has serious risks. There is

---

*Fasting means abstention but usually not total food deprivation. Most often the religious injunction is to abstain from meals before a specified time of day or to omit one component (e.g., meat). During his fasts, Gandhi took fruit juices and sometimes dried fruits, a sensible procedure because some carbohydrate offsets the more serious effects of fasting.

marked loss of sodium with depletion of extracellular fluids, and the kidneys do not remove adequately the nitrogenous end product, uric acid. Some patients have developed gout and a few have died of heart and liver failure in the course of such treatment.

Malnutrition and Infection

Well-nourished people do not escape infection, in the sense that good nutrition confers any sort of immunity. It is true that nutrition must be satisfactory to maintain the skin and internal membranes that are the first barrier to invading organisms, and secondary infections do follow deficiency of vitamin A, for example (Chapter 9). Specific nutrients are needed for formation of the antibodies that are the body's internal protection, and suppression of antibody formation has been reported in some species deficient in some nutrients, but not in all. In the case of some viruses, including the leukemia virus, animals deficient in nutrients are more, not less, resistant to invasion. Experimental immunizations in men who were deficient in selected B vitamins showed little evidence that immune mechanisms fail due to nutritional deficits. Children with severe malnutrition in poor communities who have very low levels of one of the plasma proteins, albumin, usually have relatively high levels of the gamma globulins that constitute the immune component, but they may still lack complete immunocompetency.

When the infection is established, however, nutritional status consistently affects the outcome. Persons who are well nourished are more likely to survive an infection than are those who are weakened because of malnutrition or whose reserves are too low to support them during a prolonged illness. In the tropics, seemingly healthy individuals often have malaria parasites in the blood or a large population of worms in the intestine. The people are able to cope with these parasites, almost to live symbiotically, as long as diets are adequate. But when nutritional status falls or a person becomes stressed because of some other factor, the disease overwhelms him.

Infection also conditions nutritional deficiency. Little children whose diets are barely adequate develop obvious cases of marasmus or kwashiorkor as a result of contracting some ordinary childhood disease such as measles, whooping cough, or a nonspecific diarrhea. Their reserves are so low that they cannot tolerate the least additional loss from the intestine, the accelerated metabolism of a mild fever, or a few days of nausea or poor intake. The child may die of malnutrition consequent to an infection.

Treatment of Undernutrition

In order to be effective, treatment must follow two courses:

1. **Location** and **removal** of the **contributory causes.**
2. **Improvement of the diet.**

Under the first heading comes a thorough study of the person's *daily program* to discover whatever faulty food and health habits there may be, and a general *medical examination* to see whether there are any physical defects which need to be corrected. These unfavorable factors, which predispose to poor nutrition, must then be remedied —bad living habits must be corrected, and physical defects and disease must receive proper treatment. Often considerable persistence may be needed to locate *all* the causes. *Overfatigue* is one of the most common causes and is easily corrected by longer hours of sleep, rest periods during the day, and reducing the activities which cause fatigue. Poverty is an important contributory factor, especially among the working poor who have hard physical work to perform and often many mouths to feed from a limited supply. Mothers of small children are often overtired and they do not eat if their children are hungry. Persons with more severe undernutrition often require continued observation and study by a physician in order to locate and treat the factors responsible for keeping the person below par physically.

Providing a suitable diet is perhaps the most important single measure for correcting undernutrition — certainly an adequate food supply is indispensable. The corrective diet may be started at once — that is, while one is in the process of locating and clearing up the unfavorable contributory factors. Supplements may be prescribed if specific deficiencies of vitamins and minerals exist. Although the body may not be able to take *full* advantage of the diet until all adverse factors are remedied, the diet given in the meantime should be best suited to the physical condition of the individual,* and this in turn may help to remedy defects and diseased conditions more quickly and to strengthen the tissues and organs so that they function better. A body which has been depleted by prolonged underfeeding requires gradually increased feeding and building up in numerous respects. Not only should new deposits of *fat* be laid down, but the muscles are in need of *protein* for repair and enlargement. Reserve stores of *vitamins* and minerals are used up or lost from the body during semistarvation, and an excess of nutrients in the diet is a help in the processes necessary for repair after undernutrition. The diet should be designed to promote gain of any needed lean tissue and a desirable amount of fat according to health and aesthetic considerations.

PLANNING THE REDUCING REGIMEN

For the ordinary overweight individual, by far the most satisfactory way to effect weight reduction is simply to cut down sharply on the concentrated energy foods (fats, alcohol, sugars, and starches), while maintaining an otherwise well balanced and adequate diet. Such a diet does not involve actually going hungry. It can be taken over fairly long periods without harm, and it can be continued into the postreducing period (by adding limited amounts of the foods of higher energy value) in order to hold the lower weight one has attained by reducing. It should be, so far as possible, a diet one likes and is willing to use indefinitely, and it should be *inadequate* for body needs *in only one respect* — its *energy* content.

The main things to plan for in any reducing diet are:

1. *Low energy content*
2. At least adequate protein
3. At least fairly low carbohydrate and fat
4. Plenty of minerals and vitamins
5. Good satiety value

LOW ENERGY INTAKE. Obviously, to accomplish its purpose, a reducing diet must have relatively *low energy content.* The rate at which stored fat is lost will depend on the magnitude of the difference between energy intake and expenditure. For best results it is desirable to increase energy need by increasing physical activity at the same time as intake is lowered. If one plans the diet to furnish 500 to 1000 kcal (2000 to 4000 kJ) less than needed, this should effect a weight loss of about 3 to 6 lb (1.5 to 3 kg) a month. The same rate of weight loss could be brought about by swimming a whole hour every day,

---

*Administration of large amounts of food to starved or semistarved persons can have disastrous consequences. The refeeding of concentration camp victims showed that small, frequent feeding of soft, nutritious foods is essential if vomiting, intestinal disturbances, and shock are to be avoided. The weakened organism cannot handle a large metabolic load. The same is true for severely undernourished children.

without altering food intake. A combination of low-energy diet plus activity accelerates weight reduction, promotes fitness, and prevents tissues from becoming flabby as fat is lost. More drastic reduction of energy intake, of course, causes a more rapid loss of weight, but diets below 1000 kcal (4000 kJ) are not recommended because they too severely limit the sources of essential nutrients in the diet. Diets above the 1600 kcal (6400 kJ) level give such slow results in weight loss that they are discouraging to the average adult woman, although men may show good weight loss at that level of intake.

Not only must the choice of foods be right (avoidance of concentrated energy foods), but the size of portions must be limited if intake is to be kept down. For instance, take the case of a woman dieting zealously but fitfully who announced she was having a low-energy breakfast of fruit. She consumed a very large glass of orange juice (10 oz), two large pears, and a bunch of grapes, which meant an intake of at least 500 kcal. One slice of toast with a *small* portion of butter, one egg, and a small glass of juice (4 oz) would have meant only half as much energy. Thus, even foods described as moderately low in energy can raise the intake considerably when taken in large portions. All foods furnish *some* energy, even vinegar, lemon juice, bouillon, tea and coffee, but in the foods just named the amount is so small as to be ignored in planning the diet.

All between-meal snacks or extras (such as cream and sugar, and salad dressings) taken in or on foods must be counted. This includes cocktails or other alcoholic beverages, because both alcohol and sugar in such drinks furnish energy. A table of approximate caloric content of alcoholic beverages is given in the Appendix (p. 575).

ADEQUATE PROTEIN. It is important that the reducing diet provide enough **protein** for the maintenance and upkeep of body tissues and that the mixture of proteins taken should provide all essential amino acids. Adults following a slimming diet should have 1 gm of protein per kilogram of body weight, and not less than 50 gm daily for the diet to be adequate. Children need a more liberal protein allowance. Naturally, if one cuts down on the foods that are high in carbohydrates and fats, a greater proportion of the calories tend to be taken as protein. A luxury diet with meat at every meal of the day is unnecessary, but a reducing diet may well include one liberal serving of meat per day, with either a *small* second serving of meat or one of eggs, fish, or poultry. This, together with milk and cheese, provides liberal protein.

LOW CARBOHYDRATE AND FAT. The exact distribution of calories among protein, carbohydrate, and fat is not critical, except that protein must be adequate and a *certain amount of carbohydrate is desirable*. Diets high in protein or fat, or low in carbohydrate, have been suggested as particularly successful in causing weight reduction, but there is no agreement among experts that any of these has special efficacy in the long run. As a practical matter, fats are usually sharply limited. They are such concentrated sources of energy ($2\frac{1}{4}$ times as much energy per gram as the other two foodstuffs) that only a small quantity can be included without raising the energy intake too high.

On a diet inadequate in energy to meet body needs, the body is constantly burning some of its stored fat. Under these conditions, fats may not be completely oxidized, and the acid intermediate products of their metabolism (keto acids) may accumulate in the body and cause an acidosis, or ketosis. Bloom and Azar found that healthy humans, when fed a diet exclusively of protein and fat, lost 2 pounds daily, but that there were large losses of nitrogen and salt in the urine and the subjects experienced symptoms due to acidosis (ketosis).[23] These symptoms disappeared promptly when carbohydrate was included in the diet.

Others[24] seem to have better success with a high protein–low carbohydrate diet. Weight loss may be more rapid at first on a low carbohydrate diet, but it makes little difference in the end whether reduction of energy intake is brought about by restriction of carbohydrate or fat, in long-term reduction programs.

If small amounts of carbohydrate are included in the reducing diet, acidosis is prevented. An intake of 70 to 100 gm of carbohydrate will suffice. Practically all the energy value of fruits and vegetables and over half that of skim milk comes from the carbohydrates they contain, so that not very much of the more concentrated carbohydrate foods (bread, cereals, and sweets) is needed.

MINERALS AND VITAMINS.   A person on a reducing diet should get his recommended allowance of the various needed *minerals and vitamins* to keep the body in condition while weight loss is going on. This means that any reducing diet should provide liberally for milk, meat, fruits (including citrus or tomatoes), and vegetables. The reduced amounts of bread and cereals taken should be whole-grain. Skim milk may be substituted for whole milk (it has only about half the energy value). It will furnish the needed calcium and B vitamins but no fat-soluble vitamins. Vitamin A may come from eggs, liver, and the provitamins in green, leafy, and yellow vegetables. These same foods, plus meats, may also serve to meet the need for iron. Many persons who have half starved in order to lose weight rapidly, or who have dieted on very one-sided diets, show the bad effects of this mistake in evidences of lack of vitamins or anemia.

SATIETY VALUE.   The satiety value of the diet is very important if hunger is to be avoided. If one took nothing but clear soups, beverages, fruits, and vegetables, he would obtain rapid weight loss but feel very unsatisfied. Meat, poultry, fish, cheese, and eggs have a high satiety value and should be dis-

tributed throughout the three meals of the day. Fatty foods, which leave the stomach most slowly and hence have the highest satiety value, must be kept down to small amounts, but a little oil in salad dressing, or a small piece of cheese, may occasionally be included. A small portion of fruit or a simple dessert taken at the end of a meal often does much toward making one feel well fed. Imaginative use of herbs and spices and inclusion of diet dressings and artificially sweetened beverages and fruits enhance appetite appeal. Some persons are less troubled with hunger if they have a snack between meals or at bedtime (such as an apple or orange, a few crackers, or skim milk), but these must of course be counted in the total day's energy allowance.

Lists of foods around which the reducing diet should be built (foods to use), and those which must be avoided if the energy intake is to be kept low enough to cause appreciable weight loss are given in Table 23–2.

Basic Pattern for Reducing Diet and How to Use It

It is entirely permissible for anyone to construct his own reducing diet, using whatever foods he has a preference for in amounts limited to keep the energy content of the diet down to a level at which satisfactory weight loss will be obtained.

In practice, it seems to place too much responsibility on the individual and to be too confusing to leave him entirely without guidance in the selection of a reducing diet. Therefore, we have thought it advisable to suggest a **definite type of meal plan** for those who desire to reduce, leaving considerable latitude for variety and choice of foods in making up individual menus. This we have endeavored to accomplish by presenting a **basic pattern** for the reducing diet (Table 23–3), with many

Table 23–2. Foods from Which the Reducing Diet Should Be Built

Foods to Use	Foods to Avoid
Clear soups	Alcoholic beverages
Tea and coffee (without sugar or cream)	Soft drinks with added
Milk (especially skim milk or buttermilk)	sugar
Fresh fruits and canned or stewed fruits	Fried foods
without sugar	Fatty meats
Watery and fibrous vegetables (especially	Rich dressings, sauces, and
leafy, green, and yellow vegetables)	gravy
Lean meats, eggs, and cottage cheese	Rich desserts and pastries
Small servings of low-energy desserts:	Nuts and dried fruits
e.g., gelatin or fruit juice	Sugar and sweets
	Cream, fats, and oils

Table 23–3. Basic Pattern for Reducing Diet
Approximately 1100 to 1400 kcal (4600–5500 kJ)

Total allowance for the day:
  2 cups of milk. Each cup of skim milk provides about 85 kcal (350 kJ). Whole milk yields 165 kcal (690 kJ) per cup. 1 oz of Cheddar cheese equals 1 cup of milk.
  5 oz of lean meat, fish, or poultry, broiled, boiled, or roasted but not fried. All visible fat should be trimmed. Each ounce supplies about 60 to 80 kcal (250–340 kJ); 1 oz of meat equals 1 egg: 3 sardines; 5 shrimp, clams, or oysters; 1/4 cup tuna fish, salmon, crabmeat, or lobster.
  2 or more servings of fruit without added sugar. One serving should be citrus or other fruit high in vitamin C. Each portion listed counts as one serving and provides about 40 to 50 kcal (170–200 kJ).

1 Small apple (2 in. diameter)	1/2 Small mango
1/2 Cup applesauce	1 Medium nectarine
2 Fresh apricots or 4 halves dried	1 Small orange or scant 1/2 cup juice
1/2 Small banana	1/3 Papaya
1 Cup berries (blackberries, rasp-	1 Medium peach
berries, strawberries)	1 Small pear
2/3 Cup blueberries	1/2 Cup cubed pineapple or 1/3 cup
1/4 Cantaloupe (6 in. diameter)	juice
10 Large cherries	2 Medium plums or prunes
2 Dates	2 Level tbsp raisins
1 Small dried fig	1 Large tangerine
1/2 Grapefruit or 1/2 cup juice	1 Cup dried watermelon or one
12 Grapes or 1/4 cup juice	slice 3 in. × 1 1/2 in.
1/4 Honeydew melon (7 in. diameter)	2 Tomatoes or 1 cup juice

  2 or more servings of vegetables. At least one serving should be dark green, leafy vegetable. An average (1/2 cup) serving yields 10 to 50 kcal (40–200 kJ). Any vegetable may be used, except peas, corn, and dried beans, which must be substituted for bread. No butter, margarine, salad oil, or regular salad dressing may be added except that included in the total allowance for the day. Lemon juice, vinegar, and low-calorie dressings are acceptable.
  3 or 4 servings of whole grain or enriched bread, or **substitutes.** One serving, providing 60 to 80 kcal (250–340 kJ), equals: one slice of bread; one muffin or biscuit (2 in. diameter); 1/2 cup cooked cereal, rice, macaroni, spaghetti, or noodles; scant 3/4 cup dry cereal; 5 saltine crackers; 2 graham crackers; scant 1/2 cup peas or cooked dried beans; 1/2 ear corn; small potato (2 in. diameter) or 1/2 cup mashed; 1 1/2 in. cube of sponge or angel food cake without icing.
  3 or 4 **small** servings of fat. One 50 kcal (200 kJ) serving equals: one-half tbsp butter, margarine, vegetable oil, or other clear fat; 1 slice of drained, crisp bacon; 2 level tbsp light cream (sweet or sour); 1 level tbsp cream cheese or French dressing; 5 olives.
Coffee, tea, bouillon, and other food items of negligible energy content may be used as desired.

of the details on how the pattern may be met left open to choice. The acceptance of a diet built around a smaller number of simple foods is of great help in making one contented on a more or less restricted diet. To be always in quest of new food combinations is likely to keep one's mind on food to such an extent that one becomes discontented even with a fairly elaborate diet. The use of a basic food pattern in planning reducing diets may be advantageous in three ways:

1. It permits choice.
2. It guides food selection.
3. It teaches desirable food habits.

All sorts of different menu combinations can be made, if desired, either by altering the foods selected from a given food group or varying the size of servings as needed to raise or lower the level of energy intake. Two sample menus for a day, which conform to the basic food pattern, are given in Table 23–4, and these are planned to meet the needs of young adults who must eat at least some meals away from home.

If the basic food pattern can be adapted so as to fit the energy level required to produce satisfactory weight loss, it will help to guard the intake of all nutrients other than energy, but it need not be followed slavishly. There will be wide variations among individuals in the restriction needed to produce weight loss, according to the body weight and degree of muscular activity. For a 165 lb man who is moderately active, the 1400 kcal (5500 kJ) level would represent a severe reduction below estimated energy needed for weight maintenance, while for a small sedentary woman 1400 kcal would be all she needed for maintaining weight and she would probably need to curtail intake even below the 1100 kcal (4600 kJ) level.

Table 23–4. Sample Menu Patterns from the Basic Reducing Diet

Pattern I	Pattern II
BREAKFAST	
Orange juice (½ c.)	Branflakes (¾ c.)
Poached egg (1)	with
on	Sliced banana (½)
Whole wheat toast (1 slice) ·	and
Coffee with skim milk (½ c.)	Milk (½ c.)
LUNCHEON	
Consommé	Tuna fish sandwich
Shrimp Louis	(¼ c. tuna fish with 2 tsp salad
(6 shrimp on large bed of mixed greens	dressing and lettuce on 2 slices whole-
with 1 tbsp. dressing)	wheat bread)
Small muffin (1)	Hard cooked egg
Cantaloupe (¼)	Dill pickle, green pepper, celery strips
Iced tea with lemon	Radish roses
	Milk (1 c.)
DINNER	
Broiled lamb chop (3 oz)	Frankfurters (2)
Small baked potato with sour cream	with
(tbsp) and chives	Sauerkraut
Buttered (½ tsp) green beans	Buttered (½ tsp) carrots
Sliced tomatoes	Strawberries (1 c.)
Cheese (1 oz) with saltine crackers (5)	with
Coffee with skim milk (½ c.)	Sponge cake (1½ in. cube)
	Coffee with evaporated milk (2 tbsp)

Varying the Energy Level of the Reducing Diet

The diet may be adjusted to any required energy level by reducing or using more liberal quantities of the foods of high or moderate energy value. After **estimating** the proper level of energy that will be required for one's individual case in order to secure weight loss (see General Rules for Reducing Regimen at end of chapter), one may plan a reducing diet at this energy level by consulting the Table of Nutritive Values of Foods in Average Servings in the Appendix, pp. 546 to 568. Foods should be selected from the different food groups as recommended in the basic pattern for a reducing diet given in Table 23–3, limiting the size or number of servings to attain the desired level of energy intake. The menus given in Table 23–4 illustrate diets ranging from 1100 to 1400 kcal (4600 to 5500 kJ).

Two other sets of menus found in Table 23–5 conform to the lower levels of energy intake frequently required for securing weight loss at a satisfactory rate—one at a 1000 kcal (4200 kJ) level and another at a 1200 kcal (5000 kJ) level. Even with such limited intake, it should be noted that the meals can be made attractive and hunger-satisfying. They will also meet body needs for most essential nutrients (except energy). Although the amounts of fat and carbohydrate are limited, each of the day's menus provides adequate protein (65-68 gm) and with the other foods used will probably meet the needs for well-known minerals and vitamins. If there is any doubt about this, some reliable vitamin and/or mineral capsule may be taken. These are only two of a wide variety of possible combinations within the food allowances. Higher levels can easily be arranged by either increasing proportions of the same type of foods or by adding other foods not permissible at lower levels of energy intake.

Some regular system of meals should be adopted, however, and strictly adhered to, for only thus does a reducing diet yield the desired results.

Some people may prefer to take a lighter breakfast and/or lunch and use the energy thus saved for a more normal meal with the family at noon or at night. Others may be better able to adhere to the slimming diet if the day's food allowance is divided into five smaller meals (or some reserved for snacks). Care must be taken that the total food taken does not exceed the day's allowance. Although the level of intake does not have to be *absolutely* the same each day, it is desirable that the meal plan be such that the fluctuations made by choice in foods used cause it to vary only within narrow limits, probably not more than 100 to 200 kcal (400 to 800 kJ) variations.

When the normal weight is achieved, foods should be added back very gradually, one at a time. Minor increase in weight that is sustained for several days indicates that the additions have been made too rapidly and the last addition should be deleted. Continuous recording of weight is essential as a motivation to keeping slim. Experience indicates that very few people who have been truly obese manage to hold to their reduced weight, but rather creep back to the same weight, or more, than they had before they began the reducing regimen. Success is greater if the weight is corrected all the way to the ideal rather than stopping short at some intermediate weight that neither satisfies the ego nor improves the health status in noticeable ways. A vigorous exercise program should be of help provided the person has found an activity he enjoys. No one knows if the common pattern of weight gain–weight loss–weight regain, etc. (the pattern that Mayer has called the "rhythm method of girth control") is harmful to man. A famine-feast regimen does shorten the life span of genetically obese mice

Table 23–5. Sample Menus for Reducing—Varying Energy Levels

Approx. 1000 kcal (4200 kJ) (1)*	kcal†	Approx. 1200 kcal (5000 kJ) (2)*	kcal†
Breakfast		*Breakfast*	
Grapefruit, ½	40	Orange juice, 6 oz	80
Egg, 1	80	Oatmeal, ⅔ c.	55
Whole wheat toast, 1 sl.	55	Milk, low fat, ½ cup	68
Margarine, 1 tsp	33	Coffee	0
Coffee	0		——
	——		203
	208		
Lunch		*Lunch*	
Consume, ¾ c.	20	Omelet, 2 eggs, w/milk	175
Salad—cottage cheese ½ c.	100	Asparagus, 6–7 spears,	
diet peaches ½ c.	40	canned	40
lettuce	10	low cal. mayonnaise, 1 tbsp	20
low cal. dressing, 1 tbsp	15	Melba toast, 2 slices	30
Rye wafers, 2	45	Apple, raw, 1 medium	90
Milk, skim, 1 glass	85	Milk, low fat, 1 glass	135
	——		——
	315		490
Dinner		*Dinner*	
Hamburger, lean ground, 4 oz	185	Onion soup, ¾ c. w/1 cracker	47
Green beans, ¾ cup	25	Broiled chicken, flesh only, 3½ oz	135
Tossed green salad–with ½ tomato	27	Potato, 1 med.	95
low cal. dressing, 1 tbsp	15	w/butter, 1 tsp	33
Whole wheat bread, 1 sl.	55	Carrots, ⅔ c., diced	30
Margarine, 1 tsp	33	Romaine w/vinegar	15
Jello w/fruit, ½ c.	80	and oil, 1 tsp	33
	——	Chocolate pudding, from mix, ½ c.	115
	420	Tea, w/lemon	0
			——
			503
Snack		*Snack*	
Cherries, Bing, about 15	70	Plum, raw, 1	25
	——		——
Total	1013	Total	1221

*Approximate distribution of energy nutrients: Diet (1), protein 65 gm, fat 24 gm, carbohydrate 85 gm; Diet (2), protein 68 gm, fat 35 gm, carbohydrate 153 gm.
†To convert kcal to kJ, multiply by 4.184.

more than if they are allowed to remain obese. In the mice, life span is prolonged by sustained weight reduction.[5]

Adjuncts and Fad Diets

Probably no type of quackery is more profitable at present than the special remedies sold to effect weight reduction and various adjuncts supposed to make weight loss easy and safe. They flourish because the American public has become conscious of the need to do something about overweight but still hopes to do it as painlessly as possible. So the public is credulous about remedies and fad diets that promise "You can eat all you want and still lose weight." Any manufacturer that makes this promise for a product is banking on the fact that his product contains something that reduces appetite. This may be a substance such as cellulose that provides little or no available energy but that helps fill the stomach and satisfy the craving to eat. This type of product is harmless but is expensive and probably ineffective, for laboratory studies indicate that about half the diet may be replaced by cellulose without reducing the voluntary energy intake of animals. Other products may contain one of the drugs that depress appetite. There are several that may be prescribed by physicians, but only one or two are allowed to be used without a doctor's prescription. The appetite-depressing drugs that can thus be used in preparations sold on the open market are not potent enough to have any marked effect on appetite, but perhaps taking them has some psychological effect. Truly effective products can be prescribed only by a physician.

Remedies that promise to reduce weight merely by the patient's lying on a vibrating "couch," or to reduce weight in special places so that unsightly bulges will disappear, are so suspect that federal agencies are prosecuting promoters for making false claims. The government holds that there is no evidence to show that general weight reduction can be effected by such means alone or that fatty tissue in certain areas can be broken down and gotten rid of by such means as massage. Systematic exercises for certain muscles may firm the muscles and, if accompanied by dietary control, may get rid of extra fat. However, urgent solicitation to enroll at cut rates for exercises or baths at various establishments for weight reduction should be resisted. There can be little or no personal supervision of the exercises and indiscriminate exercising for an overweight individual who is unused to it and may have back troubles or other ailments can do harm. Baths, including steam baths, can effect little weight reduction except through loss of water from the body, and this can quickly be regained merely by drinking water. The only type of bath that can be a useful adjunct to weight reduction is the cold shower or plunge. This increases the basal metabolism considerably for some time, provided the individual reacts well after a cold shower, but it is rather "heroic" treatment for a fat person to undergo. Swimming in cold water is an effective way of increasing heat loss and of providing beneficial exercise to improve muscular tone.

Although it is entirely possible to get all the nutrients needed in a well planned reducing diet, supplementary vitamins and minerals may well be a safeguard for persons on drastic or long-continued reducing diets. This is especially true of the fat-soluble vitamins, because fats are sharply curtailed and some persons will not take large amounts of leafy vegetables. In this case, it is better to buy a reputable vitamin preparation, so that the dosage may be known and controlled.

Special diets for reducing are quite in vogue. Popular magazines have all been carrying such planned diets, with menus for a week to a full month. It seems remarkable that people should be so eager to follow menu plans made out by someone who cannot know their food preferences or circumstances, or what foods one may be able to obtain readily in local markets. Usually such diets include some less used foods, or foods prepared in unusual ways. They may be relatively expensive and cause extra work, especially if the rest of the family does not wish to eat the same foods as the reducer. The good ones of these diets are no more effective than any well planned reducing diet, though they may suggest variety and avoid monotony in the diet.

For other persons, there is a special appeal in diets that involve a minimum of preparation, such as the so-called "formula diets," which can be bought already mixed in drugstores and food shops. One may lose weight fairly rapidly by subsisting entirely on such a formula (chiefly milk with some sugar added) or the formula diet may be substituted for one or two meals a day, the other meals composed of a variety of foods appropriate to a reducing diet.

However, with a bit of planning, one may select a less monotonous and less expensive diet that has the additional advantage of encouraging the improved food habits so necessary for long-term weight control. A breakfast consisting of an ordinary serving of cereal or a slice of toast, a glass of skim milk, and a small glass of fruit juice is easily prepared, better nutritionally, and yields no more energy than does one can of most of the formula preparations.

There are also the peculiar diets based on only a few foods, such as the all-fruit diet, the green-vegetable diet, the pineapple and lamb chop diet, the raw tomato and hard boiled egg diet, etc. These appeal to some people either as short cuts in reducing or as giving distinction by their unusualness. Such diets are not only monotonous to take but are so one-sided that they are sure to be too low in some of the various nutrients. On any of these diets, the size of portions must be limited (i.e., the total energy intake must be kept down) in order to effect weight reduction.

GENERAL RULES FOR REDUCING REGIMEN

1. Those who should reduce —
Normal persons who are 15 percent or more overweight.
Persons 10 percent overweight, if they have a tendency to heart disease, kidney disease or diabetes, should reduce to normal weight, or even slightly less.

2. How to find out the proper level of food intake to use for reducing.
Calculate your maintenance level (i.e., the energy intake necessary to maintain weight with normal activity), thus:
Look up (Table 23–1 on p. 512) the theoretical normal or desirable weight for your height and body build at 25 or 30 years of age.
Multiply this *ideal* weight (in pounds) by 15 if sedentary, and by 20 if active (adults require 15 to 20 kcal per lb per day) (135 to 185 kJ/kg).
This gives the supposed maintenance level of energy intake.
Plan the diet to yield 500 to 1000 kcal (2000 to 4000 kJ) per day *less* than the maintenance level, depending on how rapidly you want to lose weight.
EXAMPLE: A woman 5 ft 5 in tall, 25 years old, and of medium

frame should weigh about 116 to 130 lbs (actually weighs 167 lbs, about 25 percent overweight, and is sedentary).

$130 \times 15 = 1950$ kcal, maintenance level.

Reduce energy intake by $\frac{1}{5} - \frac{1}{3}$ of maintenance level.

$1950 - 400 = 1550$ kcal.

$1950 - 650 = 1300$ kcal.

Reducing diet for this individual should furnish 1300 to 1550 kcal.

3. *How to determine how much to reduce food level in order to get a certain rate of weight loss.*

One ounce of body fat represents approximately 230 kcal (335 kJ/ 100 gm) of food.

If you cut down food intake 500 kcal below maintenance level, you should lose about $\frac{3}{4}$ lb of fat per week, or 3 lb per month.

A reduction of 1000 kcal below maintenance level should cause weight to be lost at rate of approximately 6 lb per month.

You may not lose exactly at the calculated rate each week, especially the first week or two, but in the long run the weight loss will average about that expected, if you stick to your diet.

4. *Weighing and best rate at which to lose.*

Weigh at least once per week, on same scales if possible, at about the same time of day, and in approximately same weight clothing. Before breakfast is a good time to take weight. Small fluctuations of weight from day to day have no significance but steady, gradual loss of weight is what to work for. Keep a written record of your weight, preferably a graph to show your progress (See Fig. 23–3).

It is not advisable to reduce more rapidly than 1 to 2 lb weight loss per week.

Too rapid reduction may cause weakness and throws a severe strain on the system for rapid readjustments. It is detrimental to looks, as skin is apt to become wrinkled after the rapid loss of subcutaneous fat. Too rapid a weight loss is hard on disposition, as the very restricted diet necessary will probably cause hunger and irritability or depression.

5. *Exercise*

It is best to begin exercise gradually, if you have been sedentary. Choose some activity that you enjoy and gradually increase the amount of time spent doing it.

Never ride an elevator less than three floors. Always park your car a short walk from your destination or, better still, ride a bicycle or walk.

6. *Necessity of keeping at lower level of food intake after reducing diet.*

It should be obvious that, if you go back to the former food level on which you gained weight, you will regain the weight which has just been lost unless you increase your physical activity to compensate.

When you have lost the desired amount of weight on a restricted diet, increase the food intake *gradually* until you are taking just enough food to maintain constant weight. Keep the food intake at this new level. If you begin to gain, cut down the diet by a small amount.

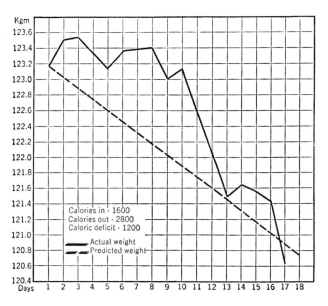

Figure 23-3. Comparison of actual and predicted weight loss in an obese patient on a reducing diet which furnished 1200 kcal less than the caloric output. During the first ten days there was little weight loss (water retention balanced loss of fat), but in the following week weight loss was so rapid that the total loss equaled the amount predicted. (Courtesy of Newburgh and Johnston.)

DIETS FOR GAINING WEIGHT

A diet suitable for building up a body which has suffered for some time from an insufficient food supply should be planned to provide:

1. *A high energy intake* — fuel in excess of body needs.

2. Liberal quantities of **high-quality protein.**

3. An **abundant** supply of **minerals and vitamins.**

The first requirement is met by including in the diet *liberal* amounts of **high-energy foods,** especially foods rich in *fats* and *starches,* such as butter or margarine, cream, salad dressings, bacon, cereals, bread, cream soups, legumes, nuts, and dried fruits — in short all foods forbidden to *overweight* individuals. Filling foods that carry little nourishment (e.g., clear soups) should be avoided. Protein of high quality for tissue building and repair is provided by including *milk, eggs,* and *meats* as freely as costs permit. Organ meats, such as liver, which are excellent sources of minerals and vitamins, should be taken frequently. Even though they may seem to increase the bulk of the diet undesirably, plenty of *fruits* and *vegetables*

should be included for their content of mineral elements and vitamins. Milk, eggs, and whole-grain bread and cereals are also valuable sources of mineral salts and vitamins. Although **high energy content** is the **main objective** of the diet, care should be taken that it provides an *abundance of all the other nutritive essentials* as well.

The diet should provide **energy in excess of body needs** by at least 500 to 1000 kcal (2000 to 4000 kJ). The intake should exceed body needs by one-half to one-third the energy required for maintenance — for example, a person who needs 2100 kcal for maintenance should take approximately 2800 to 3100 kcal when trying to gain weight. It is often necessary to force one's self to take food in excess of one's appetite. It is probably easier to accomplish this if the food is divided into more frequent meals, about five to seven a day, taken by clock time rather than by hunger or appetite.

It is easy to increase the energy intake considerably by such devices as an extra square of butter or fortified margarine at each meal (about 220 kcal), liberal use of cream, bacon, and salad dressings (1 tbsp mayonnaise, 2 tbsp thick cream,

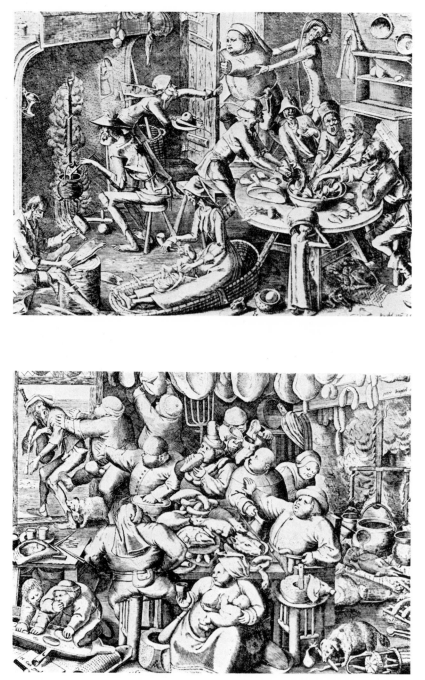

Figure 23–4.   **Top,** Starvation. **Bottom,** Gluttony. Engravings by Peter Breughel, 1563. (From Sigerist, H. E.: *Civilization and Disease.* Chicago, University of Chicago Press, 1943.)

Table 23–6.   Sample Menu for a Woman Who Wishes to Gain Weight

Breakfast	
Orange juice, 6 oz	80
Oatmeal (²/₃–³/₄ c. cooked), with sliced banana (¹/₂)	115
Cream, (half and half) ¹/₄ cup	80
Poached or soft boiled egg	77
Bacon, 3 slices	155
Whole wheat toast, 2 slices	120
Butter or margarine, 1 tbsp	100
Jam, 1 tbsp	55
Coffee, with sugar	45
	827
Midmorning	
Apple, 1 (medium)	90
Lunch	
Lettuce wedge, with sliced tomato and avocado (¹/₄)	95
French dressing, 1 tbsp	60
Creamed chicken (³/₄ cup), on slice of toast (1)	370
Hard roll, whole wheat, 1	60
Butter or margarine, 2 tsp	66
Ice cream, ¹/₂ cup	137
Sweetened strawberries	50
Milk, 8 oz	165
	1003
Midafternoon	
Chocolate milk, 1 cup	190
Dinner	
Cream of asparagus soup, ³/₄ cup	130
Crackers, 2	45
Cottage cheese (¹/₄ cup) and fruit cocktail (¹/₂ cup) salad, with	
2 tsp mayonnaise	165
Roast lamb, 4 oz	212
Mint jelly, 1 tbsp	55
Baked potato, 1 (medium)	95
Butter, 1 tbsp	100
Peas, ¹/₂ cup	55
Lemon meringue pie (¹/₆ of 9″ pie)	360
Coffee, with sugar	45
	1262
Evening	
Milk	165
Sugar cookie	90
	255
Total—approximately	3600

or 2 heaping tbsp whipped cream each furnishes about 100 kcal) and supplementary nourishment between meals and at bedtime.

The best foods to use for the **midmorning or midafternoon lunch** are *dairy products and fruit juices.* These can be served in many combinations—for example, plain cold milk enriched with cream, hot malted milk or milk flavored with chocolate or cocoa, eggnog, or beaten egg in fruit juice, and fruit juice plain or with extra calories added in milk sugar or malt sugar (which are not very sweet).

An *illustrative menu* is given in Table 23–6. The approximate amount of energy furnished is included to show how rapidly the fuel value of the diet mounts when fats and concentrated starchy foods are included in any considerable quantities. The meals alone, as planned in this diet, furnish over 3100 kcal, or 1000 kcal in excess of the energy needs of a 58 kg young woman (2100 kcal) without seeming unduly bulky. Supplementary nourishment between meals (as indicated) may be used to further increase the fuel intake by 500 kcal.

The success of any regimen for increasing weight depends chiefly on getting the individual to take a high energy diet, while he simultaneously cuts down muscular activity and tenseness by extra rest and relaxation. Those who have little appetite, or who have developed fears that foods cause digestive distress, must often force themselves to take food in excess of their natural desires at first. If this is done, the general condition usually improves to such an extent that both the appetite and digestion return to normal. Taking vitamins in tablet form may stimulate appetite and improve well being if the diet has previously been deficient in those nutrients as well as being inadequate in energy.

Rapid gains in weight should not be the main objective of the program, as such gains are usually due solely to the deposition of *fat* in the body, whereas it is greatly desired that the muscle tissues should also be built up. *Muscle development* is favored by a more gradual gain in weight on a diet containing plenty of the best quality protein (milk, eggs, and meat). *Out-door life* and some form of light, but regular, *exercise* are the best aids to building up the muscle tissues.

QUESTIONS AND PROBLEMS

1. Give four reasons why persons become overweight. How do you tell how much overweight a person is, and what are the dangers and difficulties of excess weight?

2. Is there any way (or ways) to reduce weight except by restriction of calories in the diet? What foods should be avoided or used only in small amounts in a reducing diet, and why? What foods may be used in quantity, and why? In which nutritive factor (or factors) must the reducing diet be low, and in which should it be adequate or better than adequate? Why? What food groups in the diet assure its adequacy?

3. Following the general meal pattern in Table 23–3, plan a reducing diet that furnishes about 1400 kcal. Revise this diet to drop out 400 kcal.

4. What are the health hazards associated with obesity: With underweight? Are fat people all well-nourished? Explain your answer.

5. What are the essential requirements for an effective diet for putting on weight? What kind of a regimen reinforces the good effects of the diet? What benefits may be expected from such a diet and regimen?

6. Plan a fattening and upbuilding diet that furnishes 3500 kcal for a person with good appetite and digestion. Modify it to give the same energy value for a person whose appetite is poor.

7. Compare your weight with the values given in Table 23–1. What percentage over- or underweight are you? How much will your weight change if you hold all other factors constant but

add on one 12-oz can of beer each day?
Play tennis for 30 minutes?

REFERENCES

1. Behnke, A. R., Jr., et al.: J. Amer. Med. Assoc., *118*:495, 498, 1942.
2. Seltzer, C. C., and Mayer, J.: A simplified criterion of obesity. Postgrad. Med., *38*:2, 1965.
3. Young, C. M., and Blondin, J.: Estimating body weight and fatness of young women. J. Amer. Dietet. Assoc., *41*:452, 1962.
4. Brozek, J.: Body composition. Science, *134*: 920, 1961.
5. Mayer, J.: *Overweight: Causes, Cost and Control.* Englewood Cliffs, New Jersey, Prentice-Hall, 1968.
6. Nisbett, R. E.: Determinants of food intake in obesity. Science, *159*:1254, 1968.
7. Hashim, S. A., and VanItallie, T. B.: Studies in normal and obese subjects with a monitored food dispensing device. Ann. N.Y. Acad. Sci., *131*:654, 1965.
8. Hirsch, J., Knittle, J. L., and Salans, L. B.: Cell lipid content and cell number in obese and non-obese human adipose tissue. J. Clin. Invest., *45*:1023, 1966.
9. Miller, D. S., and Payne, P. R.: Weight maintenance and food intake. J. Nutr., *78*:255, 1962.
10. Miller, D. S., and Mumford, P.: Overeating low protein diets by adult man. Proc. Nutr. Soc. Gt. Brit., *23*:xliii, 1964.
11. Cohn, C.: Feeding frequency and body composition. Ann. N. Y. Acad. Sci., *110*:395, 1963.
12. Fabry, P.: Metabolic consequences of the pattern of food intake. In Code, D. F. (ed.): *Handbook of Physiology*, Section 6, Vol. 1, Chapter 3. Baltimore, Williams and Wilkins for the American Physiological Society, 1967.
13. Trulson, M. F., et al.: Comparison of siblings in Boston and Ireland. J. Amer. Dietet. Assoc., *45*:225, 1964.
14. Paffenbarger, R. S., Laughlin, M. E., Gima, A. S., and Black, R. A.: Work activity of longshoremen as related to death from coronary heart disease and stroke. New Eng. J. Med., *282*:1109, 1970.
15. Morris, J. N.: Epidemiology and cardiovascular disease of middle age. I. Mod. Concepts Cardiovasc. Dis., *29*:625, 1960.
16. Frederickson, D. S., et al.: *Dietary Management of Hyperlipoproteinemia: A Handbook for Physicians.* Bethesda, Maryland, Natl. Heart and Lung Inst., Natl. Inst. Health, 1970.
17. Kaufmann, N. A., Paznanski, R., Blondheim, S. H., and Stein, Y.: Comparison of effects of fructose, sucrose, glucose and starch on serum lipids in patients with hypertriglyceridemia and normal subjects. Amer. J. Clin. Nutr., *20*:131, 1967.
18. Schroeder, H. A.: Cadmium hypertension in rats. Amer. J. Physiol., *207*:62, 1964.
19. Crawford, M. D., Gardner, J. J., and Morris, J. N.: Mortality and hardness of local water-supplies. Lancet, *1*:827, 1968.
20. Knowles, H. C., Jr.: Prevalence and development of diabetes. Fed. Proc., *27*:945, 1968.
21. Sharkey, T. P.: Recent research developments in diabetes mellitus—Part IV. J. Amer. Dietet. Assoc., *52*:108, 1968.
22. Keys, A. B. et al.: *The Biology of Human Starvation*, 2 vols. Minneapolis, University of Minnesota Press, 1950.
23. Bloom, W. L., and Azar, G. J.: Similarities of carbohydrate deficiency and fasting. Arch. Int. Med., *112*:333, 338, 1963.
24. Young, C. M., Scanlan, S. S., Sook Im, H., and Lutwak, L.: Effect on body composition and other parameters in obese young men of carbohydrate level of reduction diet. Amer. J. Clin. Nutr., *24*:290, 1971.

SUPPLEMENTARY READING

Albrink, M. J. (ed.): Symposium: Endocrine aspects of obesity. Amer. J. Clin. Nutr., *21*: 1397, 1968.
American Health Foundation: Position statement on diet and coronary heart disease. Prevent. Med., *1*:256, 1972.
Bray, G. A.: Effect of caloric restriction on energy expenditure in obese patients. Lancet, *2*:397, 1969.
Bray, G. A.: The myth of diet in the management of obesity. Amer. J. Clin. Nutr., *23*:1141, 1970.
Brown, H. B.: Food patterns that lower blood lipids in man. J. Amer. Dietet. Assoc., *58*: 303, 1971.
Bullen, B. A., Reed, R. B., and Mayer, J.: Physical activity of obese and nonobese adolescent girls appraised by motion picture sampling. Amer. J. Clin. Nutr., *14*:211, 1964.
Consolazio, C. F., et al.: Thiamin, riboflavin, and pyridoxine excretion during acute starvation and calorie restriction. Amer. J. Clin. Nutr., *24*:1060, 1971.
Drenick, E. J., and Alvarez, L. C.: Neutropenia in prolonged fasting. Amer. J. Clin. Nutr., *24*:859, 1971.
Durnin, J. V. G. A.: Basic physiological factors affecting calorie balance. Proc. Nutr. Soc. Gt. Brit., *20*:52, 1961.
Finkelstein, B., and Fryer, B. A.: Meal frequency and weight reduction of young women. Amer. J. Clin. Nutr., *24*:465, 1971.
Forbes, G. B.: Weight loss during fasting. Amer. J. Clin. Nutr., *24*:287, 1971.
Goldblatt, P. B., Moore, M. E., and Stunkard,

A. J.: Social factors in obesity. J. Amer. Med. Assoc., *192*:1039, 1965.

Greenfield, N. S., and Fellner, C. H.: Resting level of physical activity in obese females. Amer. J. Clin. Nutr., *22*:1418, 1969.

Hammar, S.: An interdisciplinary study of adolescent obesity. J. Pediat., *80*:373, 1972.

Inter-Society Commission for Heart Disease Resources: Primary prevention of atherosclerotic diseases. Circulation, *42*:A55, 1970.

Johnson, H. L., et al.: Metabolic aspects of calorie restriction: Nutrient balances with 500-kilocalorie intakes. Amer. J. Clin. Nutr., *24*:913, 1971.

Konishi, F.: Food energy equivalents of various activities. J. Amer. Dietet. Assoc., *46*:186, 1965.

Levy, R. I., Bonnell, M., and Ernst, N. D.: Dietary management of hyperlipoproteinemia. J. Amer. Dietet. Assoc., *58*:406, 1971.

Lincoln, J. E.: Weight gain after cessation of smoking. J. Amer. Med. Assoc., *210*:1765, 1969.

Linton, P. H., Conley, M., Kuechenmeister, C., and McClusky, H.: Satiety and obesity. Amer. J. Clin. Nutr., *25*:368, 1972.

Mayer, J., ed.: Special issue on obesity. Postgrad. Med., *51*:May 1972.

McNamara, J., Molot, M. A., Stremple, J. F., and Cutting, R. T.: Coronary artery disease in combat casualties in Vietnam. J. Amer. Med. Assoc., *216*:1185, 1971.

Rose, H. E., and Mayer, J.: Activity, calorie intake, fat storage and the energy balance of infants. Pediatrics, *41*:18, 1968.

Schauf, G. E.: Diet and management of obesity. Amer. J. Clin. Nutr., *24*:287, 1971.

Seltzer, C. C., and Mayer, J.: Body build and obesity. Who are the obese? J. Amer. Med. Assoc., *189*:677, 1964.

Selvaraj, R. J., and Seetharam Bhat, K.: Phagocytosis and leucocyte enzymes in protein-calorie malnutrition. Biochem. J., *127*: 255, 1972.

Simon, R. I.: Obesity as a depressive equivalent. J. Amer. Med. Assoc., *183*:208, 1963.

Stirling, J. L., and Stock, M. J.: Metabolic origins of thermogenesis induced by diet. Nature, *220*:801, 1968.

Swenseid, M. E., Mulcare, D. B., and Drenick, E. J.: Nitrogen and weight loss during starvation and realimentation in obesity. J. Amer. Dietet. Assoc., *46*:276, 1965.

Vitale, J. J. (ed.): Symposium: Nutrition and infection. Amer. J. Clin. Nutr., *24*:248, 1971.

Nutrition Reviews

Comparison of an 800 to 1,000 calorie diet with fasting in weight reduction. *24*:6, 1966.

Body weight and coronary heart disease. *25*:270, 1967.

Protein and insulin secretion in diabetes. *26*:15, 1968.

Epidemic cardiac failure in beer drinkers. *26*:173, 1968.

Measles and malnutrition. *26*:232, 1968.

Cardiovascular mortality and soft drinking water. *26*:295, 1968.

Fasting for obese children. *26*:335, 1968.

Diet therapy of gastrointestinal disorders. *27*:49, 1969.

Overweight and hypertension. *27*:168, 1969.

Experimental epidemiology: Nutrition and infection. *27*:306, 1969.

Cholesterol absorption versus cholesterol synthesis in man. *28*:11, 1970.

Sugar and coronary heart disease. *28*:228, 1970.

Infantile obesity and respiratory infections. *29*: 112, 1971.

Cellular growth in the fat adolescent. *29*:158, 1971.

Adipose cell size and number in experimental human obesity. *30*:60, 1972.

Appendix

CONTENTS

Table 1A. Recommended Daily Dietary Allowances, Food and Nutrition Board, National Research Council, Revised 1968*

	AGE† (years) From Up to	WEIGHT (kg)	WEIGHT (lbs)	HEIGHT cm	HEIGHT (in.)	kcal	Protein (gm)	FAT-SOLUBLE VITAMINS Vitamin A Activity (IU)	Vitamin D (IU)	Vitamin E Activity (IU)
Infants	0–1/6	4	9	55	22	kg × 120	kg × 2.2¶	1500	400	5
	1/6–1/2	7	15	63	25	kg × 110	kg × 2.0¶	1500	400	5
	1/2–1	9	20	72	28	kg × 100	kg × 1.8¶	1500	400	5
Children	1–2	12	26	81	32	1100	25	2000	400	10
	2–3	14	31	91	36	1250	25	2000	400	10
	3–4	16	35	100	39	1400	30	2500	400	10
	4–6	19	42	110	43	1600	30	2500	400	10
	6–8	23	51	121	48	2000	35	3500	400	15
	8–10	28	62	131	52	2200	40	3500	400	15
Males	10–12	35	77	140	55	2500	45	4500	400	20
	12–14	43	95	151	59	2700	50	5000	400	20
	14–18	59	130	170	67	3000	60	5000	400	25
	18–22	67	147	175	69	2800	60	5000	400	30
	22–35	70	154	175	69	2800	65	5000	—	30
	35–55	70	154	173	68	2600	65	5000	—	30
	55–75+	70	154	171	67	2400	65	5000	—	30
Females	10–12	35	77	142	56	2250	50	4500	400	20
	12–14	44	97	154	61	2300	50	5000	400	20
	14–16	52	114	157	62	2400	55	5000	400	25
	16–18	54	119	160	63	2300	55	5000	400	25
	18–22	58	128	163	64	2000	55	5000	400	25
	22–35	58	128	163	64	2000	55	5000	—	25
	35–55	58	128	160	63	1850	55	5000	—	25
	55–75+	58	128	157	62	1700	55	5000	—	25
Pregnancy						+200	65	6000	400	30
Lactation						+1000	75	8000	400	30

*From Food and Nutrition Board: *Recommended Dietary Allowances.* Publ. 1694. 7th Ed. Washington, D.C., National Academy of Sciences, 1968. Designed for the maintenance of good nutrition of practically all healthy people in the U.S.A. The allowance levels are intended to cover individual variations among most normal persons as they live in the United States under usual environmental stresses. The recommended allowances can be attained with a variety of common foods, providing other nutrients for which human requirements have been less well defined. See text for more-detailed discussion of allowances and of nutrients not tabulated.

†Entries on lines for age range 22–35 years represent the reference man and woman at age 22. All other entries represent allowances for the midpoint of the specified age range.

Table 1A. Recommended Daily Dietary Allowances, Food and Nutrition Board, National Research Council, Revised 1968* (Continued)

	WATER-SOLUBLE VITAMINS						MINERALS			
Vitamin C (mg)	Folacin‡ (mg)	Niacin (mg equiv)§	Riboflavin (mg)	Thiamin (mg)	Vitamin B-6 (mg)	Vitamin B-12 (μg)	Calcium (g)	Phosphorus (g)	Iodine (μg)	Iron (mg)
35	0.05	5	0.4	0.2	0.2	1.0	0.4	0.2	25	6
35	0.05	7	0.5	0.4	0.3	1.5	0.5	0.4	40	10
35	0.1	8	0.6	0.5	0.4	2.0	0.6	0.5	45	15
40	0.1	8	0.6	0.6	0.5	2.0	0.7	0.7	55	15
40	0.2	8	0.7	0.6	0.6	2.5	0.8	0.8	60	15
40	0.2	9	0.8	0.7	0.7	3	0.8	0.8	70	10
40	0.2	11	0.9	0.8	0.9	4	0.8	0.8	80	10
40	0.2	13	1.1	1.0	1.0	4	0.9	0.9	100	10
40	0.3	15	1.2	1.1	1.2	5	1.0	1.0	110	10
40	0.4	17	1.3	1.3	1.4	5	1.2	1.2	125	10
45	0.4	18	1.4	1.4	1.6	5	1.4	1.4	135	18
55	0.4	20	1.5	1.5	1.8	5	1.4	1.4	150	18
60	0.4	18	1.6	1.4	2.0	5	0.8	0.8	140	10
60	0.4	18	1.7	1.4	2.0	5	0.8	0.8	140	10
60	0.4	17	1.7	1.3	2.0	5	0.8	0.8	125	10
60	0.4	14	1.7	1.2	2.0	6	0.8	0.8	110	10
40	0.4	15	1.3	1.1	1.4	5	1.2	1.2	110	18
45	0.4	15	1.4	1.2	1.6	5	1.3	1.3	115	18
50	0.4	16	1.4	1.2	1.8	5	1.3	1.3	120	18
50	0.4	15	1.5	1.2	2.0	5	1.3	1.3	115	18
55	0.4	13	1.5	1.0	2.0	5	0.8	0.8	100	18
55	0.4	13	1.5	1.0	2.0	5	0.8	0.8	100	18
55	0.4	13	1.5	1.0	2.0	5	0.8	0.8	90	18
55	0.4	13	1.5	1.0	2.0	6	0.8	0.8	80	10
60	0.8	15	1.8	+0.1	2.5	8	+0.4	+0.4	125	18
60	0.5	20	2.0	+0.5	2.5	6	+0.5	+0.5	150	18

‡The folacin allowances refer to dietary sources as determined by *Lactobacillus casei* assay. Pure forms of folacin may be effective in doses less than $1/4$ of the RDA.

§Niacin equivalents include dietary sources of the vitamin itself plus 1 mg equivalent for each 60 mg of dietary tryptophan.

¶Assumes protein equivalent to human milk. For proteins not 100 percent utilized factors should be increased proportionately.

Table 1B.   Comparative Dietary Standards of Selected Countries and UN Agencies*

COUNTRY	SEX	AGE (years)	WEIGHT (kg)	ACTIVITY	ENERGY (Kcal)	PROTEIN (gm)	CALCIUM (gm)	IRON (mg)	VITAMIN A ACTIVITY (IU)	THIAMIN (mg)	RIBOFLAVIN (mg)	NIACIN EQUIV. (mg)	VITAMIN C (mg)
U.S.A.	M	22	70	*	2800	65	0.8	10	5000	1.4	1.7	18	60
	F	22	58	*	2000	55	0.8	18	5000	1.0	1.5	13	55
FAO	M	25	65	*	3200	46	0.4–0.5		*	1.3	1.8	21.1	
	F	25	65	*	2300	39	0.4–0.5		*	0.9	1.3	15.2	
Australia	M	25	70	*	2900	70	0.4–0.8	10	2500	1.2	1.5	18	30
	F	25	58	*	2100	58	0.4–0.8	10	2500	0.8	1.1	14	30
Canada	M	25	72	*	2850	50	0.5	6	3700	0.9	1.4	9	30
	F	25	57	*	2400	39	0.5	10	3700	0.7	1.2	7	30
C.A. and Panama	M	25	55	Moderate activity	2700	65	0.45	10	*	1.1	1.6	17.8	60
	F	25	50	Moderate activity	2000	60	0.45	10	*	0.8	1.2	13.2	50
Colombia	M	20–29	65	Moderate activity	2850	68	0.5	10	5000	1.1	1.7	13.8	50
	F	20–29	55	Moderate activity	1900	60	0.5	15	5000	0.8	1.1	12.5	50
France	M	25	65	Moderate activity	3000	90							
	F	25	55	Moderate activity	2400	75							
India	M	25.4	55	Moderate activity	2800	55							
	F	21.5	45	Moderate activity	2300	45							
Japan	M	26–29	56	Moderate activity	3000	70	0.6	10	2000	1.5	1.5	15	65
	F	26–29	49	Moderate activity	2400	60	0.6	10	2000	1.2	1.2	12	60
Netherlands	M	20–29	70	Light activity	3000	70	1.0	10	5500	1.2	1.8	12	50
	F	20–29	60	Light activity	2400	60	1.0	12	5500	1.0	1.5	10	50
Norway	M	25	70	None given	3400	70	0.8	12	2500	1.7	1.8	17	30
	F	25	60	None given	2500	60	0.8	12	2500	1.3	1.5	13	30
Philippines	M	None	53	Moderate activity	2400	53	0.5	*	5000	1.2	1.2	*	70
	F	Specified	46	Moderate activity	1800	46	0.5	*	5000	0.9	0.9	*	70
S. Africa	M	None	73	Moderate activity	3000	65	0.7	9	4000	1.0	1.6	15	40
	F	Specified	60	Moderate activity	2300	55	0.6	12	4000	0.8	1.4	12	40
U.K.	M	20 up	65	Medium activity	3000	87	0.8	12	5000	1.2	1.8	12	20
	F	20 up	56	Moderate activity	2500	73	0.8	12	5000	1.0	1.5	10	20
U.S.S.R.	M			Moderate activity					5000	2.0	2.5	15	70
	F			Moderate activity					5000	2.0	2.5	15	70
E. Germany	M	18–35		Light work	2700	85	0.8	10	5000	1.6	1.5	18	70
	F	18–35		Light work	2300	75	0.8	15	5000	1.4	1.3	15	70
W. Germany	M	25	72	Sedentary activity	2550	72	0.8	10	5000	1.7	1.8	18	75
	F	25	60	activity	2200	60	0.8	12	5000	1.5	1.8	14	75

*For all footnotes, see original table in Food and Nutrition Board: Recommended Dietary Allowances. Publ. 1694. 7th Ed. Washington, D.C., National Academy of Sciences, 1968, pp. 69-71.

Table 1C. FAO/WHO Recommended Intakes of Selected Nutrients*

RECOMMENDED DAILY INTAKES OF VITAMIN C, VITAMIN D, VITAMIN B-12 AND FOLACIN

		VITAMIN C (mg)	VITAMIN D[2] (μg)[3]	VITAMIN B-12 (μg)	FOLACIN (μg)
Infants,	0– 6 months[1]	20	10	0.3	40
	7–12 months	20	10	0.3	60
Children,	1– 3 years	20	10	0.9	
	4– 6 years	20	10	1.5	100
	7– 9 years	20	2.5	1.5	
	10–12 years	20	2.5	2.0	
Boys Girls	13–19 years	30	2.5	2.0	200
Adults,	men women	30	2.5	2.0	200
	pregnancy	50[4]	10[4]	3.0	400
	lactation	50	10	2.5	300

[1]It is accepted that for infants aged 0–6 months breast-feeding by a well-nourished mother is the best way to satisfy the requirements of vitamin C, vitamin B-12 and folacin, but not of vitamin D.

[2]Adequate exposure to sunlight may partially or totally replace dietary vitamin D.

[3]2.5 μg of cholecalciferol are equivalent to 100 IU of vitamin D.

[4]For 2nd and 3rd trimesters.

RECOMMENDED DAILY INTAKES OF IRON

		RECOMMENDED INTAKE ACCORDING TO TYPE OF DIET		
		less than 10 % of calories from animal foods (mg)	10–25% of calories from animal foods (mg)	more than 25 % of calories from animal foods (mg)
Infants,	0– 4 months	[1]	[1]	[1]
	5–12 months	10	7	5
Children,	1–12 years	10	7	5
Boys,	13–16 years	18	12	9
Girls,	13–16 years	24	18	12
Adults,	men	9	6	5
	non-menstruating women	28	19	14
	menstruating women pregnancy lactation	See original source, p. 52		

[1]Breast feeding is assumed to be adequate.

*From FAO/WHO: *Requirements of Ascorbic Acid, Vitamin D, Vitamin B$_{12}$, Folate, and Iron.* WHO Technical Report Series No. 452. Geneva, WHO, 1970.

Table 1C.   FAO/WHO Recommended Intakes of
Selected Nutrients* *(Continued)*

RECOMMENDED DAILY INTAKES OF THIAMIN, RIBOFLAVIN, AND NIACIN*

AGE	THIAMIN (mg)	RIBOFLAVIN (mg)	NIACIN[1] EQUIVALENTS (mg)
0–6 months[2]	—	—	—
7–12 months	0.4	0.6	6.6
1 year	0.5	0.6	7.6
2 years	0.5	0.7	8.6
3 years	0.6	0.8	9.6
4–6 years	0.7	0.9	11.2
7–9 years	0.8	1.2	13.9
10–12 years	1.0	1.4	16.5
13–15 (boys)	1.2	1.7	20.4
(girls)	1.0	1.4	17.2
16–19 (boys)	1.4	2.0	23.8
(girls)	1.0	1.3	15.8
Adults (man)	1.3	1.8	21.1
(woman)	0.9	1.3	15.2

*From FAO/WHO: *Requirements of Vitamin A, Thiamine, Riboflavine, and Niacin.* Geneva, World Health Organization Tech. Rep. Series No. 362, 1967. Recommendations are based on the following intakes per 1000 kcal: thiamin: 0.4 mg; riboflavin: 0.55 mg; niacin equivalents: 6.6.

[1]A niacin equivalent is 1 mg niacin or 60 mg L-tryptophan.

[2]For children 0 to 6 months it is accepted that breast feeding by a well-nourished mother is the best way to satisfy the nutritional requirements for thiamin, riboflavin and niacin.

EXPLANATORY NOTES ON TABLES
2A and 2B

The source of most of the figures in Tables 2A and 2B, Nutritive Values of Foods (pp. 546 to 568), is the Agriculture Handbook No. 8, *Composition of Foods—Raw, Processed, Prepared*, compiled by the Agricultural Research Service, United States Department of Agriculture, revised and published in December, 1963. Figures for a few cooked foods are taken from Bowes and Church, *Food Values of Portions Commonly Used* (9th Ed., 1963 for Table 2A; 11th Ed., 1970 for Table 2B). Unless otherwise indicated, the values given are for only the parts of the food commonly eaten (E.P., edible portion). The abbreviation *A.P.* indicates *as purchased* (e.g., for artichokes).

As used in these Tables, a dash (−) indicates lack of reliable data for a constituent believed to be present, usually in variable or negligible amounts; *tr.*, or trace, means a value too small to be measured accurately, usually less than 0.05 mg; a zero (*0*) denotes the absence of a particular nutrient.

It should be understood that there is considerable variation in composition between different samples of the same food. The figures given here represent average or mean values—that is, those most likely to be approximated in a majority of cases. Because there is now general agreement that under these circumstances it is impossible to attain accuracy within certain limits, the figures for food energy (kcals) have been rounded off to the nearest 5 kcal. Those for water, fat, and total carbohydrate are rounded off to the nearest 1 gm and for protein to the nearest 0.5 gm. Figures for calcium, iron, and the vitamins (except total vitamin A activity, which is stated in International Units) are given in milligrams. If it is desired to convert milligrams to grams, simply move the decimal point three places to the left—for example, 800 mg of calcium equals 0.8 gm. To convert milligrams of vitamins to micrograms (whole numbers), move decimal point three places to the right—for example, 0.12 mg of thiamin equals 120 mcg.

Table 2A. Nutritive Values of Foods in Average Servings or Common Measures

Food	Weight gm	Approximate Measure	Energy Kcal	Protein gm	Fat gm	Total Carbohydrate gm	Water gm	Minerals Calcium mg	Iron mg	Total Vitamin A Activity IU	Vitamins Thiamin mg	Riboflavin mg	Niacin mg	Vitamin C mg
Almonds, shelled	15	12–15 nuts	90	3.0	8.0	3	1	35	0.7	0	0.04	0.14	0.5	tr.
Apples Fresh, E.P.	150	1 med. large, 3 in. diam.	90	0.3	0.9	22	127	11	0.5	140	0.05	0.03	0.2	6
Baked, unpared	115	1 large, 2 tbsp. sugar	195	0.5	0.2	49		12	0.6	180	0.04	0.05	0.3	2
Apple juice, fresh or canned	100	1/2 cup, scant	50	0.1	tr.	12	88	6	0.6	–	0.01	0.02	0.1	1
Applesauce Sweetened	125	1/2 cup	115	0.3	0.1	30	95	5	0.6	50	0.03	0.01	tr.	1
Unsweetened	125	1/2 cup	50	0.3	0.3	13	111	5	0.6	50	0.03	0.01	tr.	1
Apricots Fresh	100	2–3 medium	50	1.0	0.2	13	85	17	0.5	2700	0.03	0.04	0.6	10
Canned, heavy syrup pack	120	4 halves, 2 tbsp. juice	105	0.7	0.1	26	92	13	0.4	1990	0.02	0.02	0.5	5
water pack	100	4 halves, 2 tbsp. juice	40	0.7	0.1	10	89	12	0.3	1830	0.02	0.02	0.4	4
Dried, sulfured, raw	30	4–6 medium halves	80	1.5	0.2	20	8	20	1.7	3270	tr.	0.05	1.0	4
unsweetened (cooked)	140	1/2 cup fruit and liquid	120	2.0	0.3	30	106	31	2.5	4200	tr.	0.07	1.4	4
Apricot nectar, canned	125	1/2 cup	70	0.4	0.1	18	106	11	0.3	1180	0.01	0.01	0.3	4
Artichokes, French, A.P.	200	1 large, cooked	50	5.5	0.4	20	173	102	2.2	300	0.14	0.08	1.4	16
Asparagus Fresh, green, cooked	100	1/2 cup cut, 6–7 spears	20	2.0	0.2	4	94	21	0.6	900	0.16	0.18	1.4	26
Canned, green	100	1/2 cup cut, 6–7 spears	20	2.0	0.4	3	93	19	1.9	800*	0.06	0.10	0.8	15
Avocados Fuerte, California	100	1/2 pear, about 4 in. long	170	2.0	17.0	6	74	10	0.6	290	0.11	0.20	1.6	14
Florida	125	1/2 pear, about 4 in. long	160	2.0	14.0	11	98	13	0.8	360	0.14	0.25	2.0	18
Bacon, broiled, drained	25	3 strips, crisp	155	8.0	13.0	0.8	2	4	0.8	0	0.13	0.09	1.3	–

*In bleached asparagus, vitamin A activity is 80 IU.

Food														
Bananas, E.P.	125	1 medium	105	1.5	0.3	28	95	10	0.9	240	0.06	0.08	0.9	12
Beans,														
Canned, with pork and tomato sauce	130	1/2 cup	160	8.0	3.0	25	92	70	2.3	170	0.10	0.04	0.8	3
Canned, with pork and sweet sauce	130	1/2 cup	195	8.0	6.0	27	86	82	3.0	–	0.08	0.05	0.7	–
Lima, fresh, boiled	80	1/2 cup, drained	90	6.0	0.4	16	57	38	2.0	220	0.14	0.08	1.0	14
Red, canned, solids and liquids	125	1/2 cup	115	7.0	0.5	21	95	36	2.3	tr.	0.06	0.05	0.8	–
Snap, green, fresh or frozen, cooked	100	3/4 cup, drained	25	1.5	0.2	5	92	50	0.6	540	0.07	0.09	0.5	12
Snap, green, canned	100	3/4 cup, drained	25	1.0	0.2	5	92	45	1.5	470	0.03	0.05	0.3	4
Soy, dry weight	30	1/2 cup, scant, after cooking	120	10.0	5.0	10		68	2.5	20	0.33	0.09	0.7	–
Bean sprouts, cooked	60	2/3 cup	15	2.0	0.1	3	55	10	0.5	10	0.05	0.06	0.4	4
Beef,														
Corned, canned	85	3 slices, 3x2x1/4 in.	185	21.5	10.0	0	50	17	3.7	–	0.02	0.20	2.9	0
hash, canned	115	1/2 cup	230	10.0	17.0	9		30	1.4	tr.	0.03	0.16	3.3	0
Dried, creamed	120	1/2 cup	210	16.0	13.0	6		106	2.1	440	0.07	0.30	1.6	0
Hamburger, broiled market ground	85	4 from pound	245	20.5	17.0	0	46	9	2.7	30	0.08	0.18	4.6	–
lean ground	85	4 from pound	185	23.0	10.0	0	51	10	3.0	20	0.08	0.20	5.1	–
Roast, chuck, braised or pot roasted	100	2 slices, 4x1-1/2x1/2in.	375	24.0	30.0	0	45	10	3.1	60	0.04	0.19	3.8	–
oven, relatively lean	100	1 slice, 4-1/2x3x1/2in.	345	23.5	27.0	0	48	10	3.1	50	0.06	0.18	4.3	–
rib, choice grade	100	1 slice, 4-1/2x3x1/2in.	440	20.0	39.0	0	40	9	2.6	80	0.05	0.15	3.6	–
Steak, round, broiled	100	1 piece, 4-1/2x3-1/2x 1/2 in.	260	28.5	15.0	0	55	12	3.5	30	0.08	0.22	5.6	–
sirloin, broiled	100	1 piece, 4-1/2x2-1/2x 1 in.	410	22.0	35.0	0	42	10	2.9	60	0.06	0.18	4.6	–
Beet greens	100	1/2 cup, boiled, drained	20	1.5	0.2	3	94	99	1.9	5100	0.07	0.15	0.3	15
Beets, cooked or canned	85	1/2 cup, drained solids	30	1.0	tr.	6	77	12	0.4	20	0.03	0.03	0.3	5
Biscuits, baking powder, from mix	100	3 biscuits, 2 in. diam.	325	7.0	9.0	52	29	68	2.3	tr.	0.27	0.25	2.0	tr.
Blackberries, dewberries, boysenberries, and youngberries, fresh	100	2/3 cup	60	1.0	0.9	13	85	32	0.9	200	0.03	0.04	0.4	21
Blueberries, fresh	100	2/3 cup	60	0.7	0.5	15	83	15	1.0	100	0.03	0.06	0.5	14

Table 2A. Nutritive Values of Foods in Average Servings or Common Measures — Continued

Food	Weight gm	Approximate Measure	Energy Kcal	Protein gm	Fat gm	Total Carbohydrate gm	Water gm	Minerals Calcium mg	Iron mg	Total Vitamin A Activity IU	Vitamins Thiamin mg	Riboflavin mg	Niacin mg	Vitamin C mg
Bread,														
Boston brown	100	3 slices, 1/2 in. thick	210	5.5	1.0	46	45	90	1.9	70	0.11	0.06	1.2	0
Corn, from mix	40	1 piece, 2 in. square	95	2.5	3.0	13	20	34	0.5	110*	0.06	0.08	0.5	tr.
French or Vienna, enriched	23	1 slice	70	2.0	0.7	13	7	10	0.5	tr.	0.06	0.05	0.6	tr.
Raisin	23	1 slice	60	1.5	0.6	12	8	16	0.3	tr.	0.01	0.02	0.2	tr.
Rye, American	23	1 slice	55	2.0	0.3	12	8	17	0.5	0	0.04	0.02	0.3	0
White, unenriched	23	1 slice	60	2.0	0.7	12	8	19	0.2	tr.	0.02	0.02	0.3	tr.
enriched	23	1 slice	60	2.0	0.7	12	8	19	0.6	tr.	0.06	0.05	0.6	tr.
Whole wheat	23	1 slice	55	2.5	0.7	11	8	23	0.5	tr.	0.06	0.03	0.7	tr.
Broccoli	100	2/3 cup, boiled, drained	25	3.0	0.3	5	91	88	0.8	2500	0.09	0.20	0.8	90
Brussels sprouts	70	5-6 sprouts, boiled drained	25	3.0	0.3	4	62	22	0.8	360	0.06	0.10	0.6	61
Butter	10	1 pat, 45 per pound	70	tr.	8.0	tr.	2	2	0	330	-	-	-	0
	14	1 tbsp.	100	tr.	11.0	tr.	2	3	0	460	-	-	-	0
Cabbage, headed														
Raw	100	1 cup, shredded	25	1.5	0.2	5	92	49	0.4	130	0.05	0.05	0.3	47
Cooked	100	1-1/3 cup	20	1.0	0.2	4	94	42	0.3	120	0.02	0.02	0.1	24
Cakes,														
Angel, from mix	40	2 in. sector of 8-in. cake	105	2.5	0.1	24	14	38	0.1	0	tr.	0.04	tr.	0
Chocolate, fudge icing	100	2 in. sector of 8-in. cake	370	4.5	16.0	56	22	70	1.0	160	0.02	0.10	0.2	tr.
Gingerbread, from mix	55	2 x 2 inches	150	1.5	4.0	28	20	50	0.9	tr.	0.02	0.05	0.4	tr.
Plain cake or cupcake, iced	100	2 in. sector of 8-in. cake or 2 medium cupcakes	370	3.5	12.0	63	21	50	0.3	200	0.02	0.07	0.1	tr.
Pound cake, plain	30	1 slice, 2-3/4x3x5/8 in.	125	2.0	6.0	16	6	12	0.2	90	0.01	0.03	0.1	tr.
Yellow cake, iced, from mix	100	2 in. sector of 8-in. cake	335	4.0	11.0	58	26	91	0.6	140	0.02	0.08	0.2	tr.

*No vitamin A activity if made with white cornmeal.

Candy,														
Caramels, plain or chocolate	30	1 oz	120	1.0	3.0	23	2	44	0.4	3	0.01	0.05	0.1	tr.
Chocolate, milk,														
plain	30	1 oz	155	2.5	10.0	17	0.3	68	0.3	80	0.02	0.10	0.1	tr.
with almonds	30	1 oz	160	3.0	11.0	15	0.5	69	0.5	70	0.02	0.12	0.2	tr.
Fudge, with nuts	30	1 oz	130	1.0	5.0	21	23	24	0.4	tr.	0.01	0.03	0.1	tr.
Hard	30	1 oz	115	0.0	0.3	29	0.4	6	0.6	0	0	0	0	0
Marshmallow	30	1 oz	100	0.6	tr.	24	5	5	0.5	0	0	tr.	tr.	0
Peanut brittle	30	1 oz	125	2.0	3.0	24	0.6	11	0.7	0	0.05	0.01	1.0	0
Cantaloupe, See Melons														
Carrots														
Raw	50	1 carrot, 5-1/2x1 in. or 1/2 cup grated	20	0.6	0.1	5	44	19	0.4	5500	0.03	0.03	0.3	4
Boiled, drained	100	2/3 cup, diced	30	0.9	0.2	7	91	33	0.6	10500	0.05	0.05	0.5	6
Cauliflower,														
Raw	100	1 cup flower buds	25	2.5	0.2	5	91	25	1.1	60	0.11	0.10	0.7	78
Boiled, drained	100	3/4 cup	20	2.5	0.2	4	93	21	0.7	60	0.09	0.08	0.6	55
Celery,														
Raw	100	2 lg. stalks or 1 cup diced	15	0.9	0.1	4	94	39	0.3	270*	0.03	0.03	0.3	9
Boiled, drained	100	3/4 cup, diced	15	0.8	0.1	3	95	31	0.2	240*	0.02	0.03	0.3	6
Cereals,														
Ready to eat														
Bran Flakes, 40%, added nutrients	30	3/4 cup	90	3.0	0.5	24	0.9	21	1.3	0	0.12	0.05	1.9	0
Corn Flakes, added nutrients	25	1 cup	95	2.0	0.1	21	1	4	0.4	0	0.11	0.02	0.5	0
Rice, puffed, added nutrients	14	1 cup	55	0.8	0.1	13	0.5	3	0.3	0	0.06	0.01	0.6	0
Wheat Flakes, added nutrients	25	1 cup	90	3.0	0.4	20	0.9	10	1.1	0	0.16	0.04	1.2	0
Wheat, puffed, added nutrients	12	1 cup	45	2.0	0.2	9	0.4	3	0.5	0	0.07	0.03	0.9	0
Wheat, shredded	40	1 large biscuit	140	4.0	0.8	32	3	17	1.4	0	0.09	0.04	1.8	0
Cooked (figured from 1 oz. dry weight)														
Cornmeal, white or yellow, unenriched	120	1/2 cup	60	1.0	0.2	13	105	1	0.2	70†	0.02	0.01	0.1	0
enriched	120	1/2 cup	60	1.0	0.2	13	105	1	0.5	70†	0.07	0.05	0.6	0

*Based on green variety; if bleached, only 140 IU.
†Based on yellow cornmeal; white cornmeal contains only a trace of vitamin A activity.

Table 2A. Nutritive Values of Foods in Average Servings or Common Measures—Continued

Food	Weight gm	Approximate Measure	Energy Kcal	Protein gm	Fat gm	Total Carbohydrate gm	Water gm	Minerals Calcium mg	Minerals Iron mg	Total Vitamin A Activity IU	Vitamins Thiamin mg	Vitamins Riboflavin mg	Vitamins Niacin mg	Vitamins Vitamin C mg
Cereals (continued)														
Corn grits, white, degerm, unenriched enriched	120	1/2 cup	60	1.0	0.1	13	105	1	0.1	tr.	0.02	0.01	0.2	0
Oatmeal	120	1/2 cup	60	1.0	0.1	13	105	1	0.4	tr.	0.05	0.04	0.5	0
Wheat, Cream of, reg. (Farina)	120	2/3 – 3/4 cup	65	2.0	1.0	12	104	11	0.7	0	0.10	0.02	0.1	0
unenriched	120	2/3 – 3/4 cup	50	2.0	0.1	10	107	5	0.2	0	0.01	0.01	0.1	0
enriched	120	2/3 – 3/4 cup	50	2.0	0.1	10	107	5	0.4	0	0.05	0.04	0.5	0
Wheat, whole meal (e.g., Ralston)	100	1/2 cup	55	2.0	0.4	11	105	8	0.6	0	0.07	0.02	0.7	0
Chard, Swiss, boiled	100	1/2 cup, stalks & leaves	20	2.0	0.2	3.0	94	73	1.8	5400	0.04	0.11	0.4	16
Cheeses, Natural														
Cheddar, American	30	1 oz or 4 tbsp., grated	120	7.5	10.0	0.6	11	225	0.3	390	0.01	0.14	tr.	0
Cottage, large or small curd, creamed	55	1/4 cup or 2 rounded tbsp.	60	7.5	2.0	2.0	43	52	0.2	90	0.02	0.14	tr.	0
uncreamed	55	1/4 cup or 2 rounded tbsp.	50	9.5	0.2	2.0	44	50	0.2	5	0.02	0.15	tr.	0
Cream	30	1 oz or 2 tbsp.	110	2.5	11.0	0.6	15	19	0.1	460	0.01	0.07	tr.	0
Swiss, domestic	30	1 oz	110	8.5	8.0	0.5	12	278	0.3	340	tr.	0.12	tr.	0
Pasteurized processed American	30	1 oz	110	7.0	9.0	0.6	12	209	0.3	370	0.01	0.12	tr.	0
Cheese food (e.g., Velveeta)	30	1 oz	95	6.0	7.0	2.0	13	171	0.2	290	0.01	0.17	tr.	0
Cheese spread, American	30	1 oz	85	5.0	6.0	3.0	15	170	0.2	260	tr.	0.16	tr.	0
Cherries,														
Raw, sweet	100	15 large, 20–25 small	70	1.5	0.3	17	80	22	0.4	110	0.05	0.06	0.4	10
Red, canned, heavy syrup	120	1/2 cup, pitted, with syrup	95	1.0	0.2	25	94	18	0.4	70	0.02	0.02	0.2	4
Red, canned, water pack	100	1/2 cup, pitted, with juice	50	1.0	0.2	12	87	15	0.3	60	0.02	0.02	0.2	3

(handwritten annotations in margins: "2-8gum to org' 60 cal."; near Cottage cheese rows: "1¼", "2g", "40g", "80%")

Food	Weight (g)	Approximate Measure	Calories	Protein (g)	Fat (g)	Carbohydrate (g)	Phosphorus (mg)	Calcium (mg)	Iron (mg)	Vitamin A (I.U.)	Thiamine (mg)	Riboflavin (mg)	Niacin (mg)	Ascorbic Acid (mg)
Chicken,														
Broiler	100	3-1/2 oz, flesh only	135	24.0	4.0	0	71	9	1.7	90	0.05	0.19	8.8	—
Canned, flesh only	100	3-1/2 oz	200	21.5	12.0	0	65	21	1.5	230	0.04	0.12	4.4	4
Creamed	177	3/4 cup	310	26.5	6.0	2	—	124	1.6	490	0.06	0.27	5.7	tr.
Fryer, breast	100	Approx. 1/2 breast, fried	205	32.5	6.0		58	12	1.7	90	0.05	0.22	14.7	—
thigh and drumstick	100	1 of each, med. size, fried	235	29.0	11.0	3	56	13	2.3	200	0.06	0.48	6.8	—
Roasted	100	3-1/2 oz, flesh and skin	250	27.0	15.0	0	57	11	1.8	420	0.08	0.14	8.2	—
Chickpeas or garbanzos, dry weight	30	1/2 cup, after cooking	110	6.0	1.0	18	—	45	2.1	15	0.10	0.03	0.6	—
Chicory or endive, curly	25	10 small leaves	5	0.5	0.1	1	23	22	0.2	1000	0.02	0.03	0.1	6
Chili con carne, canned														
With beans	250	1 cup	335	19.0	15.0	31	181	80	4.3	150	0.08	0.18	3.3	—
Without beans	250	1 cup	500	26.0	37.0	15	167	95	3.5	380	0.05	0.30	5.5	—
Chocolate (beverage), all milk	220	1 cup, small, 6 oz milk	210	7.0	8.0	32	—	222	0.5	295	0.08	0.32	0.1	1
Chocolate, bitter or baking	30	1 oz or 1 square	150	3.0	16.0	9	1	23	2.0	20	0.02	0.07	0.5	0
Clams, canned, solids and liquid	100	1/2 cup	50	8.0	0.7	3	86	55	4.1	—	0.01	0.11	1.0	—
Cocoa (beverage), all milk	200	1 cup, small, 6 oz milk	174	7.0	9.0	20	—	224	0.9	295	0.08	0.34	0.3	2
Cola type beverages, See Soft Drinks														
Coconut, dried, sweetened	15	2 tbsp., shredded	80	0.5	6.0	8	1	2	0.3	0	0.01	tr.	0.1	—
Collards, boiled, drained	100	1/2 cup	30	2.5	0.6	5	91	152	0.6	5400	0.14	0.20	1.2	46
Cookies, assorted, commercial	25	3 small or 1 large, 3 in. diameter	120	1.5	5.0	18	1	9	0.2	20	0.01	0.01	0.1	tr.

Table 2A. Nutritive Values of Foods in Average Servings or Common Measures — Continued

Food	Weight gm	Approximate Measure	Energy Kcal	Protein gm	Fat gm	Total Carbo-hydrate gm	Water gm	Minerals Calcium mg	Iron mg	Total Vitamin A Activity IU	Vitamins Thia-min mg	Ribo-flavin mg	Niacin mg	Vitamin C mg
Corn, sweet														
Fresh	100	1 small ear, cooked	90	3.5	1.0	21	74	3	0.6	400*	0.12	0.10	1.4	9
Canned, drained	100	1/2 cup, scant	85	2.5	0.8	20	76	5	0.5	350*	0.03	0.05	0.9	4
Cream style, canned	100	1/2 cup, scant	80	2.0	0.6	20	76	3	0.6	330*	0.03	0.05	1.0	5
Cornmeal, See under Cereals														
Corn syrup, light or dark	20	1 tbsp.	60	0	0	15	5	9	0.8	0	0	0	0	0
Cowpeas or blackeye peas,														
Immature, fresh	160	1 cup, cooked	170	13.0	1.0	29	115	38	3.4	560	0.48	0.18	2.2	27
Mature, dried	125	1/2 cup, cooked	95	6.5	0.4	17	100	21	1.6	12	0.20	0.05	0.5	-
Crabmeat, canned or cooked	100	5/8 cup	100	17.5	3.0	1	77	45	0.8	-	0.08	0.08	1.9	-
Crackers,														
Graham, plain	7	1 cracker, 2-1/2 in. sq.	25	0.6	0.7	5	0.4	3	0.1	0	tr.	0.01	0.1	0
Ry-Krisp	13	2 wafers, 1-7/8x3-1/2in.	45	1.5	0.2	10	0.8	7	0.5	0	0.04	0.03	0.2	0
Saltines	4	1 cracker, 2 in. square	17	0.4	0.5	3	0.2	1	0.1	0	tr.	tr.	tr.	0
Soda, plain or oyster	10	2 crackers, 2-1/2 in.sq. or 10 oyster	45	0.9	1.0	7	0.4	2	0.2	0	tr.	0.01	0.1	0
Cranberry, jelly, sweetened														
Sauce, unstrained	20	1 level tbsp.	30	tr.	tr.	8	12	1	tr.	4	tr.	tr.	tr.	tr.
	15	1 level tbsp.	25	tr.	tr.	7	8	1	tr.	3	tr.	tr.	tr.	tr.
Cream,														
Half-and-half	60	1/4 cup or 4 tbsp.	80	2.0	7.0	3	48	65	tr.	290	0.02	0.10	0.1	1
Heavy or whipping	60	1/4 cup or 4 tbsp.	210	1.5	23.0	2	34	45	tr.	920	0.01	0.07	tr.	1
Light, coffee or table	60	1/4 cup or 4 tbsp.	130	2.0	12.0	3	43	61	tr.	500	0.02	0.09	0.06	1

*Yellow corn. White corn has trace only.

Food	Measure	Weight												
Cucumbers, raw, pared	1/2 medium	50	7	0.3	0.1	2	48	9	0.2	tr.	0.02	0.02	0.1	6
Custard, See under Puddings														
Dandelion greens, boiled	1/2 cup, drained	100	35	2.0	0.6	6	90	140	1.8	11700	0.13	0.16	–	18
Dates, dried or fresh	1/2 cup pitted or 12 average	100	275	2.0	0.5	73	23	59	3.0	50	0.09	0.10	2.2	0
Doughnuts, Cake type	1 average	30	120	1.5	6.0	15	7	12	0.4	24	0.05	0.05	0.4	tr.
Yeast	1 average	30	125	2.0	8.0	11	9	11	0.5	20	0.05	0.05	0.4	0
Eggs, Raw, whole, E.P.	1 large, 24 oz per doz.	50	80	6.5	6.0	0.5	37	27	1.2	590	0.06	0.15	0.1	0
white	1 white	32	16	3.5	tr.	0.3	29	3	tr.	0	tr.	0.09	tr.	0
yolk	1 yolk	18	64	3.0	5.5	0.1	9	24	0.9	580	0.04	0.07	tr.	0
Omelet or scrambled	2 small eggs with milk	100	175	11.0	13.0	2.0	72	80	1.7	1080	0.08	0.28	0.1	0
Eggplant, raw	2 slices or 1/2 cup pieces	100	25	1.0	0.2	6	92	12	0.7	10	0.05	0.05	0.6	5
Fats, Cooking, vegetable, solid or oil	1/2 cup	100	885	0	100.0	0	0	0	0	–	0	0	0	0
	1 tbsp.	12.5	110	0	13.0	0	0	0	0	–	0	0	0	0
Figs, Fresh	2 large or 3 small	100	80	1.0	0.3	20	78	35	0.6	80	0.06	0.05	0.4	2
Canned, heavy syrup	3 figs and 2 tbsp. syrup	100	85	0.5	0.2	22	77	13	0.4	30	0.03	0.03	0.2	1
Dried	1 large	20	55	0.9	0.3	14	5	25	0.6	20	0.02	0.02	0.1	0
Fish, Cod, steak, baked	4 oz, before cooking	100	170	28.5	5.0	0	65	31	1.0	180	0.08	0.11	3.0	–
Fish sticks	5 sticks, or 4 oz, cooked	110	195	18.0	10.0	7	72	12	0.4	0	0.04	0.08	1.8	–
Flounder or sole	4 oz, before cooking	100	200	30.0	8.0	0	58	23	1.4	–	0.07	0.08	2.5	2
Haddock, cooked, fried	4 oz, before cooking	100	165	19.5	6.0	6	66	40	1.2	–	0.04	0.07	3.2	2
Halibut, broiled	3-1/2 oz, cooked	100	171	25.0	7.0	0	67	16	0.8	680	0.05	0.07	8.3	–
Mackerel, Atlantic	3-1/2 oz, cooked with butter	100	235	22.0	16.0	0	62	6	1.2	530	0.15	0.27	7.6	–
Salmon, fresh, broiled	3-1/2 oz, cooked	100	180	27.0	7.0	0	63	–	1.2	160	0.16	0.06	9.8	0
Canned, pink	1/2 cup	110	155	23.0	7.0	0	78	216	0.9	80	0.03	0.20	8.8	–
Canned, sockeye or red	1/2 cup	110	190	22.0	10.0	0	74	285	1.3	250	0.04	0.18	8.0	–

Table 2A. Nutritive Values of Foods in Average Servings or Common Measures—Continued

Food	Weight gm	Approximate Measure	Energy kcal	Protein gm.	Fat gm	Total Carbo-hydrate gm	Water gm	Minerals Calcium mg	Iron mg	Vitamins Total Vitamin A Activity IU	Thia-min mg	Ribo-flavin mg	Niacin mg	Vitamin C mg
Fish (continued)														
Sardines, Atlantic, packed in oil	85	3 oz, drained solids	175	20.5	9.0	—	52	371	2.5	190	0.03	0.17	4.6	—
Swordfish, broiled	100	3-1/2 oz, cooked with butter	175	28.0	6.0	0	65	27	1.3	2050	0.04	0.05	10.9	—
Tuna, canned, in oil	100	5/8 cup, drained	195	29.0	8.0	0	61	8	1.9	80	0.05	0.12	11.9	—
water pack	100	5/8 cup, solids and liquids	125	28.0	0.8	0	70	16	1.6	—	—	0.10	13.3	—
Flours,														
Rye, light	80	1 cup, sifted	285	8.0	0.8	62	9	18	0.9	0	0.12	0.06	0.5	0
Wheat, patent, all purpose, unenriched	110	1 cup, sifted	400	11.5	1.0	84	13	18	0.9	0	0.07	0.06	1.0	0
enriched	110	1 cup, sifted	400	11.5	1.0	84	13	18	3.2	0	0.48	0.29	3.9	0
whole grain	120	1 cup, stirred	400	16.0	2.0	85	14	49	4.0	0	0.66	0.14	5.2	0
Fruit cocktail (heavy syrup)	100	1/2 cup, scant	75	0.4	0.1	20	80	9	0.4	140	0.02	0.01	0.4	2
Gelatin, dry, plain	10	1 tbsp.	35	8.5	tr.	0	1	—	—	—	0.02	—	—	—
Gelatin dessert,														
Plain	120	1/2 cup	70	2.0	0.0	17	101	—	—	—	—	—	—	—
With fruit	120	1/2 cup	80	1.5	0.1	20	98	—	—	—	—	—	—	4
Grapefruit,														
Raw, pulp only	100	1/2 med, 4-1/4 in. diam.	40	0.5	0.1	11	88	16	0.4	80	0.04	0.02	0.2	38
Canned, in syrup	100	1/2 cup, scant, solids and liquid	70	0.6	0.1	18	81	13	0.3	10	0.03	0.02	0.2	30

Food	Weight (g)	Measure													
Grapefruit juice, canned,															
Unsweetened	180	6 oz, 3/4 cup	75	0.9	0.2	18	161	14	0.7	20	0.05	0.04	0.4	61
Sweetened	180	6 oz, 3/4 cup	95	0.9	0.2	23	155	14	0.7	20	0.05	0.04	0.4	56
Grapes,															
American type (slip-skin)	100	22–24 avg. size	70	1.5	1.0	16	82	16	0.4	100	0.05	0.03	0.3	4
European type (adherent skin)	100	22–24 avg. size	65	0.6	0.3	17	81	12	0.4	100	0.05	0.03	0.3	4
Grape juice	195	6 oz, 3/4 cup	130	0.4	tr.	32	162	21	0.6	-	0.08	0.04	0.4	tr.
Griddle cakes, from mix, with milk	25	1 med., 4 in. diam.	50	1.5	1.0	8	14	55	0.2	30	0.04	0.06	0.2	tr.
Ham, smoked															
Cooked	100	3-1/2 oz, 2–3 small slices	290	21.0	22.0	0	54	9	2.6	0	0.47	0.18	3.6	-
Canned	100	3-1/2 oz	195	18.5	12.0	0.9	65	11	2.7	0	0.53	0.19	3.8	-
Heart, beef, braised	85	3 oz	160	27.0	5.0	0.6	52	5	5.0	30	0.21	1.04	6.5	1
Honey, strained	20	1 tbsp.	60	0.1	0	16	3	1	0.1	0	tr.	0.01	0.1	tr.
Ice cream, plain, factory pack	100	3/4 cup (12 % fat)	205	4.0	13.0	21	62	123	0.1	520	0.04	0.19	0.1	1
Ice milk (dessert)	100	2/3 cup	150	5.0	5.0	22	67	156	0.1	210	0.05	0.22	0.1	1
Ices, water, lime	100	1/2 cup	80	0.4	tr.	33	67	tr.	tr.	0	tr.	tr.	tr.	1
Jams, jellies, preserves, marmalade	20	1 tbsp.	55	0.1	tr.	14	6	4	0.2	tr.	tr.	0.01	tr.	tr.
Kale, boiled, drained	55	1/2 cup, leaves only	20	2.5	0.4	3	48	103	0.9	4570	0.06	0.10	0.9	51
Kidney,															
Beef, raw	100	3-1/2 oz	130	15.0	7.0	0.9	76	11	7.4	690	0.36	2.55	6.4	15
Lamb, raw	100	3-1/2 oz	105	17.0	3.0	0.9	78	13	7.6	690	0.51	2.42	7.4	15
Kohlrabi, boiled, drained	75	1/2 cup diced	20	1.5	0.1	4	69	25	0.2	15	0.05	0.02	0.2	32

Table 2A. Nutritive Values of Foods in Average Servings or Common Measures—Continued

Food	Weight gm	Approximate Measure	Energy kcal	Protein gm	Fat gm	Total Carbo-hydrate gm	Water gm	Minerals Calcium mg	Iron mg	Vitamins Total Vitamin A Activity IU	Thia-min mg	Ribo-flavin mg	Niacin mg	Vitamin C mg
Lamb, (choice grade)														
Chop, loin, broiled														
lean and fat	100	1 avg., 3-1/2 oz, 3/4 in. thick	360	22.0	29.0	0	47	9	1.3	—	0.12	0.23	5.0	—
lean only	66	2.4 oz	125	19.0	5.0	0	41	8	1.3	—	0.10	0.18	4.0	—
Leg, roasted														
lean and fat	100	3-1/2 oz, 2 sl. 4x3x 1/4 in.	280	25.5	19.0	0	54	11	1.7	0	0.15	0.27	5.5	—
lean only	85	3 oz	160	24.0	6.0	0	53	11	1.9	—	0.14	0.26	5.3	—
Shoulder, roasted														
lean and fat	100	3-1/2 oz	340	22.0	27.0	0	50	10	1.2	—	0.13	0.23	4.7	—
lean only	75	2.7 oz	155	20.0	8.0	0	46	9	1.4	—	0.11	0.21	4.3	—
Lard	110	1/2 cup	990	0	110.0	0	0	0	0	0	0	0	0	0
	14	1 tbsp.	125	0	14.0	0	0	0	0	0	0	0	0	0
Lemon juice	100	1/2 cup, scant	25	0.5	0.2	8	91	7	0.2	20	0.03	0.01	0.1	46
	15	1 tbsp.	5	0.1	tr.	1	14	1	tr.	tr.	0.01	tr.	tr.	7
Lemonade concentrate, frozen	250	1 cup, diluted as directed	110	0.3	tr.	29	221	3	tr.	tr.	tr.	0.02	0.2	18
Lentils, dried, cooked	100	1/2 cup	105	8.0	tr.	19	72	25	2.1	20	0.07	0.06	0.6	0
Lettuce, raw														
Compact head	50	2 lg. or 4 small leaves	7	0.5	0.1	1	48	17	1.0	485	0.03	0.03	0.2	4
Iceberg type	90	1/5 head, 4-3/4 in. diam.	12	0.8	0.1	3	86	18	0.5	300	0.05	0.05	0.3	5
Loose leaf	50	2 lg. or 4 small leaves	9	0.7	0.2	2	47	34	0.7	950	0.03	0.04	0.2	9
Liver,														
Beef, fried	75	2 slices 3x2-1/4x3/8 in.	170	20.0	8.0	4	42	8	6.6	40050	0.20	3.14	12.4	20
Lamb, broiled	75	2 slices 3x2-1/4x3/8 in.	195	24.0	9.0	2	38	12	13.4	55880	0.37	3.83	18.7	27
Pork, fried	75	2 slices 3x2-1/4x3/8 in.	180	22.0	9.0	2	41	11	21.8	11180	0.26	3.27	16.7	17
Lobster, canned or cooked	100	2/3 cup meat	95	18.5	2.0	0.3	77	65	0.8	—	0.10	0.07	—	—

Food	Weight (g)	Approximate measure	Food energy (cal.)	Protein (g)	Fat (g)	Carbohydrate (g)	Water (g)	Calcium (mg)	Iron (mg)	Vitamin A (I.U.)	Thiamin (mg)	Riboflavin (mg)	Niacin (mg)	Ascorbic acid (mg)
Loganberries,														
Fresh	100	2/3 cup	60	1.0	0.6	15	83	35	1.2	200	0.03	0.04	0.4	24
Canned, juice pack	100	1/2 cup, scant, solids and juice	55	0.7	0.5	13	86	27	1.2	150	0.02	0.03	0.3	12
Macaroni or Spaghetti,														
Unenriched, tender	140	1 cup, cooked 14–20 min.	155	5.0	0.6	32	101	11	0.6	0	0.01	0.01	0.4	0
Enriched, tender	140	1 cup, cooked 14–20 min.	155	5.0	0.6	32	101	11	1.3	0	0.20	0.11	1.5	0
Baked with cheese	220	1 cup	475	19.0	24.0	44	128	398	2.0	950	0.22	0.44	2.0	tr.
Margarine, fortified*	10	1 pat, 1/45 lb	70	0.1	8.0	tr.	2	2	0	330	—	—	—	0
	14	1 tbsp.	100	0.1	11.0	0.1	2	3	0	460	—	—	—	0
Melons, E.P.														
Cantaloupe or muskmelons	100	1/2 of 4-1/2 in. melon	30	0.7	0.1	8	91	14	0.4	3400	0.04	0.03	0.6	33
Casaba	100	3-1/2 oz., 1 avg. serving	35	0.8	0.3	8	91	14	0.4	40	0.04	0.03	0.6	23
Watermelon	100	1/2 cup, balls or cubes	25	0.5	0.2	6	93	7	0.5	590	0.03	0.03	0.2	7
	900	1/16 of 10x16 in. melon	235	4.5	2.0	58	833	63	4.5	5310	0.27	0.27	1.8	63
Milk,														
Whole, fresh	244	8 oz, 1 cup or full glass	160	8.5	9.0	12	213.0	285	tr.	370	0.07	0.41	0.2	2
2% Milk	250	1 cup	150	10.5	5.0	13	221	358	tr.	200	0.10	0.53	2.80	2
Skim or buttermilk	246	1 cup	90	9.0	0.2	13	223.0	298	tr.	tr.	0.10	0.44	0.2	2
Half and Half	242	1 cup	325	8.0	28.0	11	193.0	261	tr.	1160	0.07	0.39	0.3	2
Evaporated	126	1/2 cup or 1 cup reconst.	170	9.0	10.0	12	93.0	318	0.1	400	0.05	0.43	tr.	1
Condensed (sweetened)	20	1 tbsp.	65	1.5	2.0	11	5.0	52	tr.	70	0.02	0.08	0.1	tr.
Dried, whole	8	1 tbsp.	40	2.0	2.0	3	0.2	73	tr.	90	0.02	0.12	0.1	1
skim (nonfat solids)	7.5	1 tbsp.	25	2.5	0.1	4	0.2	98	tr.	tr.	0.03	0.14	tr.	1
Malted, plain, dry	8	1 tbsp.	35	1.0	0.7	6	0.2	23	0.2	80	0.03	0.04	0.2	0
Chocolate drink commercial	250	1 cup (skim milk used)	190	8.0	6.0	27	207.0	270	0.5	200	0.10	0.40	0.3	3
Yogurt, low-fat	246	1 cup	125	8.5	4.0	13	219.0	295	tr.	170	0.10	0.44	0.2	2
Molasses,														
Light	20	1 tbsp.	50	—	—	13	5	33	0.9	—	0.01	0.01	tr.	—
Medium	20	1 tbsp.	45	—	—	12	5	58	1.2	—	-	0.02	0.2	—
Blackstrap	20	1 tbsp.	40	—	—	11	5	137	3.2	—	0.02	0.04	0.4	—
Muffins,														
Bran	35	1 medium	90	2.5	3.0	15	12	50	1.3	80	0.05	0.08	1.4	tr.
Cornmeal (yellow, enriched)	45	1 medium	140	3.0	5.0	21	15	47	0.8	140	0.09	0.10	0.7	tr.
White flour, enriched	40	1 medium	120	3.0	4.0	15	15	42	0.6	40	0.07	0.09	0.6	tr.

*Almost all margarines now on sale are fortified to contain 15,000 IU of vitamin A activity per pound.

Table 2A. Nutritive Values of Foods in Average Servings or Common Measures — Continued

Food	Weight gm	Approximate Measure	Energy kcal	Protein gm	Fat gm	Total Carbohydrate gm	Water gm	Minerals Calcium mg	Iron mg	Total Vitamin A Activity IU	Vitamins Thiamin mg	Riboflavin mg	Niacin mg	Vitamin C mg
Mushrooms, raw	100	3-1/2 oz	30	2.5	0.3	4	90	6	0.8	tr.	0.10	0.46	4.2	3
Mustard greens, boiled, drained	100	2/3 cup	25	2.0	0.4	4	93	138	1.8	5800	0.08	0.14	0.6	48
Mustard, prepared, brown or yellow	15	1 tbsp.	11	1.0	1.0	1	12	13	0.3	—	—	—	—	—
Noodles, egg Unenriched	100	2/3 cup, cooked	125	4.0	2.0	23	70	10	0.6	70	0.03	0.02	0.4	0
Enriched	100	2/3 cup, cooked	125	4.0	2.0	23	70	10	0.9	70	0.14	0.08	1.2	0
Nuts, mixed, shelled	15	8-12 average nuts	95	2.5	9.0	3	—	14	0.5	tr.	0.09	0.02	0.6	tr.
Oils, salad or cooking	110	1/2 cup	970	0	110.0	0	0	0	0	—	0	0	0	0
	14	1 tbsp.	125	0	14.0	0	0	0	0	—	0	0	0	0
Okra, boiled, drained	100	9 pods, 3 in. long	30	2.0	0.3	6	91	92	0.5	490	0.13	0.18	0.9	20
Olives, E.P. Green	5	1 large or 2 small	5	tr.	0.6	0.1	4	3	0.08	15	—	—	—	—
Ripe (Mission)	5	1 large or 2 small	10	0.1	1.0	0.2	4	5	0.09	5	tr.	tr.	—	—
Onions, green (scallions), raw	8.5	1 medium, without tops	5	0.1	tr.	0.9	7	3	0.05	tr.	tr.	tr.	0.03	2
Onions, mature, dry Raw	100	1 onion, 2-1/2 in. diam.	40	1.5	0.1	9	89	27	0.5	40	0.03	0.04	0.2	10
	10	1 tbsp., chopped	4	0.2	tr.	0.9	9	3	0.05	5	tr.	tr.	0.02	1
Boiled, drained	100	1/2 cup, 3-4 small	30	1.0	0.1	7	92	24	0.4	40	0.03	0.03	0.2	7
Oranges, raw, E.P.	150	1 medium, 3 in. diam.	75	1.5	0.3	18	129	62	0.6	300	0.15	0.06	0.6	75
Orange juice, Fresh or canned	185	6 oz, 3/4 cup, 1 sm. glass	80	1.0	0.4	19	163	20	0.4	370	0.17	0.06	0.7	93
Frozen, concentrate (as diluted)	185	6 oz, 3/4 cup, 1 sm. glass	80	1.0	0.2	20	163	17	0.2	370	0.17	0.02	0.6	83

Food	Weight (g)	Measure												
Oysters, raw Eastern Pacific and Olympia	120 120	5–8 medium 5–8 medium or 3-1/2 oz Olympia	80 110	10.0 13.0	2.0 3.0	4 8	102 95	113 102	6.6 8.6	370 –	0.17 0.14	0.22 –	3.0 1.6	– 36
Oyster stew (1 part oysters, 3 parts milk)	230	1 cup, 3–4 oysters	200	11.0	12.0	11	193	269	3.2	640	0.14	0.41	1.6	–
Pancakes. See Griddle cakes														
Papayas, raw	100	1/2 cup, cubed	40	0.6	0.1	10	89	20	0.3	1750	0.04	0.04	0.3	56
Parsley, raw	3.5	1 tbsp., chopped	2	0.1	tr.	0.3	3	7	0.2	300	tr.	0.01	tr.	6
Peaches, Raw, yellow, E.P. Canned, heavy syrup water pack	115 120 120	1 med. peach, 2 in. diam. 2 halves, 2 tbsp. juice 1/2 cup, sliced, with liquid	45 95 40	0.7 0.5 0.5	0.1 0.1 0.1	11 24 10	103 95 109	10 5 5	0.6 0.4 0.4	1530 520 540	0.02 0.01 0.01	0.06 0.02 0.04	1.2 0.7 0.7	8 4 4
Dried, sulfured, cooked, unsweetened	135	1/2 cup, 5–6 halves, 3 tbsp. liquid	110	1.5	0.3	29	103	20	2.6	1650	tr.	0.08	2.0	3
Peanuts, shelled, roasted	15	15–17 nuts (without skins)	90	4.0	8.0	3	tr.	11	0.3	–	0.05	0.02	2.6	0
Peanut butter	16	1 tbsp.	90	4.0	8.0	3	tr.	10	0.3	–	0.02	0.02	2.4	0
Pears, Raw, including skin Canned, heavy syrup water pack	180 120 120	1 pear, 3x2-1/2 in. diam. 2 halves and 2 tbsp. syrup 2 halves and 2 tbsp. juice	110 90 40	1.5 0.2 0.2	0.7 0.2 0.2	28 24 10	148 96 109	14 6 6	0.5 0.2 0.2	40 tr. tr.	0.04 0.01 0.01	0.07 0.02 0.02	0.2 0.1 0.1	7 1 1
Peas, Green, fresh or frozen Canned, drained Split, dry, cooked	80 80 125	1/2 cup, boiled, drained 1/2 cup 1/2 cup (from 1 oz dry wt.)	55 65 145	4.5 4.0 10.0	0.3 0.3 0.4	10 12 26	65 63 88	18 20 14	1.4 1.4 2.1	430 550 50	0.22 0.09 0.19	0.09 0.05 0.11	1.8 0.8 1.1	16 6 –
Peas and carrots, frozen, cooked	75	1/2 cup	40	2.5	0.2	8	64	19	0.8	6980	0.14	0.05	1.0	6
Pecans	15	12 halves or 2 tbsp. chopped	105	1.0	11.0	2	1	11	0.4	20	0.13	0.02	0.1	tr.

Table 2A. Nutritive Values of Foods in Average Servings or Common Measures—Continued

Food	Weight gm	Approximate Measure	Energy kcal	Protein gm	Fat gm	Total Carbohydrate gm	Water gm	Minerals Calcium mg	Minerals Iron mg	Total Vitamin A Activity IU	Vitamins Thiamin mg	Vitamins Riboflavin mg	Vitamins Niacin mg	Vitamin C mg
Peppers,														
Green, raw, E.P.	65	1 medium shell	15	0.8	0.1	3	61	6	0.5	270	0.05	0.05	0.3	83
	10	1 tbsp., chopped	5	0.1	tr.	0.5	9	1	0.1	40	0.01	0.01	tr.	13
Red, canned (pimientos)	40	1 medium	10	0.4	0.2	2	37	3	0.6	920	0.01	0.02	0.2	38
Pickles, cucumber														
Dill	135	1 large, 4x1-3/4 in.	15	0.9	0.3	3	126	35	1.4	140	tr.	0.03	tr.	8
Sweet	20	1 pickle, 2-3/4x3/4 in.	30	0.1	0.1	7	12	2	0.2	20	tr.	tr.	tr.	1
Relish, sweet or mixed	13	1 tbsp.	20	0.1	0.1	4	8	3	0.1	0	0	0	0	0
Pies,														
Apple	160	1/6 of 9 inch pie	410	3.5	18.0	61	76	13	0.5	50	0.03	0.03	0.6	2
Blackberry	160	1/6 of 9 inch pie	390	4.0	18.0	55	82	30	0.8	140	0.03	0.03	0.5	6
Cherry	160	1/6 of 9 inch pie	420	4.0	18.0	61	75	22	0.5	700	0.03	0.03	0.8	tr.
Chocolate meringue	160	1/6 of 9 inch pie	405	7.5	19.0	54	77	110	1.1	300	0.05	0.19	0.3	tr.
Custard	160	1/6 of 9 inch pie	350	10.0	14.0	37	93	154	1.0	370	0.08	0.26	0.5	0
Lemon meringue	140	1/6 of 9 inch pie	360	5.0	14.0	53	66	20	0.7	240	0.04	0.11	0.3	4
Mince	160	1/6 of 9 inch pie	435	4.0	18.0	66	69	45	1.6	tr.	0.11	0.06	0.6	2
Pumpkin	150	1/6 of 9 inch pie	320	6.0	17.0	37	89	77	0.8	3710	0.05	0.15	0.8	tr.
Pineapple,														
Raw	100	2/3 cup, no sugar	50	0.4	0.2	14	85	17	0.5	70	0.09	0.03	0.2	17
Canned, crushed, heavy syrup	130	1/2 cup, solids and liquid	95	0.4	0.1	25	104	14	0.4	70	0.10	0.03	0.3	9
sliced	120	2 small or 1 large slice, 2 tbsp. juice	90	0.4	0.1	23	96	13	0.4	60	0.10	0.02	0.2	8
water pack	100	2 small or 1 large slice, 2 tbsp. liquid	40	0.3	0.1	10	89	12	0.3	50	0.08	0.02	0.2	7
Pineapple juice, canned, unsweetened	185	6 oz, 3/4 cup, 1 sm. glass	100	0.7	0.2	25	158	28	0.6	90	0.09	0.04	0.4	17
Pineapple and grape-fruit juice	185	6 oz, 3/4 cup	100	0.4	tr.	25	159	9	0.4	20	0.04	0.02	0.2	30

Food	Weight (g)	Measure												
Pinenuts, Piñon	15	2 tbsp.	95	2.0	9.0	3	1	2	0.8	5	0.19	0.03	0.7	tr.
Plums,														
Raw, hybrid type	100	2 medium	50	0.5	0.2	12	87	12	0.5	250	0.03	0.03	0.5	6
Canned, purple (Italian) heavy syrup	120	3 med., 2 tbsp. syrup	100	0.5	0.1	26	93	11	1.1	1450	0.02	0.02	0.5	2
Popcorn, with oil and salt	15	1 cup	70	2.0	3.0	9	1	1	0.3	–	–	0.01	0.3	0
Pork,														
Chops, broiled, E.P. lean and fat	66	1 medium thick chop (from above serving)	245	15.0	20.0	0	30	7	1.9	0	0.33	0.15	3.2	–
lean only	48		110	13.5	6.0	0	28	6	1.8	0	0.29	0.13	2.6	–
Loin, roasted lean and fat	90	2 slices, 3-1/2x3-1/4 in. (from above serving)	335	20.0	28.0	0	41	9	2.6	0	0.45	0.21	4.4	–
lean only	70		165	20.0	9.0	0	40	8	2.5	0	0.43	0.20	3.9	–
Potatoes,														
Baked	100	1 medium	95	2.5	0.1	21	75	9	0.7	tr.	0.10	0.04	1.7	20
Boiled, pared before cooking	100	1 medium	65	2.0	0.1	15	83	6	0.5	tr.	0.09	0.03	1.2	16
French-fried	100	20 pieces, 2x1/2x1/2 in.	275	4.5	13.0	36	45	15	1.3	tr.	0.13	0.08	3.1	21
frozen (reheated)	100	20 pieces, 2x1/2x1/2 in.	220	3.5	8.0	34	53	9	1.8	tr.	0.14	0.02	2.6	21
Mashed, milk and table fat added	100	1/2 cup	95	2.0	4.0	12	80	24	0.4	170	0.08	0.05	1.0	9
Potato chips	20	10 chips, 2 in. diam.	115	1.0	8.0	10	tr.	8	0.4	tr.	0.04	0.01	1.0	3
Prunes, dried														
Softened	32	4 prunes, medium	80	0.7	0.2	22	9	16	1.2	510	0.03	0.05	0.5	1
Cooked, unsweetened	135	8-9 med., 2 tbsp. juice	160	1.5	0.4	42	90	32	2.4	1010	0.04	0.09	0.9	1
Prune juice, canned	180	6 oz, 3/4 cup	140	0.7	0.2	34	144	25	0.7	–	0.02	0.02	0.7	4
Puddings,														
Apple Brown Betty	100		150	1.5	4.0	30	65	18	0.6	100	0.06	0.04	0.4	1
Chocolate, cooked or instant (from mix)	130	1/2 cup	160	4.5	4.0	30	91	133	0.4	170	0.03	0.20	0.1	tr.
Custard	100	1/2 cup	115	5.5	6.0	11	77	112	0.4	350	0.04	0.19	0.1	tr.
Junket (mix) with milk	130	1/2 cup	125	4.0	5.0	17	104	152	tr.	200	0.04	0.21	0.1	1
Prune whip	65	1/2 cup	100	3.0	0.1	24	37	14	0.8	300	0.01	0.09	0.3	1
Rice, with raisins	145	2/3 cup	210	5.0	5.0	39	95	142	0.6	160	0.04	0.20	0.3	tr.
Tapioca, cream	100	1/2 cup	135	5.0	5.0	17	72	105	0.4	290	0.04	0.18	0.1	1
Vanilla, home recipe, with starch	130	1/2 cup	145	5.0	5.0	21	99	152	tr.	210	0.04	0.21	0.1	1

Table 2A. Nutritive Values of Foods in Average Servings or Common Measures — Continued

Food	Weight gm	Approximate Measure	Energy kcal	Protein gm	Fat gm	Total Carbohydrate gm	Water gm	Minerals Calcium mg	Iron mg	Total Vitamin A Activity IU	Vitamins Thiamin mg	Riboflavin mg	Niacin mg	Vitamin C mg
Pumpkin, canned	120	1 cup	40	1.0	0.4	10	108	30	0.5	7680	0.04	0.06	0.7	6
Radishes, raw, common	40	4 small	7	0.4	tr.	1	38	12	0.4	5	tr.	tr.	0.1	10
Raisins, natural unbleached	40	1/4 cup	115	1.0	0.1	31	7	25	1.4	4	0.02	0.01	0.1	tr.
	10	1 tbsp.	30	0.1	tr.	8	2	6	0.3	1	tr.	tr.	tr.	tr.
Raspberries														
Black, fresh	100	2/3 cup	75	2.0	1.0	16	81	30	0.9	tr.	0.03	0.09	0.9	18
Red, fresh	100	2/3 cup	55	1.0	0.5	14	84	22	0.9	130	0.03	0.09	0.9	25
Red, canned, water pack	100	1/2 cup, solids and liquid	35	0.7	0.1	9	90	15	0.6	90	0.01	0.04	0.5	9
Rhubarb, cooked, with sugar	135	1/2 cup, fruit and syrup	190	0.7	0.1	49	85	105	0.8	110	0.03	0.07	0.4	8
Rice,														
Brown, cooked	100	2/3 cup	120	2.5	0.6	26	70	12	0.5	0	0.09	0.02	1.4	0
White, enriched, cooked	100	2/3 cup	110	2.0	0.1	24	73	10	0.9	0	0.11		1.0	0
Precooked, instant	100	2/3 cup	110	2.0	tr.	24	73	3	0.8	0	0.13		1.0	0
Rolls and buns (enriched)														
Plain (pan rolls)	28	1 small	85	2.5	2.0	15	9	21	0.5	tr.	0.08	0.05	0.6	tr.
Hamburger bun	38	1 large	115	3.0	2.0	20	12	28	0.7	tr.	0.11	0.07	0.8	tr.
Hard	52	1 large	160	5.0	2.0	31	13	24	1.2	tr.	0.14	0.12	1.4	tr.
Rutabagas, boiled, drained	80	1/2 cup, diced (yellow turnip)	30	0.7	0.1	7	72	47	0.2	440	0.05	0.05	0.6	21
Rye wafers, See Crackers														

Food	Measure	Weight (g)	Food energy (cal.)	Protein (g)	Fat (g)	Carbohydrate (g)		Calcium (mg)	Iron (mg)	Vitamin A (I.U.)	Thiamine (mg)	Riboflavin (mg)	Niacin (mg)	Ascorbic acid (mg)
Salad dressings, avg. commercial														
Blue Cheese	1 tbsp.	16	80	0.8	8.0	1.0	5	13	tr.	30	tr.	0.02	tr.	tr.
French	1 tbsp.	15	60	0.1	6.0	3.0	6	2	0.1	–	–	–	–	–
low-calorie	1 tbsp.	15	15	0.1	0.6	2.0	12	2	0.1	–	–	–	–	–
Mayonnaise	1 tbsp.	14	100	0.2	11.0	0.3	2	3	0.1	40	tr.	0.01	tr.	–
Salad dressing (mayonnaise type)	1 tbsp.	15	65	0.2	6.0	2.0	6	2	tr.	30	tr.	tr.	tr.	–
low-calorie	1 tbsp.	15	20	0.2	2.0	0.7	12	3	tr.	30	tr.	tr.	tr.	–
Thousand Island	1 tbsp.	15	75	0.1	8.0	2.0	5	2	0.1	50	tr.	tr.	tr.	tr.
Salad dressings, Boiled, home recipe	1 tbsp.	17	30	0.7	2.0	3	12	15	0.1	80	0.01	0.03	tr.	tr.
Sauces, Butterscotch sauce	2 tbsp.	44	205	0.5	7.0	41	–	41	1.4	300	tr.	tr.	tr.	tr.
Cheese sauce	2 tbsp.	38	65	3.0	5.0	2	13	88	0.1	210	0.01	0.08	0.1	tr.
Chocolate syrup, thin	2 tbsp.	40	100	0.9	0.8	25	13	7	0.6	tr.	0.02	0.03	0.2	0
Fudge type	2 tbsp.	50	165	3.0	7.0	27	–	64	0.7	80	0.01	0.11	0.2	tr.
Custard sauce, avg.	2 tbsp.	36	40	2.0	2.0	5	–	39	0.2	120	tr.	0.12	0.1	tr.
Hard sauce	2 tbsp.	21	95	0.1	6.0	12	–	2	tr.	230	0.03	tr.	tr.	0
Hollandaise, true	1/4 cup, scant	50	180	2.5	19.0	0.4	7	23	0.9	1030	tr.	0.04	tr.	tr.
Tartar sauce	1 tbsp.	20	105	0.3	12.0	0.8	–	4	0.2	40	–	tr.	tr.	tr.
Tomato catsup or chili sauce	1 tbsp.	17	20	0.3	0.1	4	12	4	0.1	240	0.02	0.01	0.3	3
White sauce, medium	1/2 cup	133	215	5.0	17.0	12	98	153	0.3	610	0.05	0.23	0.3	tr.
Sauerkraut, canned	2/3 cup, solids and liquid	125	20	1.0	0.3	5	116	45	0.6	60	0.04	0.05	0.3	18
Sausages, Bologna, all meat	1 oz, 1 slice 4-1/4 × 1/8 in.	30	85	4.0	7.0	1	17	–	–	–	–	–	–	–
Frankfurter	1 average, cooked	50	150	6.0	14.0	0.8	29	3	0.8	–	0.08	0.10	1.3	–
Liverwurst, fresh	1 oz	30	90	5.0	8.0	0.5	16	3	1.6	1910	0.06	0.39	1.7	–
Luncheon meat, pork, cured, canned or pkg.	1 oz	30	90	5.0	8.0	0.4	17	3	0.7	0	0.09	0.06	0.9	–
Pork sausage, link, cooked	3 links	60	285	11.0	27.0	tr.	21	4	1.4	0	0.47	0.20	2.2	–
Salami, dry	1 oz	30	135	7.0	11.0	0.4	9	4	1.1	–	0.11	0.08	1.6	–
Vienna sausage, canned	2 oz, 1/2 can	60	145	8.5	12.0	0.2	38	5	1.3	–	0.05	0.08	1.6	–
Scallops, Raw	3-1/2 oz	100	80	15.5	0.2	3	80	26	1.8	–	–	0.06	1.3	–
Frozen, breaded, fried	3-1/2 oz, reheated	100	195	18.0	8.0	11	60	–	–	–	–	–	–	–

Table 2A. Nutritive Values of Foods in Average Servings or Common Measures—Continued

Food	Weight gm	Approximate Measure	Energy kcal	Protein gm	Fat gm	Total Carbohydrate gm	Water gm	Minerals Calcium mg	Iron mg	Total Vitamin A Activity IU	Vitamins Thiamin mg	Riboflavin mg	Niacin mg	Vitamin C mg
Sherbet, orange	100	1/2 cup	135	0.9	1.0	31	67	16	tr.	60	0.01	0.03	tr.	2
Shrimp, canned	85	3 oz, meat only	100	20.5	0.9	0.6	60	98	2.6	50	0.01	0.03	1.5	—
Sirup, table, cane and maple	20	1 tbsp.	50	0	0	13	7	3	tr.	0	0	0	0	0
Soft Drinks,														
Cola type	170	1 bottle, 6 oz	65	0	0	17	153	—	—	0	0	0	0	0
Dietary drink (less than 1 Cal./oz.)	170	1 bottle, 6 oz	—	0	0	—	170	—	—	0	0	0	0	0
Ginger Ale	170	1 bottle, 6 oz	50	0	0	14	156	—	—	0	0	0	0	0
Root Beer	170	1 bottle, 6 oz	70	0	0	18	152	—	—	0	0	0	0	0
Soups, canned, diluted, ready to serve														
Asparagus or celery cream of, made with water	190	3/4 cup	70	1.0	4.0	7	175	38	0.4	150	0.02	0.04	tr.	tr.
made with milk	190	3/4 cup	130	5.0	7.0	12	163	154	0.6	300	0.04	0.21	0.6	2
Bean, with pork	185	3/4 cup	125	6.0	4.0	16	156	46	1.7	480	0.09	0.06	0.7	2
Bouillon, broth or consomme	180	3/4 cup	20	4.0	0	2	172	tr.	0.4	tr.	tr.	0.02	0.9	—
Chicken, cream of,	190	3/4 cup	75	2.5	5.0	6	175	19	0.4	320	0.02	0.04	0.4	tr.
with rice	185	3/4 cup	40	2.5	0.9	4	175	6	0.2	110	tr.	0.02	0.6	—
Clam chowder (Manhattan)	190	3/4 cup	60	2.0	2.0	10	175	27	0.8	680	0.02	0.02	0.8	—
Mushroom, cream of	190	3/4 cup	105	2.0	8.0	8	170	32	0.4	60	0.02	0.10	0.6	tr.
Pea, split	185	3/4 cup	110	7.0	2.0	16	158	22	1.1	330	0.19	0.11	1.1	tr.
Tomato	185	3/4 cup	65	1.5	2.0	12	167	11	0.6	760	0.04	0.04	0.9	9
Vegetable beef	185	3/4 cup	60	4.0	2.0	7	170	9	0.6	2040	0.04	0.04	0.7	—
Soups, dehydrated, add water as directed														
Chicken noodle	185	3/4 cup	40	1.5	1.0	6	175	6	0.2	40	0.06	0.04	0.4	tr.
Onion	185	3/4 cup	30	1.0	0.9	4	177	7	0.2	tr.	tr.	tr.	tr.	2

Food	gm	Measure												
Spaghetti, canned, in tomato sauce, with Cheese	100	2/3 cup	75	2.0	0.6	15	80	16	1.1	370	0.14	0.11	1.8	4
Meat balls	100	2/3 cup	100	5.0	4.0	11	78	21	1.3	400	0.06	0.07	0.9	2
Spinach, fresh or frozen, boiled	90	1/2 cup, drained	20	3.0	0.3	3	83	84	2.0	7290	0.06	0.13	0.5	25
Squash, Summer, boiled, drained	100	1/2 cup	15	0.9	0.1	3	96	25	0.4	390	0.05	0.08	0.8	10
Winter, baked	100	3-1/2 oz (yellow)	65	2.0	0.4	15	81	28	0.8	4200	0.05	0.13	0.7	13
boiled, drained	100	1/2 cup	40	1.0	0.3	9	89	20	0.5	3500	0.04	0.10	0.4	8
Starch, pure (arrowroot, corn, etc.)	8	1 tbsp.	30	tr.	tr.	7	1	0	0	0	0	0	0	0
Strawberries, Fresh	100	2/3 cup	35	0.7	0.5	8	90	21	1.0	60	0.03	0.07	0.6	59
Frozen, sweetened, whole	100	3-1/2 oz	90	0.4	0.2	24	76	13	0.6	30	0.02	0.06	0.5	55
Sugar, Brown	110	1/2 cup, firmly packed	410	0	0	106	2	94	3.7	0	0.01	0.03	0.2	0
White, granulated	100	1/2 cup	385	0	0	100	1	0	0.1	0	0	0	0	0
	12	1 tbsp. or 3 level tsp.	45	0	0	12	tr.	0	tr.	0	0	0	0	0
powdered	128	1 cup, stirred before meas.	495	0	0	127	1	0	0.1	0	0	0	0	0
loaf	8	1 tbsp.	30	0	0	8	tr.	0	tr.	0	0	0	0	0
	7	1 cube or domino	30	0	0	7	tr.	0	tr.	0	0	0	0	0
Sweet potatoes, cooked, Baked, skinned	100	1 small	140	2.0	0.5	33	64	40	0.9	8100	0.09	0.07	0.7	22
Boiled in skin	100	1/2 medium	115	2.0	0.4	26	71	32	0.7	7900	0.09	0.06	0.6	17
Candied	100	1/2 medium	170	1.5	3.0	34	60	37	0.9	6300	0.06	0.04	0.4	10
Canned, vacuum pack	100	1/2 cup	110	2.0	0.2	25	72	25	0.8	7800	0.05	0.04	0.6	14
Tomatoes, Fresh	150	1 medium, 2x2-1/2 in.	35	1.5	0.3	7	140	20	0.8	1350	0.09	0.06	1.1	35
Canned or cooked	120	1/2 cup, solids and liquid	25	1.0	0.2	5	124	7	0.6	1080	0.06	0.04	0.8	20
Tomato juice, canned	180	6 oz, 3/4 cup	35	1.5	0.2	8	169	13	1.6	1440	0.09	0.05	1.4	29
Tomato purée, canned (sauce)	120	1/2 cup	50	2.0	0.2	11	104	16	2.0	1920	0.11	0.06	1.7	40

Table 2A. Nutritive Values of Foods in Average Servings or Common Measures — Continued

Food	Weight gm.	Approximate Measure	Energy kcal	Protein gm	Fat gm	Total Carbohydrate gm	Water gm	Minerals Calcium mg	Minerals Iron mg	Total Vitamin A Activity IU	Vitamins Thiamin mg	Vitamins Riboflavin mg	Vitamins Niacin mg	Vitamins Vitamin C mg
Tongue, Beef, fresh, simmered Canned or cured, beef, lamb, etc.	100	3-1/2 oz., cooked	245	21.5	17.0	0.4	61	7	2.2	–	0.05	0.29	3.5	–
	100	3-1/2 oz., cooked	265	19.5	20.0	0.3	57	–	–	–	–	–	–	–
Tuna, See Fish.														
Turkey, roasted (flesh only) Light meat	100	3-1/2 oz, 3 slices (3-1/2x2x2-1/4 in.)	175	33.0	4.0	0	62	–	1.2	–	0.05	0.14	11.1	–
Dark meat	100	3-1/2 oz	205	30.0	8.0	0	61	–	2.3	–	0.04	0.23	4.2	–
Turnips, white, boiled, drained	75	1/2 cup, diced	20	0.6	0.2	4	70	26	0.3	tr.	0.03	0.04	0.2	17
Turnip greens, boiled, drained	75	1/2 cup	15	2.0	0.2	3	70	138	0.8	4730	0.11	0.18	0.5	52
Veal, Cutlet, broiled	100	3-1/2 oz	215	27.0	11.0	0	60	11	3.2	–	0.07	0.25	5.4	–
Shoulder, oven braised	100	3-1/2 oz	235	28.0	13.0	0	59	12	3.5	–	0.09	0.29	6.4	–
Vinegar, cider	15	1 tbsp.	5	tr.	0	0.9	14	1	0.1	–	–	–	–	–
Waffles (from mix), with milk and eggs	75	One, 4-1/2x5-1/2x 1/2 in.	205	6.5	8.0	27	31	179	1.0	170	0.11	0.17	0.7	tr.
Walnuts, English	100	1 cup, halves	650	15.0	64.0	16	4	99	3.1	30	0.33	0.13	0.9	2
	15	2 tbsp., chopped	100	2.0	10.0	2	1	15	0.5	10	0.05	0.02	0.1	tr.
Watercress, raw	10	10 average sprigs	2	0.2	tr.	0.3	9	15	0.2	490	0.01	0.02	0.1	8

Watermelon, See Melons.

		10	35	2.5	1.0	5	1	7	1.0	0	0.20	0.07	0.4	0
Wheat germ, crude	1 tbsp., rounded	10												
Yeast,														
Baker's, moist	1 cake, compressed	12	10	1.5	0.1	1	9	2	0.6	tr.	0.09	0.20	1.3	tr.
dry, active	1 tbsp.	8	20	3.0	0.1	3	tr.	4	1.3	tr.	0.19	0.43	2.9	tr.
Brewer's (debittered)	1 tbsp.	8	23	3.0	0.08	(3)	tr.	(17)	1.4	tr.	1.24	0.34	3.0	tr.

Yogurt, See Milk.

For source, see Explanatory Notes, p. 545.

Table 2B. Nutritive Value of Representative Snack and Ethnic Foods*

Food	Weight gm	Approximate measure	Energy kcal	Protein gm	Fat gm	Total Carbohydrate gm	Water gm	Minerals		Total Vitamin A Activity IU	Vitamins			
								Calcium mg	Iron mg		Thiamin mg	Riboflavin mg	Niacin mg	Vitamin C mg
Bamboo shoots	100	3/4 cup	25	2.6	0.3	5	91	13	0.5	20	0.15	0.07	0.6	4
Cheese fondue	100	2/3 cup	265	14.8	18.3	10	54.2	317	1.2	880	0.06	0.34	0.2	tr.
Chow mein, chicken	100	2/3 cup	100	12.4	4.0	4	78.0	23	1.0	110	0.03	0.09	1.7	4
Corn fritters	100	3-1/2 oz	380	7.8	21.5	40	29.1	64	1.7	400	0.16	0.20	1.6	2
Dasheen (Japanese taro)	100	1-1/3 corms	100	1.9	0.2	24	73	28	1.0	20	0.13	0.04	1.1	4
Frog legs	100	4 large legs	75	16.4	0.3	0	81.9	18	1.5	0	0.14	0.25	1.2	—
Hominy grits, enriched, cooked	100	2/3 cup	50	1.2	0.1	11	87.1	1	0.3	60	0.04	0.03	0.4	0
Kumquat	100	5-6 medium	65	0.9	0.1	17	81.3	63	0.4	600	0.08	0.10	—	36
Lychee nuts, raw	100	3-1/2 oz	65	0.9	0.3	16	81.9	8	0.4	—	—	0.05	—	42
Mango	100	1/2 medium	65	0.7	0.4	17	81.4	10	0.4	4800	0.05	0.05	1.1	35
Octopus, raw	100	3-1/2 oz	75	15.3	0.8	0	82.2	29	—	—	0.02	0.06	1.8	—
Okra, cooked	100	8-9 pods	30	2.0	0.3	6.0	91.1	92	0.5	490	0.13	0.18	0.9	20
Pakchoy (Chinese cabbage)	100	2/3 cup	15	1.4	0.2	2	95.2	148	0.6	3100	0.04	0.08	0.7	15
Pizza, cheese	100	1/6 of 14" pizza	235	12.0	8.3	28	48.3	221	1.0	630	0.06	0.20	1.0	8
sausage	100	1/6 of 14" pizza	235	7.8	9.3	30	50.6	17	1.2	560	0.09	0.12	1.5	9
Plantain	100	1, 5" long	120	1.1	0.4	31	66.4	7	0.7	—	0.06	0.04	0.6	14
Pretzels	25	8 3-ring pretzels	100	2.4	1.1	19	1.1	5.5	0.4	0	tr.	tr.	0.2	0
Prickly pear	100	3-1/2 oz	40	0.5	0.1	11	88.0	20	0.3	60	0.01	0.03	0.4	22
Sesame seeds, hulled	100	3-1/2 oz	580	18.2	53.4	18	5.5	110	2.4	—	0.18	0.13	5.4	0
Soybean curd (tofu)	100	3-1/2 oz	70	7.8	4.2	2	84.8	128	1.9	0	0.06	0.03	0.1	0
Sunflower seed kernels	100	3-1/2 oz	560	24.0	47.3	20	4.8	120	7.1	50	2.0	0.23	5.4	—
Sweet potato pie	160	1/6 of medium pie	340	7.2	18.2	38	95.5	110	0.8	3840	0.08	0.19	0.5	6
Tamales	110	1/4 can; 3.9 oz	155	5.0	7.9	16	81.0	22	1.3	—	—	—	—	—
Tortilla, corn	30	8" diam.	65	1.5	0.6	14	13.1	60	0.9	6	0.04	0.02	0.3	—
Water chestnuts	100	16 water chestnuts	80	1.4	0.2	19.0	78.3	4	0.6	0	0.14	0.20	1.0	4

*For source, see Explanatory Notes, p. 545.

Table 3. Examples of Vitamin B-6, Pantothenic Acid, Folacin, and Vitamin B-12 Content of Average Servings of Foods*

Food	Weight gm	Approximate Measure	Vitamin B-6 mg	Pantothenic Acid mg	Folacin mcg	Vitamin B-12 mcg
Almonds, shelled	15	12-15 nuts	0.02	0.07	6.75	0
Apples, raw, unpared	150	1 medium-large, 3-inch diameter	0.04	0.16	3.00	0
Applesauce, canned, sweetened	125	1/2 cup	0.04	0.11	—	0
Asparagus,						
Fresh	100	1/2 cup, 6–7 spears	0.15	0.62	109.00	0
Canned, green	100	1/2 cup, 6–7 spears	0.06	0.20	27.00	0
Avocados	100	1/2 pear, about 4 in.	0.42	1.07	30.00	0
Bacon, cured	25	3 strips	0.03	0.08	0.50†‡	0
Bananas	125	1 medium	0.64	0.32	12.12	0
Beans						
Canned, with pork and tomato sauce	130	1/2 cup	—	0.12	—	—
Canned, with pork and sweet sauce	130	1/2 cup	—	0.08	—	0
Lima, frozen	80	1/2 cup, drained	0.12	0.19	27.20	0
Snap, green, canned	100	3/4 cup, drained	0.04	0.08	12.00	0
Snap, green, frozen	100	3/4 cup, drained	0.07	0.14	27.50	0
Beef, fresh, without bone	100	2 slices, 4 × 1-1/2 × 1/2 inch	0.33	0.47	10.50	1.40
Beet greens	100	1/2 cup	0.10	0.25	60.00	0
Beets, red, canned	85	1/2 cup, drained	0.04	0.08	2.38	0

*Values for vitamin B-6, pantothenic acid, and vitamin B-12 are from Orr, M. L.: Pantothenic Acid, Vitamin B₆, and Vitamin B₁₂ in Foods. Home Ec. Res. Rep. No. 36. Washington, D.C., U.S. Department of Agriculture, 1969. Values for folacin are from Hardinge, M. G., and Crooks, H.: Lesser known vitamins in foods. J. Amer. Dietet. Assoc., 38:240, 1961, unless otherwise noted. Values are based on the edible portion of the raw product, unless otherwise noted. For more folacin values, see Hoppner, K., Lampi, B., and Perrin, D. E.: J. Inst. Can. Sci. Technol. Aliment., 5:60, 1972.
†Hurdle, A. D. F., Barton, D., and Searles, I. H.: A method for measuring folate in food and its application to a hospital diet. Amer. J. Clin. Nutr., 21:1202, 1968.
‡Fried.

Table 3.   Examples of Vitamin B-6, Pantothenic Acid, Folacin, and Vitamin B-12 Content of Average Servings of Foods* (Continued)

Food	Weight	Approximate Measure	Vitamin B-6 mg	Pantothenic Acid mg	Folacin mcg	Vitamin B-12 mcg
Beverages, alcoholic						
Beer	226	8 oz glass	0.14	0.18	16.95	0
Wine	100	3-1/2 oz glass	0.04	0.03	–	0
Breads						
French or Vienna	23	1 slice	0.01	0.09	–	0
White, made with nonfat dry milk	23	1 slice	0.01	0.10	3.4	0
Whole wheat	23	1 slice	0.04	0.18	6.9	0
Broccoli	100	2/3 cup, drained	0.19	1.17	53.5	0
Cabbage	100	1 cup, shredded	0.16	0.20	32.3	0
Carrots	50	1 carrot, 5-1/2 × 1 in. or 1/2 cup grated	0.08	0.14	4.0	0
Cauliflower	100	1 cup flower buds	0.21	1.00	22.20	0
Cereals						
Ready to eat						
Cornflakes	25	1 cup	0.02	0.05	1.40	0
Puffed rice	14	1 cup	0.01	0.05	1.06	0
Puffed wheat	12	1 cup	0.02	–	–	0
Shredded wheat	40	1 large biscuit	0.10	0.28	22.00	0
40% bran flakes	30	3/4 cup	0.12	0.26	30.00	0
Cooked (figured from 30 gm dry weight)						
Cornmeal	120	1/2 cup	0.08	0.17	2.70	0
Farina	120	2/3–3/4 cup	0.02	0.15	–	0
Whole wheat	100	1/2 cup	0.12	0.26	14.70	0
Oatmeal	120	2/3–3/4 cup	0.04	0.45	9.90	0
Cheeses						
Cheddar	30	1 oz or 4 tbsp. grated	0.02	0.15	4.5	0.30
Cottage	55	1/4 cup or 2 rounded tablespoons	0.02	0.12	17.05	0.55

Food	Serving	Grams				
Cream	1 oz or 2 tbsp.	30	0.02	0.08	—	0.07
Swiss	1 oz	30	0.02	0.11	—	0.54
Processed cheddar	1 oz	30	0.02	0.12	3.10	0.24
Chicken						
Breast	1/2 breast	100	0.68	0.80	3.00	0.45
Thigh, drumstick	1 of each, med. size	100	0.32	1.00	2.80	0.40
Boned, canned	3-1/2 oz	100	0.30	0.85	—	0.79
Chickpeas, dry weight	1/2 cup, after cooking	30	0.16	0.38	37.50	0
Chili con carne with beans, canned	1 cup	250	0.26	0.35	—	—
Corn, sweet						
Fresh	1 small ear	100	0.16	0.54	28.00	0
Canned	1/2 cup, drained	100	0.20	0.22	7.70	0
Crab, cooked or canned	5/8 cup	100	0.30	0.60	0.40	10.00
Cream, light (coffee or table)	1/4 cup or 4 tbsp.	60	0.02	0.19	—	0.15
Cucumbers	1/2 medium	50	0.02	0.12	7.00	0
Eggs, whole, fresh	1 large, 24 oz/doz	50	0.06	0.80	2.50	1.00
Fish						
Halibut	3-1/2 oz	100	0.43	0.28	—	1.00
Mackerel, Pacific	3-1/2 oz	100	0.50	0.24	0.60	0.90
Atlantic	3-1/2 oz	100	0.66	0.85	—	9.00
Salmon, fresh	3-1/2 oz	100	0.70	1.30	—	4.00
canned	1/2 cup	110	0.33	0.60	0.55	7.58
Tuna, canned	5/8 cup	100	0.43	0.32	1.80	2.20
Heart, beef	3 oz	85	0.21	2.12	—	9.35
Honey	1 tbsp.	20	tr.	0.04	0.60	0
Kale, fresh	1/2 cup	55	0.16	0.55	38.50	0
Kidney, beef	3-1/2 oz	100	0.43	3.85	—	0
Lettuce	2 large or 4 small leaves	50	0.03	0.10	10.50	0
Liver, beef	2 slices 3 × 2-1/4 × 3/8 inch	75	0.63	5.78	220.50	60.00

Table 3.   Examples of Vitamin B-6, Pantothenic Acid, Folacin, and Vitamin B-12 Content of Average Servings of Foods* (Continued)

Food	Weight	Approximate Measure	Vitamin B-6	Pantothenic Acid	Folacin	Vitamin B-12
	gm		mg	mg	mcg	mcg
Milk						
Buttermilk	246	1 cup	0.09	0.76	—	0.54
Whole, fresh	244	8 oz, 1 cup or glass	0.10	0.83	1.50	1.00
Skim, fresh	246	1 cup	0.10	0.91	—	0.98
Evaporated, reconstituted	100	1 cup	0.06	0.78	1.70	0.20
Dried, skim	7.5	1 tbsp.	0.03	0.27	0.50	0.02
Molasses	20	1 tbsp.	0.04	0.07	1.90	0
Mushrooms, fresh	100	3-1/2 oz	0.12	2.20	24.00	0
Mustard greens	100	2/3 cup	—	0.21	60.00	0
Orange juice						
Fresh	185	6 oz, 3/4 cup, 1 small glass	0.07	0.35	4.07	0
Frozen, as diluted	185	6 oz, 3/4 cup, 1 small glass	0.05	0.30	4.07	0
Peaches						
Fresh	115	1 medium peach, 2 in. diameter	0.03	0.20	4.60	0
Canned	120	2 halves, 2 tbsp. juice	0.02	0.06	0.60	0
Peanuts, shelled, roasted	15	15–17 nuts	0.06	0.32	8.50	0
Pears						
Fresh	180	1 pear, 3 × 2-1/2 in. diameter	0.03	0.13	—	0
Canned	120	2 halves, 2 tbsp. juice	0.02	0.03	8.40	0
Peas						
Fresh, shelled	80	1/2 cup	0.13	0.60	20.00	0
Frozen	80	1/2 cup	0.10	0.25	20.00	0
Canned	80	1/2 cup	0.04	0.12	8.24	0
Pepper, green	65	1 medium	0.17	0.15	—	0
Pie, apple	160	1/6 of 9 in. pie	—	0.18	—	0

Food	Measure	Weight				
Pineapple						
Fresh	2/3 cup, no sugar	100	0.09	0.16	6.00	0
Canned, sliced	2 small or 1 large slice	120	—	0.17	0.96	0
Juice, frozen, as diluted	6 oz, 3/4 cup 1 small glass	185	0.14	0.23	1.85	0
Popcorn, popped, plain	1 cup	15	0.03	—	—	0.
Pork, fresh, without bone	2 slices, 3-1/2 × 3-1/4 inch	90	0.32	0.54	2.16	0.50
Potato						
Fresh	1 medium	100	0.25	0.38	6.80	0
Frozen, French-fried	20 pieces, 2 × 1/2 × 1/2 inch	100	0.18	0.54	—	0
Chips	10 chips, 2-in. diam.	20	0.04	—	—	0
Prunes, dried	4 med. prunes	32	0.08	0.15	1.73	0
Radishes	4 small	40	0.03	0.07	—	0
Raisins, golden seedless	1 tbsp.	10	0.04	0.01	1.00	0
Rice, dry						
Brown	1/2 cup when cooked	30	0.33	0.16	6.00	0
White, regular	1/2 cup when cooked	30	0.16	0.05	4.80	0
White, parboiled	1/2 cup when cooked	30	0.27	0.13	5.70	0
Sauerkraut, canned	2/3 cup	125	0.16	0.12	—	0
Sausages						
Bologna	1 oz, 1 slice	30	0.03	—	—	—
Frankfurter, all meat	1 average size	50	0.07	0.22	—	0.65
Liverwurst	1 oz	30	0.06	0.83	—	4.17
Salami	1 oz	30	0.04	—	—	0.42
Pork sausage links	3 links	60	0.10	0.41	6.90§	0.32
Vienna, canned	2 oz, 1/2 can	60	0.05	—	—	—
Soybeans, raw	1/2 cup when cooked	30	0.24	0.51	67.20	0
Spinach, fresh	1/2 cup	90	0.25	0.27	26.10	0
Squash, fresh						
Summer	1/2 cup	100	0.08	0.36	17.00	0
Winter	1/2 cup	100	0.15	0.40	12.0	0

§As purchased.

Table 3. Examples of Vitamin B-6, Pantothenic Acid, Folacin, and Vitamin B-12 Content of Average Servings of Foods* (Continued)

Food	Weight	Approximate Measure	Vitamin B-6 mg	Pantothenic Acid mg	Folacin mcg	Vitamin B-12 mcg
Strawberries, fresh	100	2/3 cup	0.06	0.34	9.00	0
Sugar, white, table	12	1 tbsp.	0	0	0	0
Sweet potatoes						
Fresh	100	1 small	0.22	0.82	12.00	0
Canned	100	1/2 cup	0.07	0.43	—	0
Tomatoes						
Fresh	150	1 medium	0.15	0.49	12.0	0
Canned	120	1/2 cup	0.11	0.28	4.40	0
Tomato juice, canned	180	6 oz, 3/4 cup	0.35	0.45	12.06	0
Tortilla	30	8 in. diameter	0.02	0.02	—	0
Veal cutlet	100	3-1/2 oz	0.34	0.90	—	1.60
Vegetable oils	14	1 tbsp.	0	0	0	0
Vegetables, mixed, frozen	75	1/2 cup	0.08	0.21	12.0	0
Walnuts	15	2 tbsp., chopped	0.11	0.14	11.50	0
Wheat flour						
Whole	120	1 cup	0.41	1.32	45.60	0
All-purpose	110	1 cup	0.07	0.51	8.80	0
Wheat germ	10	1 tbsp., rounded	0.12	0.12	30.50	0
Yeast						
Baker's, dry, active	8	1 tbsp.	0.16	0.88	—	0
Brewer's, debittered	8	1 tbsp.	0.20	0.96	161.80	0
Yogurt	246	1 cup	0.11	0.77	—	0.27

Table 4. Alcoholic Beverages, Caloric Values and Alcoholic Content of Portions Commonly Used*

	Approximate Measure	Weight gm	Energy kcal	Carbohydrate gm	Alcohol† gm
Distilled liquors					
Liqueurs					
Anisette	1 cordial glass	20	75	7.0	7.0
Apricot brandy	1 cordial glass	20	65	6.0	6.0
Benedictine	1 cordial glass	20	70	6.6	6.6
Creme de menthe	1 cordial glass	20	67	6.0	7.0
Curaçao	1 cordial glass	20	55	6.0	6.0
Brandy	1 brandy glass	30	73		10.5
Gin, dry	1 jigger, 1½ oz	45	105		15.1
Rum	1 jigger, 1½ oz	45	105		15.1
Whiskey, rye	1 jigger, 1½ oz	45	119		17.2
Whiskey, Scotch	1 jigger, 1½ oz	45	105		15.1
Wines					
California, red	1 wine glass	100	85		10.0
California, sauterne	1 wine glass	100	85	4.0	10.5
Champagne, domestic	1 wine glass	120	85	3.0	11.0
French vermouth or					
Madeira	1 wine glass	100	105	1.0	15.0
Port or muscatel	1 wine glass	100	158	14.0	15.0
Sherry, dry, domestic	1 wine glass	60	85	4.8	9.0
Vermouth, Italian	1 wine glass	100	167	12.0	18.0
Malt liquors (American)					
Ale, mild	Large glass, 8 oz	230	100	8.0	8.9
Ale, mild	1 bottle, 12 oz	345	148	12.0	13.1
Beer, avg.	Large glass, 8 oz	240	114	10.6	8.9
Beer, avg.	1 bottle, 12 oz	360	175	15.8	13.3
Mixed drinks, cocktails					
(approx. from recipes)					
Daiquiri	1 cocktail glass	100	125	5.2	15.1
Egg nog, Christmas					
type	1 punch cup, 4 oz	123	335	18.0	15.0
Gin rickey	1 glass	120	150	1.3	21.0
High ball	1 glass, 8 oz	240	165		24.0
Manhattan	1 cocktail glass	100	165	7.9	19.2
Martini	1 cocktail glass	100	140	0.3	18.5
Mint julep	1 glass, 10 oz	300	212	2.7	29.2
Old fashioned	1 glass, 4 oz	100	180	3.5	24.0
Planter's punch	1 glass	100	175	7.9	21.5
Rum sour	1 glass	100	165		21.0
Tom Collins	1 glass, 10 oz	300	180	9.0	21.5

*Figures chiefly from Bowes and Church: *Food Values of Portions Commonly Used*, 11th Ed., Lippincott, 1970.

†The caloric value of alcohol is approximately 7 kcal per gram, but the body has limited capacity to oxidize it. This gives a physiological reason for sipping rather than gulping down such beverages.

Table 5.   Conversion Factors for Weights and Measures*

TO CHANGE	TO	MULTIPLY BY
Inches	Centimeters	2.54
Feet	Meters	.305
Miles	Kilometers	1.609
Meters	Inches	39.37
Kilometers	Miles	.621
Fluid ounces	Cubic centimeters	29.57
Quarts	Liters	.946
Cubic centimeters	Fluid ounces	.034
Liters	Quarts	1.057
Grains	Milligrams	64.799
Ounces (av.)	Grams	28.35
Pounds (av.)	Kilograms	.454
Ounces (troy)	Grams	31.103
Pounds (troy)	Kilograms	.373
Grams	Grains	15.432
Kilograms	Pounds	2.205
Kilocalories	KiloJoules	4.184
Kilocalories	MegaJoules	.004

*Also see Chapter 1, Table 1–2.

Table 6. Minimum Daily Requirements of Certain Vitamins and Minerals*†

	Infants Under 1 Year	Children 1–5	Children 6–11	Children 12 Years and Over	Adults	Pregnancy or Lactation
Calcium, gm	—	0.75	0.75	0.75	0.75	1.5
Phosphorus, gm	—	0.75	0.75	0.75	0.75	1.5
Iron, mg	—	7.5	10.0	10.0	10.0	15.0
Iodine, mg	—	0.1	0.1	0.1	0.1	0.1
Vitamin A, IU	1500	3000	3000	4000	4000	—
Thiamin, mg	0.25	0.5	0.75	1.0	1.0	—
USP units	238	167	250	333	—	—
Riboflavin, mg ‡	0.6	0.9	0.9	1.2	1.2	—
Niacin, mg	5.0	5.0	7.5	7.5	10.0	—
Vitamin C, mg	10.0	20.0	20.0	30.0	30.0	—
USP units	200	400	—	600	—	—
Vitamin D, IU	400	400	400	400	400	—

*Reprinted from Title 21, Code of Federal Regulations, and 21 CFR, 1959 supplement.

†As established by U.S. Food and Drug Administration in 1958 and found on some labels (though obsolete).

‡Amendment published in Federal Register, June 1, 1957; 22 F. R. 3841; amendment effective July 1, 1958.

Table 7. Approximate Loss of Nutrients During Preparation and Cooking of Foods—Percent Loss from Raw Product*

Food Group	Thiamin	Riboflavin	Niacin	Vitamin C
Milk, cream, ice cream, cheese	—	—	—	—
Bacon, salt pork	55	—	—	—
Eggs	15	5	—	—
Meat, poultry, fish	25	5	10	—
Dry beans, peas, and nuts	—	—	—	—
Potatoes, sweet potatoes	25	20	20	35
Citrus fruits, tomatoes	—	—	—	15
Leafy, green, and yellow vegetables	45	40	40	50
Other vegetables and fruits	20	20	20	25
Sugar, other sweets	—	—	—	—
Flour and uncooked cereals	10	—	10	—

*From Harris, R. H., and von Loesecke, H. (eds.): *Nutrition Evaluation of Food Processing.* New York, John Wiley & Sons, 1960, p. 484.

Table 8.   Percentiles* for Height and Weight for Boys 0–18 years†

AGE	BODY WEIGHT, KG			HEIGHT, CM		
	3*	50*	97*	3*	50*	97*
0–3 months	3.72	4.56	6.01	51.55	55.50	59.15
3–6 months	5.58	6.65	8.44	59.90	63.40	67.05
6–9 months	6.94	8.32	10.25	65.35	68.80	73.15
9–12 months	7.96	9.57	11.72	69.50	73.20	78.10
1–2 years	9.57	11.43	14.29	77.50	81.80	88.20
2–3 years	11.43	13.61	16.78	86.90	92.10	99.50
3–4 years	12.93	15.56	18.82	94.30	99.80	106.50
4–5 years	14.33	17.42	21.50	100.60	106.70	114.30
5–6 years	16.56	20.68	25.92	105.30	114.40	122.85
6–7 years	18.48	23.22	29.71	111.25	120.80	129.80
7–8 years	20.64	25.90	33.86	116.80	127.10	136.80
8–9 years	22.79	28.62	38.38	121.90	132.80	142.75
9–10 years	24.78	31.30	43.04	126.45	137.90	147.80
10–11 years	26.90	33.93	48.02	131.05	142.30	152.35
11–12 years	29.26	36.74	53.50	135.75	146.90	158.15
12–13 years	31.57	40.23	59.47	140.15	152.30	165.70
13–14 years	34.43	45.50	65.46	144.30	158.90	173.30
14–15 years	38.80	51.66	70.80	149.05	165.30	180.95
15–16 years	44.16	56.65	75.32	154.10	169.70	183.70
16–17 years	48.51	60.33	78.50	157.75	172.70	186.10
17–18 years	50.69	62.41	80.42	159.30	174.10	187.10

*The percentile refers to the percent of subjects below the given weight or height.
†From Nelson, W. E., et al. (eds.): *Textbook of Pediatrics.* 9th Ed. Philadelphia, W. B. Saunders Co., 1969.

Table 9.   Percentiles* for Height and Weight for Girls 0–18 years†

AGE	BODY WEIGHT, KG			HEIGHT, CM		
	3*	50*	97*	3*	50*	97*
0–3 months	3.54	4.49	5.51	51.45	54.85	58.35
3–6 months	5.10	6.44	7.92	58.45	62.35	65.95
6–9 months	6.30	7.98	10.02	63.25	67.65	71.45
9–12 months	7.24	9.23	11.64	67.15	72.15	76.45
1–2 years	8.80	11.11	14.02	74.90	80.90	86.70
2–3 years	10.70	13.43	17.33	84.50	91.40	98.70
3–4 years	12.47	15.38	20.55	92.00	99.50	108.00
4–5 years	13.98	17.46	23.09	98.10	106.80	116.20
5–6 years	16.08	19.96	25.06	105.30	112.80	121.70
6–7 years	17.30	22.41	28.58	111.00	119.10	128.55
7–8 years	19.64	25.04	33.16	116.55	125.20	134.55
8–9 years	21.41	27.67	38.28	121.35	130.50	140.40
9–10 years	23.20	30.44	43.50	125.65	135.80	146.35
10–11 years	25.20	33.79	48.72	130.00	141.70	153.35
11–12 years	27.56	37.74	54.56	135.05	148.10	161.00
12–13 years	30.80	42.37	61.24	140.75	154.30	166.50
13–14 years	35.22	47.04	66.48	145.95	158.40	169.55
14–15 years	39.03	50.35	69.40	149.20	160.40	171.15
15–16 years	41.00	52.30	70.96	150.50	161.70	171.80
16–17 years	42.12	53.57	71.94	150.90	162.40	172.10
17–18 years	42.73	54.20	72.62	151.00	162.50	172.00

*The percentile refers to the percent of subjects below the given weight or height.
†From Nelson, W. E., et al. (eds.): *Textbook of Pediatrics.* 9th Ed. Philadelphia, W. B. Saunders Co., 1969.

Table 10.   Average Weights of Men*

Graduated Weights (in indoor clothing) in Pounds

Age Groups

Height	15–16	17–19	20–24	25–29	30–39	40–49	50–59	60–69
5' 0''	98	113	122	128	131	134	136	133
1''	102	116	125	131	134	137	139	136
2''	107	119	128	134	137	140	142	139
3''	112	123	132	138	141	144	145	142
4''	117	127	136	141	145	148	149	146
5''	122	131	139	144	149	152	153	150
6''	127	135	142	148	153	156	157	154
7''	132	139	145	151	157	161	162	159
8''	137	143	149	155	161	165	166	163
9''	142	147	153	159	165	169	170	168
10''	146	151	157	163	170	174	175	173
11''	150	155	161	167	174	178	180	178
6' 0''	154	160	166	172	179	183	185	183
1''	159	164	170	177	183	187	189	188
2''	164	168	174	182	188	192	194	193
3''	169	172	178	186	193	197	199	198
4''	†	176	181	190	199	203	205	204

*Excerpted from *Build and Blood Pressure Study*, Society of Actuaries, October 1959.
†Average weights omitted in classes having too few cases.

Table 11.   Average Weights of Women*

Graduated Weights (in indoor clothing) in Pounds

Age Groups

Height	15–16	17–19	20–24	25–29	30–39	40–49	50–59	60–69
4'10''	97	99	102	107	115	122	125	127
11''	100	102	105	110	117	124	127	129
5' 0''	103	105	108	113	120	127	130	131
1''	107	109	112	116	123	130	133	134
2''	111	113	115	119	126	133	136	137
3''	114	116	118	122	129	136	140	141
4''	117	120	121	125	132	140	144	145
5''	121	124	125	129	135	143	148	149
6''	125	127	129	133	139	147	152	153
7''	128	130	132	136	142	151	156	157
8''	132	134	136	140	146	155	160	161
9''	136	138	140	144	150	159	164	165
10''	†	142	144	148	154	164	169	†
11''	†	147	149	153	159	169	174	†
6' 0''	†	152	154	158	164	174	180	†

*Excerpted from *Build and Blood Pressure Study*, Society of Actuaries, October 1959.
†Average weights omitted in classes having too few cases.

Table 12. Structure and Melting Points of Some Common Fatty Acids

No. of Carbon Atoms	Fatty Acids		Melting Point in °C.
Saturated			
4	Butyric	C_3H_7COOH	−7.9
6	Caproic	$C_5H_{11}COOH$	−3.4
10	Capric	$C_9H_{19}COOH$	31.6
16	Palmitic	$C_{15}H_{31}COOH$	62.9
18	Stearic	$C_{17}H_{35}COOH$	69.6
Unsaturated			
18	Oleic	$CH_3(CH_2)_7CH=CH(CH_2)_7COOH$	16.3
18	Linoleic	$CH_3(CH_2)_4CH=CHCH_2CH=CH(CH_2)_7COOH$	−5.0
18	Linolenic	$CH_3CH_2CH=CHCH_2CH=CHCH_2CH=CH(CH_2)_7COOH$	−11.0
20	Arachidonic	$CH_3(CH_2)_4(CH=CHCH_2)_4(CH_2)_2COOH$	−49.5

Table 13. Structural Formulas of the Most Common Amino Acids*

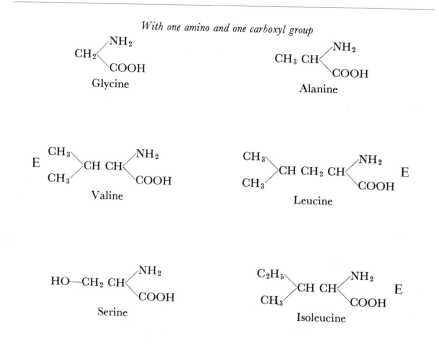

With one amino and one carboxyl group

Glycine

Alanine

Valine

Leucine

Serine

Isoleucine

*Each of the essential amino acids is indicated by an *E*. Histidine and perhaps arginine are needed only by growing children, not by adults (see Chap. 5).

Table 13.   Structural Formulas of the Most Common Amino Acids— *Continued*

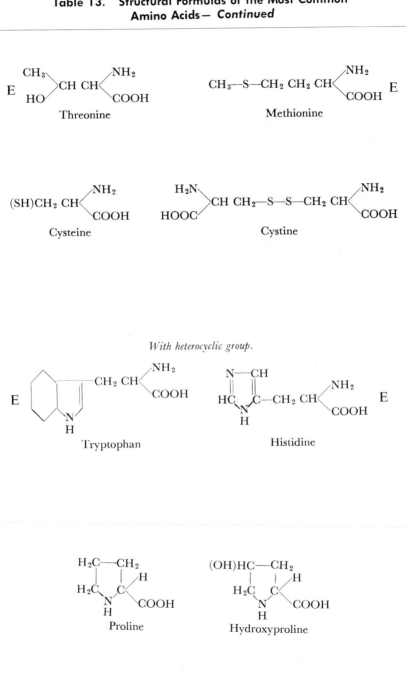

E $\underset{HO}{\overset{CH_3}{\diagdown}}$ CH CH $\underset{COOH}{\overset{NH_2}{\diagup}}$

Threonine

CH_3—S—CH_2 CH_2 CH $\underset{COOH}{\overset{NH_2}{\diagup}}$ E

Methionine

(SH)CH_2 CH $\underset{COOH}{\overset{NH_2}{\diagup}}$

Cysteine

$\underset{HOOC}{\overset{H_2N}{\diagdown}}$ CH CH_2—S—S—CH_2 CH $\underset{COOH}{\overset{NH_2}{\diagup}}$

Cystine

With heterocyclic group.

Tryptophan

Histidine

Proline

Hydroxyproline

Table 13.   Structural Formulas of the Most Common
Amino Acids — Continued

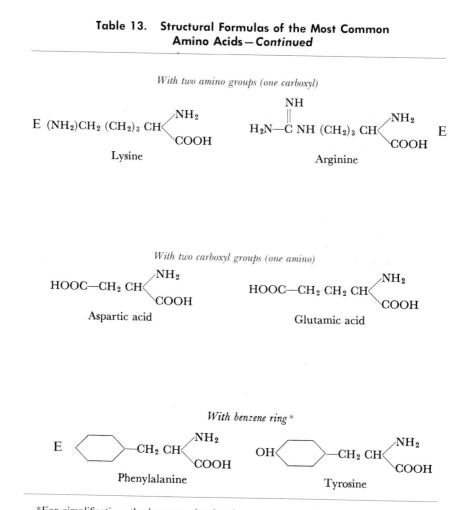

With two amino groups (one carboxyl)

E (NH₂)CH₂ (CH₂)₃ CH⟨ NH₂ / COOH

Lysine

H₂N—C NH (CH₂)₃ CH⟨ NH₂ / COOH   E
   ‖
   NH

Arginine

With two carboxyl groups (one amino)

HOOC—CH₂ CH⟨ NH₂ / COOH

Aspartic acid

HOOC—CH₂ CH₂ CH⟨ NH₂ / COOH

Glutamic acid

With benzene ring *

E ⬡—CH₂ CH⟨ NH₂ / COOH

Phenylalanine

OH⬡—CH₂ CH⟨ NH₂ / COOH

Tyrosine

---

*For simplification, the benzene ring is often represented by a hexagon. It should be understood that there is a carbon atom (C) at each of the six points of the hexagon with hydrogen atoms attached, except where the valence bond is attached to the remainder of the molecule. The benzyl radical may also be represented as:

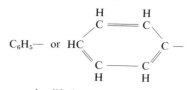

C_6H_5— or

In the heterocyclic groups, simplified representations of which are used in formulas on the following page, there are also carbon atoms at each point unless otherwise indicated (e.g., N), with hydrogen atoms attached as needed to satisfy valences.

Table 14.   Structures of Water-Soluble Vitamins

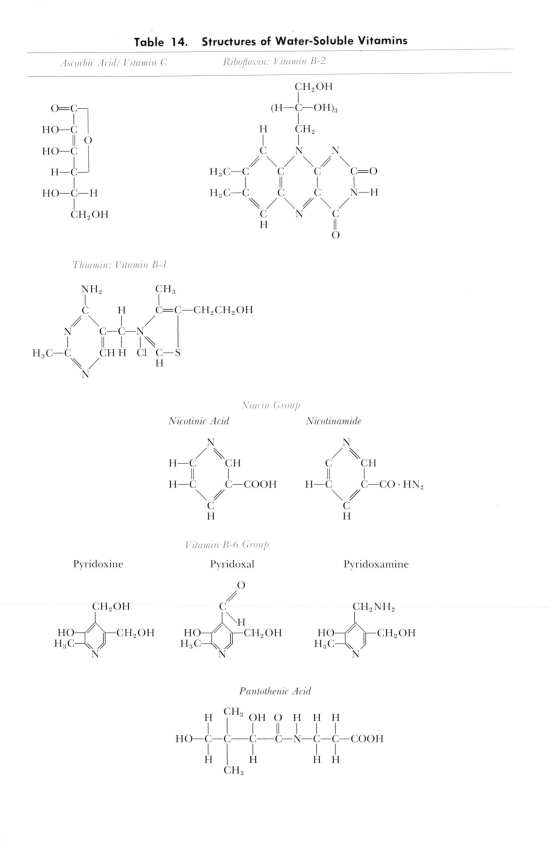

Ascorbic Acid: Vitamin C

Riboflavin: Vitamin B-2

Thiamin: Vitamin B-1

Niacin Group

Nicotinic Acid

Nicotinamide

Vitamin B-6 Group

Pyridoxine

Pyridoxal

Pyridoxamine

Pantothenic Acid

Table 14.   Structures of Water-Soluble Vitamins (Continued)

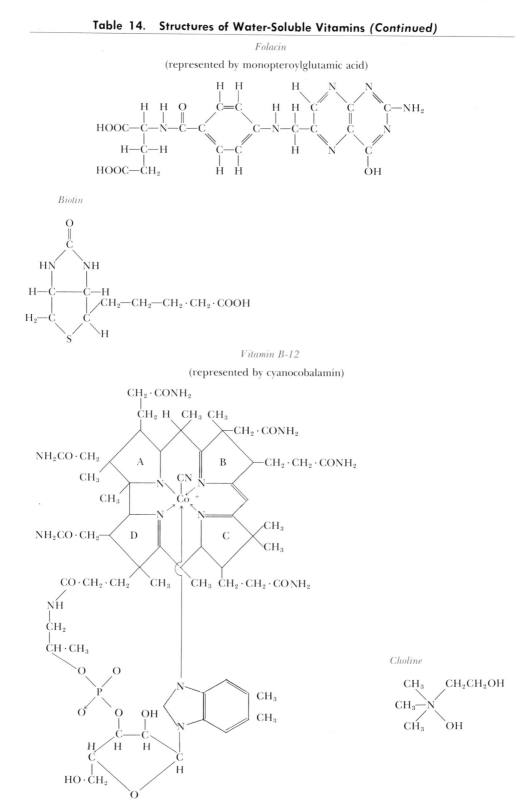

Folacin

(represented by monopteroylglutamic acid)

Biotin

Vitamin B-12

(represented by cyanocobalamin)

Choline

Table 15.   Structures of Fat-Soluble Vitamins

Vitamin A (represented by retinol)

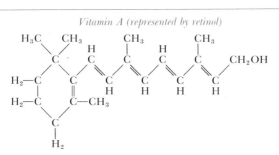

Vitamin D (represented by cholecalciferol, vitamin D_3)

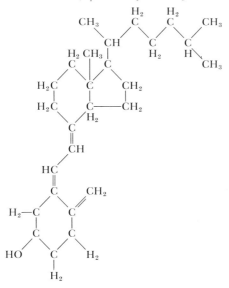

Vitamin E (represented by alpha tocopherol)

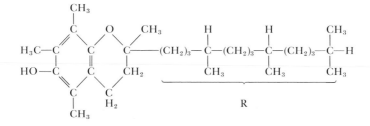

Vitamin K (represented by phytylmenaquinone, vitamin K_1)

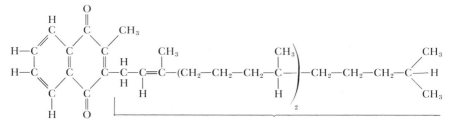

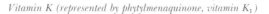

Index